In the Shadow of

FDR

BY THE SAME AUTHOR

Flood Control Politics

The Perils of Prosperity, 1914–32

Franklin D. Roosevelt and the New Deal, 1932–1940

New Deal and Global War

The Great Age of Change

Franklin D. Roosevelt: A Profile

The New Deal: A Documentary History

The Growth of the American Republic, with Samuel Eliot Morison and
Henry Steele Commager

A Troubled Feast

In the Shadow of
FDR

FROM HARRY TRUMAN
TO RONALD REAGAN

William E. Leuchtenburg

REVISED EDITION

Cornell University Press

ITHACA AND LONDON

First published 1983 by Cornell University Press.

Second printing, 1984.

First printing, revised edition, Cornell Paperbacks, 1985.

International Standard Book Number (cloth) 0-8014-1387-7
International Standard Book Number (paper) 0-8014-9303-X
Library of Congress Catalog Card Number 83-45147
Printed in the United States of America
*Librarians: Library of Congress cataloging information
appears on the last page of the book.*

*The paper in this book is acid-free and meets the guidelines
for permanence and durability of the Committee on Production
Guidelines for Book Longevity of the Council on Library Resources.*

Contents

Preface

In the summer of 1939 I was sixteen, just graduated from a mammoth high school in the borough of Queens in New York City, and, though I had my heart set on going to Cornell University, resigned to spending the next four years riding a subway to a municipal college while living at home in a claustrophobic apartment. Tuition at Cornell was $400 a year, a sum far beyond anything that my family, with all the goodwill in the world, could hope to provide. But early in August I returned from a brief vacation on my grandparents' farm in the Delaware Valley to find the mailbox bulging with congratulatory letters from my high school teachers. Out of one envelope fell a newspaper clipping announcing that I had won a Regents scholarship of $100 a year for four years. Out of another tumbled a clipping saying that I was also one of six students in Queens to win a Cornell scholarship of $200 a year for four years. Overnight I had $300 of the money I needed. But if I did not come up with the remaining $100, still a formidable amount, I would never get to see the campus above Cayuga's waters. So, though it was already late summer and work was hard to get, I found a job wheeling a Good Humor ice cream cart through the streets of Sunnyside.

Unhappily, a Good Humor cost a dime, twice as much as any other ice cream bar, and in this tenth year of the Great Depression, most people felt they could not afford one. Day after day I pedaled my cart from early morning until after dark, but came little nearer my goal. Often I returned with my ice cream compartment almost as full as when I had started out, and registration in Ithaca was only a few weeks away.

Then one stifling day a middle-aged man who drove a Good Humor truck went out of his way to let me know that on the farthest reach of town there was a huge and hungry crowd—because Franklin D. Roosevelt was expected to dedicate an extension of Queens Boulevard. I pedaled my bike many, many blocks, and when I got to the site I was able to sell every ice cream bar in my cart. That day's sales gave me just enough money to pay the Cornell tuition, and on a memorable September morning I set off for Ithaca.

Even with this problem solved, and with help from my generous and overextended family, I still needed to work my way through college and I had no idea how I was going to do it. But when I arrived on campus, I was told of the opportunities offered by one of the Roosevelt agencies, the National Youth Administration, and on that first day at Cornell I was assigned to cleaning test tubes at thirty cents an hour. From that day on, the NYA sustained me throughout my years at Cornell.

I never did get to see President Roosevelt, either on that summer day at Queens Boulevard, when I was on the outer edge of a milling throng, or on any other day. But, in September 1939, like millions of other Americans who never saw him, I was powerfully aware of his influence on us; in the very month that World War II began, the New Deal and his conduct of foreign affairs were transforming our lives.

In the spring of 1980 I returned to Cornell to examine the shadow cast by FDR not on the nation but on the Democrats who followed him in the White House. I was honored to be invited to give the Becker Lectures, named after the distinguished historian Carl Becker, who could still be seen about the Cornell campus in 1939. On successive days I spoke on the meaning of Franklin D. Roosevelt for Harry Truman, John F. Kennedy, and Lyndon B. Johnson. Over the next two years I amplified these accounts by drawing on a wealth of manuscript sources, especially those at the presidential libraries in Hyde Park, Independence, Boston, and Austin. In addition, after research trips to such archives as the Eisenhower Library in Abilene, I wrote chapters on FDR's influence on the presidents I had not discussed at Cornell, not least Ronald Reagan, who was still months away from the Oval Office when I delivered the Becker Lectures.

For most of his successors Franklin Roosevelt was a formidable presence. Like the Pelew Island god described by Sir James George Frazer, FDR became a kind of deity only a short time after his death. Though he was not the victim of an assassin, Roosevelt was often perceived as Lincoln had been—as a deity who gave his life for his people. During the post-1945 era he was even regarded, in some respects, as still the president, much as French medieval kings were thought to continue to reign, however briefly, after death. At a ceremony of homage to FDR at Itamaraty, Brazil, in May, 1945, Ambassador Adolf Berle declared:

> Great men have two lives: one which occurs while they work on this earth;
> a second which begins at the day of their death and continues as long as

their ideas and conceptions remain powerful. In this second life, the conceptions earlier developed exert influence on men and events for an indefinite period of time. Now, only a month after his death, we are seeing the beginning of his second, and perhaps greater, life. None of us can prophesy what its results will be; but few will deny that there is a continuing and beneficent spirit which will not cease to speak to a world in pain.[1]

More than two decades later the *Time-Life* correspondent Hugh Sidey wrote of a White House gathering that drew a number of Washington dignitaries to honor FDR: "You could stand on this Tuesday afternoon in February of 1967 and look out over the faces in the East Room of the White House and suddenly understand that Franklin Roosevelt still owned Washington. His ideas prevailed. His men endured. The government that functioned now was his creation perhaps more than that of any other single man." From the White House, Sidey recorded, "you looked out down the Mall and saw the gray Federal buildings that stood there and they were monuments to that amazing man. . . . So much had happened and yet so much was the same."[2]

Roosevelt left his mark on his successors in a great many ways. Three of the first four presidents who came after him—Truman, Eisenhower, and Johnson—were men whose careers he had advanced, and the other, Kennedy, had first gained familiarity with Washington when Roosevelt named his father to high office. No one before Roosevelt had so dominated the political culture of his day, if for no better reason than that no one before him had been in the White House for so long, and in the process he created the expectation that the chief executive would be a primary shaper of his times—an expectation with which each of his successors has had to deal. He bequeathed them not only the legacy of the New Deal but that of a global foreign policy, as well as all those instrumentalities that emerged during the years when he was Dr. Win the War. The age of Roosevelt set the agenda for much of the postwar era, whose debates centered on such questions as whether price controls should be maintained, how far social security was to be extended, to what level the minimum wage ought to be raised, and how large the domain of public power should be. Long after FDR was gone, New Deal agencies such as the TVA and the SEC continued to administer statutes drafted in his first term, and the Fair Deal, the New Frontier, and the Great Society all drew heavily on the Roosevelt experiments.

"All contemporary national politics descend from Franklin Roosevelt," Theodore White has observed. The first Democrat in eighty years to enter the White House with a popular majority, Roosevelt helped bring about a fundamental realignment of American politics. He created an "FDR coalition" that combined traditional Democratic sources of strength in the Solid South with lower-income ethnic groups in the great cities and appealed, as one survey found, to those "cosmopolitans and statists" who approved of the twentieth-century trend toward modernization. In no election after FDR's final victory in 1944 did the South remain solid, and the alliance became frayed in several other ways, too. Nonetheless, as late as 1980 an observer noted that two shrewd election experts had "likened the demise of the FDR coalition to the death of theater in New York City. There have been decades of rhetoric about its death, but if you venture into Manhattan's theater district the lights are bright. So it is with the FDR coalition. For 47 months we hear about how it is breaking up, yet, on Election Day, presto, there it is again."[3]

Roosevelt's success as the architect of a new political era encouraged subsequent Democratic presidents, and even some Republicans, to identify with FDR. They fought off usurpers who claimed that they were the true heirs to the Roosevelt legacy, campaigned in the image of FDR, and year in, year out recited Roosevelt's sayings. They appointed to posts in their administrations men and women who had served under FDR, and made use of Roosevelt's approaches in coping with the problems of their own day.

They did all of these things not only out of conviction but also out of necessity, for they had a vivid sensation of being watched. They knew that their performances were monitored for any sign of deviation from the true faith by a corps of inspectors—by Mrs. Roosevelt, who sometimes behaved like a Chinese empress dowager; by the late president's sons, who had their own notions of how far the FDR legacy might take them; by all those bright young men of the 1930s who still had advice to give in the 1980s; and by the large body of liberal activists for whom FDR was an idol.

These critics asked not whether Roosevelt's successors dealt adequately with contemporary problems but whether they equaled FDR. They were required not merely to quote Roosevelt and replicate his policies but to do so with conspicuous ardor, not only to put through a program of similar magnitude but to carry it off with the same flair. Each was expected to have a rubric—to be known by three initials like FDR, to be the progenitor of a catch phrase like *New Deal*. When they ran for office, it was asked why they fell so far short of the Great Campaigner, and at the end of each successor's first hundred days, observers compared the score with FDR's. Even their wives had to bear the onus of contrast to Eleanor Roosevelt.

To be sure, much that American presidents did in the ensuing decades owed little or nothing to FDR. A Kennedy or a Johnson often responded to a pressing problem with no thought of Roosevelt. Each relied upon his own instincts or was driven by forces that emerged well after Roosevelt's death. Nor was FDR the only predecessor who was recalled. We need not take literally Lyndon Johnson's claim that he "walked with Lincoln every night" to recognize that there were other chief executives whose influence was pertinent.[4] Not even direct citations of Roosevelt offer incontrovertible proof of his influence, for his successors sometimes cited him only ritualistically and used him selectively for their own purposes.

Moreover, the postwar presidents had to bear in mind that the public was deeply divided about Franklin Roosevelt. If there was a large cult of FDR-worshipers, millions of other Americans loathed him—for upsetting class relations, for showing disrespect toward venerated institutions such as the Supreme Court, for creating the leviathan state, and for leading the nation into a war that cost the lives of thousands of young men. Many others were not quite sure what they thought about him—he seemed to have brought both good and ill—and hence he was an uncertain model for his successors to emulate. A commission set up in 1946 to approve a memorial to Roosevelt encountered so many difficulties that by the summer of 1981 it had become the longest-running single-purpose commission in U.S. history.[5]

Still, no one doubted that FDR was a protean figure. From 1945 to the present, historians have unfailingly ranked him with Washington and Lincoln, and the men who succeeded him found one question inescapable: How did they measure up to FDR? They were expected to tread in the rows that he had furrowed, even, like those who sought a sign of grace from a Chinese emperor, to exhibit the quality of *hsiao*, of filial piety.[6] Little wonder that they sometimes felt much like the Athenian who voted to exile Aristides because he had wearied of hearing him called "the Just."

I welcome the opportunity to acknowledge the help I have received in writing this book. David Burner and Thomas West, who devoted an extraordinary amount of energy to reading the manuscript, made many trenchant suggestions. Richard Polenberg, a most congenial host on my visit to Ithaca, submitted astute reports on each chapter to Cornell University Press. I have benefited from the counsel of scholars who read the entire manuscript—Otis L. Graham, Jr., Dewey W. Grantham, Thomas Guinsburg, and Arthur Schlesinger, Jr.—as well as from that of Michael Beschloss, William H. Chafe, Robert Dallek, Robert Divine, and Richard Kirkendall, who read selected chapters.

The Becker Lectures were written when I was Mellon Senior Fellow at the National Humanities Center in North Carolina, and I appreciate the assistance at that early stage of fellows and staff of the center, in particular Charles Bergquist, Geoffrey Blodgett, Muriel Bradbrook, John Kasson, Sanford Lakoff, Gertrud Lenzer, Michael Lofaro, David Lowenthal, Stephen Marcus, Marvin Meyers, Kent Mullikin, James Olney, John Opie, Ákos Östör, R. R. Palmer, Merrill Peterson, Deborah and John Sitter, Rebecca Sutton, Alan Tuttle, John Wall, Edward Williams, David Wills, and Edith Wyschogrod.

Others who in a variety of ways gave me aid along the way include Diane Alampi, Meade Alcorn, James L. Baughman, Stephen B. Baxter, Lawson Bolling, John W. Chambers, Amy Davis, Gary M. Fink, Richard Fried, Robert Greene, Hendrik Hertzberg, Harry Jeffrey, my sons Christopher, Joshua, and Thomas Leuchtenburg, Peter Levy, David McCullough, Cathy Mitten, John Mundy, James T. Patterson, Scott Pitts, James W Rowe, Jr., Kathy Slobogin, Morton Sosna, Laura Sunderlin, Myron Waldman, Christopher Williams, and Bernard Wishy.

I have profited from questions raised by audiences who have heard segments of the book presented in lectures given in widely scattered locations—from the University of South Carolina to the University of Arizona, from Smith College to Colorado State University, from the living room of Congressman Stephen J. Solarz in Virginia to an ancient Florentine great hall in Italy.

Lawrence Malley and the staff of Cornell University Press have shown an inspiriting faith in this book, and the staffs of a great many manuscript archives, notably those at the presidential libraries, have been most resourceful in responding to my inquiries.

By far my greatest debt is to Jean Anne Williams, who nurtured this book from the first word to the last, who improved it immeasurably by her exceptional editorial skills, who cheered me in moments of adversity and shared times of joy.

WILLIAM E. LEUCHTENBURG

Chapel Hill, North Carolina

PREFACE TO THE PAPERBACK EDITION

In addition to incorporating minor alterations in the original text, this paperback edition carries the story of the impact of FDR on his successors through the 1984 election and its aftermath.

W. E. L.

In the Shadow of
FDR

[1]

Harry Truman

I

On the afternoon of April 12, 1945, Vice-President Harry Truman was presiding in the Senate over a long, dull debate on a water treaty. When the session ended, about five o'clock, he made his way over to the office of Speaker Sam Rayburn to join his friends for their afternoon round of bourbon and tap water. No sooner had his drink been poured than the vice-president was told to call the White House. The president's press secretary, Stephen Early, wanted him to come down right away, quickly and quietly. Truman raced through an underground tunnel to the Capitol, ordered a car, and, unescorted, rode down Pennsylvania Avenue to the White House. By the time he got there, it was nearly twilight. Upon entering the executive mansion, he took an elevator to the second floor, walked down a corridor, and entered a study. There Mrs. Roosevelt came up to him, put her arm on his shoulder, and said softly, "Harry, the President is dead." Franklin D. Roosevelt had died that afternoon in Warm Springs, Georgia. After a moment of shock, Truman recovered himself to ask Mrs. Roosevelt: "Is there anything I can do for you?" She replied: "Is there anything we can do for you? For you are the one in trouble now."[1]

That was an odd remark to make to someone who had just ascended to the highest office in the land, but Truman grasped immediately that he was indeed "in trouble," for Roosevelt had so embodied everyone's notion of who "the president" was that it seemed incomprehensible that anyone else could be president of the United States. A member of the White House staff later said of April 12: "It was all so sudden, I had completely forgotten about Mr. Truman. Stunned, I realized that I simply couldn't comprehend the Presidency as something separate from

Roosevelt. The Presidency, the White House, the war, our lives—they were all Roosevelt." One journalist wrote of Truman, "For a time he walked, as completely as did the smallest laborer who had been a 'Roosevelt man,' in the long shadow of the dead President."[2]

Many Americans could not remember when there had been anyone in the White House but Roosevelt, and they had assumed without thinking about it that he would be there forever. During the 1944 campaign, the *Chicago Daily News* wrote of Roosevelt, "If he was good enough for my pappy and my grandpappy, he is good enough for me." According to one story that year, a man said to a loyal Democrat who had just become father of a baby boy, "Maybe he'll grow up to be president." "Why?" the man snarled. "What's the matter with Roosevelt?"[3]

So hard was it to visualize Truman in Roosevelt's chair that some could not even say his title when speaking to him. One Washington correspondent has recalled that "it was difficult, unnatural to address this man as 'Mr. President,' so we skirted around the edges by prefacing our questions with the word 'Sir' or by not using any form of address at all." On the night of April 12 Secretary of Agriculture Claude Wickard wrote in his diary: "I have resolved that I would be very careful when I addressed the new President to call him 'Mr. President' . . . but much to my surprise and somewhat to my disgust I shook hands with him and said, 'Harry, we want to help you all we can.'"[4]

The secretaries who had served under FDR found it especially hard to accept the transition. Lela Stiles was shocked at what seemed indecent haste in swearing in the new president, and Grace Tully could not understand what Harry Truman was doing walking into the Pullman car that had been built for Roosevelt. Lela Stiles has written: "Roosevelt had been regarded by millions as indispensable to winning the war. Now he was gone, and you could hear people on the street murmuring to themselves, 'President Truman, President Truman.' They were trying to get used to the name." When at noon on the first morning of Truman's tenure a messenger cried, "The President is coming out," one secretary was stunned for a moment, then burst into tears and ran into her office. Sobbing, she said, "I thought he meant the President—I mean President Roosevelt."[5]

At Roosevelt's funeral, the old New Dealers regarded Truman as a sorry substitute. Rexford Tugwell, a charter member of the 1932 Brain Trust, had some sympathy for the new president, but he noted that when Truman affirmed that he would be wholly devoted to carrying out FDR's policies, "the dry Missouri voice, it was sad to say, was a disastrous declination from the Roosevelt oratory which had familiarized Americans with a richness they had come to take for granted and now realized had been a golden gift they had not sufficiently valued." Years later Truman recalled that on the funeral train to Hyde Park, "every place we stopped there'd be a crowd just as if . . . well, you'd think the world had come to an end, and I thought so, too." He added, "On the way back I heard old Harold Ickes carrying on about how the country would go to hell now that Roosevelt was gone. He said there wasn't any leadership anymore, something like that. He went on and on. He was a man who carried on a good deal." "Did he know that you could hear him?" Truman was asked. "I think yes, I think that is what he had in mind, that I'd hear him."[6]

When Roosevelt's body arrived back in Washington on the funeral train from Warm Springs, Truman once more took second rank. As the procession moved through the crowded streets of Washington from Union Station to the White House, the eyes of the thousands of onlookers massed on the sidewalks focused not on the new president but on the caisson. Truman later wrote:

> I shall never forget the sight of so many grief-stricken people. Some wept without restraint. Some shed their tears in silence. Others were grim and stoic, but all were genuine in their mourning. It was impossible now to tell who had been for him and who had not. Throughout that enormous throng all of them were expressing their sense of loss and sadness at the passing of a remarkable man. . . . When the cortege passed along Constitution Avenue, most of those who lined the streets were in tears.[7]

At the White House, two hundred FDR loyalists were there to pay Roosevelt homage, Harry Hopkins, his face a "dreadful cold white," looking as though he no longer had anything to live for. When President Truman entered the room, nobody rose.[8]

Often Truman did not receive even the minimal respect due a man who held the same office that Roosevelt had adorned. On his second morning in the White House, he phoned Jesse Jones, administrator of the Reconstruction Finance Corporation, to report that the president had appointed a St. Louis man to be a federal loan official. "Did he make the appointment before he died?" Jones asked. "No," Truman replied. "He made it just now."[9]

So much did Roosevelt dominate the Truman years that one of FDR's former advisors put forth the novel claim that Roosevelt continued to be president of the United States beyond the grave. On the first anniversary of FDR's death, Samuel Rosenman wrote:

> One year later, it is well to recall a fact too easily overlooked. That fact is that, although Franklin D. Roosevelt died before the fighting in World War II had ended, he left a mark upon the post-war world which has not

been erased, and never will be. He was not only a pre-war President, and later a war President; he was also, in a very real and practical sense, a post-war President.

No one believed that more strongly than Harry Truman. As one commentator has noted, "He did not visualize himself in the robes of greatness and he approached power with a disbelieving look." Five months after he took office, he was still writing Mrs. Roosevelt, "I never think of anyone as the President, but Mr. Roosevelt."[10]

II

From the very beginning, FDR and his circle had been a problem for Truman. He had won the Democratic nomination for U.S. senator in 1934 after a campaign in which he said he was "heart and soul for Roosevelt," and when he came to Washington he voted as the White House wished on every measure. Yet Truman rarely got to see the president. It took five months even to schedule an appointment with Roosevelt, and when he did get to talk to him, the meeting lasted only seven minutes. Many in the capital perceived Truman as merely a nondescript minion of the Kansas City boss, Tom Pendergast—in the words of the *St. Louis Post-Dispatch,* "Ambassador in Washington of the defunct principality of Pendergastia."[11]

Some of the disdain for Truman derived from the fact that, in contrast to the eloquent FDR, he made so little mark as a public speaker that he was "definitely classed among the Senatorial Mutes." In the years when FDR was winning the admiration of millions, Truman rarely rose from his seat. A newsreel crew dispatched to record one of his speeches was so exasperated by the number of retakes required that the cameraman yelled at him, "Senator, speak up!" As they left, Truman heard the sound man say in disgust, "He ain't no Roosevelt."[12]

Truman got so little respect from Roosevelt and the White House staff that they made him angry. When the administration prevailed upon Pendergast to bring pressure on him to switch his vote in a Senate leadership contest, Truman was irate. "I'm tired of being pushed around and having the President treat me like an office boy," he told a newspaperman on Capitol Hill. "They better learn downtown right now that no Tom Pendergast or anybody else tells Senator Truman how to vote."[13]

The White House paid no attention. The very next year, when Truman's vote was needed to break a tie, a state highway trooper overtook his car while he was driving to Missouri and fetched him back to Washington. Hopping mad, Truman told FDR's press secretary, "This is the third time I've come back here to bail you guys out on a vote. You tell that to the President!" No matter. The administration continued to ignore Truman on federal patronage and funneled it instead through the senior senator from Missouri, even though Bennett Champ Clark was hostile to Roosevelt's aims. Exasperated, Truman announced that he opposed a third term for the president.[14]

In 1940 the relationship between Truman and Roosevelt sank still further. As Truman's term was expiring, the governor of Missouri, Lloyd Stark, came to the senator to assure him that he had no political aspirations. The moment Stark walked out of his office, Truman said to an aide, "That son of a bitch is gonna run against me." Stark had made himself welcome in Roosevelt circles by being a vocal advocate of a third term for FDR, and the president, to pave the way for Stark's senatorial ambitions, tried to get Truman to step aside by offering him an appointment to the Interstate Commerce Commission. "Tell them to go to hell," Truman instructed an aide. Undeterred by FDR's coolness, Truman announced his candidacy with the comment "Just the other day I spent a very pleasant hour with the President at the White House, discussing various bills pending in Congress, and he expressed the hope that I would come back to the Senate next year." Despite the handicap of Roosevelt's hands-off posture, Truman survived the primary contest and went on to gain reelection in November to another six-year term.[15]

During World War II Truman and Roosevelt continued to have difficulties. No longer an obscure backbencher, Truman did not hesitate to scold the chief executive: "Mr. President, the White House and Capitol are not connected by a one-way street." Roosevelt, for his part, was infuriated by Truman's blunder in carelessly approving the draft of a ghostwritten article excoriating the administration for inefficiency. Months went by after "We Can Lose the War in Washington" appeared before the president would agree to a reconciliation.[16]

On balance, however, World War II proved to be the making of Truman as a public figure and did much to bring him closer to Roosevelt. As chairman of the Senate Committee to Investigate the National Defense Program, Truman took pains to avoid interfering with the president's conduct of the war as the Joint Committee of Fifteen had intruded on Lincoln during the Civil War. Afterward, he reflected, "I am happy to say that so far as I know our committee did not make any of those mistakes. We were never an embarrassment to Roosevelt, not at any time."[17]

Truman's constructive role in World War II led to his choice as FDR's running mate in 1944, though that decision could hardly have been made more grudgingly or inconsiderately. Roosevelt said that if he were a delegate, he would vote not for Truman but for Vice-President Henry Wallace (though he did nothing further to promote Wallace's chances), and even when he agreed that Truman would be acceptable, he indicated that he preferred Justice William O. Douglas. The president never extended Truman the courtesy of a personal invitation to join the ticket. Informed that Truman was balking at running for vice-president, he replied, in a telephone conversation designed for Truman to overhear, "Well, you tell him if he wants to break up the Democratic party in the middle of a war, that's his responsibility," then slammed down the phone. Shaken by this unceremonious invitation, Truman, though recognizing that he had no option save to say yes, asked, "Why the hell didn't he tell me in the first place?"[18]

In the eighty-two days he was vice-president, Truman had so little contact with Roosevelt that he cannot be said to have received any tutelage at all. "I don't think I saw him but twice as Vice President except at Cabinet meetings," Truman subsequently acknowledged. Not once did he see the inside of the map room at the White House, where battle strategy was reviewed, and Roosevelt failed to keep him abreast of diplomatic developments for he was viewed as altogether too insignificant a subaltern to be trusted with secrets of state. (Roosevelt appears never to have entertained seriously the possibility that he would die.) When Roosevelt went to Yalta, he informed the vice-president that he could send dispatches via the map room only if they were "*absolutely urgent*"; and if Truman's messages ran too long, the map room officer would have the discretion to refuse to radio them. A week before FDR's death, the vice-president was reduced to writing, "Hate to bother you but I have a suggestion to make." As Truman later told his daughter, "He never did talk to me confidentially about the war, or about foreign affairs or what he had in mind for the peace after the war." Incredibly, Truman never even met the secretary of state, Edward R. Stettinius, Jr.[19]

Truman sometimes denied that Roosevelt had not taken him into his fold (though he admitted as much to his daughter), either because it was too humiliating or because he wanted so desperately to be thought of as FDR's heir. After a talk with Truman in August 1945, Rex Tugwell recorded:

> He embarrassed me a little by suggesting that perhaps he felt less at home in the White House than I. My familiarity with the White House, I told

him, was a little old now: his own relations with President Roosevelt must, in late years, have had something of the same nature as my own earlier ones. He spoke then, at some length, and with feeling, of the way in which, after it became apparent to President Roosevelt that they thought alike, he had been turned to for confidences in the most important matters. There was much more of this, he said, than anyone knew; and he was very grateful for it now, since it had given him a start in a job which otherwise might have overwhelmed him.[20]

Years later, when Merle Miller, in his extensive interviews with him, mentioned that Truman had seen Roosevelt only twice between FDR's fourth inauguration and his death, Truman responded, "There were more meetings than that. Those were *scheduled* meetings, but there were other times . . . several other times when I wouldn't go in the front way at the White House, but I went. . . . When I saw Roosevelt, it was usually about something that was coming up in the Senate." Miller persisted: "Mr. President, some historians feel that you might have been better prepared for the Presidency and some of the enormous problems that you inherited if Roosevelt had told you more about them, had been more frank." Miller notes: "Mr. Truman's mouth became a very thin line, and he said, 'He did all he could. I've explained all about that, and I told you that's all there is to it, and it is.'"[21]

A single episode at the end of his first cabinet meeting reveals how poorly informed Truman actually had been during his apprenticeship. As the cabinet members filed out, Secretary of War Henry Stimson moved to the chair next to Truman's. When they were alone, Stimson confided that the government had been working secretly on an explosive of "exceptional force" that no one in Congress knew about. That was all that the man Franklin Roosevelt had appointed to the cabinet felt free to tell the president of the United States at that time. Truman did not even grasp that Stimson was talking about the atomic bomb. On the following day the president learned a bit more, but nearly two weeks would go by before Stimson spelled out in detail what was happening, and Truman still appears to have been kept in ignorance of the meaning of the phrase "Manhattan Project" more than a month after he succeeded FDR.[22]

III

In his first months in office Truman would point to FDR's portrait and say, "I'm trying to do what he would like." That would be the theme of all of Truman's first term—that he was nothing more than the executor of Roosevelt's estate. It was not an assignment he cherished. One night in the fall of 1944 he had awakened from a nightmare in a cold sweat; he had dreamed that Roosevelt had died and he would have to take his place. But now that he was seated in FDR's chair, he sensed that his one hope for success was to persuade the nation that he was faithful to his liege's memory. As one historian has observed, "Truman fairly peppered his speeches with references to his immediate predecessor—'the greatest President this country has ever had.' His reiterated praise for Roosevelt must have confused some of his less literate following about just who was head of the Democratic party during the postwar years."[23]

During the summer of 1945, Truman decided on a bold plan to identify himself with Roosevelt's aspirations for a postwar New Deal. In a cabin aboard ship on his way home from the Potsdam conference, Truman told Samuel Rosenman that he wanted to send Congress a message on domestic policy right away instead of waiting for the State of the Union occasion in January. As Rosenman, who had been one of FDR's favorite speechwriters, picked up a pad and pencil, Truman surveyed the Roosevelt programs of the 1930s and outlined his own plans for the future. "You know, Mr. President," Rosenman said, when Truman had concluded, "this is the most exciting and pleasant surprise I have had in a long time." "How is that?" Truman asked. Rosenman responded:

> Well, I suppose I have been listening too much to rumors about what you are going to do—rumors which come from some of your conservative friends, and particularly from some of your former colleagues up on Capitol Hill. They say you are going to be quite a shock to those who followed Roosevelt—that the New Deal is as good as dead—that we are all going back to "normalcy" and that a good part of the so-called "Roosevelt nonsense" is now over. . . . I never really believed any of that in view of your long voting record in the Senate. . . . But this seems to settle it. This really sets forth a progressive political philosophy and a liberal program of action.[24]

On September 6 Truman startled Congress with a twenty-one-point message that drew abundantly on the draft prepared by FDR's former counsel and that consisted largely of Roosevelt's unfinished agenda. He called for a series of New Deal–style reforms, such as increased social security payments and additional projects modeled on the Tennessee Valley Authority, and stated:

> The objectives for our domestic economy which we seek in our long-range plans were summarized by the late President Franklin D. Roosevelt over a

year and a half ago in the form of an economic bill of rights. Let us make the attainment of those rights the essence of postwar American economic life.[25]

Republican conservatives treated Truman's twenty-one-point message as a twenty-one-gun salute to their ancient enemy, Franklin Roosevelt. They had thought that they were rid of him at long last, and here he had reappeared, for Truman seemed Roosevelt redivivus, if not worse. A GOP congressman from Tennessee denounced the president's message as a "fly-specked dish of New Deal hash," while the minority leader in the House, Joseph Martin, expostulated: "Now, nobody should have any more doubt. Not even President Roosevelt ever asked so much at one sitting. It is just a case of out–New Dealing the New Deal." So fierce was the opposition that it was unlikely that much of the program could be enacted. But Truman's intention had been less to put through a program than to establish himself as heir to Roosevelt, and in this, at least for the moment, he had succeeded admirably.[26]

Few contributed more to this effort, in foreign as well as domestic policy, than two of FDR's former associates, Judge Rosenman and ambassador Harriman, each of whom helped legitimate Truman's claims. Though Roosevelt had shown little zeal for Truman's nomination in 1944, Rosenman insisted that FDR had singled Truman out. "Harry S. Truman was picked by Franklin D. Roosevelt and by no one else," Rosenman declared. Averell Harriman served Truman in a similar capacity in foreign affairs. As ambassador to Russia, a post to which he had been appointed by Roosevelt, he was gratified that Truman did not waver from what he perceived to be Roosevelt's no-nonsense attitude toward Moscow. Not long after FDR's death, Harriman told Truman, "Frankly, one of the reasons that made me rush back to Washington was the fear that you did not understand, as I had seen Roosevelt understand, that Stalin is breaking his agreements."[27]

Some critics of the administration's foreign policy questioned whether Harriman was interpreting FDR's legacy properly, but Truman never doubted that he was being true to Roosevelt, a view that many of his supporters upheld. When, some time after he left office, a student asked him whether his impression of Stalin differed from FDR's, Truman replied, "President Roosevelt thought the same as I. The only thing was that we found Stalin such a blooming liar." Truman's defenders pointed out that Roosevelt had told Stalin of his "bitter resentment" of "vile representations," and that on the last day of his life he had written Winston Churchill, "We must be firm." Nor, they said, could Truman be blamed for dropping the atomic bomb. "I know FDR would have used it in a minute," Admiral William Leahy declared, "to prove that he had not wasted two billion dollars."[28]

Though such advisers as Harriman and Rosenman were helpful, Truman understood that if he was to win acceptance as FDR's heir, he needed to please one person beyond all others: Eleanor Roosevelt. Hence he took pains not to do anything to antagonize her. Early in his administration the chief White House secretary, Eddie McKim, a sergeant in Truman's World War I artillery battery, put this association in jeopardy when he came upon White House stenographers answering the thousands of condolence letters Eleanor Roosevelt had received. "So this is 'My Day,'" he said. "Mrs. Roosevelt is no longer riding the gravy train. Stop it!" He discharged the stenographers and ordered the work halted. The story got out, and people who cherished Mrs. Roosevelt were incensed. Truman reversed the order and eased McKim out of the White House.[29]

Truman showed extraordinary deference to the former first lady. Out of consideration for her, he did not exercise his prerogative of moving immediately into the White House, but took quarters across the street at Blair House, where he and his family lived for several weeks. Truman began his presidency, Joseph and Stewart Alsop noted, "by regularly telephoning his predecessor's widow, to inquire anxiously 'what *he* would have done' about this or that great problem." The president "humbly consulted Mrs. Roosevelt as he might have consulted a medium." Three days after he moved into the White House, Truman wrote her an eight-page letter in longhand. She was "very touched" by the trouble he had taken, she replied, and she responded with several pages of advice. It was especially important, she said, to get on good terms with Churchill. "If you talk to him about books and let him quote to you from his marvelous memory everything on earth from Barbara Frietchie to the Nonsense Rhymes and Greek tragedy, you will find him easier to deal with on political subjects," she counseled. He should also talk to her son Elliott, who got on well with the Soviets, and he should try to get the Russians to laugh ("That was where Franklin usually won out.")[30]

Through the remainder of 1945 Truman continued to woo Mrs. Roosevelt, whom he called "First Lady." When he received the news of the Japanese surrender in August, one of his first acts was to phone Eleanor Roosevelt to say that he wished that it had been her husband rather than he that had been in the White House to tell the American people the news. (She was sure that FDR was there, Mrs. Roosevelt answered.) That fall Truman informed Secretary of State James F. Byrnes that only two people were essential to his political team—Henry Wallace, because of his labor following, and Mrs. Roosevelt, because blacks looked up to her. Henry he could "take care of," but he wanted Byrnes to figure out how to get Mrs. Roosevelt aboard his administration. A week later, at Byrnes's suggestion, he invited her to become delegate to the United Nations Assembly in London, and much to his delight she accepted. She agreed to take the post because she thought, a close friend explained, "that someone connected with F.D.R. could by her presence in London keep the Assembly's sights high," and when in 1948 the president of the Assembly paid her a tribute, he said, "She has raised a great name to an even greater honor."[31]

Despite all of the attention he showered upon her, Mrs. Roosevelt sometimes constituted a problem for the president, not least because of the contrasts that were drawn with his wife, of whom he felt fiercely proud. Early in 1945, when Eleanor Roosevelt was still first lady, a short, plump, gray-haired woman made her way into the White House. "Ma'am, your name?" the chief usher asked. "Mrs. Truman," the woman answered. As Mrs. Roosevelt's successor, Bess Truman made little more impression than she had when, as wife of the vice-president of the United States, she went unrecognized. People were constantly comparing her to the former first lady, usually unfavorably. Reporters objected that, unlike Mrs. Roosevelt, she held no press conferences, and that as a public figure she lacked force; on one occasion, when called upon to christen a C-54, she weakly struck the nose of the plane nine times without cracking the champagne bottle. At first she was not even accepted as mistress of her own home. When she commented on the condition of the White House rooms, the housekeeper retorted, "Mrs. Roosevelt never complained."[32]

More significant, Mrs. Roosevelt did not always approve of the administration's policies, and she frequently made her attitude plain in her nationally syndicated newspaper column. She told Henry Wallace that she thought Churchill had taken terrible advantage of Truman on his visit to America in 1946, and when the president announced the Truman Doctrine, she said that it would undermine the United Nations. One of her columns expressed apprehension over the growing influence of the military in the Truman administration, as exemplified by naval maneuvers in the Mediterranean. "I must say it did not fill me with great joy to have the planes from the carrier Franklin D. Roosevelt writing the ship's initials in the sky over Greece at a time when many people wondered just what was going to happen in that country," she told her readers. It is not surprising that on occasion the president found her trying. After a conference with Truman, his budget director set down in his diary what the president had told him—"that she was a great woman although she did at times aggravate him."[33]

Yet Truman never faltered in his endeavor to convince Mrs. Roosevelt that he was a worthy successor to her husband. In May 1947 he wrote her somewhat pathetically, "As you know, my only effort has been to carry out what I thought were the wishes of the late President." In an address the following winter Truman demonstrated that nearly three years in the White House had not changed his perspective. Eleanor Roosevelt, he declared, had "made a wonderful contribution to the welfare of this nation since the President died." Then he paused as if to reflect upon what he had just revealed about himself, looked out at the audience, and said, "He's the only one I ever think of as President."[34]

IV

Though Truman started out with the keenest sense of being a stand-in for Roosevelt, he also understood that eventually he would have to be his own man. "From my reading of American history I knew that there was no cut-and-dried answer to the question of what obligations a President by inheritance had in regard to the program of his predecessor—especially a program on which a great President had recently been re-elected for the fourth time," he wrote later. "Fortunately that program was no problem for me. . . . I believed in it firmly and without reservation." Yet as he looked about the cabinet table on his first afternoon in office, he also had other thoughts. "I always fully supported the Roosevelt program—both international and domestic—but I knew that certain major administrative weaknesses existed," he subsequently noted. "President Roosevelt often said he was no administrator. He was a man of vision and ideas, and he preferred to delegate administration to others—sometimes to others who were not ideally suited to carry out what he had in mind. I was well aware of this, and even on that first day I knew that I would eventually have to make changes, both in the Cabinet and in administrative policy."[35]

Truman had hardly taken office when he revealed that he intended to depart from FDR's New Deal emphases. On April 24 he said to Senator Pepper of Florida, "You know Claude I was for Roosevelt before he became President and supported him in the Senate but now I am responsible for the unity and harmony of the country and I suspect most of the time you will find me about in the middle of the road."

[12]

Pepper noted in his diary: "I told him I did not quarrel with his taking that position as president but I knew he would not expect me as Senator to quit advocating those causes in which I believed. He smiled, put his hand on my shoulder and said 'That is just what I want you to do and I'll be with you whenever I can.'"36

The new president also attempted to cope with the suffocating sense that everywhere he turned in the White House, the Roosevelts were still there. On his first day in office Truman sat down to work at his predecessor's desk in the oval study only to find that FDR's mementos covered much of the desk and his naval prints and ship models put his personal stamp on the room. When the Trumans moved into the White House in May, it seemed "like a ghost house. The walls of the second floor rooms were streaked with dust and faded around the outlines of all Mrs. Roosevelt's pictures." At the outset, the president tried to disturb the possessions of the former occupants as little as possible. But even on the first day Truman swept FDR's mementos from his desk, and after a time he had the desk itself shipped to Hyde Park and did his work at Herbert Hoover's old desk, a change that to some of the New Dealers seemed symptomatic.37

Only six weeks after he entered the White House, Truman did something that left the FDR circle wondering whether he was friend or enemy. An aide noted in his diary:

> The President said he was going to tell us something he had done last night on his own—and we might all throw bricks at him. He said he was . . . studying the food situation—the European food situation—and he decided to write a note to Herbert Hoover. So he said he wrote one out himself, in longhand, signed it and mailed it, suggesting he would be glad to see and talk to him sometime.
>
> Steve Early seemed a little upset. He went on to say that during the Roosevelt term, Hoover never came to the White House to pay his respects.38

Truman later acknowledged that Hoover was "to the right of Louis the Fourteenth," but he thought that as a former president Hoover deserved more respect than he had received from FDR. Hoover himself could not credit the notion that he might be welcome in a Democratic administration. "You know very well they don't let me come to the White House," he told Clinton Anderson, a congressman Truman had asked to be secretary of agriculture. "There's bitterness between the friends of Franklin Roosevelt and me, and though Franklin Roosevelt is dead, that bitterness seems to linger on." At Truman's behest, however, Anderson returned, saying, "Mr. Hoover, the President says to come on over here and that he runs the White House now, not these old friends of Mr. Roosevelt." Truman put Hoover to work as a troubleshooter, and he made the significant symbolic gesture of reversing FDR's action in changing the name of Hoover Dam to Boulder Dam. "Roosevelt couldn't stand him and he hated Roosevelt," Truman commented afterward. "But . . . he can do some things. No reason to treat him other than with respect." The FDR followers, though, were indignant that Truman had violated the rule that Hoover was never again to set foot in the White House. Henry Wallace, who was keeping close watch on the new president, said FDR would turn over in his grave.[39]

In some respects Truman appeared to be calculatedly repudiating the Roosevelt model. Jonathan Daniels, who served in the White House under both men, was to write of Truman: "In Roosevelt's chair he made no image of the great prince which Roosevelt even in his lightest moments was to those around him. Sometimes Truman seemed almost deliberately to shatter such an image by use of a barnyard vocabulary." Another White House aide has suggested that Truman's reluctance to badger Congress to adopt legislation derived from his experience in the Senate, when there had been so much resistance to Roosevelt's presumption. When an interviewer recalled an instance of Roosevelt's strong-arm methods when Truman was senator, Truman acknowledged, "Oh, yes. I was angry, and I was hurt." He resolved that he himself would be more courteous in the Oval Office. He thought, too, that he could do a better job of administering the government. FDR's policy of trying to run the State Department, he told an American ambassador, had been hopeless.[40]

Truman diverged from FDR most conspicuously in his attitude toward the officials Roosevelt had bequeathed him. He later wrote his biographer:

> I wonder if you have thought to go into the background and ability of each member of the cabinet and those who sat with the cabinet which I inherited on April 12, 1945. . . . As I look back on that situation it makes me shudder. I am sure that God Almighty had me by the hand. He must have had a personal interest in the welfare of this great Republic.
>
> There was Stettinius, Sec. of State—a fine man, good looking, amiable, cooperative, but never an idea new or old; Morgenthau, block head, nut—I wonder why F.D.R. kept him around. . . . Then Henry Wallace, Sec. of Commerce, who had no reason to love me or be loyal to me. Of course he wasn't loyal. "Honest" Harold Ickes who was never for anyone but Harold, would have cut F.D.R.'s throat—or mine for his "high minded" ideas of a headline—and did. Agriculture's Wickard, a nice man, who never learned how his department was set up. Then there was Leo

Crowley, whose sense of honor was minus and Chester Bowles, price control man, whose idea of administration was conversation with crazy columnists. . . .

There was not a man in the list who would talk frankly at a Cabinet meeting! The honest ones were afraid to and the others wanted to fool me anyhow.

In a subsequent interview, he added, "I don't know how I ever got out of that mudhole. Stettinius was as dumb as they come. Morgenthau didn't know shit from apple butter."[41]

President Truman took a particularly jaundiced view of the Roosevelt liberals who continued to pay homage to the fallen leader. As one national correspondent noted, "He had an inborn and articulate distrust of and distaste for the Georgetown New Dealer—the pipe-smoking, tweed-jacketed martini-and-salad man who frequented this self-consciously tony and relatively Bohemian part of Washington while the Truman type of administrator went his unterrified way with his bourbon and cigar." His aide Clark Clifford remembers Truman's telling him, "Most of the people Roosevelt had close around him were 'crackpots and lunatic fringe.' I want to keep my feet on the ground. . . . I don't want any experiments; the American people have been through a lot of experiments and they want a rest from experiments." Truman, Clifford adds, disliked the very words "progressive" and "liberal." Even when Truman recorded in his diary, "There should be a real liberal party in this country," he added, "and I don't mean a crackpot professional one."[42]

Truman made short work of ridding himself of most of the Roosevelt holdovers in his cabinet. Some Truman fired; others decided voluntarily to take their autographed pictures of FDR down from the wall and leave town. A White House aide informed Attorney General Francis Biddle that he had twenty-four hours to vacate his post. (Biddle insisted that the president tell him that to his face. When Truman did, Biddle gave him a pat on the back and said, "Now, Harry, that wasn't so bad, was it?") Unable to get from Truman the broad authority he wanted, Secretary of the Treasury Henry Morgenthau, Jr., left the cabinet with a farewell letter that began, "When Franklin D. Roosevelt came to Washington, he asked me to come with him, stating that when he was through we would go back to Dutchess County together." After Secretary of Labor Frances Perkins departed, Henry Wallace wrote her, "You and Henry Morgenthau had been such old-time friends of the President's that it seems now as though the Roosevelt flavor has completely gone out of the Cabinet." (To Wallace, as to Truman, only FDR was "the President.")[43]

[15]

In his first four months in office, Truman either forced out or accepted the resignations of all but two of the members of the cabinet he had inherited from Roosevelt. At the Gridiron Club dinner that year, an impersonator of one of the departing officials, Frances Perkins, sang a parody to the tune of "The Whiffenpoof Song":

> To the old Blue Eagle's feathers,
>   To the horse and buggy days—
> To the Felix and the Cork we loved so well,
>   Sing the old New Deal survivors
> Who are scattered far and wide
>   Since the magic of our music lost its spell.
> Yes, the alphabet of magic,
>   And the tricks we did so well—
> NRA and Triple A among the best;
>   Oh we had our day of glory,
> Although it could not last—
>   So we'll pass—and be forgotten with the rest!
>
> We're little New Dealers who've lost our way—
>   Baa! Baa! Baa!
> We're little New Dealers who've gone astray—
>   Baa! Baa! Baa!
> Little New Dealers, after the spree,
>   Damned from Kansas to Kankakee,
> Lord have mercy on such as we—
>   Baa! Baa! Baa!

So disgruntled were the Roosevelt followers that it became of the greatest importance for Truman to hold on to the two cabinet officers from the FDR era who remained: Harold Ickes and Henry Wallace.[44]

Secretary of the Interior Ickes would have made Job impatient. A man jealous of his reputation as "Honest Harold" and determined that no Teapot Dome scandal would ever besmirch his administration, he had spent no small part of his long tenure under FDR threatening to resign if he could not have his way, and he was even more testy after Roosevelt died. Truman had been in office only a few weeks when Ickes gave him a piece of his mind, and the president had to do his best to mollify him. In June 1945 Henry Wallace noted in his diary: "When Harold called on Truman, the President started out by saying to Ickes, 'I want you to feel perfectly free to come over here at any time and call me any kind of an s.o.b. you want to.' This had cheered up Harold enormously."[45]

Before Truman had even settled in at the White House, though, he had raised Ickes' suspicions. Both Ickes and Wallace had been disturbed to see Edwin Pauley, the California oilman and Democratic national treasurer, in Truman's private car on the Roosevelt funeral train. Wallace recorded in his diary:

Knowing Pauley's oil record in California and his activities at the Chicago convention, I also knew that an era of experimental liberalism had come to an end—and that trouble lay ahead. Having worked with a man who in his prime had genuine spiritual lifting power, I was overcome with sadness at the thought of what the Pauleys would do to a man like Truman.[46]

Early in 1946 Truman unwittingly precipitated a showdown by nominating Pauley to be undersecretary of the Navy, a first step toward making him secretary of defense when that office was created. "I wanted the hardest, meanest son of a bitch I could get," Truman later explained. At subsequent hearings, Ickes said that on the FDR funeral train Pauley had told him that he could raise huge sums for the party if Ickes would call off a suit establishing federal title to tidelands oil, the "rawest proposition ever made to me." When Truman stood behind his nominee, Ickes wrote a brusque letter of resignation, and Truman not only accepted it but told him he had three days to clear out.[47]

Truman later summed up the episode in a memo he wrote for his own satisfaction: "I had to accept the resignation of Harold Ickes because he wanted me to be Franklin Roosevelt—and I could not be." He found it hard to comprehend the charge that in nominating Pauley he was betraying FDR, for Roosevelt had asked him to help get Pauley confirmed. Yet the choice of Pauley and the dismissal of Ickes persuaded the Roosevelt circle that Truman wanted to rid the government of all traces of FDR's influence. Of Roosevelt's original cabinet, Wallace alone remained.[48]

The only thing surprising about the final rupture between Wallace and Truman is that it took so long to happen. From the beginning Wallace was worried about the influence in the new administration of such military figures as General Leslie Groves, "a Roosevelt hater and a Mrs. Roosevelt scorner." (Wallace had been told that "Groves in 1943 at Los Alamos had called Roosevelt a son-of-a-bitch and had told two off-color stories about Mrs. Roosevelt.") Truman in turn always had the uncomfortable feeling that the secretary of commerce thought he should be sitting in his chair at the White House. Yet they stuck together until September 1946, when in a talk to a left-wing rally at Madison Square Garden Wallace stated that "the danger of war is much less from communism than it is from imperialism—whether it be of the United States or England." He also said that China, despite its long border with the Soviet Union, should be free of outside influence, and the leftish audience hissed. When he interpolated, "And I know of my own positive knowledge that that was in Roosevelt's heart and mind," he was hissed again. But on balance the address was seen as a criticism of the administration's "get tough" foreign policy, and as a consequence, after some hours of shuffling his feet, Truman fired him.[49]

V

Long before he discharged Henry Wallace, the president heard the din of a raucous chorus chanting the same harsh lyric: Truman is no FDR. As Jonathan Daniels, the first of his biographers, was shortly to observe, the decline of Truman's popularity in the year after he succeeded Roosevelt paralleled almost precisely the downturn of Andrew Johnson's reputation in the months after he took over from Lincoln. Observers did not ask what kind of president Truman was but rather whether he was comparable to FDR. In the first months of his presidency, a single question was heard again and again: "What would Roosevelt do if he were alive?" And, as increasingly the new president failed to measure up to FDR, or at least to the heroic FDR as he was remembered, the question became more bitter: "What would *Truman* do if he were alive?"[50]

Those who had admired Roosevelt could not summon up the same respect for a man who lacked the Groton panache and was a Mason, Shriner, Moose, Elk, and lapsed haberdasher. There was more than a touch of Eastern seaboard snobbery in the letter the journalist Joseph Alsop wrote his cousin Eleanor Roosevelt from Washington. In FDR's day, he said, the White House had reflected the magisterial qualities of the chief executive; Truman's White House, on the other hand, was like "the lounge of the Lion's Club of Independence, Missouri, where one is conscious chiefly of the odor of ten-cent cigars and the easy laughter evoked by the new smoking room story."[51]

But, as another writer later remembered, people in a small town in East Texas responded in much the same fashion:

Somehow we just couldn't accept the haberdasher in the king's chair. A Midwestern machine politician . . . posturing as leader of the western world, sitting alongside such titans as Churchill and Stalin, while his big-bellied cronies, men whose horizons did not soar beyond a gravel contract or a patronage job for a ne'er-do-well brother-in-law, elbowed aside the elite of Mr. Roosevelt's New Deal. Most of us in Marshall missed Mr. Roosevelt, the only President we had ever known. The day he died people stood around the courthouse square and cried, and the preachers had special church services that evening so that we could pray for him.

But Truman? Common people, I fear, distrust their very own. One looked at Truman and saw not a President of Rooseveltian stature, but a man as ordinary as Mr. Bradbury, who ran the men's wear store in Marshall, or Sam Hall, the Harrison County judge. Imaginations would stretch, but not so far as to put either of these men in the White House. So why Truman?[52]

Those who had been close to FDR, especially the New Deal liberals, found the turn of events all but intolerable. The head of the Tennessee Valley Authority, David Lilienthal, on learning of Roosevelt's death, recorded his "consternation at the thought of that Throttlebottom, Truman. 'The country and the world doesn't deserve to be left this way.'" Two weeks later, Lilienthal, on a plane taking him away from Washington, reflected on a White House conference:

It somehow didn't seem like the President's office, though I had gone through that familiar door so many times in the past twelve years. President Truman seemed a long way away and rose to greet me. . . . It made a pang go through me to realize what a difference it made that *he could walk* and move about, and how little of the magnificence that President Roosevelt had he has. Not even in the President's office. To succeed a man who had acquired such an aura is a tough break for anyone.[53]

Others shared this perception. When Dorothy Rosenman, the wife of the presidential speechwriter, went to the White House for the first time in the Truman era, she immediately sensed that something was wrong. Then she recognized what it was: she had never before known a president who could walk. Six weeks after FDR's death, a leading progressive said of a meeting with Truman: "The sense of loss was terrific. FDR was crippled and never could rise to greet you. Nevertheless, rooted to his chair he created an impression of greater strength than Harry Truman did, alert and lively, striding to meet us with his hand out."[54]

Though Lilienthal admired the president's pluck, he regretted the deterioration in style. After hearing Truman wisecracking in the doorway of his office one September day in 1945, Lilienthal commented in his diary:

This remark epitomizes the humor of the Middle West, its barbershops and filling stations where men pass the time of day, but can you imagine a Groton President saying that? F.D.R.'s humor had a different kind of expression. Also, F.D.R. laughed; Truman grins broadly and he does laugh, but it is so fleeting that it is hardly a laugh at all—a chuckle, or more the sound effect of a grin.[55]

Those who compared Truman's conduct at press conferences with that of his predecessor also gave the new chief executive much lower scores on style. They noted that under the misapprehension that Roosevelt's success at these sessions reflected total artlessness, Truman answered every question that came to him and allowed reporters to put words like "red herring" and "police action" in his mouth. A man who served in the White House under both presidents later commented:

FDR treated his press conferences like a poker game, while Truman kept exposing his hand. . . . FDR was always in control, tossing out trial balloons for public opinion, chiding reporters for asking silly questions and deftly turning aside subjects that he felt shouldn't be brought up. Truman was always direct—a question deserved an answer; he let the reporters take advantage of his low boiling point and his general willingness to please.[56]

Yet the disaffection from Truman rested on more than a contrast in style. The Roosevelt followers sensed that however liberal some of Truman's policies might be, he was not one of them; he did not share their openness to further innovations or take the same pride in their accomplishments. At one press conference he referred repeatedly to the Tennessee Valley Authority as the TWA. Even where laughter ran through the press corps, he persisted. At last a newspaperman asked, "Don't you mean TVA, Mr. President? The TWA is an airline." Though the Roosevelt loyalists had some reason for disappointment, they were not always fair-minded. As James H. Rowe, Jr., who had been one of FDR's White House aides, recalled, "The atmosphere was such that the New Dealers thought Roosevelt was perfect and therefore no matter who went in—if God had replaced him, He wouldn't have satisfied them."[57]

Senator Pepper registered the response of many other left-wing Democrats. "O Fatal day!" he scrawled in his diary across the top of the page for April 12. After hearing the news of Roosevelt's death, he wrote, "What a tragedy for the Nation and the World!" On the next day he issued a statement expressing confidence that Truman would carry on, but three days later, on listening to the new president address Congress for the first time, Pepper commented in his diary, "He didn't praise Pres. R. quite enough to suit me." A week later he talked to Mrs. Roosevelt and her son Elliott at the White House. "I told them that I was one of those enlisted for the duration with the Roosevelt cause and the duration meant my life," he recorded. By the time a month had gone by he was reflecting, "We simply have no leader in State dept. or White House big enough to handle this big job the way it should be handled. Roosevelt is not here in body or spirit."[58]

Truman outraged the liberals not only by removing FDR's officeholders, but by appointing successors who seemed a sorry lot, out of sympathy with the Roosevelt aspirations. "To attempt to contrast any or all of them with their opposite numbers during the New Deal is almost too painful to consider," observed two contemporary critics. "There is no one in the Truman 'gang' who has the ingenuity and political savvy of Tom Corcoran, the brilliant legal mind of Ben Cohen, the literary flair of Adolf Berle, the public relations sagacity of Steve Early, the shrewd economic mind of Isador Lubin, or the charm of Harry Hopkins." It was bad enough that Truman would replace a cabinet official such as Attorney General Francis Biddle with a plodder such as Tom Clark. Even more distressing, he named to the White House staff, and elevated to the rank of major general, a foul-mouthed old army buddy, Harry Vaughan, a "flap-mouthed dunderhead" with the face of "a slack, vacuous St. Bernard." General Vaughan explained to a group of Presbyterian women the difference between the Roosevelt and Truman governments: "After a diet of caviar, you like to get back to ham and eggs." It was such appointments that led one observer to remark, "It is more important to have a connection with Battery D, 129th Field Artillery, than with Felix Frankfurter."[59]

The freelance radical journalist I. F. Stone summed up the dismay at the transition in the capital from Roosevelt to Truman:

> The little name plates outside the little doors . . . began to change. In Justice, Treasury, Commerce and elsewhere, the New Dealers began to be replaced by the kind of men one was accustomed to meet in county courthouses. . . . The composite impression was of big-bellied, good-natured guys who knew a lot of dirty jokes, spent as little time in their offices as possible, saw Washington as a chance to make useful "contacts," and were anxious to get what they could for themselves out of the experience. They were not unusually corrupt or especially wicked—that would have made the capital a dramatic instead of a depressing experience for a reporter. They were just trying to get along. The Truman era was the era of the moocher. The place was full of Wimpys who could be had for a hamburger.[60]

Critics charged Truman and his appointees with reversing FDR's policies, especially with respect to the Soviet Union. As early as May 1945, a group of congressmen sent a public letter to Secretary of State Stettinius expressing concern that the United States had "begun to lose the position which President Roosevelt struggled to win and maintain for our country, as an independent mediator among the great powers, friendly to all and a partisan to none." Over the ensuing months these apprehensions deepened. A year and a half later, a left-wing union convention cheered Claude Pepper when he stated, "If Roosevelt were alive we'd be getting on better with Russia."[61]

For those who, like the chairman of the British Labour party, Harold Laski, were unhappy with the administration's policies, invoking the memory of FDR served as a way to lash out at Truman. In an article published in *The Nation* in the spring of 1946 titled "If Roosevelt Had Lived," Laski wrote: "Had he lived, I am confident that the distrust between the Anglo-Saxon powers and Soviet Russia would never have been permitted to assume its present and unnecessary proportions." After cataloguing a number of other errors that Roosevelt would have avoided but Truman had not, Laski presented his main argument: "If a foreigner may venture an opinion, one of the most tragic consequences of Franklin Roosevelt's death is the evident disintegration of the liberal forces which he made a coherent whole. I do not mean that there are fewer liberals in the United States than when he was in the White House. Rather do I mean that there is not the same focal point about which men and women of liberal views can gather."[62]

Many Americans agreed with Laski's judgment that Truman had fallen short on domestic policy, too, notably with respect to handling the transition from a wartime to a peacetime economy. The fight over reconversion pitted such Roosevelt men as Chester Bowles against such Truman appointees as John Snyder, and in the ferociously fought engagements Bowles's partisans frequently accused Truman of failing to approach problems in the spirit of FDR. When in December 1945 Truman called for new labor legislation and urged unions to defer strikes, the head of the CIO denounced him for "a very serious departure" from FDR's policies, while the United Automobile Workers deplored his attitude as a "retreat from economic democracy as furthered under the courageous leadership of Franklin D. Roosevelt."[63]

Like Andrew Johnson, to whom he was often compared, Truman faced all the difficulties his predecessor had bequeathed him, especially all the vexatious problems of reconversion from a war to a peacetime economy, and he received the blame for anything that misfired, blame that Roosevelt, by his timely death, escaped. Truman inherited the many consequences of the pressure-group state that had grown up under Roosevelt and had to operate it in a less auspicious time. As Barton J. Bernstein has observed, "Whereas the politics of depression generally allowed the Roosevelt Administration, by bestowing benefits, to court interest groups and contribute to an economic upturn, the politics of inflation required a responsible government like Truman's to curb wages, prices, and profits and to deny the growing expectations of rival groups." Furthermore, the farmer-labor coalition of 1936 that had provided much of the basis of FDR's support had become badly strained by 1946.[64]

The 1946 midterm elections brought out all of the swirling discontents over the shortcomings of Truman as FDR's successor. By the final stage of the 1946 campaign, Truman's stock had fallen so low that the Democratic national chairman, Robert Hannegan, told the president to stay out of sight, and the party turned to recordings of Roosevelt's voice to arouse the FDR faithful. In one of a series of nine-minute radio commercials, a discussion of the meat shortage, a voice said, "Here's what President Roosevelt had to say about it," although the shortage had developed after FDR was in his grave. The radio audience then heard Roosevelt discoursing on the leading problem of the Truman presidency. The Republican national chairman denounced this ploy as "one of the cheapest and most grisly stratagems in the history of American politics."[65]

Humiliated at having had to take second place to a dead man, Truman also got the blame for the outcome of the elections, in which the Republicans won control of Congress for the first time in sixteen years. The 1946 results appeared to lead to one overwhelming conclusion—that, having been routed in the first test in sixteen years without Roosevelt at the helm, the party could not survive the loss of FDR. When immediately after the elections it was seriously suggested that Truman resign from office, like a British prime minister who had lost a vote of confidence, a number of people in the Roosevelt circle, including Harold Ickes, rushed to endorse the idea. (The notion originated with Senator William Fulbright; henceforth, Truman always referred to him as Senator Halfbright.)[66]

In the aftermath of the 1946 elections, as the 80th Congress set out to dismantle the New Deal brick by brick, his fellow Democrats sought to lay all of the onus for the debacle on Truman. National Democratic officials who sought cooperation in reconstructing the party ward by ward were told by local political leaders that the responsibility for the poor prospects of their party lay not with them but with Truman, "because he didn't have the magic voice that Roosevelt had had." In the years when FDR's mellifluous tones were heard across the land, they had not been required to perform grubby precinct work, and they would not have to do so now if only there were a Roosevelt in the White House. In late 1946 a prominent liberal said of Truman, "I look at him, and I say to myself, 'Yes, he is in Roosevelt's chair, yes he is, yes he is.' And then I say, 'Oh, no, no, my God, it's impossible.'"[67]

"Mr. Truman has not merely been accused of failing to resemble his predecessor," the political editor James Wechsler noted early in 1947. "He has been blamed for everything that has gone wrong since Mr. Roosevelt died." He added:

> We are told that Mr. Roosevelt's survival would have ushered in a golden age and that Mr. Truman has set out deliberately to repudiate the works of his predecessor. . . . We are told that Roosevelt had found the path to permanent peace and that Truman has brought us to the brink of atomic war, that Roosevelt could have created a postwar New Deal while Truman has invited the money-changers back into the temple. And some liberals, pondering the legend, either pray for a Second Coming or give themselves up to black despair, cursing the fate that struck so cruelly in April 1945.[68]

In truth, FDR was rapidly becoming a cult figure. On the first anniversary of his death, a right-wing daily, noting the attention paid to the event, complained that Roosevelt was the only president with two commemorative days, marking the anniversaries of both his birth and his death. Often the homage he received had a religious element. His life ended only months before World War II had concluded in victory, Roosevelt was likened to Moses, who was permitted a glimpse of the Promised Land before he died. He had a particular appeal on college campuses and at gatherings of New Deal liberals, some of whom came to think of themselves almost as members of a government in exile. Less than two weeks after FDR's death, a new college was named after him in Chicago (it would subsequently be called Roosevelt University), and each year at Roosevelt Day dinners in scores of cities around the country Democratic politicians told liberals what they wanted to hear—that the world would be a better place if FDR were still around. In 1947, as Truman sifted the ashes of the 1946 defeat, Fiorello La Guardia said of Roosevelt, "How we miss him. Hardly a domestic problem or an international situation today but what we say, 'Oh, if F.D.R. were only here.'"[69]

VI

Almost everyone agreed that Truman would be a one-term president. The Republicans looked forward confidently to victory in 1948 because for the first time in twenty years they did not have to confront Franklin D. Roosevelt. All they had to do was to rerun Thomas E. Dewey, whom FDR had defeated in 1944, against a much easier mark. Surveys showed how far Truman fell short of reaching Roosevelt's stature. A 1948 poll asked, "Considering all the men in America who have been prominent in public affairs during the past 50 years, which one or two have you admired the most?" Respondents put FDR far ahead with 43 percent; the next nearest figure got 17 percent, and Harry Truman only 3 percent. Moreover, Truman's popularity with the Roosevelt faithful declined alarmingly in the first four months of 1948. In January he had the backing of two-thirds of those who had voted for FDR in 1944; in April, less than half.[70]

With no dissent, writers agreed that Truman was doomed to lose because he lacked FDR's magic. A memo by the columnist Drew Pearson, written as "the Truman dark comes down on the Roosevelt period," noted Ickes' conviction "that Truman simply did not have the brains around him to run the kind of government that the Roosevelt reforms envisaged and the international situation required." An article by Raymond Moley in the March 8, 1948, issue of *Newsweek* was no less somber. The former member of Roosevelt's Brain Trust wrote:

> On the 15th anniversary of its rise to power, the Democratic party is returning to the primeval chaos from which FDR lifted it. . . . Truman simply does not have what it takes to bring masses of city voters enthusiastically, almost fanatically, to vote Democratic. The vast majorities in the big Northern cities were not voting Democratic in the past 15 years. They were voting Roosevelt.[71]

It seemed particularly improbable that Truman could elicit the same degree of support from black voters. During the 1944 campaign a leading black journal had charged Truman with being a member of the Klan and Republicans had circulated a rumor through Harlem: "Roosevelt is old and may die and you will then have a Ku Klux Klansman in the White House." At Roosevelt's funeral Truman noted particularly "an old Negro woman with her apron to her eyes as she sat on the curb. She was crying as if she had lost her son." "I am speaking for 13 million Negroes," a woman wrote Steve Early a short while later. "You know what Mr. Rosevlet ment to Negroes. the think I am riting you for, is will you try to make clear to Mr. Trueman what the Negroes want. and that is first class citicinship. we know Mr. Rosevelt wuld have give us that. . . . Most Negroes believe Mr. Trueman is a Negro Hater. the town he came from is very unfair to Negroes. I feail you can explain to him that God crated all men Equal."[72]

Truman quieted the doubts of many blacks by moving well beyond what Roosevelt had done, though partly under pressure from FDR liberals and at no little risk to his political future. By serving as vice-chairman of the President's Committee on Civil Rights, Franklin D. Roosevelt, Jr., provided a visible link to the past, but the report of Truman's committee was so much bolder than anything FDR had advocated that a sizable number of southern whites threatened to leave the party. At the 1948 Democratic convention Truman attempted to placate the dissidents by urging the delegates to reaffirm the civil rights plank on which Roosevelt had run in 1944, and his representatives scoffed at the efforts of such men as Hubert Humphrey to ram through a much more outspoken commitment. "Who is this pipsqueak who knows more than Franklin Roosevelt knew about Negro rights?" an administration senator asked. When the Humphrey forces prevailed, thirty-five delegates from the Deep South walked out of the hall. This was the climactic episode in the creation of the States' Rights party, which was to take four southern states from the Democrats in the fall. Why were they doing this? a reporter asked the leader of the bolters, J. Strom Thurmond of South Carolina. After all, FDR had run on a program of equal rights and there had been no party split. "I agree," the governor answered. "But Truman really means it."[73]

Strongly challenged by the Republicans, seriously weakened by the secession of the Dixiecrats, Truman suffered what appeared to be a crippling blow when idolators of Franklin Roosevelt flocked to the standard of yet another defector, Henry Wallace. Much like courtiers on the Continent seeking to win the throne for an exiled prince, many viewed Wallace as the legitimate heir to the Roosevelt succession and Harry Truman as a usurper. Even those who did not share this fantasy had no doubt that Wallace, not Truman, was the embodiment of FDR's ideals. Moments after learning of Roosevelt's death, the young mayor of Minneapolis, Hubert Humphrey, who later would have second thoughts, had written Wallace, "I simply can't conceal my emotions. How I wish you were at the helm." At the same time, Mrs. Roosevelt wrote Wallace, "I feel that you are peculiarly fitted to carry on the ideals which were close to my husband's heart." In June 1945, Claude Pepper called him "the greatest living spokesman of Rooseveltianism." By the first anniversary of FDR's death, Wallace had become, as Truman's biographer later observed, "the well-loved of many groups which felt a peculiar loneliness in the Democratic Party when Roosevelt died." When Truman fired Wallace, he gave left-wing critics of the cold war a leader around whom they could rally. A conference of progressives meeting right after Wallace was dismissed called upon him to "carry on with the confidence that you have the support of the millions upon millions who believe in the program of Franklin Roosevelt," and almost exactly a year later, another gathering of progressives was told, "There is only one man who can take FDR's place and that man is Henry A. Wallace."[74]

Such claims served to intensify an already overheated dispute about who was the proper interpreter of the FDR canon. Remarking on "the performance of some liberal and left-wing leaders who have claimed to be the exclusive owners of Franklin D. Roosevelt's testament," James Wechsler commented, "Nothing quite like this has happened since the turbulent debate over Lenin's will." Some of their statements seemed more appropriate to a séance. "Senator Pepper has told us with great certitude what Mr. Roosevelt would have said and done in every crucial problem that has confronted Mr. Truman," he noted. "Mr. Wallace, once distinguished for his humility, boasts equally clear communion with the departed President."[75]

The acrimonious controversy had been precipitated by the publication in 1946 of Elliott Roosevelt's *As He Saw It,* a memoir that charged that the peace his father had crafted was being sabotaged by Truman and his cronies. A critical piece on *As He Saw It* by Joseph Alsop brought a personal rebuke from Mrs. Roosevelt, who told the columnist that she was "quite horrified" by what he had said. "You may or may not think that Elliott is an admirable person," she wrote him. "I happen to know that he has ideals and that he is doing what he is today from an idealistic feeling about his Father and his Father's policies." She ended her letter with the biting sentence: "Writing for money is no sin, which you well know, only dishonest writing is a sin."

Unpersuaded, Alsop replied to his "Cousin Eleanor":

As a public personality, I consider that Elliott has no existence independent of yourself and his father. . . . Elliott is using his close relationship to the President to confer authenticity upon a thoroughly dangerous and unpleasant kind of attack on his father's memory. In this case, he is, in fact, the attacker. I began my work as a political observer without either deep belief or strong feeling, except the feeling so common among people educated as we have been, that politics is a dirty business and that the people are a set of boobs. By slow stages (and to the day of my death I shall feel guilty that they were so slow), the President's example infused a certain meaning and seriousness into my work. I have a sense of personal gratitude to him which I shall never lose, and his memory means a great deal to me—as it does to many millions of other Americans. Consequently, what Elliott has done fills me with inexpressible distaste.[76]

In sum, Alsop insisted that he was a better interpreter of what FDR meant than the late president's son.

As Wallace edged toward running as a third-party candidate in 1948, Elliott Roosevelt's challengers took to the field to question the legitimacy of the new pretender. When Wallace toured England in the spring of 1947, Joseph Alsop and Arthur M. Schlesinger, Jr., wrote *The Times* of London to deny "that Mr. Wallace has any right to represent himself, or to permit his friends to represent him, as the heir of Franklin Delano Roosevelt. . . . As to Mr. Wallace's claim to carry on the Roosevelt foreign policy, it is grossly, though no doubt unconsciously, false." It was true, they agreed, that there had been a break with the policies FDR had pursued as late as Yalta, but the shift would have come many months sooner if he had lived, for he was determined to deal sternly with the Russians. Unhappily, FDR's death had "left an empty space," for Roosevelt, like a upas tree, "stunted or destroyed the political growth around him." Into the barren forest that remained, they said, had walked such men as Henry Wallace, "feebly parroting superficial, left-over slogans as their domestic program, and as a foreign policy pleading for woolly acquiescence in the designs of the Soviet Union."[77]

Curiously, the one man who could have sustained the view that he was not FDR's faithful vassal was Wallace himself. When Wallace took over the *New Republic* in order to further his presidential ambitions, a member of the staff, Theodore White, made an astonishing discovery—"that Wallace literally loathed Franklin Roosevelt," for he had been the man who had made it possible for Truman to be in the seat of power that rightfully belonged to him. In an interview years later, Wallace said, "While you're in the Cabinet of a President you feel that you owe a great loyalty to the President, until that President does something to forfeit that loyalty. Obviously I couldn't have the same feeling of loyalty to Roosevelt as his fourth term began as I had before."[78]

These sentiments did not deter Wallace from making the most of his association with FDR when he took to the field in 1948 as the Progressive party candidate, a race that pitted Roosevelt's choice for vice-president in 1940 against his selection in 1944. In West Virginia Wallace's followers threw away all the pamphlets and mimeographed handouts they had prepared and relied on a single document—an address by President Roosevelt praising Wallace. At the Progressive party convention, the delegates held a memorial service for Roosevelt and, to the tune of "I've Got Sixpence," sang that a vote for Wallace, "our guiding star," meant achieving "all the dreams we shared with F.D.R." Wallace began his acceptance speech by saying, "Four years and four days ago, . . . I rose to second the nomination of Franklin Roosevelt." FDR, he stated, had given the nation "a vision of peace" and hope for an economic bill of rights. He added:

It was the dream that all of us had, and Roosevelt put it into words, and we loved him for it.
　　Two years later the war was over and Franklin Roosevelt was dead. And what followed was the great betrayal. . . .
　　In Hyde Park they buried our President—and in Washington they buried our dreams.
　　One day after Roosevelt died Harry Truman entered the White House. And forty-six days later Herbert Hoover was there.[79]

With both wings of his party broken off, Truman seemed so certain a loser that a vigorous effort was launched by the Roosevelt element to deny Truman the presidential nomination. As Hubert Humphrey was later to say, "Much of the pressure came from people associated with Franklin Roosevelt." Eleanor Roosevelt called Humphrey more than once to talk over the advisability of jettisoning the president. In March FDR's choice to head the Office of Price Administration, Chester Bowles, confided, "I have been trying to stimulate some others to organize a 'Let's Get Rid of Truman' movement," and in April Senator Pepper wrote in his diary, "The sooner the President goes the better." When Americans for Democratic Action, an organization composed largely of Roosevelt liberals, endorsed General Dwight Eisenhower and Justice William O. Douglas as replacements for Truman, it pointed out that Douglas had "stood shoulder to shoulder with FDR." On a small Minnesota campus that spring, a college freshman put a Douglas button on his lapel because, Fritz Mondale's biographer has written, he was "yearning for a liberal hero to pick up Roosevelt's mantle."[80]
　　Two of the Roosevelt boys played especially prominent roles in the "dump Truman" movement. At a Jefferson-Jackson Day dinner in Los Angeles, the toastmaster, James Roosevelt, received sustained applause when he proposed drafting General Eisenhower as the Democratic presidential candidate, while the party's national chairman was booed for lauding Truman. Shortly thereafter it became known that on the

other side of the continent Franklin D. Roosevelt, Jr., planned to join the draft-Eisenhower movement. At Truman's behest, General George C. Marshall persuaded the secretary of defense, James Forrestal, to ask Eisenhower to phone FDR, Jr., to tell him not to speak out. But Franklin, Jr., persisted. At the Democratic National Convention, he solicited New York support for Ike at the same time that his brother Jimmy, as chairman of the California delegation, was the most conspicuous leader of the dump-Truman forces.

The effort met resistance from a good number in the FDR circle, notably David Lilienthal, who had long since ceased thinking of Truman as a "Throttlebottom." Though Roosevelt is said to have decided that he could not risk antagonizing the powerful senator from Tennessee, Kenneth McKellar, by reappointing Lilienthal as chairman of the TVA, Truman had shown no hesitation in doing so. In the following year, again over savage opposition from McKellar and from conservatives who called the TVA chairman a radical, Truman named Lilienthal to the Atomic Energy Commission. In a private memo, the president wrote, "If Mr. L is a Communist so am I."[81]

This experience left its mark. On July 5, 1948, Lilienthal wrote in his diary:

> I am simply aghast at the unfair way in which President Truman is being "judged," if the current lynch-law atmosphere can be called "judging." And the attitude of liberals and progressives, now whooping it up for Eisenhower or Douglas, is the hardest to understand or be other than damn mad about.
>
> Truman's *record* is that of a man who, facing problems that would have strained and perhaps even floored Roosevelt at his best, has met these problems head on in almost every case. The way he took on the aggressions of Russia; the courage in calling a special session of an antagonistic Congress controlled by the opposition to put through an extensive program for the restoration of Europe; his civil rights program, upon which he hasn't welched or trimmed—my God! What *do* these people want?
>
> If it is said that he wobbled on veterans' housing or Palestine or this or that, did F.D.R. never wobble? Don't be funny; F.D.R. wobbled through the Neutrality Act and Arms Embargo (isolation of the very worst and blindest kind); he wobbled on economic matters all the time. . . .
>
> As for ultra-conservative appointments, . . . who was it who put Forrestal and Harriman and Lovett (about whom they complain, foolishly for the most part) into public life in the first place but F.D.R. himself?[82]

Once Truman had beaten back this effort and won the nomination, most of the Roosevelt liberals rallied to him. Harold Ickes, despite his earlier feud with the president, announced that he was backing his old foe, though in private he confided, "I am supporting as my candidate for President a man who is as fully equipped for that office as would be Adam's off ox." In California, the FDR faction in the movie industry turned out a pro-Truman film that was screened in motion picture theaters across America, and Jimmy Roosevelt declared that he would cast his ballot for the president.[83]

The Roosevelt contingent proved particularly useful to Truman in offsetting the Wallace appeal. The New Deal senator Robert Wagner, deploring Wallace's deviation from the party of FDR, made obvious reference to Franklin Roosevelt when he said, "Yes, the angels are weeping and there is a great man and good friend of Henry Wallace who, I am sure, weeps with them." Under the aegis of Americans for Democratic Action, a group of prominent FDR associates, including Tommy Corcoran, Abe Fortas, Harold Ickes, and Jim Rowe, issued a statement denouncing the Progressive party as "a repudiation of the methods and purposes of Franklin D. Roosevelt" and urging "all followers of Franklin D. Roosevelt to oppose Henry Wallace [and] . . . vote on November 2 for Harry S. Truman."[84]

The Roosevelt family turned out in force to deny that Wallace and the Progressive party were carrying on FDR's program. Eleanor Roosevelt, who said that Wallace's attitude toward Moscow was the "same as Chamberlain's with Herr Hitler," declared that "any use of my husband's name in connection with that party is . . . entirely dishonest," and FDR, Jr., asserted, "No one has or ever will inherit the mantle of Franklin D. Roosevelt, and most certainly not Henry Wallace in pursuit of his present dangerous adventure." Jimmy Roosevelt was even more emphatic. The California Democratic chairman stated:

> Mr. Wallace and his backers claim to be the sole inheritors of and believers in the policies of Franklin D. Roosevelt. By what right? Look close and you will find among these people some with strong personal grudges, some who follow a totalitarian line and some Republican propagandists. Most of them wouldn't know or support a Roosevelt policy if they saw one.[85]

The FDR liberals gravitated toward Truman in the summer and fall of 1948 in good part because, on the advice of his counselors, Truman calculatedly based his 1948 campaign on an appeal to memories of Franklin Roosevelt. A memorandum from Clark Clifford, most of which originated with Jim Rowe, emphasized the importance of attracting "the progressives who followed Roosevelt for four elections but are increasingly restive under President Truman." The progressive coalition included organized labor, which had been "inspired by Roosevelt"; blacks, who had switched to the Democrats "after intensive work by President Roosevelt"; and freelance reformers in such organizations as Americans for Democratic Action, "where most of the Roosevelt New Dealers have found haven." In accord with these recommendations, Truman told the delegates to the Democratic National Convention in July, "Labor never had but one friend in politics, and that is the Democratic Party and Franklin D. Roosevelt," and he wound up his acceptance speech by asserting, "The battle cry is just the same now as it was in 1932."[86]

In the ensuing give-'em-hell-Harry circuit, Truman lost no opportunity to remind voters of what Roosevelt had done for them. He crisscrossed the country on the Ferdinand Magellan, an armor-plated Pullman car with bulletproof glass that the railroad industry had constructed for Roosevelt, and at one whistle stop after another he warned the citizenry that the Republicans were "waiting eagerly for the time when they can go ahead and do a real hatchet job on the New Deal." "Think it over when you go into the voting booths next month," he would say. "Think of the gains you've obtained in the last sixteen years—higher wages, social security, unemployment compensation, federal loans to save your homes and a thousand other things." Like Roosevelt, he campaigned less against his Republican rival than against Herbert Hoover, and again and again he pointed out that the country had been rescued from the Hoover Depression by "a great and true lover of democracy—Franklin Roosevelt."[87]

But without Eleanor Roosevelt's endorsement, Truman had faint hope of winning those last few votes he needed, and it was obvious that she had no enthusiasm for her husband's successor. "I must write you a very frank and unpleasant letter," she told the president in March, for she thought he was letting down the United Nations and she was also dissatisfied with his domestic policies. "Believe me, Sir, it is going to be impossible to elect a Democrat if it is done by appealing to the conservatives," she scolded him. Despite repeated requests, she refused to make a forthright endorsement. Only after hearing that it was being reported that she favored Dewey could Mrs. Roosevelt bring herself to write Truman, "I am unqualifiedly for you as the Democratic candidate." But she enclosed that statement in a covering letter to Frances Perkins that said, "I haven't actually endorsed Mr. Truman because he has been such a weak and vacillating person and made such poor appointments."[88]

Not until the last week of the campaign did she go any further, after a party official phoned her in Paris to say that, despite reports of a certain Dewey victory, Truman could win if he could take the critical state of New York. "I think, Mrs. Roosevelt, that you are the key to the situation," he told her. "I think your influence could elect President Truman. Without you . . . well, we may fail." In order to have the maximum impact, Mrs. Roosevelt got up in the middle of the night to deliver a six-minute address in support of Truman for which ABC, reluctantly, interrupted its hit show, Bert Parks's "Stop the Music." It was aired less than thirty-six hours before the polls opened.[89] To the very end, Truman was in bondage to the Roosevelts.

But when Truman caught almost everyone by surprise by winning a dramatic come-from-behind victory in November, he appeared finally to be out from FDR's shadow. To be sure, he had won with the help of the Roosevelt clan and others in Roosevelt's orbit. Yet he now had his own identity, that of a scrapper who against all odds had made it by himself. "I glory in his spunk," said one southern senator. After the 1948 election, Truman, it seemed, would become president in his own right for the first time.[90]

VII

It was not to be. He could no more escape FDR's presence in his second term than in his first. John Hersey, the author of a profile of Truman well into his second term, noted that in the White House "on the wall, to his right, to make him feel the weight of the mantle on his shoulders, was a portrait of Roosevelt, caped for the sea and storm-blown." In Truman's second term, Washington correspondents still wrote such sentences as "When Franklin Roosevelt died in 1945 and Harry Truman took his place, it was as if the star of the show had left and his role had been taken by a spear carrier from the mob scene." Even in Truman's final year in office, the news analyst Elmer Davis, who had headed a World War II agency under FDR, said, "What I miss about Roosevelt means of course what I miss in Truman—what people will miss this summer in the good major-leaguer who tries to take Joe Di Maggio's place. He will try to do the same things, with considerable success; he will have devotion, industry, talent, everything but the touch of genius."[91]

Election analysts insisted that the surprise outcome in 1948 should be credited not to Truman's grit but to FDR's perspicacity. "Harry Truman won this election because Franklin Roosevelt had worked so well," the *New Republic* declared, while Walter Lippmann concluded, "It can

[33]

be said with much justice that of all Roosevelt's electoral triumphs this one in 1948 is the most impressive." Truman, it was noted, had run behind his party at the same time that Democratic congressional candidates were reproducing almost to the decimal point FDR's margin in 1944, his last race. One commentary went so far as to say, "The vote in 1948 was a testament to a dead man's vision." It explained, "Despite all of Truman's bungling and reactionary mistakes from 1945 to 1947, once he rededicated himself to the Roosevelt program, the political coalition Roosevelt had formed proved inherently strong enough to stagger in again. This alone pulled Truman through." One of Winston Churchill's American correspondents held a similar view. The victory, the British leader was told, was no political upset, as the newspapers claimed, but rather the natural consequence "of the policies which had been in effect for the last sixteen years." The author of the letter: Harry Truman.[92]

Truman, though, no longer viewed himself as a caretaker chief executive who was, as he notes in his autobiography, merely "serving out the term of Roosevelt." Long afterward he explained, "I always knew that from April, 1945, until January, 1949, what I would really be doing was filling out the fourth term of Roosevelt, who was a great President, but I had some ideas of my own, and in order to carry them out I had to run for reelection and be reelected, and that is exactly what happened." Sam Rosenman, who had become one of Truman's most trusted advisers, recalled a marked change. In his first term Truman had been committed to the idea that he had become president only because Roosevelt had chosen him and that he was obliged to recognize that it was FDR's policies the people had endorsed in 1944. Rosenman added:

> He was very conscious of those facts; and every time he took a step he would say to himself: "I wonder what Roosevelt would have done? Would he think this is the right thing?" You know, he had a picture on the wall of Roosevelt that he could see just by turning, and he frequently said to me, "I'm trying to do what he would like." And he'd look to me because he knew that I knew what Roosevelt would have liked. This lasted until his reelection in 1948. After that I never heard him say that again. He was then President on his own, after a very bitter and uphill fight; and while I'm sure he often thought of President Roosevelt, it was never in terms of saying "What would he have done?"[93]

Truman's attempt to dissociate himself from FDR appears to have been disadvantageous. The managing editor of the Gallup Poll pointed out that Truman's popularity in his elected term "was actually below that of his first term when he was serving out Roosevelt's mandate." He explained:

His identification with FDR is significant. . . . So long as he was wearing the mantle of the late President, he fared pretty well with the voters. In many respects, the combination of voting blocs forged by FDR . . . had a lot to do with bringing Truman his victory in 1948. When Truman tried to go it alone, however, his performance with the public was likely to suffer—it seemed that he was much more popular as a substitute Roosevelt than as a real-life Truman.[94]

Whatever the public perception may have been, Washington commentators never let up in comparing Roosevelt and Truman, almost always in FDR's favor. Truman could not even get through his inauguration without such a contrast being drawn. Drew Pearson observed:

In a way, his swearing in ceremony was like Truman's administration in the past and a portent of what it will be in the future—nice, mediocre, and bungling. Roosevelt, despite the fact that he couldn't walk, appeared with great dignity, took the oath of office, gave his speech, and left. There were no waits, no false moves, no bad timing.[95]

In 1949 Truman sought to establish his own identity by offering a program under a different rubric, "the Fair Deal," but analysts regarded it as little more than a warmed-over New Deal. Though calling Truman's State of the Union message "magnificent," a Washington correspondent characterized it as a "restatement of the entire Roosevelt program, reassembling and codifying the abandoned social legislation of the bombed-out New Deal decade." He noted how an Associated Press writer had dated the origins of a number of Truman's recommendations: "a government department covering health, education, and social security—Roosevelt, 1937; St. Lawrence seaway—Roosevelt, 1934; Department of Labor reorganization and expansion—Roosevelt, special message, 1938; federal aid to education—Roosevelt platform, 1934; price support for farmers—Roosevelt, 1933, on a Hoover precedent; rural electrification and soil conservation—Roosevelt, 1935; expand TVA principle—Roosevelt asked Congress to set up seven valley authorities."[96]

The Alsops took a much harsher view. Calling the Fair Deal "a New Deal without intellectual content," they stated:

Where Roosevelt consciously intended his measures to alter the pattern of American society, Truman really does not want to change anything at all. . . . Instead, Truman simply sees his health and housing, education and labor policies and all the others as convenient ways of helping large groups of citizens, not essentially very different from the veterans' bonus after the first World War.[97]

[35]

Observers also attributed the difficulties of the Truman administration in the McCarthy era to the fact that it lacked the political acumen of FDR and his circle. The outspoken former Texas congressman Maury Maverick told Truman's secretary of state, Dean Acheson, "If Harold Ickes got caught in a whorehouse at three A.M. killing a woman, a lot of people would go to bail him out. But not you, you've got no friends." Drew Pearson commented in his diary:

> Franklin D. Roosevelt was a past master of public opinion, knew that his only hold on Congress was to be stronger with the country than they were. Once Congress knew that they were stronger than he, they were ready to turn on him like a pack of wolves on a lame steer.
>
> Neither Harry Truman nor Dean realized that. That is why Congress has turned on them now.[98]

Despite all of these exasperating comparisons, Truman continued to identify with FDR. A few days after the Republican victory in 1952, one of Truman's aides recorded his reflections:

> He said that . . . many people in this country do not know what it means to have the Republicans in control and that perhaps it would be well for them to experience it. . . . The President expressed the idea that it might be a good thing for these people to learn for themselves what President Roosevelt and he had been trying to do.[99]

VIII

Yet when the attacks on him for failing to measure up to Roosevelt persisted into his new term, Truman took a much more questioning look at the FDR legacy, about which he already had strong misgivings. Several years after he left the White House, Truman told an interviewer that after Roosevelt announced his program, "I went crazy about him and stayed that way until he died."[100] No doubt he meant that, at least to an extent. But he also nurtured resentment about how he had been treated by FDR and the Roosevelt loyalists, and that animus increasingly became manifest.

Toward the end of 1949 the Alsops observed that "at the Truman White House . . . connections with the Rooseveltian past have become a positive disadvantage." They explained:

> In part, of course, this is the natural reaction of any man who is condemned to live in the permanent shadow of an invidious comparison. Was

not Elisha so irritable that he caused she-bears to tear and rend the poor children who mocked his bald spot? And did not his inward sourness probably derive from his dislike of being endlessly compared with Elijah? Yet this is not sufficient explanation of the great change in Truman. . . .

The truth is that Harry S. Truman . . . is now firmly convinced that the Fair Deal is a great improvement over the New Deal.[101]

The sense of grievance had been building for a long time. Truman did not care for the way the White House had dealt with him in the 1930s, and he appreciated even less that he had been let into the presidency through the servants' entrance. A personal memo of September 1945 indicates that he blamed FDR for the fix he was in. "This terrible job was virtually crammed down my throat in Chicago," he complained. He was later to observe of the 1944 convention: "Was finally forced into the nomination by the president [phoning] from San Diego. He'd never told *me* what he wanted." Confronted with the obligation to fill out Roosevelt's term, he sometimes had uncharitable thoughts. In June 1946, when attempting to cope with FDR's old nemesis, John L. Lewis of the United Mine Workers, Truman made a desk note to let off some steam: "Lewis ought to have been shot in 1942, but Franklin didn't have the guts to do it."[102]

The *Chicago Tribune*'s Walter Trohan, whose testimony is not always reliable, has recalled an episode when Clark Clifford drafted a speech for the president:

He did a thing which I considered strange. . . . He finished reading it, and Clark raised up his right hand and said, "May God wither this hand if I ever write the name of the cadaver again." (The cadaver was Franklin D. Roosevelt.) And Truman said, "And may he split this tongue if I ever use the name again," because Mr. Truman . . . was not really too fond of Mr. Roosevelt, for the way he had been treated, and he had a right to his point of view.[103]

As Truman campaigned for election in 1948, at a time when the Roosevelt family was doing all it could to expel him from the White House, ill feeling toward the head of the clan rose to the surface. In May 1948 he noted in his diary, "I was handicapped by lack of knowledge of both foreign and domestic affairs—due principally to Mr. Roosevelt's inability to pass on responsibility. He was always careful to see that no credit went to anyone else for accomplishment. . . . All Roosevelts want the personal aggrandizement. Too bad." Two months later he wrote: "I don't believe the USA wants any more fakirs—Teddy and Franklin are enough."[104]

The president would not forgive the Roosevelt boys for their part in the "dump Truman" movement of 1948. In the following year he informed his biographer, "Mrs. Roosevelt called me up once and said I am so disgusted I can hardly talk. Three of my sons are here to tell me I ought to come out for Eisenhower. I am ashamed of them." On a trip west, he added, he had "told off" James Roosevelt. "I got him into a corner and told him 'you're one hell of a fellow. Here I am trying to do everything I can to carry out your father's policies. You've got no business trying to pull the rug out from under me.'" The interviewer noted Truman's further thoughts: "Says Franklin came in and made amends. Thinks Elliott has no sense. And does not have a very high opinion of Jimmie."[105]

Thirteen years after the election, when asked what he thought of the actions of FDR's sons, he responded:

> Well, their father was a great politician, but none of his sons seem[s] to have inherited his abilities in that line. They just never seem to have what it takes to get people to vote for them. I told one of them, James I think it was, and I was out in California making a speech. I told him he was a goddam fool for trying to get rid of somebody who was just carrying out his father's policies. Trying to anyway.
>
> Of course, later, after the convention, he came around and supported me, but I never did forget what went on earlier.
>
> I never did anything about it, but the old man never forgets.[106]

Nor did Truman have any higher opinion of the New Deal luminaries. Persuaded against his will to invite William O. Douglas to be his running mate, Truman took the unusual step of preparing a memorandum to set down his thoughts:

> I call him, tell him I'm doing to him what FDR did to me. He owes it to the country to accept.
>
> He belongs to that crowd of Tommy Corcoran, Harold Ickes, Claude Pepper crackpots whose word is worth less than Jimmy Roosevelt's. I hope he has a more honorable political outlook. No professional liberal is intellectually honest. That's a real indictment—but true as the Ten Commandments. Professional liberals aren't familiar with the Ten Commandments or the Sermon on the Mount.
>
> Most Roosevelts aren't either![107]

Truman aimed his sharpest arrows not at liberals in general but at his predecessor's family in particular. He continued:

Then we have them whose definition of loyalty is loyalty to themselves—
that is it is a one way street.

Take the Roosevelt clan as an example. As long as Wm. Howard Taft
was supporting Teddy he was a great man—but when Taft needed support
Teddy supported Teddy. The present generation of Franklin's is something on that order.[108]

The course of Truman's relations with Eleanor Roosevelt ran no
more smoothly after 1948 than before. Mrs. Roosevelt became riled
when the president failed to mention her husband in an address to the
United Nations and infuriated when in California he endorsed the
Democratic candidate for the U.S. Senate, Helen Gahagan Douglas,
but said nothing about her son Jimmy, who was running for governor.
She even contemplated resigning from her post at the UN. In 1956 the
two clashed when Truman made an aborted attempt to deny Adlai
Stevenson the Democratic presidential nomination. At a massive press
conference at the Chicago convention, she said condescendingly that
Stevenson would start out "better equipped" to lead the nation in
foreign affairs than Harry Truman had been when he entered the White
House.[109]

When Truman thought the time had come for him to make the most
significant political decision of his final term, he related it once more to
his perception of Roosevelt. In one of those memoranda that he wrote
with an eye toward the historian, Truman stated:

There is a lure in power. It can get into a man's blood just as gambling and
lust for money have been known to do.

This is a Republic. The greatest in the history of the world. I want this
country to continue as a Republic. Cincinnatus and Washington pointed
the way. When Rome forgot Cincinnatus its downfall began. When we
forget the examples of such men as Washington, Jefferson and Andrew
Jackson, all of whom could have had a continuation in the office, then will
we start down the road to dictatorship and ruin. I know I could be elected
again and continue to break the old precedent as it was broken by F.D.R.
It should not be done.[110]

IX

The country's preoccupation with Roosevelt served to deprive Truman of the recognition that he and his admirers thought he merited.
There was hardly a program or policy of the Truman years that did not

owe at least something to his predecessor—from the postwar reconversion to the seizure of the steel mills, from the first conference of the United Nations to the intervention in Korea. Yet Truman made distinctive contributions, too—the Marshall Plan, the Berlin airlift, Point Four, the dismissal of General MacArthur, the emergence of the civil rights issue—and he had reason to think that there were other ways that history might judge him than merely as FDR's successor. David Lilienthal thought that "the thing to do was not to complain that T. wasn't highly articulate as F.D.R. was, but to see that he had other qualities perhaps quite as good but different." That was a perspective few shared. A journalist summed up the core of Truman's difficulty: "His deepest misfortune was to replace a Roosevelt—rather than a Harding—and to face each day the exacting challenge of comparison with his predecessor."[111]

Years later, Truman made a one-sentence comment that encapsulated his experience: "Heroes know when to die." He was speaking of the greatness of Abraham Lincoln, but in a way that left his interviewer with a question: "Was he making an analogy between Lincoln's death and that of Franklin Roosevelt?" It became clear that this was exactly what he was doing when Truman began to talk about Lincoln's trouble-plagued successor, Andrew Johnson, a man with whom he clearly identified. "It took about eighty years for the truth about Andrew Johnson to come out, but it finally did, and now people know what kind of President he was," Truman said. Johnson had gotten into such trouble, he went on, for one reason: he tried to carry out his predecessor's policy. "There never was a man in the White House who was more thoroughly and completely mistreated than Johnson," Truman contended. Yet for all the undeserved abuse for adhering to the program of his predecessor, Johnson had proved himself to be a man of courage. The interviewer pressed on with another question: What would have happened if Lincoln had lived? The question embraced a different but similar inquiry: What would have happened if Roosevelt had lived? Truman's response provided the answer to both queries, the explicit one and the implicit one. "If Lincoln had lived, he would have had the same experience," Truman stated, "but like I said, heroes know when to die."[112]

[2]

First Republican Interlude:
Dwight D. Eisenhower

I

When Franklin Roosevelt went to Cairo in November 1943 for a summit meeting with Winston Churchill and Chiang Kai-shek, he knew he could no longer postpone the choice of a general to command OVERLORD, the cross-Channel invasion of the European continent. Both Churchill and Stalin favored the same man, George Catlett Marshall, the universally respected United States Army chief of staff. So did FDR's aide Harry Hopkins and Secretary of War Henry Stimson, for Marshall had earned, in Stimson's words, "a towering eminence of reputation as a tried soldier and as a broad-minded and skillful administrator." Marshall had his heart set on the assignment, and the president had indicated he was to have it. Toward the end of the Cairo conference, Roosevelt summoned Marshall to his quarters to dispatch a message to Stalin announcing his decision. As the president dictated, Marshall wrote down the words: "The immediate appointment of General Eisenhower to command of Overlord operation has been decided upon." In this idiosyncratic, even callous manner, Roosevelt let it be known that it would not be Marshall who would lead the Allied Expeditionary Forces, but Dwight David Eisenhower.[1]

For a long time to come, the world would think of Dwight Eisenhower as FDR's chosen one, and the general was to be overshadowed by the president. At the start of World War II, it was an altogether uneven match. Eisenhower was an obscure officer, one of many, while Roosevelt was the leader not only of the United States of America but of an Allied coalition locked in a death struggle with the Axis powers.

As late as the North African campaign Roosevelt all but obliterated Eisenhower. No one was more devoted to Eisenhower than the attractive young Irishwoman Kay Summersby, his wartime chauffeur, but she was to write of her first glimpse of FDR at El Aaouina: "His personality positively crackled, without as much as a word. That famous smile magnetized every eye. Even General Eisenhower, usually prominent in the foreground, seemed to fade away with the others into a gray backdrop which permitted the spotlight to shine on only one person. To every person standing there, President Roosevelt was the only man in the airstrip."[2]

So luminous was Eisenhower's personality that it was inevitable that he would find his own place, but he never escaped the FDR connection. As the general emerged as a world figure, people often thought of him in conjunction with Roosevelt—two confident, benign men who smiled easily and were at home with themselves, forming a combination chosen, it seemed, by some grand design to provide leadership appropriate to a democratic war. Afterward Eisenhower was perceived to be FDR's heir, a man admirably equipped to legitimize the New Deal and carry it further. In fact, Eisenhower, though he had a grudging admiration for his commander in chief in World War II, did not like the New Deal, and as much as he dared, he sought to stifle it. He liked Roosevelt as a person even less. Yet even at the zenith of his renown in the 1950s, on which in his own way he put his imprint as surely as Roosevelt dominated the 1930s, Eisenhower found that he could not dismantle what Roosevelt had built and that FDR remained a formidable presence.

II

FDR's message to Stalin on OVERLORD did not mark the first time that Roosevelt had singled Eisenhower out for preferment. Indeed, the story of Eisenhower's rise to prominence during FDR's third term would defy belief if we did not know that it was true. As late as September 1941, Eisenhower was still a colonel, unknown to the country and even to many of his fellow officers. Though he distinguished himself in the massive military maneuvers in Louisiana that month, he had absolutely no combat experience. His wildest hope was that before the war ended he might lead a division into battle. But in short order he was jumped over 366 senior officers. By March 1942 Eisenhower, already a brigadier general, had been promoted to major general (temporary), and hardly six months after Pearl Harbor he was in command of U.S. forces for the entire European theater.[3]

Roosevelt had still more honors to bestow. In August 1943 Eisenhower was elevated to a permanent post of major general and awarded the Distinguished Service Medal. A month later, in appreciation of his performance in North Africa and in Sicily, he received the Oak Leaf Cluster. To put Eisenhower on a par with the top-ranking British generals, Roosevelt gave him his fourth star, though his forces were still bogged down in Africa. Even Eisenhower could not believe what was happening to him. He had arrived in Europe with two stars on his shoulders, an American staff officer no one in Britain had ever heard of. Eighteen months later FDR, with many able officers to choose from, picked Eisenhower out from all the others to command the Allied invasion of the Continent.[4]

Though Marshall was much more responsible than FDR for Eisenhower's swift rise, Roosevelt approved each of his promotions, and it was Roosevelt that made the critical OVERLORD appointment; and he saw to it that for the rest of the war the world viewed the president and the general in tandem. From their second meeting he called Eisenhower "Ike." On his way to Cairo the president stopped off at Oran, on the Barbary Coast, to see Eisenhower, and together the two men toured the battlefields of Tunis. There FDR delighted his companion by his speculations about the Battle of Zama of 202 B.C. (After ruminating about whether any of the Punic wars had been fought on the same mountainous terrain on which the battles of World War II had been waged, Roosevelt concluded that it was more likely that the Carthaginians had confined their elephants to the plains.) On his homeward journey the president again stopped off in Tunis in order to tell Eisenhower personally that he had been named supreme commander of the Allied Expeditionary Forces. "Well, Ike," he said casually, "you are going to command OVERLORD." By 1944 Eisenhower's name was so closely linked to Roosevelt's that a gossip columnist-broadcaster reported that if the Republicans nominated Douglas MacArthur, the president would choose Ike as his running mate.[5]

Roosevelt took pains to identify himself with the general's skyrocketing career. In a talk at the annual dinner of the White House Correspondents' Association in 1943, he said: "I spent many hours in Casablanca with this young general—a descendant of Kansas pioneers. I know what a fine, tough job he has done and how carefully and skilfully he is directing the soldiers under him. I want to say to you tonight— and to him—that we have every confidence in his leadership." Two years later, in his final annual message to Congress, the president, in discussing the Battle of the Bulge, declared: "General Eisenhower has faced this period of trial with admirable calm and resolution and with steadily increasing success. He has my complete confidence."[6]

General Eisenhower, for his part, spoke on more than one occasion of his esteem for Roosevelt. The general did not serve merely in a military capacity—at one point he drafted a message to Chiang Kai-shek for FDR's signature—and he was grateful for FDR's support in the much-criticized Darlan deal in North Africa. "My recent visit to your Headquarters was, for me, an uplifting experience and one that I know will be reflected in increased efficiency in my own operations," he wrote the president early in 1943. "I cannot tell you how much I appreciated the kind words you had to say about our efforts." He recognized how much Roosevelt meant to the people of the free world, and what a hero he was to the beleaguered British. Toward the end of 1943 Eisenhower requested a signed photograph of the president for a soldier in the British Motor Transport Corps who had been FDR's driver in Tunisia, Kay Summersby.[7]

Eisenhower never ceased to marvel at the retentiveness of FDR's mind. In his account of their meeting in North Africa, he wrote, "I was struck with his phenomenal memory for detail. . . . He repeated entire sentences, almost paragraphs, from the radiogram I had sent home to explain the Darlan matter." A wartime conference in Washington left a similar impression. "As always he amazed me with his intimate knowledge of world geography," Eisenhower recalled. "The most obscure places in faraway countries were always accurately placed on his mental map."[8]

To the end of his days Eisenhower expressed gratification for the performance of FDR as commander in chief. During his final illness he wrote: "Any President, if he is to be effective, must be able to inspire people. It is an essential quality of leadership. I have often thought how fortunate it was that the two great Allies of World War II were led by two men—Churchill and Franklin D. Roosevelt—who had that ability and used it masterfully." He said of Roosevelt:

I admired him greatly as a war leader. The man exuded an infectious optimism; indeed, the thought of defeat apparently never crossed his mind, despite the fact that we were fighting two great wars simultaneously on opposite sides of the earth. This was true even during the dark days of our early reverses in the Pacific. Somehow, he was able to convey his own exuberant confidence to the American people, just as Churchill did to his people in Britain's even darker hours. As a result, during the war years, despite often justified political opposition on domestic measures, F.D.R. had the nation almost solidly behind him in his conduct of the war.[9]

The news of FDR's death on April 12, 1945, reached Eisenhower at the end of a particularly grueling day, and added to the sense of foreboding that day had brought. For it was on April 12 that Eisenhower had first witnessed the horror of an internment camp. "I never dreamed that such cruelty, bestiality, and savagery could really exist in this world!" he wrote his wife. Weary, shaken, he was not able to turn in until after midnight at a house that had been the residence of a Nazi commandant, and even then there was no rest. Shortly after midnight Patton and Bradley awakened him to relay a radio report of the president's death in Warm Springs. One of his biographers has written: "The supreme commander would never forget the stunned grief of that moment, the sense of enormous personal loss. Whatever his faults, the President's buoyant personality had been through twelve years of unparalleled crisis one of the positive assets of the whole Western world. It was as though a great mountain from which one had been accustomed to taking his bearings had suddenly crumbled into dust." In his memoirs Eisenhower put it more simply: "We went to bed depressed and sad."[10]

Eisenhower doubted that anyone could lead America through the crisis of war as well as Roosevelt, and he made no secret of his consternation. The day after learning of the president's death, he wrote Harry Hopkins, "I bitterly regret that he could not have been spared to see the final day of victory," and he referred to "the tragic loss I feel." Two months later he told the House of Representatives, "From his strength and indomitable spirit I drew constant support and confidence in the solution of my problems." In 1947 he was still saying, "I knew him solely in his capacity as leader of a nation at war—and in that capacity he seemed to me to fulfill all that could possibly be expected of him."[11]

So closely was Eisenhower associated with Franklin Roosevelt that when people began to talk seriously about Ike as a presidential prospect, right-wing Republicans dismissed him as FDR Redux. As early as 1947, Archibald Roosevelt (of the Oyster Bay branch of the clan) sent General MacArthur what he called an "indiscreet" political analysis:

The Willkie Group. This is a small, wealthy, and very vociferous group. It is very new-dealish, and somewhat pro-communist. It gets great support from the Herald-Tribune, and Helen Reid. The Democratic New Deal, oddly enough[,] has great influence with them and they love Eleanor Roosevelt, & so forth.

They started out supporting Stassen, & have now switched to Eisenhower—encouraged largely by Democratic New Dealers who want a candidate with as little different policies from Truman & Franklin as possible. Then they can say, keep the original, and don't buy a substitute. Just as they did with Willkie and Franklin.[12]

In the following year, at the height of the acrimonious struggle over the GOP presidential nomination, Army's football coach, Red Blaik, expressed similar sentiments. "How can anyone believe that Eisenhower, endorsed by the Roosevelts, James and Elliot[t], the Deweycrats, Senator Morse and his ilk, and probably Truman himself, represents anything but a political mongrel?" he asked MacArthur. "If there is no war, are we to succumb under a glorified military WPA program in operation both abroad and at home?"[13]

However excessive Blaik's communication was, he stood on firm ground in claiming that Ike found special favor among members of FDR's family. As early as 1943, Eisenhower had noted in his diary, "I have seen quite a bit of Colonel Elliott Roosevelt who is apparently quite close to the President in family councils," and in 1948 Elliott had joined two of his brothers in attempting to draft the general for the Democratic presidential nomination. In March 1948 Franklin D. Roosevelt, Jr., stated:

In times of crisis the Democratic party has provided such great leaders as Jefferson, Jackson, Wilson, and Franklin D. Roosevelt. In keeping with this tradition, I am convinced that the Democratic party will again mirror the overwhelming will of the American people, when its leaders meet at the Democratic national convention in Philadelphia, and will draft General Dwight D. Eisenhower for President.[14]

Though liberals were guilty of overreaching in claiming that Eisenhower shared their outlook, pollsters found that he did inherit some of FDR's following. In the spring of 1948, a *Newsweek* writer reported:

For thirteen years, the Majority Man remained faithful to Franklin D. Roosevelt. Times changed and policies shifted, but the Man followed Roosevelt because, for better or worse, he relied on the Roosevelt judgment and was willing to submit to the Roosevelt leadership. . . .

What he is really looking for, as the enthusiasm for Eisenhower has shown, is someone to fill the seat of the Great White Father vacated by Franklin D. Roosevelt, someone to take him by the hand and lead him through the maze of events toward peace and security. By a curious combination of impressions and moods and mental images, he has come to believe that Eisenhower is the man to do it.[15]

The relationship of Dwight's brother Milton to FDR also made Republican conservatives uneasy. Milton was known to be one of FDR's intimates, trusted to carry out a number of confidential assignments for Roosevelt. "We became fast friends," Milton later wrote. "I developed a genuine liking for him." Roosevelt in turn only wished that there were more than one Milton Eisenhower so that he could fill several slots at the same time. When General Eisenhower first met FDR, he was unnerved by the president's opening sentence: "I'm having an awful lot of trouble with your brother Milton." Eisenhower was about to leap to his brother's defense when Roosevelt added disarmingly, "Four different government departments want him and I have to decide where he is to go."[16]

The presentiment that Ike was an FDR man under the skin did not die when he won the GOP presidential nomination in 1952. Only after a summit conference on Morningside Drive, where Eisenhower was presiding over Columbia University, was Senator Taft prepared to say of his party's candidate:

> A good many of my friends have been concerned because so many of his editorial and columnist supporters, and other individuals who have heretofore always taken the New Deal line, have been urging him to repudiate the Republican platform, approve New Deal policies and purge everyone who fought hard for Republican principles against . . . the left-wingers. . . .
>
> I am completely satisfied that General Eisenhower will give the country an Administration inspired by the Republican principles of continued and expanding liberty for all as against the continued growth of New Deal socialism.[17]

Even after Eisenhower entered the White House, the Republican right still saw him as a closet Roosevelt follower, in part because he was so frequently likened to FDR. "Eisenhower and 1952 have a great deal in common with Roosevelt and 1932," wrote one columnist, while another noted in his diary, "In many respects Eisenhower reminds me of F.D.R.—the same contagious charm, the same ability to talk, and the same tendency toward pleasant-sounding generalities."[18] The Old Guard responded predictably. When the Democrats regained control of Congress after the 1954 elections, Representative Clarence Brown blamed the president for not rejecting the Roosevelt system. "You know it seems to me that Ike is trying to follow Harry Hopkins and rake leaves across the road and back the next day," a former GOP minority leader wrote to an upstate New York congressman in 1957. "It seems to me our Republican administration is getting about as interested in a Christmas tree for all the people of the world as our old friend President Roosevelt."[19]

Eisenhower contributed to the conservatives' unease by the care he took never to attack Franklin Roosevelt in any public statement. In a 1952 campaign speech in Indianapolis, he spoke of "1945, when the present mess in Washington began," implying that he was absolving FDR. He was no less reticent in foreign affairs. When Republicans in Congress clamored for a resolution denouncing the Yalta agreements, Eisenhower refused to oblige them. He had campaigned on the iniquity of the compact reached by Roosevelt, Stalin, and Churchill in 1945, but once elected he sent Congress a resolution reprimanding the USSR for subverting the agreements, thereby placing the blame not on FDR but on Stalin. He did so in good part because he was advised that it was in America's national interest and because he needed Democratic support for his foreign policy, but also because he was unsympathetic with the desire of the Republican right to make Roosevelt a villain. In private, he might say of Yalta, "Our commander in chief didn't have to be so indiscreet and crazy," but, as one of his aides has commented, with only slight exaggeration, "in public utterances, throughout his life, Eisenhower remained impeccably correct about Roosevelt, the man who had assured his place in history by giving him command." When, early in 1955, the State Department proposed to release the Yalta papers, which were expected to tarnish FDR's image, Sherman Adams told Undersecretary of State Walter Bedell Smith, "Now, Beetle, you know how the Boss feels: he doesn't want to throw any rocks at Roosevelt."[20]

The Taft wing of the Republican party complained that Eisenhower declined to condemn FDR's foreign policy not merely out of respect for his former chief but because he shared Roosevelt's outlook. That seemed to be obvious in regard to Latin America. The president's special ambassador, Milton Eisenhower, was an admirer of the Good Neighbor Policy, which he was later to call "a bold and imaginative step that eliminated much of the enmity toward the United States that had been building up over a long period of years."[21] Observers sensed that even when Eisenhower did not acknowledge that he was FDR's legatee, he had the same internationalist aspirations. Indeed, as John Foster Dulles boarded yet another plane to yet another remote landing field, he seemed bent on carrying fealty to Roosevelt's globalism to the point of absurdity.

In domestic matters, also, Eisenhower, it was said, carried on FDR's policies. It quickly became a staple of political commentary to observe that Eisenhower's chief contribution was to make the New Deal permanent by incorporating it in a bipartisan consensus. Under Eisenhower, it was noted, the principles of the Social Security Act were safeguarded and even amplified, and in 1956 a liberal critic puzzled over the fact that the administration was "so New Dealish in its welfare program." When Eisenhower's archconservative brother Edgar upbraided him for carrying on liberal policies, the president replied angrily, "Should any political party attempt to abolish social security and eliminate labor laws and farm programs, you would not hear of that party again in our political history." In short, to the consternation of some and to the delight of others, Eisenhower seemed, as much as a Republican in a decade of moderation could, to be perpetuating the programs of the man who, at a critical stage in his career, had sent the surprising letter to Stalin and toward whom he had every reason to feel the greatest friendliness.[22]

III

In truth, though, no matter what his public affirmations and in spite of whatever fidelity he felt toward Roosevelt as his commander, Eisenhower did not care much for FDR. On numerous occasions Eisenhower told his aides that he held a low opinion of him. He often said that his predecessor had "usurped" the powers of Congress, and he could understand why the legislators felt deprived, Emmet Hughes has recorded. Another of his confidants has emphasized that his disesteem extended beyond policy matters. "Roosevelt's only idea of humor was a practical joke at some poor fellow's expense," Arthur Larson reports Eisenhower's saying to him. "Then came the shocker: 'Roosevelt was essentially a cruel man.'"[23] Still more explicit is the testimony of another assistant, William Bragg Ewald. He recounts Eisenhower's telling a stag dinner audience that as a fairly young officer he had been called upon to help put FDR to bed because he had drunk too much. "I like a highball or two myself," he added, "but I'll tell you one thing: nobody's ever going to have to put *me* into bed." (It is hard to know what to make of this tale, since Roosevelt is known to have been a moderate drinker.) Most revealing of Eisenhower's feelings toward FDR is a remark he let slip in the course of defending the president against criticism of his controversial wartime agreements. "For those things I don't blame Roosevelt one damn bit," he said sharply, "much as I didn't like him."[24]

Eisenhower thought even less of Eleanor Roosevelt, especially after Perle Mesta told him that Mrs. Roosevelt had said something offensive at a dinner party. Her friends were sure that Mrs. Roosevelt would never have made any personal remarks, and they ascribed his attitude to her criticism of him for not defending General Marshall or to his wish to appease the McCarthyites by getting rid of her. In fact, his accusation may not have been baseless. Early in 1954 Mrs. Roosevelt wrote a columnist:

> I felt it was not quite right to appear there when the President had never invited me to the White House. I had been told he had a special feeling of animosity against me because he thought that I had said Mrs. Eisenhower drank! Needless to say I did nothing of the kind but in Paris rumors were rife to the effect and I once asked Mrs. Mesta later in New York whether there was any truth in this rumor.[25]

Long before then Mrs. Roosevelt had been cut off from any contact with the president. She had stated flatly during the 1952 campaign that if the general were elected, she would not want to serve under him, and she strained relations further by taking her time about submitting her resignation from her UN post. At the end of the year she received a cool note from Eisenhower accepting her resignation, and through all of his eight years in office, she was out in the cold. At Eleanor Roosevelt's graveside one of her closest friends asked Eisenhower, "How could it happen that you did not make use of this lady? We had no better ambassador." Eisenhower shrugged and walked away.[26]

Dwight Eisenhower came naturally by his antipathy to the Roosevelts. His father was of the Republican persuasion, and other members of his family were ferociously hostile to the New Deal. In 1934 four of the brothers met in Washington and argued for hours about the Roosevelt administration. Two of them, Milton and Earl, though critical, saw something to be said for it, while Dwight joined his brother Edgar, described as late as the 1950s as "violent[ly] anti-Roosevelt," in denouncing it. His brother Arthur, a Kansas City banker, told an interviewer in President Eisenhower's first term, "During the early days of the Roosevelt administration, it seemed to me that the President blamed bankers for all the troubles, troubles which clearly were not of their making. Evidently the purpose was to divert attention away from other causes or circumstances. Anyway, we were constantly bombarded with criticism. There is none of that today." Dwight himself was opposed to FDR in 1932 and 1936 and especially disapproved of his bid for a third term in 1940. He did favor Roosevelt's return to office in 1944, but only because he did not want to break up a winning team in wartime.[27]

Still, Eisenhower's response to the age of Roosevelt probably reflected less antagonism than detachment. He did not vote in any of the contests in which FDR was a candidate because he thought Army officers should be nonpartisan, and even in 1944 he expressed his pleasure in the outcome of the election in the most guarded manner. Late in November of that year he ended a long communication to Marshall by saying, "A personal matter: I have carefully avoided sending the President any message, verbal or otherwise, concerning the results of the recent Election. However, if you deem it appropriate, I should be glad for you to let him know, informally, of my sense of satisfaction that our war leadership is permitted to continue uninterruptedly to the completion of its task. If you consider this inappropriate, please forget it."[28] Eisenhower was fifty-eight years old before he cast his first vote.

In an article published in the spring of 1953, the Washington correspondent Joseph C. Harsch observed:

> The whole story of the first Hundred Days of Eisenhower makes coherent sense only if one can first appreciate the unusual fact that Mr. Eisenhower's own personal emotions were never engaged in the great controversies of the New Deal–Fair Deal period. He had no part in that collective experience of the rest of the American people. It is as though he walked out of the United States when he entered the Army forty years ago, and back into it in June of 1952. He has been as remote from, and as emotionally untouched by, the great American civil conflicts of the past twenty years as William of Orange was remote from the wars between Cavaliers and Roundheads which slid into history when William set sail for England in 1688.[29]

Removed from the fray as he was, he shared none of the enthusiasms of the FDR followers, and insofar as he did relate to the events of the times, he developed an inchoate animus against Roosevelt.

Eisenhower's direct experience with FDR came wholly in the military sphere, and though his assessment of the president's performance in World War II was unmistakably positive, he found much to disapprove of even there. Eisenhower was said to have described Roosevelt's decision to land in North Africa as perhaps the "blackest day in history," and he thought that at Casablanca FDR's attitude toward military problems was almost "frivolous." When Roosevelt tried to tell him what to do in North Africa, Eisenhower reminded him that he was the general in charge of all of the Allied forces, not merely an American officer, and that he could not answer to an order from the president that was only a personal directive. So insistent was Eisenhower in his objections to FDR's plan to partition Germany that Roosevelt had to tell him to mind his own business and leave political questions to his superiors. Years later Eisenhower spoke of his irritation with Roosevelt's stubbornness and the president's unwillingness to follow proper procedure on such questions as interallied cooperation. "No matter how much you explained to FDR," Eisenhower said, "he never understood that in matters that big you just have to go through channels."[30]

The complaint about Roosevelt's failure to go through channels indicates that Eisenhower entered the White House with a very different perception of the presidency from Roosevelt's and with very different aspirations. Richard Neustadt has written: "Eisenhower wanted to be President, but what he wanted from it was a far cry from what F.D.R. had wanted. Roosevelt was a politician seeking personal power; Eisenhower was a hero seeking national unity. He came to crown a reputation not to make one."[31] Ike's speech writer, Emmet Hughes, emphasized this point even more forcefully:

> The Eisenhower who rose to fame in the 1940s, under the wartime presidency of Franklin Roosevelt, brought to the White House of the 1950s a view of the presidency so definite and so durable as to seem almost a studied retort and rebuke to a Roosevelt. Where Roosevelt had sought and coveted power, Eisenhower distrusted and discounted it: one man's appetite was the other man's distaste. Where Roosevelt had avidly grasped and adroitly manipulated the abundant authorities of the office, Eisenhower fingered them almost hesitantly and always respectfully—or generously dispersed them. Where Roosevelt had challenged Congress, Eisenhower courted it. Where Roosevelt had been an extravagant partisan, Eisenhower was a tepid partisan. Where Roosevelt had trusted no one and nothing so confidently as his own judgment and his own instinct, Eisenhower trusted and required a consensus of Cabinet or staff to shape the supreme judgments and determinations. Where Roosevelt had sought to goad and taunt and prod the processes of government toward the new and the untried, Eisenhower sought to be both guardian of old values and healer of old wounds.[32]

Though more recent scholarship has suggested that Eisenhower exercised power with more relish than his contemporaries surmised, it cannot be doubted that he thought of FDR's reign as having set a series of bad examples. He resented the precedent Roosevelt had set in scheduling regular press conferences. He was dismayed, too, that anyone had ever succeeded to the presidency so unprepared as FDR had left Truman, and as a consequence he told his choice for vice-president, Nixon, that he would make him a member of the policy-making councils of the new administration. When Eisenhower was urged to fling himself into the 1954 campaign to avert the strong likelihood that he would have to run the government with a Democratic Congress, he refused to do so, and not merely because he thought it unbecoming. He explained: "I think that history proves that no President, regardless of his popularity, can pass that popularity on to a Party or to an individual. Conspicuous failures were Wilson and the second Roosevelt."[33]

In conversations at the White House Eisenhower made clear how arrogant he thought Roosevelt had been. Early in 1954 he recalled one episode: "I asked Roosevelt in Egypt if he had the right to make decisions on subjects that should properly be in the peace treaty and he replied—rather annoyed—'why yes—eh yes!'"[34] Two years later, after reading a laudatory editorial about his presidency, Eisenhower said, "*This* is what I mean to people—sense and honesty and fairness and a decent amount of progress. I don't think the people *want* to be listening to a Roosevelt, sounding as if he were one of the Apostles."[35] How, then, could he explain his fulsome tribute to FDR in 1945? Easily, Eisenhower replied; Marshall had put him up to it.[36]

Though during the Eisenhower years commentators frequently said that the president was carrying on the New Deal, that is a misreading of the record. In his careful study of the Eighty-third Congress, Gary Reichard has concluded that Eisenhower was "far from a Republican New Dealer," and Richard Dalfiume has written, "Eisenhower was basically a conservative on domestic matters, and any tribute to him for consolidating the New Deal–Fair Deal seems unrealistic." Such, too, was the judgment of Emmet Hughes. "There is some unrealism in any tribute to Eisenhower for ratifying or consolidating the social gains of the New Deal and Fair Deal," he wrote. Eisenhower "held an antipathy toward TVA—and at least a tolerance toward right-to-work laws—scarcely reminiscent of the basic social attitudes of the New Deal. There was exceedingly little . . . to suggest the labor of a President who was *trying* to be a farsighted consolidator of past social legislation. And it is not easy to assign historic credit to a man for achievements he never attempted."[37]

Eisenhower's hostility to Roosevelt's programs had evolved over a number of years. It first came to public notice after he assumed the presidency of Columbia University. When in 1949 he delivered a commencement address on Morningside Heights assailing "the modern preachers of the paternalistic state," a newspaper three thousand miles away wrote that this "must have shocked any devotees of the New Deal." Nor was that the only such talk he gave that year. As Eisenhower noted in his diary, by 1951 the pressure for him to be a presidential candidate came more from Republicans than from Democrats, because many Republicans remembered his speech to the American Bar Association in September 1949 and "felt that as opposed to the New Deal—Fair Deal philosophies of the thirties and forties, it was sound Republicanism."[38]

Three years later he ran for the presidency in part in order to call a halt to the continuation of Roosevelt's policies. When Republican leaders flew to Europe to urge him to become a candidate, he consented because, one of his advisers later explained, he feared a Democratic victory "would mean more New Dealism and the like." In a reflective entry in his diary less than a month after taking office, Eisenhower explained his candidacy for the presidency in 1952: "I was persuaded that I had a duty to turn to another task, that of offering myself as a political leader to unseat the New Deal—Fair Deal bureaucracy in Washington."[39]

Eisenhower subsequently elaborated on why, after long rejecting the idea, he eventually agreed to run:

> I think the argument that began to carry for me the greatest possible force was that the landslide victories of 1936, 1940, 1944 and Truman's victory over Dewey in 1948 were all achieved under a doctrine of "spend and spend, and elect and elect." It seemed to me that this had to be stopped or our country would deviate badly from the precepts on which we had placed so much faith—the courage and self-dependence of each citizen, the importance of opportunity as opposed to mere material security, and our belief that American progress depended upon the work and sweat of all our citizens, each trying to satisfy the needs and desires of himself and his family—and that instead we were coming to the point where we looked toward a paternalistic state to guide our steps from cradle to grave.[40]

This attitude persisted throughout his years in the White House. In 1958 Eisenhower scolded Congress, "I am concerned over the sudden upsurge of pump-priming schemes, such as the setting up of huge federal bureaucracies of the PWA or the WPA type."[41]

More than once Eisenhower vented his hostility toward the public power projects Roosevelt had fostered, especially the Tennessee Valley Authority. In June 1953 he stunned observers by referring to the TVA as an example of "creeping socialism." When an Associated Press writer phoned in Eisenhower's remark, the AP office called him back to ask: "He didn't really say that, did he now?" Gordon Clapp, the head of the TVA, was aghast. "What a shocking smear on one of the greatest American achievements in this century," he wrote his predecessor, David Lilienthal. In the following month, Eisenhower told his cabinet, "By God, if ever we could do it, before we leave here, I'd like to see us *sell* the whole thing, but I suppose we can't go that far." He did, though, over the next several years, float the ill-fated Dixon-Yates scheme to circumscribe the TVA, veto a bill to give greater independence to the Rural Electrification Administration, and sign legislation to limit the TVA's potential for growth. With good reason, Eisenhower could boast, "No one has worked harder than I have to stop the expansion of TVA."[42]

To carry out his program Eisenhower surrounded himself with men who abhorred the age of Roosevelt. Secretary of Agriculture Ezra Taft Benson, proud that his father had been the last man in the county to sign up for wheat quotas under FDR, forced Claude Wickard, who had been Roosevelt's secretary of agriculture, out of his job as REA administrator, though he had a ten-year tenure. When another veteran of the FDR years, the economic analyst Louis Bean, returned from abroad, he found that Benson had moved a stranger into his office and he had no place even to hang his hat. The head of the U.S. Information Agency, Arthur Larson, praised by Eisenhower for articulating the president's own approach to government, declared that "throughout the New and Fair Deals, this country was in the grip of a somewhat alien philosophy, imported from Europe." Both Sherman Adams and John Foster Dulles sought to avoid the pattern set by FDR's lieutenants, and in advocating advanced public works planning the chairman of the Council of Economic Advisers, Arthur F. Burns, told the president, "The millions of dollars spent on 'leaf raking' projects by the W.P.A. during the depression of the thirties presents a shocking example of the results of unpreparedness."[43]

It comes as no surprise that Eisenhower and those in his circle employed "New Dealer" as a term of opprobrium. The president was in office less than a month when he said approvingly of a man recommended for an ambassadorship, "We would find a proper post for him, because he is a most able and devoted career man. Moreover, there is nothing New Dealish about him." Similarly, his press secretary, James Hagerty, fell readily into using "New Dealer" as an epithet. Hagerty's resort to this terminology, though, did not match the language of the Republican floor leader, Charles Halleck. Hagerty entered in his diary: *"Halleck on pinks and New Dealers in regional offices*—'They have loaded those offices with nits, bedbugs and lice.'"[44]

Eisenhower chose for secretary of state a man who had disliked Roosevelt and whom Roosevelt had detested. A conservative New York lawyer, John Foster Dulles had accused FDR of seeking to regiment business and destroy the Supreme Court, as well as of pushing the country toward an altogether unnecessary war with Nazi Germany. Dulles had deprecated the Atlantic Charter as "tentative and incomplete," and he had carped, too, about the preparations for Dumbarton Oaks. In January 1945 he censured Roosevelt "for disliking to take sides on issues that passionately divide much of our electorate," and as one "who prefers lofty generalities." When Dulles was eventually named an adviser to the United Nations founding conference at San Francisco, it was only after strenuous resistance from Roosevelt, who resented Dulles' faultfinding during the 1944 campaign as he had never taken exception to what had been said against him in any previous contest.[45]

No one made clearer that he was not intent on carrying on FDR's policies than Eisenhower himself. When at a 1954 press conference a correspondent noted that "some people have characterized your legislative program as an extension of the New Deal," the president replied, "I do think that all the way along we have showed the difference between . . . the philosophy of this Government, and that of the New Deal." That same year Hagerty recorded in his diary that Eisenhower had said, "Can't give way to every damn pressure group that bombards Congress. That's New Deal stuff." Even more compelling were his remarks to a Republican club in Indianapolis in the fall of 1954: "We have got to stir up and obtain the same kind of enthusiasm we had in 1952. And I admit it is not as easy. Because then we had always a symbol. Here was the New Deal standing up there and doing things to us we didn't like, and we really got busy and girded up our loins and went into battle. That is what we have got to do again."[46]

In seeking to exploit anti–New Deal sentiment, Eisenhower and his political aides took advantage of fissures in the FDR coalition created by disapproval of Roosevelt's policies and his style of leadership. Antipathy toward FDR was particularly noticeable among southern whites. A Virginia lawyer told his friend Senator Byrd, "It is my humble belief the Democratic Party no longer exists as a national party except as a label to elect certain people at election time. The Democratic Party nationally has been in a continuous process of deterioration since the advent of Franklin Roosevelt." But it could be discerned elsewhere, too. In the Great Depression FDR had no more fervent admirer than the columnist John Franklin Carter. But in 1953 he wrote, "We've had our bellyfull of great leaders—Stalin, Hitler, Mussolini, Churchill and Roosevelt—and the hecatombs of World War II are melancholy monument to this principle of life."[47]

Many who had once supported Roosevelt had reached the conclusion that Eisenhower's "modern Republicanism" suited an age of affluence better than FDR's depression-born ideology. As the 1956 election approached, the political analyst Samuel Lubell observed, "The New

Deal generation, once so zealous to make America over, devotes its evenings to wrestling with mortgage payments and inculcating a respect for tradition and discipline in overly progressive children." Some Democrats who had formed their attachments in the Great Depression switched their affiliation as their circumstances changed. In *The Ninth Wave,* a novel published in 1956, Eugene Burdick told his readers of "Joe Wilson of Burlingame, San Francisco Peninsula, who was once Jere Wilzweski of Pittsburgh." As he moved from the blast furnaces to a white-collar job and then to an executive position, he detected "that everyone in the block, all of the barbecue-pit owners, the mechanical lawn-mower owners, the Chrysler and Mercury owners, the commuters, the Peninsulates, the *Fortune*-reading people, were Republican." So he and his wife unobtrusively changed their registration to the Grand Old Party, "and, finally, even began to reconstruct their memory of Roosevelt and remembered him as a socialist, father of much-marrying children, fomenter of discontent, upsetter of the peace, and heard and believed that Eleanor had never loved him."[48]

IV

Yet despite the shift in sentiment in the 1950s and the hostility of the administration to the age of Roosevelt, Eisenhower discovered that FDR still cast a shadow. Liberal Democrats continued to turn out for ADA's Roosevelt Day dinners across the land, and each year on FDR's birthday or on the anniversary of his death the halls of Congress rang with tributes to the Illustrious Departed. Sometimes the demonstrations were more tangible, as when plans were laid for the Franklin Delano Roosevelt Bridge to link the coasts of Maine and New Brunswick, site of his summer home in Campobello. Little more than a year after Eisenhower took office, the historian Eric Goldman defined a contemporary liberal as one who "measures politicians by the memory of Franklin Roosevelt."[49]

In April 1955 members of both houses of Congress paid homage to FDR on the tenth anniversary of his death. No fewer than twenty-three senators rose to speak, cutting across a wide spectrum from liberal Richard Neuberger of Oregon to conservative Strom Thurmond of South Carolina. Even the Old Guard Republican Alexander Wiley of Wisconsin joined in the panegyrics. "I did not agree with much of his philosophy," Wiley said. "I find, however, as the years go on and as I look back that much that he stood for has influenced our times tremendously. What has been said so eloquently today by many of the distinguished Senators on the other side of the aisle, regarding his fear-lessness, his hope and his willingness to adventure in new fields to meet the problems, is correct." Paul Douglas of Illinois had a particular reason for lauding Roosevelt: "He had the discernment to appoint George Marshall, who was 33d on the list, to be Commanding General of the Armies; and he picked out an obscure lieutenant colonel and made him commander of the forces of the field in Europe, thus starting Dwight D. Eisenhower on the road to fame."[50]

Some of the comments indicated that only a decade after his death Roosevelt was well on his way to being canonized. Barratt O'Hara of Illinois told his colleagues in the House: "As the prophet Isaiah came to a stricken Israel to lift from misery and despond to a new exaltation by faith and courage and the dignified charity of brotherhood, so did Franklin Delano Roosevelt in our day come to the suffering people in the cities, the hamlets, and the regions of sparse population." That "great soul" had achieved so much though "every physical movement was attended by pain as agonizing at times as that which must have attended the Christ with ugly spikes nailing Him to the cross." Not to be outdone, Senator Robert Kerr of Oklahoma declared:

> I am reminded that 2,000 years ago the most flaming personality of all times gave utterance to one of the most inspiring sentences I have ever read: "I am come that they might have life, and that they might have it more abundantly." . . .
>
> Those words come to us from One who, divine in origin, frequently was human in achievement. When we reflect upon that noble statement of His purpose, Mr. President, I wish to state that in my judgment no man of our generation has done more to make it a living reality in this day and time than has Franklin D. Roosevelt.[51]

These rituals could not have seemed out of the ordinary to Eisen-hower, for he received repeated promptings that FDR offered a model for him, and the advice came not only from Democrats. As Eisenhower prepared to take office, Henry Cabot Lodge had told him: "You should maintain the honeymoon atmosphere as long as possible. Roosevelt maintained it all the time. Although there was a small group that hated him, he never had a long period of sour bad feeling among the masses of people as Hoover did. You can do the same." Lodge also recom-mended that the president-elect follow FDR's example as a party leader. "Franklin D. Roosevelt's political activities had permanently strength-ened the Democratic party and had made the word 'Democrat' a real political asset—of particular help to unpopular candidates," Lodge wrote later. "Eisenhower, I thought, could do the same for the word 'Republican.'"[52]

After he took office, Eisenhower continued to be measured by FDR's standard, and he did not always fare well. In the summer of 1956 Congressman Herman P. Eberharter of Pennsylvania told his colleagues in the House: "The Roosevelt administrations show up like shining beacons of imagination and forthright action when compared to this Republican record of inaction and timidity. Just imagine Roosevelt attacking the depression the way Eisenhower 'attacked' the 1953–54 recession: that is, by sitting and waiting for it to go away."[53]

More important than such partisan sniping was the attitude of newspapermen, some of whom did not cotton to Eisenhower as they had to Roosevelt. Unlike FDR, he appeared to be insecure around them, stiffer, more remote. "Mr. Roosevelt seemed to go out of his way to learn about people's troubles, whether it amounted to a news man's hangover or the poker losses of a press photographer," noted a veteran *New York Times* correspondent. Eisenhower "seems to like people the way a five-star general would be expected to like his troops—in a detached sort of way." At the "Little White House" in Augusta, reporters were kept at a far remove; at the press cottage in Warm Springs, FDR's staff had mingled with journalists and "Mr. Roosevelt himself was known to put in an appearance and to lend his baritone to the barber shop harmony that featured the soirees."[54]

Like every chief executive in the post-Roosevelt era, Eisenhower found that the press insisted on grading him at the end of his "First Hundred Days" and that his mark did not equal FDR's. Even a Republican senator who was one of his keenest admirers conceded, "There has been nothing spectacular. People who expected the world to be changed in a minute or that Ike's Administration would assume its full stature the first month, as Athena sprang from the forehead of Jove, are sadly disappointed, as some of my letters indicate."[55] Joseph C. Harsch was more cutting. He wrote:

> Dwight D. Eisenhower's public performance during the First Hundred Days of his Presidency has been so at variance with his adherents' more extravagant campaign forecasts of a "new broom" sweeping out "the rascals" in a vast purge of the personalities and policies of the past that the net result almost seems to be a man whanging golf balls at the White House back fence while history flows around him.
>
> The memory of Franklin Roosevelt's voracious seizure and joyous exercise of Presidential power twenty years earlier contributes to a companion illusion of a man who slipped into the White House by the back door on January 20, 1953, and hasn't yet found his way to the President's desk.[56]

FDR left his mark in still another manner. During all of Eisenhower's presidency the Democrats held a 2-to-1 edge in registered voters, and for six of the eight years they controlled Congress. That served fair warning that the Roosevelt coalition was still strong enough to recapture the White House, thereby leaving the Eisenhower reign merely an interlude in an era of Democratic dominance rather than, as the general hoped, the beginning of a Republican epoch. This situation, concluded a prominent political analyst, reflected not the imperatives of the time but FDR's enduring impact on the political culture of the 1950s. "This Roosevelt appeal to the 'forgotten man' in the dark depression days of the early 1930s is an appeal that the Republicans are still forced to battle," he declared. "It is the main reason why the GOP is the minority party in United States politics." That judgment was confirmed by the token black in the Eisenhower White House. In 1956 E. Frederic Morrow, Ike's administrative officer for special projects, wrote in his diary, "This generation of Negroes will never forget the desperate depression of the thirties, and the fact that the President at that time was Roosevelt, and that they were fed and given job opportunities through various work programs has caused them to be eternally grateful to him and to the party he represented."[57]

The most vivid evidence, though, of the shadow Roosevelt cast on Eisenhower came in a series of polls Gallup conducted. Asked in 1956 "What THREE United States Presidents do you regard as the GREATEST?" respondents placed Roosevelt first with 69 percent, ahead even of Lincoln and Washington. Though Eisenhower came in fourth, he had less than half of FDR's ballots. Still more striking was a survey taken by Gallup a year earlier, when he pitted Roosevelt against Eisenhower in a hypothetical contest. At a time when Eisenhower was at the very peak of his popularity, FDR handed him a bad drubbing. This was hardly surprising, given the revelations of yet another survey. In May 1958 Gallup put the question "If you could invite any three famous persons in history—from the present or past—to your home for dinner, which three would you most like to have?" Respondents placed FDR second (Lincoln was first), two rungs ahead of George Washington. Eleanor Roosevelt finished sixth, Jesus eleventh.[58]

Eisenhower never fell under the Roosevelt shadow to the extent that Truman did, but for those close to him the contrasts drawn grated nonetheless. Two decades after he left the White House, Sherman Adams said:

I'm very distressed at this tendency of academics to look down their noses at the Eisenhower administration. It's a common sort of thing with the intelligentsia. It's just typical. Look at Mr. Roosevelt. He's a great favorite with the academics, and he's probably a great man. But he lost a lot of battles, didn't he? The NRA was struck down. He lost the battle over the Supreme Court. Then he got us into World War II. Well, we may not have done as much, may not have been as spectacular in terms of our willingness to break with the past, but we didn't lose a lot of battles either. A lot of our most important accomplishments were negative—things we avoided. We maintained a peaceful front and adjudicated a lot of issues that seemed ominous and threatening at the time. Eisenhower didn't claim to be a purveyor of miracles. He never represented himself to do things he couldn't do.[59]

In alleging that scholars rated FDR more highly than Eisenhower, Adams knew what he was talking about. A poll of American historians published a year after Eisenhower left office put Franklin Roosevelt in the "great" category but assigned Eisenhower to the nether reaches of "average," a notch below Chester Arthur.[60] So long as Eisenhower's ranking rested on his performance as measured against that of the presidents who had gone before him, especially the imposing FDR, he would not do well. It required experience with the performance of his successors—with a disastrous war, a noxious scandal, and economic woes more troublesome than those of the 1950s—to put Eisenhower's presidency in a different light.

More clearly than anyone else, Eisenhower saw that his place in history would be determined by how long Roosevelt's ideas endured. In an "afterthought" to his memoirs he stated that the historical significance of his presidency rested on a single question: whether the American people accepted the FDR legacy or rejected it. If they turned away from the emphases of the age of Roosevelt, he wrote, "then the future would hold encomiums for my administration as the first great break with the political philosophy of the decades beginning in 1933. The years of my two terms would be counted as some of the most meaningful during our national existence." If they did not, then "the growth of paternalism to the point of virtual regimentation would so condition the attitude of future historians that our time in office would be represented as only a slight impediment to the trend begun in 1933 under the New Deal."[61] In sum, so long as the shadow of FDR still fell on the land, his years in the White House would have small significance.

If historians were reluctant to give Eisenhower a high grade, he scored much better with the American people, though even in that regard he encountered a reminder of Roosevelt's influence. So popular was Eisenhower that despite all of the vicissitudes of his final year in the presidency, he could almost certainly have been elected to a third term.

It is by no means clear that he would have been willing to serve again even if that had been possible, but if he had, his historical stature would have risen considerably, for he and Roosevelt would have gone down in the history books together as the only chief executives to have held office for more than eight years. Indeed, no other presidents since Andrew Jackson were well enough thought of to fill out three full terms. But there was no possibility for Eisenhower to act out this scenario. The Twenty-second Amendment, adopted in good part out of a desire to chastise Franklin Roosevelt for violating the taboo against more than two terms, stood as an insurmountable barrier in Eisenhower's path, much to the rueful discomfiture of his admirers.[62] In this unintended, altogether capricious manner, the shadow of FDR fell on his favorite field general to Eisenhower's very last day in the White House.

[3]

John F. Kennedy

I

Ten days after Franklin Roosevelt was inaugurated in March 1933, a prominent financier wrote him: "I just stopped off at Providence to see my oldest daughter at the Sacred Heart Convent. The Mother Superior of the convent, a real saintly woman, said the nuns were praying for you and then made a remarkable statement for a religious woman to make 'That since your inauguration peace seemed to come on the earth; in fact it seemed like another resurrection.'"[1] The financier who sent Roosevelt this report was Joseph P. Kennedy.

Five years later, when a former secretary of state met with Joe Kennedy, he discerned a very different attitude. Henry Stimson noted in his diary: "Speaking of the effect of all this [the New Deal] upon himself, Kennedy said that a few years ago he thought he had made money enough to provide for his children. He now saw it likely to be all gone and he lay awake nights over it."[2]

These two episodes indicate the conflicting perceptions of FDR that John F. Kennedy absorbed as a young man, and they go far toward explaining why he did not feel the infatuation of others of his generation toward Roosevelt. Through most of his days, Jack Kennedy, having received confusing signals at the formative period of his life, would be ambivalent toward Roosevelt and his legacy and detached from the enthusiasms of FDR's admirers. Eventually, though, he was to learn that he could not ignore the power of the Roosevelt heritage.

II

It is striking how little impact Roosevelt had on Jack Kennedy in his youth. Much of the time he was at school, cut off from the events of the

Great Depression and the New Deal. "Please send me the Litary [sic] Digest," he wrote from the Canterbury School in the fall of 1930, "because I did not know about the Market Slump until a long time after, or a paper. Please send me some golf balls."[3] More important, he displayed surprisingly little interest in national affairs as his schooling continued.[4]

To be sure, as a result of the influence of his father, Jack Kennedy could not escape an awareness of FDR, if to little effect. He was fifteen when Roosevelt came to power, sixteen when his father became chairman of an important New Deal agency and hence was linked to the president in any newspaper Jack was likely to read. Furthermore, Joe Kennedy ran an extraordinary dinner table. "I can hardly remember a mealtime," Robert Kennedy later said, "when the conversation was not dominated by what Franklin D. Roosevelt was doing or what was happening around the world."[5] Yet in the 1936 campaign, when his father was whipping up support for Roosevelt's reelection, Jack Kennedy, then a freshman at Harvard, gave no evidence of sharing the national ardor for FDR.[6]

During his Harvard years, he did come to develop an appreciation for the New Deal and for Roosevelt, but a subdued one. In 1937 he wrote his father that though it was probably true that a Franco victory would be better for Spain, "yet at the beginning the government was in the right morally speaking as its program was similar to the New Deal."[7] His chum Charles Spalding has said that Kennedy was keen about what the New Deal sought to achieve and studied closely FDR's political success. "But I don't recall that there was any idolatry on the part of . . . Kennedy for President Roosevelt, as a young man, the way there was for so many people," he added. "There just wasn't anything about President Roosevelt that stirred . . . Kennedy emotionally, as there was about Churchill." Spalding's shrewdest comment on Kennedy's attitude toward Roosevelt is: "Well, it must have been colored there by the relationship that his father had, and that was full of ups and downs."[8] If Jack Kennedy felt even intermittent excitement about FDR, it found no public expression. Though Harvard in these years was churning with discussions of the New Deal, he shunned the Harvard Liberal Union and the Young Democrats and never spoke out in favor of the Roosevelt reforms.

John Kennedy's slowly focusing attention to public affairs derived not from the New Deal but from events abroad, a development that owed much to the fact that his father was ambassador at a time when Hitler's ambitions were shaking the globe. When, after a trip to Prague in the midst of the Nazi invasion of March 1939, he returned to Harvard in the fall, he chose as the title of his senior thesis "Appeasement at Munich."[9] With considerable editorial assistance from Arthur Krock, Washington correspondent of the *New York Times,* young Kennedy managed to fashion the manuscript for publication. Joe Kennedy received two copies of the book by airmail; one he sent to the prime minister, the other to the British writer Harold Laski, who unobligingly told him that he regretted that the ambassador had permitted his son to publish so immature a work. "I don't honestly think any publisher would have looked at that book of Jack's if he had not been your son, and if you had not been Ambassador," Laski added.[10] *Why England Slept* appeared with a foreword by Henry Luce stating that Roosevelt was "glib," "sanctimonious," and lacked frankness, honesty, and courage.[11] To the world in 1940, Jack Kennedy had no identity save as his father's son, and his father by that year had moved more and more into the vortex of the FDR demonologists, though he had once dwelt in quite a different universe.[12]

III

Joseph Kennedy first ran into Franklin D. Roosevelt during World War I. As assistant general manager of the Bethlehem Shipyards, south of Boston, Kennedy had more than one encounter with the young and determined assistant secretary of the Navy. Once when Kennedy refused to release two battleships from his yards until payment was received, Roosevelt sent navy tugs to tow them away. "Roosevelt was the hardest trader I'd ever run up against," Kennedy was to say about one engagement. "When I left his office, I was so disappointed and angry that I broke down and cried." But if Roosevelt infuriated Kennedy, he also earned his respect as a resourceful, tough-minded official, a memory Kennedy carried with him through the 1920s.[13]

After the Wall Street crash, Joe Kennedy, a self-made multimillionaire whose concerns were no longer confined to the business world, hopped on the bandwagon to make Franklin Roosevelt president of the United States. He had survived 1929 remarkably well, but, as he later recalled, he brooded about the future. He told a writer:

Long before the stock market crash, back at the peak of the boom, when Jack was nine or ten years old, I had established million dollar trust funds for each of our children. After the Crash, I began to wonder if those trust funds were going to be worth a damn. I was really worried. I knew that big, drastic changes had to be made in our economic system and I felt that

Roosevelt was the one who could make those changes. I wanted him in the White House for my own security, and for the security of our kids, and I was ready to do anything to help elect him.[14]

The story is plausible, but insufficient. Once Kennedy became interested in politics, he was looking for a growth stock and he knew he had one in FDR. Furthermore, in the waning months of prohibition it did not hurt to be associated with the president's son James, who accompanied him to England. There they secured the American franchise for Gordon's gin, Ron Rico rum, and three brands of Scotch—Haig & Haig, John Dewar, and King William—which they contrived to import "for medicinal purposes."[15]

In 1932 Joe Kennedy donated large sums to FDR's campaign and made himself useful in other ways. He later said, "I was the first man with more than $12 in the bank who openly supported him." Kennedy also helped win the backing of the newspaper titan William Randolph Hearst at a critical juncture in the 1932 Democratic convention. "Isn't it wonderful!" his mother-in-law cried. "My son-in-law Joe Kennedy made Franklin Roosevelt President!" The claim was exaggerated, and there were other men backing Roosevelt who had more than $12 in their accounts. Still, his contributions—financial and political—were large enough so that Kennedy was able to ride on the campaign train and get prominent recognition as a likely cabinet nominee.[16]

Kennedy, however, did not conceal his patronizing, almost contemptuous view of the candidate. In the summer of 1932, Roy W. Howard, head of the Scripps-Howard newspaper chain, wrote FDR's defeated rival for the Democratic nomination, Newton D. Baker, of an interview with the financier: "He, himself, is quite frank in his very low estimate of Roosevelt's ability, as evidenced by his statement to me yesterday that he intends to keep constant contact with Roosevelt." Though "Kennedy was very frank in his expressions of understanding of Roosevelt's immaturity, vacillation, and general weak-kneed character," he nonetheless anticipated that he would "be able to go a long way toward molding Roosevelt's thought processes and policies along lines agreeable to him." As "a very energetic Irishman of about forty years," Kennedy, Howard concluded, was "enjoying his Warwick role."[17]

The relationship between Joe Kennedy and Franklin Roosevelt seldom ran smoothly, and FDR's first term had hardly begun before Kennedy had cause for resentment. Confident that he would be named secretary of the Treasury, he waited in vain for a call from Washington. Having promised to expel the moneychangers from the temple, the president, his adviser Louis Howe told him, should not put a moneyed man in the Treasury post. The most Kennedy could get from Roosevelt was a request to "be sure to let us know when you are going through Washington and stop off and see us." Kennedy was so angry that he threatened to sue the Democratic party for money he had lent it. The Brain Truster Raymond Moley, who stayed with him in Palm Beach, has reported, "There I heard plenty of Kennedy's excoriation of Roosevelt, of his criticisms of the President-elect, who, according to Kennedy, had no program—and what ideas he had were unworthy of note. There must have been hundreds of dollars in telephone calls to provide an exchange of abuse of Roosevelt between Kennedy and W. R. Hearst." But when Kennedy finally went to Washington, Roosevelt exuded so much charm that the financier was mollified. "Where have you been all these months?" the president asked him. "I thought you'd got lost." When Kennedy left the White House, he reckoned that his time for preferment could not be far off.[18]

He was right. In June 1934 Roosevelt named him chairman of the newly created Securities and Exchange Commission. It was a highly controversial appointment.[19] Liberals were appalled at the choice of a Wall Street plunger to head an agency that was supposed to keep watch on the Street. One commentator called the selection "grotesque," and another described Kennedy as an "antisocial gambler, a blundering wrecker of corporations, a tool of other capitalists, and a conscienceless market manipulator to boot." Years later, Joe's son Teddy took advantage of this episode to poke fun at President Nixon. Senator Edward Kennedy told a Gridiron Club gathering in 1971:

> I don't want to seem too critical of the administration, but once in a while even its friendliest observers have to stand up and protest. For instance, can you imagine a President of the United States trying to get away with appointing to the Securities and Exchange Commission, in fact to the chairmanship of that commission, a man who has been involved in all kinds of litigation, investigations, and alleged manipulations? Nothing like that has happened since 1934, when FDR appointed my father to the chairmanship of the SEC.[20]

Kennedy's detractors, however, underestimated his determination to do a good job, and in the end they had to eat their words. At a meeting in the White House with Roosevelt before the appointment, Moley had said bluntly to Kennedy, "If anything in your career in business could injure the President, this is the time to spill it." Moley has related Kennedy's response: "With a burst of profanity he defied anyone . . . to point to a single shady act in his whole life. The President did not need to worry about that. . . . What was more, he would give his critics—and here again the profanity flowed freely—an administration of the S.E.C. that would be a credit to the country, the President, himself, and his family—clear down to the ninth child." And so he did. A historian of the SEC has concluded, "Kennedy ideally served as . . . the first domesticator of the bulls and bears."[21]

Joe Kennedy and Franklin Roosevelt rapidly developed a unique association. No one else dared speak to the president as the SEC chairman did. In telephone conversations Kennedy would begin courteously with "Yes, Mr. President; yes Sir; yes Sir," but quickly revert to "Now listen to me, boy." When Roosevelt told Kennedy that he would have to break off his liaison with Gloria Swanson, Kennedy replied that the president would first have to stop consorting with his secretary, Missy Le Hand. Roosevelt even paid him the honor of a president's calling on a private citizen by going to Joe Kennedy's Washington home, Marwood, to swim, debate policy, and view the latest movies. (Marwood, which Kennedy called "the Hindenburg Palace," had a large theater, and, to accommodate FDR, a specially constructed elevator.)[22]

The two men also had family ties. Kennedy helped the President's son, Jimmy, with his insurance business, and Rose Kennedy was a fan of FDR's.[23] Kennedy's father-in-law, John F. Fitzgerald, provided another link. A legendary Boston politician, "Honey Fitz" was especially renowned for breaking into "Sweet Adeline" with no prompting. On one occasion, he was run down by a truck at a Fourth of July baseball game. Before he would permit himself to be taken to the hospital, he insisted on sitting up and singing "Sweet Adeline" so that everyone would know he was all right. Roosevelt had once heard Honey Fitz give a rendition of the song in Spanish in South America, and when Jack Kennedy was taken by his grandfather to visit Roosevelt, the president flung out his arms and exclaimed, "El Dulce Adelino!"[24]

In September 1935 Kennedy resigned as chairman of the SEC, but with expressions of fealty to Roosevelt which he made good on in the months to come. "You know how deeply devoted I am to you personally," he wrote the president. In 1936 Kennedy aided FDR's bid for reelection by making another sizable contribution, lining up business support, and reproving men of wealth who failed to appreciate Roosevelt. "We are witnessing the strangest hatred of history," Kennedy told a reporter. "The American bourgeoisie could have searched far and wide before finding a more devoted and effective champion of their cause." Kennedy also wrote a campaign tract with a title that said it all, *I'm for Roosevelt.*[25]

Kennedy's fidelity to the president carried into the start of the new term. Roosevelt named him chairman of the new Maritime Commission in February 1937, the same month he introduced his Court-packing plan, and Kennedy in turn not only supported the much-criticized scheme but continued to annoy his fellow businessmen by extolling FDR. At his twenty-fifth Harvard reunion in 1937, Joe Kennedy drew boos from his classmates when he praised Roosevelt, and in December 1937 he said, "I looked to Washington as a great enthusiast of the New Deal. I still am an enthusiast of the New Deal."[26]

By that time, though, Joe Kennedy's disapproval of many of FDR's policies had become increasingly manifest. Even in Roosevelt's first term Kennedy had dared to offend the president by opposing both the Wealth Tax Act and FDR's pet remedy of a death sentence for utility holding companies, a feature the SEC chairman said he would not want to administer. If some tories thought of Kennedy as, like Roosevelt, a traitor to his class, others knew better. "You asked about Joe Kennedy," a prominent Old Guard Republican wrote a member of the House of Lords. "I am sorry to see him leave Washington because he was a vigorous upholder of a conservative course; was courageous and candid in his contact with the president; and persuaded the latter to moderate his methods. You may wonder at the statement, but things might have been worse." In the fall of 1938 Senator Claude Pepper, after a talk with Roosevelt, recorded in his diary: "Asked about Kennedy. Hadn't he got a bit high hat? What had he said? I told him what K. said. Nobody in the show worth a damn. . . . Election made the Pres. so stubborn nobody could tell him anything and that R's policies were screwy and doomed to failure."[27] For Jack Kennedy, then starting his senior year at Harvard, it must have been hard to know what he was to think about President Roosevelt.

The signals Jack Kennedy received became especially perplexing after December 1937, when the president appointed his father ambassador to Great Britain. Roosevelt had bestowed a singular honor on an Irish Catholic of rude origins by naming him his country's envoy extraordinary and plenipotentiary to the Court of St. James's. ("Well, Rose," Jack's father said to his mother as they dressed for a dinner with the king and queen in their suite at Windsor Castle, "this is a helluva long way from East Boston, isn't it?") The president allegedly made the appointment, however, in order to get this "very dangerous man" out of the country, and viewed his mission as "the greatest joke in the world." He told Henry Morgenthau that he had arranged to have his ambassador "watched hourly." Kennedy soon revealed that he bore watching, for as Roosevelt concentrated on alerting the nation to the menace of fascism, Kennedy bent his efforts toward keeping America out of war at any cost, even if it meant appeasement of Hitler.[28]

Before long Roosevelt had lost faith in Joe Kennedy. He believed that, like America's envoy in World War I, Walter Hines Page, Kennedy had been gulled by British governing circles and made himself an object of ridicule. "Who would have thought that the English could take into camp a red-headed Irishman," he asked at the time of the Munich crisis. "The young man needs his wrist slapped rather hard."[29] During a stag party at the White House at the outset of the war in Europe, Harold Ickes said that Neville Chamberlain, notorious as an "appeaser," had decided to augment his cabinet to make a place for Joe Kennedy. Ickes noted in his diary, "The President threw back his head and had a good laugh at this."[30]

Even worse, Joe Kennedy proved to be disloyal to the president. The White House received repeated reports that Kennedy spoke savagely of the president and did not care who heard him, whether British servants or hostile American publishers.[31] Roosevelt gave full credence, too, to information that Kennedy was telling people in England that the Jews were running America and that FDR would be beaten in 1940. Still, he kept him on, in part because he anticipated that the ambassador would not last long, since he had a habit of quitting when the going got tough.[32]

Roosevelt had added reason to suspect the loyalty of the Kennedy clan. At the Democratic national convention Joseph Kennedy, Jr., who at twenty-four was being groomed by his father for a political career, sought to impede the president's ambition to be drafted for a third term by voting for the Irish Catholic James A. Farley, never more than a lukewarm New Dealer. "Junior, it was clear, was doing what the Ambassador could, at that point, not do openly," one historian has written. Even when Roosevelt was nominated overwhelmingly on the first ballot, Joe Kennedy, Jr., alone of the Massachusetts delegates, opposed the motion to make FDR's nomination unanimous. After the convention, Joe Kennedy wrote Jim Farley about Joe, Jr.: "I had heard about the struggle to get him to change his vote and was delighted he took stand he did. After all if he is going into politics he might just as well learn now that the only thing to do is stand by your convictions."[33]

The president knew, too, that for some time past rumors had been circulating that Joe Kennedy would be Roosevelt's successor in 1940, or that he would be the president's running mate that year. In their column in the *New York Daily News,* John O'Donnell and Doris Fleeson wrote late in 1937, "Irish-Catholic Joseph Patrick Kennedy, hard-boiled, sophisticated trouble-shooter of the New Deal, emerged tonight as the Crown Prince of the Roosevelt regime, as the man F.D.R. thinks will best fit the nation's requirements when the time comes in the next Democratic National Convention to name the man who will lead the Democratic Party in the national campaign." The account gives signs of having been a planted story, but that could not be said of an item in Ickes' diary the following summer. The secretary of the interior commented:

> A feeling in some quarters that there may be an understanding between [Vice-President John Nance] Garner and Farley looking to a ticket consisting of these twain in 1940 has led to the suggestion that in such an event the President might have to turn to Joe Kennedy as a candidate for Vice President. This would match a Roman Catholic against a Roman Catholic. While Farley would have certain undoubted political advantages, Kennedy would be able to command the great conservative business support and his campaign would be well financed, since he himself is a very rich man.

Roosevelt had no intention of accepting Kennedy as his running mate, however, let alone of stepping aside for him. Kennedy, whose experience with FDR had sharpened his awareness of the power of the Oval Office, would have to satisfy himself instead vicariously through his sons.[34]

Far from regarding Kennedy as a partner, Roosevelt viewed him as a menace who had to be scotched, for he had heard from sources in both Britain and America that Kennedy was planning to return to the United States to denounce him as a warmonger and back his Republican opponent. In London, Kennedy had boasted to English friends that he could "put twenty-five million Catholic votes behind Wendell Willkie to throw Roosevelt out," and if this was bombast, the White House had no doubt that the ambassador could do a world of mischief. The administration counterattacked. Stephen Early, FDR's press chief, got a Washington correspondent to write "a nasty story" about Kennedy, and the State Department conspired to keep him in England, out of harm's way. When Kennedy would not be put off any longer, Roosevelt arranged to have him met at the airport by one of his lieutenants and Rose Kennedy. On the way to Washington, she said, "Now, Joe, don't forget that you are Irish, Roman Catholic, the very first to become Ambassador to the Court of St. James's. President Roosevelt did that for you; and I want you to remember that when you are talking to him."[35]

Whatever Kennedy intended, Roosevelt outfoxed him. On the day

[71]

the ambassador returned to America, the president was lunching with the young Texas congressman Lyndon Johnson when the phone rang. "Ah, Joe, old friend, it is good to hear your voice," Roosevelt said. "Please come over to the White House tonight for a little family dinner. I am dying to talk to you. You have been doing a wonderful job." Then he hung up the phone, looked at Johnson, and "drew his forefinger across his throat like a razor."[36] That night, at dinner at the White House, the President was at his most beguiling, as he hinted at public honors that lay ahead, even, Joe Kennedy may have thought, the 1944 presidential nomination.[37]

The tactics worked. Two nights later, in the final week of the campaign, a network of 114 CBS radio stations broadcast a speech that Kennedy paid for himself in which he said: "My wife and I have given nine hostages to fortune. Our children are more important than anything else in the world. The kind of America that they and their children will inherit is of grave concern to us all. In the light of these considerations I believe that Franklin D. Roosevelt should be reelected president of the United States." The following evening at Boston Garden, the lair of Irish Catholic isolationists, Roosevelt welcomed home "that Boston boy, beloved by all of Boston and a lot of other places, my ambassador to the Court of St. James's, Joe Kennedy."[38]

Kennedy, instead of waiting to see if he would reap any benefit from his eleventh-hour exertion, promptly did himself in.[39] A few days after the election, he gave Boston newspapermen an indiscreet interview in which he spoke scornfully of England and said of Eleanor Roosevelt, "She's always sending me a note to have some little Susie Glotz to tea at the embassy." After the *Boston Globe* published an account by Louis Lyons of his remarks, which he claimed had been off the record, Kennedy was finished. But he did not leave without firing a parting shot. "You will either go down as the greatest President in history, or the greatest horse's ass," he told Roosevelt. There was a third possibility, the president returned. "I may go down as the President of an unimportant country at the end of my term."[40]

Joe Kennedy sat out the war a bitter man, waiting for a call from Roosevelt that never came. "In this great crisis all Americans are with you," he wired the president on hearing the news of Pearl Harbor. "Name the battle post. I'm yours to command." No response. Four months later he tried again: "I don't want to appear in the role of a man looking for a job for the sake of getting an appointment, but Joe and Jack are in the service and I feel that my experience in these critical times might be worth something." Roosevelt came up with nothing but a trivial assignment, which Kennedy turned down flat, and he remained "a private citizen without portfolio" seething with resentment. "I am so damn well fed up with everything and so disgusted at sitting on my fanny at Cape Cod and Palm Beach when I really believe I could do something in this war effort," he confided to a columnist friend. However, "I am still in the leper colony."[41]

That should not have surprised him, for in 1942 Joe Kennedy had gone out of his way to frustrate the president's aims by persuading his father-in-law to run against an FDR follower in the Democratic senatorial primary in Massachusetts, though Honey Fitz was almost eighty.[42] Among those who donated to Honey Fitz's campaign was John F. Kennedy. It is hardly out of the ordinary that he would give a hand to a member of his family, but it is noteworthy that Jack Kennedy's first political activity was to contribute to an effort to defeat a Roosevelt favorite. As a prominent Boston political commentator observed, "In Washington, this contest is regarded as a fight between Joseph P. Kennedy and the Roosevelt administration."[43]

Worse was still to come. Joe Kennedy, Jr., the apple of his father's eye, was killed over the Bay of Biscay while flying explosives to the Continent, and Joe Kennedy never forgave Roosevelt for it. (In one of those incredible coincidences that would seem contrived in a Gothic novel but sometimes do happen, the glare from the midair explosion that took the life of Kennedy's son momentarily blinded a crew member in the flight escort: FDR's son Elliott.)[44] In 1944 Joe Kennedy asked Senator Truman, Roosevelt's running mate, "Harry, what the hell are you doing campaigning for that crippled son of a bitch that killed my son Joe?"[45] Roosevelt sent condolences on the death of Joe, Jr., but not until Joe Kennedy was reported ready to endorse FDR's Republican rival in 1944 did the president summon his former envoy to the White House. It was the last time they ever met. If the president was defeated, Kennedy told him, the blame would lie with his advisers, who had surrounded him with "Jews and Communists."[46]

Not many months later the death of Roosevelt plunged the nation into grief, but not Joe Kennedy. From Palm Beach he issued the expected sort of encomium: "A greater love hath no man than he who gives his life for his country. . . . We can best show our devotion to the President's memory by working to see that his ideals shall not fail." But to his daughter he wrote that though there was "real sorrow" for two or three days, "there is also no doubt that it was a great thing for the country." Little less revealing was the reaction of the young naval lieutenant John F. Kennedy. Asked later how he had responded to the news of Roosevelt's death, an event that saddened and frightened many men in the service, he replied drily, "I had no deeply traumatic experience."[47]

IV

Twenty-one months after FDR's death, John Kennedy took his seat in the U.S. House of Representatives, still very much his father's son. In June 1948 Congressman Kennedy told the Polish-American Citizens Clubs in Roxbury that Franklin Roosevelt "did not understand the Russian mind." The next day, the *Boston Herald* headlined his speech:

KENNEDY SAYS
ROOSEVELT SOLD
POLAND TO REDS

Early in 1949 he assailed Roosevelt again in a one-minute speech on the floor of the House, and five days later he told an audience in Salem:

> At the Yalta Conference in 1945 a sick Roosevelt, with the advice of General Marshall and other Chiefs of Staff, gave the Kurile Islands as well as the control of various strategic Chinese ports, such as Port Arthur and Dairen, to the Soviet Union.
> According to former Ambassador Bullitt, in *Life* magazine in 1948, "Whatever share of the responsibility was Roosevelt's and whatever share was Marshall's, the vital interest of the United States in the independent integrity of China was sacrificed, and the foundation was laid for the present tragic situation in the Far East."[48]

Another of Joe Kennedy's boys, Jack's younger brother Robert, shared these sentiments. As a law student at the University of Virginia in 1950–51, he wrote a seminar paper on Yalta that accused Franklin Roosevelt and his lieutenants of espousing a "bankrupt" philosophy of accommodation with the immoral Soviet Union, a philosophy that "spelled death and dishonor for the world" and brought America "everlasting dishonor." In 1954 he once more attacked FDR. In an exchange of letters in the *New York Times* he referred to the Yalta agreements as disastrous and condemned Roosevelt for negotiating with the Russians "with inadequate knowledge and without consulting any of the personages, either military or political, who would ordinarily have had the most complete knowledge of the problems involved."[49]

[74]

Much of the world continued to think of the Kennedy boys as creatures of their father, and when Jack Kennedy ran for the U.S. Senate in 1952, he found his father's record in the Roosevelt years an embarrassment. His opponents circulated leaflets with quotations from captured German documents in which a Nazi official relayed what he claimed to be Ambassador Kennedy's anti-Semitic notions. According to one particularly damaging document, Joe Kennedy had said that "very strong anti-Semitic tendencies existed in the United States and that a large portion of the population had an understanding of the German attitude toward the Jews." With the ballots of Jewish voters and of those who abhorred anti-Semitism in jeopardy, the Kennedy forces flew Congressman Franklin Delano Roosevelt, Jr., into Boston to put FDR's cloak around Kennedy. "Jack was in serious trouble in the Jewish districts because of the rumors that the old man was anti-Semitic," Roosevelt later recalled. "I went in and Congressman John McCormack told me afterwards that I swung the Jewish vote over big to Jack and it was just about the margin of victory." The triumph opened wider horizons for Jack Kennedy, but he remained under not FDR's influence but Joe Kennedy's, not just in foreign affairs but in domestic policy.[50]

Either because of the ambiguous signals he had received from his father as he was reaching political maturity or because of his temperament, Kennedy showed a conspicuous lack of inclination to identify himself as a New Deal liberal. To be sure, his voting record was not far out of line with that of representative New Deal–style Democrats, but that was to be expected of a member of Congress from a highly urbanized northern industrial state. In such matters as public housing, he even took some initiative. But he did not seem to feel much empathy for the plight of the poor, and he voted to slash funds for that archetypal New Deal project, the Tennessee Valley Authority.[51] Even when he agreed that New Deal reforms were valuable, he thought of them as artifacts of the far-distant past. In 1953 he published a ghostwritten article that referred to "a law that's as dated as silent movies—Social Security."[52]

Kennedy cast one of his first votes as congressman in favor of the Twenty-second Amendment, to limit a president to two terms, though this amendment was widely perceived to be aimed at FDR. "My God, can't they let the man rest in peace?" a Democratic congressional leader asked.[53] Kennedy later claimed that he had backed the amendment not as a rebuke to Roosevelt but out of conviction that no chief executive ought to be expected to have the stamina to remain in office more than eight years. This belief, however, came directly from the Roosevelt example. Kennedy had talked to one of FDR's physicians, who told him that Roosevelt had run for reelection in 1944 against his doctors' advice, with fatal results. Whatever his motivations, in voting as he did, Kennedy joined those who, according to critics, were using the amendment as "a retrospective act of petty symbolic revenge against the recently deceased Franklin D. Roosevelt."[54]

These departures in his voting record bothered liberals less than his attitude. The problems of American society, they gathered, did not arrest him. On one occasion in 1953, he asked his chief assistant, Theodore Sorensen, what cabinet posts he would choose if he had the opportunity. "Justice, Labor and Health-Education-Welfare," Sorensen answered. "I wouldn't have any interest in any of those," Kennedy returned emphatically, "only Secretary of State or Defense."[55] Liberals sensed that he was not one of them, that even when he voted "correctly," he did not care as they cared.

Interviewers pursued him with questions designed to ferret out why he seemed so detached, and Kennedy tried to oblige them. "Some people have their liberalism 'made' by the time they reach their late twenties," he once observed. "I didn't. I was caught in cross currents and eddies. It was only later that I got into the stream of things." Asked in 1956 to account for "the somewhat emotionless quality of his liberalism," Kennedy replied, "In 1946 I really knew nothing about these things. I had no background particularly; in my family we were interested not so much in the ideas of politics as in the mechanics of the whole process. Then I found myself in Congress representing the poorest district in Massachusetts. Naturally, the interests of my constituents led me to take the liberal line; all the pressures converged toward that end."[56]

These statements say less and reveal more than Kennedy could have intended. He "knew nothing about these things" despite having grown to manhood in the Great Depression and gone to Harvard and served in the war during the age of Roosevelt. He "had no background" though his father had headed two of the New Deal regulatory commissions. Even in the 1950s there was no sense of compassion or involvement, only of "pressures" that compelled him "to take the liberal line." Particularly suggestive is his remark about "cross currents," possibly an allusion to the pulls toward and away from Roosevelt he felt in his own home. His simplest explanation probably hews closest to the truth: "I'd just come out of my father's house at the time, and these were the things I knew."[57]

In the 1950s Kennedy wanted to make one thing clear: he was not to be taken for a "liberal." He did not wish to be placed at any point in the ideological spectrum, but to be thought of only as a "Massachusetts

Democrat." Called upon to respond to those who criticized him for not being a "true liberal," Kennedy retorted, "I'd be very happy to tell them I'm not a liberal at all. I never joined the Americans for Democratic Action or the American Veterans Committee. I'm not comfortable with those people."[58]

If Kennedy expressed disregard for the Roosevelt liberals, they returned it in full measure. As one writer has said:

> The tendency among the sensible-shoe, twilight-burnished New Deal liberals of the period—the Eleanor Roosevelts, the Thomas Finletters and Paul Butlers and Archibald MacLeishes—was to see this standard-bearer of a second-generation bid for political power as callow and opportunistic, able to summon up a little too self-consciously a suitable ironic aside or a moderately recherché text insert from Burke or Stendhal or Dante or Duff Cooper: the lacquer peeled readily, the sealer of a gentleman's education had never penetrated deeply enough to insure a true and necessary preoccupation with individual liberties or social concern more profound than the giveaway proposal before Congress at any calendar moment.[59]

The Roosevelt liberals had one grievance in particular against Kennedy: his performance on McCarthyism. Though he cast some votes contrary to Joe McCarthy's wishes, he never put himself on record against the excesses of the Wisconsin senator. He was accused variously of being insensitive to the civil liberties issue, of sharing McCarthy's belief in widespread subversion going back to the Roosevelt era, of truckling to his Irish Catholic constituents, or of being influenced unduly by his father, a McCarthy partisan.[60] Early in 1953, the columnist Drew Pearson wrote in his diary:

> Lunched with Jack Kennedy, the new Senator from Massachusetts. He has the makings of a first-class Senator or a first-class fascist—probably depending on whether the right kind of people take the trouble to surround him. His brother is now counsel for McCarthy's committee and he himself has been appointed on McCarthy's committee, though Jack claims against his wishes. There was a time when I didn't quite understand why F.D.R. broke with Joe Kennedy. But the more I see of Jack, the more I can understand it.[61]

Much to his discomfort, Kennedy had one particularly sharp critic— Eleanor Roosevelt. For all her magnanimity, Mrs. Roosevelt was not altogether free of hostility toward the Catholic church, and her feelings were exacerbated when in 1949, in the midst of an acrimonious dispute over her opposition to federal aid to parochial schools, Cardinal Spellman accused her of anti-Catholic prejudice "unworthy of an American mother." This outrageous statement provided some of the setting for her conflict with Congressman Kennedy, a running battle that would last for a decade. In 1950 she announced that she was "certainly opposed" to a Kennedy bill authorizing public funds for Catholic institutions. She did relent enough to give her blessing to a more modest Kennedy proposal to appropriate federal money to bus pupils to Catholic schools, but that may have been because Kennedy's bill was cosponsored by Franklin D. Roosevelt, Jr. (Throughout the next decade, she had to bear in mind that in finding fault with Kennedy, she was setting herself against two of her sons, FDR, Jr., and often James.) The school-bill episode, however, added to her distrust of Kennedy. Herbert Parmet has observed:

> Given Eleanor Roosevelt's experience with the Kennedys, that was simply another black mark on their record. Jack's father had provided several: his attitude toward the Germans and the war, his relations with the Roosevelt White House, and, especially as far as Mrs. Roosevelt was concerned, his crude remarks about her as reported by Louis Lyons. Now she was seeing Joe Kennedy's son in action. What else could she have expected?[62]

Mrs. Roosevelt took particular exception to Kennedy's failure to speak out against McCarthy. As one of her confidants later said:

> I think she just thought that the man lacked, at that point in his career, the courage to do something and he had the margin of safety in his constituency to do it, because he was very popular and he had influence. It was Boston, and Irish Catholics and Polish Catholics generally, who were very much involved in the politics of revenge which McCarthy represented and that Kennedy could have done something about.[63]

When Kennedy sought the vice-presidential nomination in 1956, he illadvisedly tried to line up the former first lady on his side in the hope that this strategy would bring him a large number of FDR admirers. Instead, Mrs. Roosevelt embarrassed him by asking him why he still had not spoken out against McCarthy. Kennedy had made himself particularly vulnerable on this question by writing a book with the title *Profiles in Courage,* which opened him to the taunt that he should have shown less profile and more courage.[64]

Kennedy ran into more opposition from Mrs. Roosevelt in 1958 as he was mounting his campaign for the Democratic presidential nomination in 1960. In an article in the *Saturday Evening Post* she repeated what she had told a friend of Kennedy's in 1956. Asked to support the senator's ambition for the vice-presidential nomination, she had replied, "I think McCarthyism is a question on which public officials must stand up and be counted. I still have not heard Senator Kennedy express his convictions. And I can't be sure of the political future of anyone who does not willingly state where he stands on that issue." The magazine featured the piece under the banner "As for the current front-runner young Senator Kennedy, she takes a dim view of him."[65]

The most important flare-up, however, resulted from her remarks on a television program in December. Save for Adlai Stevenson, no aspirant for the Democratic presidential nomination in 1960 had "yet shown a spark of the greatness I think we need," she told an interviewer. What, then, would she do if she were faced with a choice "between a conservative Democrat like Kennedy and a liberal Republican [like] Rockefeller?" She answered, "I would hope very much that that particular problem would not come up. I would do all I possibly could, I think, to have us nominate someone at least for President who we felt did not have any of the difficulties that possibly might come up if Senator Kennedy were nominated." In an acerbic comment on the author of *Profiles in Courage,* Mrs. Roosevelt said that she "would hesitate to place the difficult decisions that have to be taken by the next President of the United States with someone who understands what courage is and admires it but has not quite the independence to have it." Moreover, she regretted the influence of the senator's father, who had been "spending oodles of money all over the country" to get his son the Democratic nomination "and probably has a representative in every state by now."[66]

Unable to join issue directly with Mrs. Roosevelt in her aspersion on his character, Kennedy took out after her doggedly on the charge of his father's intervention. "Because I know of your long fight against the injudicious use of false statements, rumors or innuendo as a means of injuring the reputation of an individual, I am certain that you are the victim of misinformation," he wrote her on December 11 in a nice sally against someone who had been raising the issue of McCarthyism against him. A week later she replied that it was "commonly accepted as fact" that his father was spending lavishly "to make his son the first Catholic President of this country." It was disappointing, Kennedy retorted, that she would accept rumor as fact, and he expected her to "correct the record in a fair and gracious manner." Though his language was carefully phrased, Kennedy understood that he was involved in a contest of wills with high stakes. He wrote Philip Graham, publisher of the *Washington Post,* to whom he forwarded copies of the correspondence, "The ball is now on her side of the net and I have no doubt her response will be another volley."[67]

The grim tennis match continued through all of January. In the first week of the new year Eleanor Roosevelt published Kennedy's latest letter in her column. Not nearly good enough, the senator told her. She still had not admitted, either publicly or in her correspondence with him, that she had no evidence to substantiate the allegations. "My informants were just casual people in casual conversation," she returned lamely. "It would be impossible to get their names because for the most part I don't even know them." If he wanted yet another column, though, she would write it—just tell her. "Many, many thanks for your very gracious letter," Kennedy wrote back. "I appreciate your assurance that you do not believe in these rumors and you understand how such matters arise. I would not want to ask you to write another column on this and I believe we can let it stand for the present." That same day, though, he wrote Graham in a very different key. It was interesting, he said, to compare Mrs. Roosevelt's denials now with her "categorical statements" on television in December. "Her performance is very curious," Graham agreed. It became even more curious a week later. Unwilling to permit the controversy to rest with Kennedy's graceful withdrawal, she sent him a wire that was at once supercilious and stinging: "MY DEAR BOY I ONLY SAY THESE THINGS FOR YOUR OWN GOOD I HAVE FOUND IN LIFETIME OF ADVERSITY THAT WHEN BLOWS ARE RAINED ON ONE, IT IS ADVISABLE TO TURN THE OTHER PROFILE."[68]

Jack Kennedy thought it unfair for Eleanor Roosevelt to blame him for the views of his father. He could not understand why she did not see that he was faithful to her husband's ideals, he told the Brandeis professor Lawrence Fuchs at a Honolulu hotel in the spring of 1959. "It's just a matter of prejudice; it's an argument she had with my father thirty years ago," he said. When Fuchs, who had been teaching classes with Mrs. Roosevelt, demurred, Kennedy insisted, "You just don't know. She hates my father." Exasperated by what he was sure was naked bias, he stormed around the room saying: "Don't you love your father? I love my father. But that doesn't mean I have to agree with him. We hardly agree on anything. Why, he's to the right of Herbert Hoover. Do you agree with your father on everything in politics?" No, Fuchs replied. "Then why the hell are they so prejudiced?" Kennedy asked. The only time his father had ever tried to influence his vote, he went on, was to get him to confirm Eisenhower's appointment of a Jew; yet liberals associated him with what was thought to be his father's anti-

Semitism. As he tossed clothes into a suitcase, his voice rose as he repeated, "Don't you love your father? I love my father."[69]

Gore Vidal, who supported John Kennedy's candidacy in 1960 but later became a waspish critic, has written:

> In 1960, after listening to [Kennedy] denounce Eleanor Roosevelt at some length, I asked him why he thought she was so much opposed to his candidacy. The answer was quick: "She hated my father and she can't stand it that his children turned out so much better than hers." I was startled at how little he understood Mrs. Roosevelt who, to be fair, did not at all understand him, though at the end she was won by his personal charm. Yet it was significant that he could not take seriously any of her political objections to him (e.g., his attitude to McCarthyism); he merely assumed that she, like himself, was essentially concerned with family, and, envying the father, would want to thwart the son.[70]

Vidal, though, has also recalled another occasion which indicates that Jack Kennedy may well have been right in thinking that he was at a disadvantage with Eleanor Roosevelt because memories of Jack's father still rankled. At Hyde Park in 1960, Mrs. Roosevelt brought up the time "when Mr. Joe Kennedy came back from London . . . to Boston and gave that *unfortunate* interview in which he was . . . well, somewhat *critical* of us." She went on:

> Well, *my* Franklin said, "We better have him down here"—we were at Hyde Park—"and see what he has to say." So Mr. Kennedy arrived at Rhinecliff on the train and I met him and took him straight to Franklin. Well, ten minutes later one of the aides came and said, "The President wants to see you right away." This was unheard of. So I *rushed* into the office and there was Franklin, white as a sheet. He asked Mr. Kennedy to step outside and then he said, and his voice was *shaking,* "I never want to see that man again as long as I live." . . . Then Franklin said, "Get him out of here," and I said, "But, dear, you've invited him for the week-end, and we've got guests for lunch and the train doesn't leave until two," and Franklin said, "Then you drive him around Hyde Park and put him on that train," and I did and it was the most dreadful four hours of my life!

After a pause, she added, "I wonder if the *true* story of Joe Kennedy will ever be known."[71] In a conversation with Congressman Richard Bolling at Hyde Park on Memorial Day, 1960, Mrs. Roosevelt confessed that her dislike of Joe Kennedy shaped her attitude toward his son. She acknowledged that the sins of a father should not be visited on a son, but she could no more exculpate Jack for his irresolution on McCarthyism than absolve Joe for his behavior as ambassador.[72]

Ironically, at the same time that Eleanor Roosevelt was venting her disapproval of him, Jack Kennedy was, for the first time, gravitating toward Franklin Roosevelt and his legacy. Dore Schary's *Sunrise at Campobello* may have provided the first impetus. When it opened in New York on January 30, 1958, on the seventy-sixth anniversary of FDR's birth, Senator Kennedy was in the audience. Afterward he went to a postperformance party at the Sherry Netherland, where he told Schary, whom he knew fairly well, that he thought the play had some very important things to say. Yes, Schary responded, especially the scene where Roosevelt talks about the right of a Catholic to run for the presidency.[73]

Whether as a consequence of Schary's play or of Ted Sorensen's fondness for historical allusions, or more likely because he was beginning to recognize that FDR liberals could further his aspiration to be president, Kennedy began to draw on the Roosevelt canon in his 1958 speaking circuit. As he made his way around the country that year and the next talking at Roosevelt Day affairs and Democratic dinners, he gave only slightly altered versions of the same speech, in which he paid tribute to "the man in whose progressive image our party must be forever molded—Franklin D. Roosevelt." He never failed to mention his favorite recollection of him—of how at Franklin Field in 1936, FDR tumbled and fell but quickly composed himself and, giving the audience no sign of what had just happened, delivered "one of his most buoyant, winning speeches." That address, Kennedy stated, set forth a standard that was still our best guide: "Governments can err, Presidents do make mistakes; but the immortal Dante tells us that divine justice weighs the sins of the cold-blooded and the sins of the warm-hearted in different scales. Better the occasional faults of a Government that lives in a spirit of charity than the consistent omissions of a Government frozen in the ice of its own indifference." (Theodore White later wrote that in the 1960s, both John and Robert Kennedy "at any time, any place, when lost for words or for specific program would go into what we reporters used to call 'the Dante sequence.'")[74]

When in 1960 Kennedy entered a contest for the presidential nomination that raised a series of rigorous challenges beginning with the Wisconsin primary, he portrayed himself as a man who would get the country moving again following years of Eisenhower torpor, just as Roosevelt had inspirited the nation in the post-Hoover era. In January 1960 Kennedy said, "Despite the increasing evidence of a lost national purpose and a soft national will, F.D.R.'s words in his First Inaugural still ring true: 'In every dark hour of our national life, a leadership of frankness and vigor has met with that understanding and support of the people themselves which is essential to victory.'"[75]

This effort to draw a contrast with his predecessor resulted in one droll episode. In a speech at Oshkosh matching his intentions to Roosevelt's performance, Kennedy quoted from a poem by Robert Sherwood:

> Plodding feet
> Tramp—tramp
> The Grand Old Party's
> Breaking camp.
> Blare of bugles, din-din
> The New Deal is moving in.

Afterward, in a hotel bar, Austin Weirwein of the *New York Times* told him that he had been "a little off" in his remarks. How so? Kennedy asked. "That line of verse," the reporter replied. "'The blare of bugles, din-din, the New Deal is moving in.' There should be another 'din' in there. 'The blare of bugles, din-*din*-din.'" Kennedy looked at him in disbelief and turned in for the night. The next morning he told an aide, "Haven't we got enough troubles without that Weirwein complaining because there ought to be another din? What am I supposed to do? Put it to music and play it for him?"[76]

Though Kennedy quoted Roosevelt, he ran not as an FDR liberal but as a man of the center, which had essentially been his position in the late 1950s even when he had been lauding FDR. For it was not the social reformer Kennedy especially admired but, as the Franklin Field parable suggested, the leader who could keep his cool. "This is the image of Roosevelt that we honor here tonight—the man of determination and steel in an hour of crisis," Kennedy said. The modern era, he emphasized, called for the valor Roosevelt had displayed in 1936, the courage to "recognize that creeping Communism is a greater enemy than creeping inflation." While seeking to make use of the FDR totem in the Cold War, Kennedy also gave some attention to social concerns. But he saw it as the duty of the Democrats "to use the impulses of liberalism without creating an impulsive party."[77]

At the same time that Kennedy paid obligatory homage to Roosevelt, he distanced himself from him. In Butte, Montana, in March 1959, he stated: "While our agenda of unfinished tasks may remind us of the 1930s, the role of our party, our Government and our nation in the years that lie ahead is certain to be completely different. For we are also challenged by problems which were never even foreseen by Franklin Roosevelt. . . . We are confronted with crises which the policies of the New Deal and the Fair Deal cannot adequately meet."[78]

Not everyone cared to hear this. Kennedy could not hope to win the 1960 Democratic nomination without gaining the confidence of the legions of Roosevelt loyalists, and in Wisconsin he began to learn that his failure to identify himself with the FDR experience reconfirmed latent doubts about how committed he was to liberal values. After a campaign talk in the auditorium of a Catholic school in Appleton, Joe McCarthy's heartland, a questioner asked him why he had not gone on record against McCarthy and quoted Eleanor Roosevelt's suggestion that he lacked courage. Bristling, Kennedy replied, "I'm not going to take criticism on that from you or Mrs. Roosevelt or anyone else." As one journalist has written, "At every turn, the shadow of Eleanor Roosevelt fell across Jack Kennedy's political fortunes."[79] Kennedy survived the Wisconsin contest, but not well enough; he needed to prove himself all over again in the West Virginia primary, a contest in an overwhelmingly Protestant state that he had to win if he was to go on. In West Virginia Kennedy was to learn how long a shadow was still cast not only by Eleanor Roosevelt but by FDR.

v

In the critical state of West Virginia Kennedy soon recognized that his only rival in the primary could advance a far better claim than he to the votes of that state's multitude of Roosevelt followers. In the tiny South Dakota town in which Hubert Humphrey was raised there was little but the merciless sun, the choking dust, and the mean chores at his father's drugstore, where he once sacked so much insecticide that he became ill. Then one day he rode in his father's Model A flivver to the edge of town to see a civic event that had everyone buzzing. To Doland, South Dakota, all the way from Washington had come men to plant the first trees for FDR's pet scheme of a shelter belt many miles wide running from the Canadian border to the Texas Panhandle as a barrier against the dust storms. The trees planted that day soon died. No matter. For Humphrey the important point was that there was a man in Washington who cared enough about the problems of a remote village to try to do something about them.[80]

Like a Jimmy Stewart come to Washington, Humphrey wore his love for his idol on his sleeve. In the summer of 1935, when Kennedy was viewing the New Deal with detachment, young Humphrey wrote of his experiences in traveling to the nation's capital with a Huron, South Dakota, Boy Scout troop: "Washington, D.C., thrills me to my very finger tips. I simply revel and beam with delight in this realm of politics and government. Oh Gosh, I hope my dream comes true—I'm going to try anyhow, but first I shall prepare myself for the task by reading and thinking always as a liberal. Roosevelt is a super-man."[81] During the following summer he actually shook hands with his hero when Roosevelt toured the dust bowl and Humphrey was county chairman of the Young Democrats in South Dakota.

As Humphrey moved out in the world, he hitched his wagon to the president's. In 1939–40, as a penurious graduate student at Louisiana State University, while his wife made sandwiches that he sold to other students for a dime each, Humphrey wrote an M.A. thesis titled "The Political Philosophy of the New Deal," an essay that applauded FDR's achievements. After working with the WPA and in war agencies in Minnesota, Humphrey took up a full-time career in politics; his first accomplishment came as state campaign director when he led the drive that resulted in Roosevelt's carrying Minnesota easily in 1944.[82]

The news of Roosevelt's death came to Humphrey in the midst of his first bid for high public office, the mayoralty of Minneapolis. Only moments after he learned of it, he wrote Henry Wallace: "I've just heard of the death of our great President. May God bless this nation and the world. I scarcely know what to say. It is as if one of my own family had passed away." A week later Humphrey addressed a labor rally at the CIO Hall in Minneapolis bedecked with a large banner announcing "A VOTE FOR HUMPHREY IS A VOTE FOR ROOSEVELT'S POLICIES" and with a backdrop of a huge spotlit portrait of FDR.[83]

In 1960 Senator Humphrey challenged Kennedy in a similar fashion. His campaign staff passed out thousands of leaflets showing him on a platform decorated with chrysanthemums and featuring a giant picture of FDR. As one of his biographers has observed, "Here was no jet age candidate gearing his words to a youthful and prosperous America, but a politician dredging up memories of the depression over 20 years before and conjuring up the fading image of Franklin Delano Roosevelt."[84]

However problematic Humphrey's appeal might have been elsewhere, it was ideally suited to West Virginia. Over and over participants in the West Virginia campaign, asked to account for the outcome, came up with the same sentence: "The name Roosevelt was *magic* in the coal fields of West Virginia." People remembered Eleanor Roosevelt's interest in the impoverished families of the hollows (one village in West Virginia even bore the name Eleanor), but even more what FDR had done. "If there was one god in West Virginia, it was Franklin D. Roosevelt," the correspondent Peter Lisagor has stated. "There were more monuments to Roosevelt in West Virginia than perhaps anywhere else. By monuments, I mean bridges, structures that were built in the Roosevelt time. And you'd go to some small mountain cabin, and about the only picture on the wall would be a picture of Franklin D. Roosevelt."[85]

A West Virginia political figure explained:

This area of the state, prior to 1933, when Franklin D. Roosevelt became President, was dominated by the coal operators. . . . With the advent of President Roosevelt, he made it possible through legislation for the coal miners to organize and to bargain collectively with their employers and, as a result, soon thereafter most of the coal miners, practically all of them, changed their political affiliation from the Republican Party to the Democratic Party. Up until 1933 . . . my County, McDowell, . . . was overwhelmingly Republican, but after the right to organize was granted, following the election of President Roosevelt, then the picture changed to where it became overwhelmingly Democratic and has remained so ever since.[86]

In a state with such an outlook, the credentials of a bona fide Roosevelt man posed so large a threat to Kennedy, who initially trailed Humphrey 60–40 in the polls, that he was compelled to rethink his strategy. A report from the pollster Louis Harris left no doubt about what he needed to do: arouse apathetic lower-income groups. There was only one way he could do that—abandon the image he had adopted in Wisconsin of appealing to all of the people and present himself instead as "an all-out New Deal Democrat." A West Virginian, asked by Robert Kennedy what his brother should stress, gave similar advice—"the 'Four F's' and only the 'Four F's'": the flag, food, family, and Franklin. "I felt that Senator Kennedy could talk about Franklin Delano Roosevelt anywhere in our state and win many, many, many, many friends and votes," he later explained.[87]

To implement this strategy, Kennedy recruited a man who was selling Italian cars in Washington—Franklin D. Roosevelt, Jr. Of all the former president's sons, FDR, Jr., looked the most like his father, and when he flashed a smile, he was the very image of him. His voice, as Humphrey was to say, "seemed a precise echo of fireside chats heard on crystal sets and Emerson radios."[88] Wherever he went in West Virginia to deliver a New Deal speech that was more persuasive than anything Kennedy could work himself up to do, Roosevelt drew the most applause when he mentioned "my father." It did not matter that Humphrey could make a far better claim than Kennedy to the line of succession, for in Franklin D. Roosevelt, Jr., Kennedy had the patriarch of liberalism incarnate. Nor did truth count. In one speech, Roosevelt said, "My daddy and Jack Kennedy's daddy were just like that!" as he raised two fingers tightly together. In addition, at Joe Kennedy's suggestion, thousands of letters with FDR, Jr.'s signature were shipped north and then mailed to West Virginia voters with the proper postmark: Hyde Park, New York.[89]

Franklin D. Roosevelt, Jr., also figured in the West Virginia primary in a different, and less seemly, way. "There's another candidate in your primary," he told West Virginia voters with regard to Hubert Humphrey. "He's a good Democrat, but I don't know where he was in World War II." Roosevelt subsequently became more explicit. He castigated Humphrey as a "draft dodger" who had busied himself seeking deferments while Kennedy was performing heroically in the Pacific. When Roosevelt was charged with hitting below the belt, Kennedy's press chief, Pierre Salinger, defended the allegations as only what was to be expected in a heated contest. Though Kennedy professed to deplore the injection of such matters into the campaign, he did so belatedly and then went on to say that no one had made "a greater contribution to the discussion of the issues" in 1960 than FDR, Jr.[90] "I am not running against Franklin D. Roosevelt, Junior," Humphrey responded. "I am running against Jack Kennedy, the son of Joe Kennedy, who was a mortal enemy of FDR, Senior." But Roosevelt's cheapjack remarks helped carry the day. To the end, the result remained in doubt, and Kennedy tried to put the best face on the possibility that he might lose West Virginia. "After all," he said, "Franklin Roosevelt didn't win all the primaries in 1932." But the contest ended in a Kennedy victory, and immediately afterward Humphrey dropped out of the race, a demonstration of Kennedy's power that proved indispensable to him in winning the presidential nomination. As one veteran of the campaign said, "He was conceived in Boston but he was born in West Virginia."[91]

Many observers credited Franklin Roosevelt, Jr., with playing the decisive role in the West Virginia primary by convincing the electorate that Kennedy "represented FDR's second coming." "People here thought there was nothing like his father when he was president," recalled a Logan County man. "They really thought there was nothing like the Roosevelts. I think he was able to get through to them on that alone." At Wellsburg Courthouse, in Brooke County, coal miners told the local Kennedy leader "that all they would like was to get close to FDR, Jr. just to touch him or just to see him." It was in the coal fields south of the Kanawha that FDR, Jr., had the greatest pull. One West Virginian explained, "The name Roosevelt is the fourth person of the blessed trinity—if there's such a thing—in the coal areas." Humphrey's cochairman believed that FDR, Jr.'s visit turned the race around. After he came in, "we had lost the lead in southern West Virginia, and from there on it seemed like a rush switching from Senator Humphrey to Senator Kennedy."[92]

A Kennedy leader agreed. He acknowledged that in the course of the campaign Kennedy had become concerned about the poverty he saw in the state, and that this feeling made his formerly "flat" speeches "increasingly alive." But he doubted that this would have sufficed. It was Roosevelt, he stated, who made the "tremendous difference." He explained: "FDR, Jr., to many people in West Virginia, was almost God's son coming down and saying that it was all right to vote for this Catholic, that it was permissible, that it wasn't something terrible to do. To me FDR, Jr. made it possible for many people to vote for Kennedy that couldn't have conceived of it as a possibility before."[93]

With Humphrey out of the race, thanks in good part to the intervention of FDR, Jr., Kennedy had a much easier road to the nomination but he continued to meet resistance from a powerful figure who even more than Humphrey epitomized the FDR legacy, Eleanor Roosevelt. For a time she would not commit herself, but when a group of liberals, among them Arthur Schlesinger, Jr., and J. Kenneth Galbraith, came out for Kennedy, she moved into open opposition.[94] "I am about to exercise the prerogative of a woman and change my mind," she declared on June 10. There was no longer any question, she went on, that the strongest possible ticket was Stevenson-Kennedy, and she thought that Kennedy should take second place because it would give him "the opportunity to grow and learn."[95]

The fact that three of her sons—James, Franklin, and Elliott—backed Kennedy made her stand all the more conspicuous. (Jimmy Roosevelt may even have thought that he was in line for the vice-presidential nomination. He told Adam Clayton Powell that Kennedy had "practically" offered him second spot on the ticket. "Get it in writing," the Harlem congressman replied.) When Jimmy Roosevelt went to the arena in Los Angeles to attend the national Democratic convention, a demonstrator yelled at him, "If Stevenson's good enough for your mother, he ought to be good enough for you."[96]

Although she preferred to stay home, Mrs. Roosevelt flew to Los Angeles in a last-ditch attempt to deny Kennedy the nomination and win it for Stevenson. "It seems absurd," she said with a twist of the knife, "to accept anyone as second best until you have done all you can to get the best." At a well-attended press conference, she raised doubts about whether Kennedy could gain essential black votes and whether anti-Catholic prejudice might not hurt him. "Just six sentences spoken almost like a grandmother," reported a Cleveland columnist, "and Senator Kennedy had been hatcheted twice." He added that when she was asked about her sons' support of Kennedy, she replied in a fashion that suggested "the plight of a mother who knows best but who like all mothers must sigh and sit back at the idiocies of youth." On the night before the balloting the indefatigable seventy-five-year-old woman made her way to no fewer than eleven caucuses. "There was Eleanor Roosevelt, fine, precise, hand-worked like ivory," reported Norman Mailer. "Her voice was almost attractive as she explained in the firm, sad tones of the first lady in this small town why she could not admit Mr. Kennedy, who was no doubt a gentleman, into her political house."[97]

Everyone in Los Angeles understood that in that political house were stored memories of the party's greatest days, and that FDR remained the leader by whom every Democrat was measured. In its convention issue, *Newsweek* featured an article, "Franklin D. Roosevelt—The Mystic Presence at L.A. in 1960." "So long as the American two-party system of government endures, there will never be a Democratic National Convention without four-time winner Franklin D. Roosevelt," it stated. "Though it is sixteen years to the month since he was last nominated by a wildly cheering convention, he is still the Democratic hero; and the mention of his name is still enough to bring a thousand delegates roaring to their feet." The young man in charge of arrangements for the Georgia delegation, only four when Roosevelt was first nominated, told *Newsweek:* "He is a legend in the South. No Southern politician, no matter what he thought of Roosevelt privately, would ever utter a word against him in public. Roosevelt created the agencies that brought the South out of economic disaster—AAA, the NRA, the TVA, the REA. He brought electricity to every farm community in the nation. He literally lit up the farm communities of the country." From a very different vantage ground, a Chicago congressman of Polish extraction declared, "The name of Franklin D. Roosevelt is still very, very much alive in my district. My people are, by and large, second generation Americans, and they still have Roosevelt's picture upon the walls of their homes. They remember the black days of the depression, and how Roosevelt led them out of it." So the legend of Roosevelt, *Newsweek* concluded, lived "in nearly every delegate's subconscious. And there was no Democrat in Los Angeles who did not quicken to his name." But the "delegates looked at the candidates on opening day this week, and saw no Roosevelt. They saw Jack Kennedy, who had some of the Rooseveltian glamour and charm, but not his maturity."[98]

Jack Kennedy did not need reminders of FDR's presence, for he and his aides showed that they were conscious of Roosevelt in much that they did at the convention. On the day before he was nominated, Kennedy called Jim Farley to his hotel suite in Los Angeles to ask him how he would run the campaign if he were doing it just as he had directed FDR's, and at a caucus of farm state delegates, Kennedy responded to the claim that no easterner could be trusted by pointing out that the easterner Franklin D. Roosevelt had been the best friend agriculture had ever had. When—to the dismay of Eleanor Roosevelt, who left the convention on the verge of tears—Kennedy won the nomination, the *Christian Science Monitor* observed that those who had written Senator Kennedy off because he was "not the warm, volatile type of an Al Smith or a Franklin Roosevelt . . . did not until late wake up to the fact that he was putting together a coalition of political forces closely resembling the one FDR managed."[99]

Though Kennedy's victory was likened to FDR's, his supporters, as well as independent observers, saw his triumph as the waning of the age of Roosevelt. One of Kennedy's top campaign officials, Larry O'Brien, told a journalist at the close of the convention, "The old generation is gone—Mrs. FDR, Truman, Stevenson. Look around you and you will see the new generation that will be running the party." A former New Deal luminary had a similar perspective. David Lilienthal was sorry to see such people as Eleanor Roosevelt leave the hall so disconsolate, but, he observed, "hanging on has nothing to do with the law of life, which is change." Lilienthal added: "Four years ago . . . I pleaded with Stevenson to tell the old heroes to go fishing; that he was running the Party and running it for the future, not to glorify the past. I don't think he believed that course a practical one. Perhaps he does now, after Kennedy has 'taken' the lot of them, Truman, Roosevelt, Lehman, and a lot of the others."[100]

Kennedy in his acceptance address treated the Roosevelt legacy as old baggage. "The New Deal and the Fair Deal were bold measures for their generations—but now this is a new generation," he declared. In the central paragraph of his speech, Kennedy emphasized:

Woodrow Wilson's New Freedom promised our nation a new political and economic framework. Franklin Roosevelt's New Deal promised security and succor to those in need. But the New Frontier of which I speak is not a set of promises—it is a set of challenges. It sums up not what I intend to offer to the American people, but what I intend to ask of them. . . . It holds out the promise of more sacrifice instead of more security.[101]

Yet no sooner had his campaign for the presidency against Richard Nixon started than, as an Eisenhower aide would write sardonically, "Kennedy began running as a reincarnation of F.D.R." In August he traveled to Hyde Park to commemorate the twenty-fifth anniversary of the Social Security Act and pledged to complete the work Roosevelt had so well begun. For weeks thereafter, at campaign stops in such places as Spring Lake, New Jersey, and Nashua, New Hampshire, Kennedy promised to live up to the heritage of Franklin Roosevelt while his assistants asked the press to refer to him as "JFK" in order to associate him with "FDR."[102]

On the last day of September 1960, Chet Huntley and David Brinkley came to his home on Cape Cod to interview him before the TV cameras, and Kennedy, in response to their questions, turned instinctively to FDR's experience. Asked what role Lyndon Johnson would play in his administration, he replied, "President Roosevelt gave his Vice President several tasks." Just as Henry Wallace had performed important administrative functions, so would Johnson. In Vietnam, as in Algeria, he would associate the United States with the worldwide desire for independence from imperial powers. "I just want to see us have the same identification with this cause we did during Roosevelt's administration," he explained. "Do you think the White House can change this emphasis from private luxury to public services?" he was asked. "Roosevelt did an awful lot in his day," Kennedy responded.[103]

Kennedy both began and concluded his debates with Richard Nixon by drawing upon FDR. In his opening statement he quoted one of Roosevelt's sentences, and in his final comments he said "that the function of the President is to set before the people the unfinished business of our society, as Franklin Roosevelt did in the thirties." Even more striking was his closing statement in the fourth debate with Nixon:

I believe that this party, Republican Party, has stood still really for 25 years; its leadership has. It opposed all the programs of President Roosevelt and others, for minimum wage, and for housing, and economic growth, and development of our natural resources, the Tennessee Valley and all the rest. And I believe that if we can get a party which believes in movement, which believes in going ahead, then we can reestablish our position in the world . . . particularly to try to reestablish the atmosphere . . . which existed in Latin America at the time of Franklin Roosevelt. . . .

Franklin Roosevelt said in 1936 that that generation of Americans had a "rendezvous with destiny." I believe in 1960 and '61 and '2 and '3 we have a "rendezvous with destiny."[104]

In part because of Kennedy's self-conscious identification with FDR, comparisons of Roosevelt and Kennedy surfaced frequently in 1960. When the senator appeared at the National Press Club, he spoke, noted one columnist, "in a clear upper-class accent that oddly recalled FDR," and when his name was placed in nomination in Los Angeles, the band broke out in Roosevelt's old theme, "Happy Days Are Here Again." Sam Rayburn called Kennedy the greatest northern Democrat since FDR, and the governor of Pennsylvania, David Lawrence, said he had not seen anything like the crowd response to Kennedy since Roosevelt. In a book published during the 1960 campaign, Arthur Schlesinger, Jr., wrote: "Like Roosevelt's polio, Kennedy's near fatal sickness in 1955 no doubt accelerated his private crisis of identity. Like Roosevelt, he emerged more focused, more purposeful, more formidable."[105]

Kennedy benefited, too, from the fact that the country perceived him to be, like Roosevelt, a patrician. To be sure, Kennedy did not boast a seventeenth-century lineage or descend from the landed gentry. Yet in other respects they were similar. Both had gone to prestigious prep schools; both were Harvard men; both had sailed the New England coast; each had a sense of *noblesse oblige*. Like Roosevelt, Kennedy was a man of inherited wealth who could, to a degree, view business from the outside. In comparing Kennedy to Roosevelt, a columnist for the *New Republic* observed: "Each had an upper-class education, found a life of public service more attractive than money-grabbing and each had a respect for the decencies. At heart, too, each had a kind of patrician reticence, an impervious private dignity." Kennedy moved easily in transatlantic society; his sister had married the Marquess of Hartington. "Jack," said a Massachusetts governor, "is the first Irish Brahmin."[106]

No matter how often he was compared to FDR or how often he cited him in his speeches, however, Kennedy could not be secure about leading a united party until he had won the endorsement of Eleanor Roosevelt. Her efforts to deny him the nomination had left bad feelings on both sides. One of Kennedy's West Virginia supporters later said, "I thought her entrance at the National Convention in Los Angeles while he was speaking was one of the rudest things I had ever seen done."[107] On the other hand, a Pittsburgh man wrote Galbraith "in protest about the damn dirty way Kennedy people in the democratic party treated Mrs. Roosevelt." He added:

After all Mrs. Roosevelt and F.D.R. did for the party do [you] not think that any fairminded person would relize [sic] that she owned a place in the

N.Y. State delegation. It must [have] made Mrs. Roosevelt a Grand Lady over 75 to shedd [sic] a few bitter tears to be frozen out because she was not for your Senator Kennedy.

In my opinion if Senator Kennedy was a man of any common decency he would have seen to it that Mrs. Roosevelt got her place back.[108]

No sooner had Kennedy won the nomination than he set out to woo her. At first she was so resentful that when Kennedy phoned her at the Los Angeles airport she refused to take his call. When she returned to New York, she would not lend her name to the national Democratic campaign. "Kennedy, relentless in his pursuit, looked upon Mrs. Roosevelt as something of a sovereign state," Fuchs has written. "If not friendship, at least he needed a treaty of alliance from her. It was time to parley."[109]

Only after a while would she agree even to talk to Kennedy. He went to Hyde Park on August 14 with some trepidation, understanding it to be a summit meeting of two sovereigns. He told a friend, "It's the raft at Tilsit," where Napoleon had confronted the tsar. When Kennedy told Mrs. Roosevelt that the party was much more fragmented than in FDR's time, she replied that he could not win without the Stevenson following in New York and California. She exacted no specific price for her support but made clear that he should lean not only on Stevenson but on another former FDR appointee, Chester Bowles. Informed that he was encouraging Stevenson to do research, she replied that more was required—he must prove himself to Adlai. On leaving, Kennedy shook his head and said, "She's really tough, isn't she?" Mollified by his promises, she agreed to be honorary chairman of the Kennedy committee in New York. "Whether I would take any trips or become more involved will depend on whether or not I am happy with the way he progresses as a person in the campaign," she wrote a friend in a letter she passed on to Kennedy.[110]

Once Mrs. Roosevelt had made her provisional commitment, the relationship prospered. Early in September, Kennedy wrote to her in Poland that the latest efforts for social legislation had failed, but asserted, "I will take this fight to the people during this campaign; and if elected, I will make the most of those 'first 100 days' to bring about these and other measures which the country needs so badly." After Mrs. Roosevelt returned to the United States, she flung herself into the campaign with no thought of her advanced age. She spoke in Cleveland, Denver, Los Angeles, and "in out of the way places, you know, crazy out of the way places, where it took a good deal of physical getting around in trains and planes." She was first on the list of speakers requested by blacks, and she served to ease the anxiety of the Stevenson crowd about the candidate's character.[111]

Toward the end of the campaign, she wrote Kennedy a letter that suggested they were drawing closer. The burden of her message was a prophetic warning: "I think it would be unwise for people to have the impression that you did expect separately to interfere in the internal affairs of Cuba." But she added: "Things at present look as though they are going pretty well. I cannot, of course, ever feel safe till the last week is over because with Mr. Nixon I always have the feeling that he will pull some trick at the last minute. On the whole, things look pretty good, however. In the meantime, good luck!" And she closed the letter "Very cordially yours."[112]

Kennedy had no doubt of the ethnic implications of Mrs. Roosevelt's willingness to serve in a titular capacity in New York. Early in September he phoned his brother Robert to say, "We should plan at the appropriate time to have an ad run which would be of particular interest to the Jewish voters to be run in the *New York Times* and the *New York Post* signed by Herbert Lehman and Mrs. Roosevelt." Nine years earlier, John Kennedy and two members of his family had traveled to Israel, where they found themselves outshone by another member of their party, Franklin D. Roosevelt, Jr. Robert Kennedy wrote home from Israel, "I have finally solved the problem as to why the Jews did not accept Jesus Christ. F.D.R., Jr. is what they have been waiting for."[113]

In a very close race, Kennedy had to win the forty-five electoral votes of New York, where Jews made up a large proportion of the population. "Many Jewish voters feel a personal revulsion against Joe Kennedy," a *New York Times* survey revealed. "They find it difficult not to transfer that dislike to the son." On the eve of the election an ad in the Manhattan press recited reports of Joe Kennedy's anti-Semitism and his influence on his son, but to no avail, for a counterforce was at work. As a biographer of Joseph Kennedy has written: "What occurred in the heavily Jewish districts of New York City on election day, 1960, deserves high rank among the classic ironies of U.S. politics. For the deep distrust of Joe Kennedy was neutralized by an even deeper nostalgia. A furrier, sunning himself on a park bench in East Flatbush, gave a hint of what would come. . . . 'Kennedy,' the furrier said, 'is another Franklin D. Roosevelt.'"[114]

In the most fundamental respect, John Kennedy owed his election as president to the shadow cast by FDR, for he campaigned as the candidate of the majority party that the Democrats had become in the Roosevelt years. Though the Kennedy electorate did not match the FDR coalition in every respect, the two were congruent enough so that in the

Midwest Kennedy carried precisely the same four states and lost the same eight states that Roosevelt did in 1944. Overall, he ran well in many of the sorts of districts that had given their ballots to Roosevelt—ethnic working-class precincts in the big cities. Furthermore, there was common ideological bedrock. The Democratic party, noted an astute political scientist, "became the majority party . . . when Roosevelt wooed an earlier generation with the program and philosophy of the New Deal. . . . The policies and programs of Democratic leaders since that time, down to and including Kennedy, were faithful to the Roosevelt tradition. If the election of 1960 were no more than an unthinking return of Democrats to the faith of their fathers, that in itself would be a mandate to the Democratic victors—to do what was expected of them, to apply the Roosevelt-born tradition to the issues of the 1960s."[115]

But now that he had been elected, was it certain that Kennedy would relate the FDR legacy to the issues of the 1960s? Some had their doubts. Kennedy, they pointed out, had taken up Roosevelt only when it was in his political interest to do so—in the West Virginia primary and in the presidential campaign. He still seemed too much the man of ironic detachment he had always been to be thought of as another FDR. Roosevelt, wrote a liberal editor, was "a man who deeply cared, who was capable of brilliant dramatization because he was fervently committed." It was not clear, he thought, that this could be said of Kennedy. The incoming president had shown himself to be well organized, but there was "a certain coolness and grayness in his very orderliness." The editor added: "It is not fair to ask Kennedy to be FDR. All the same his success turns on showing he cares, cares passionately, and doing it before the elite turn against him and begin to hate him for saving them."[116]

Mrs. Roosevelt, on the contrary, was losing her skepticism. At the end of the campaign, she "expressed herself with absolutely unprecedented enthusiasm about you," Schlesinger informed Kennedy. She had told Schlesinger:

> I don't think anyone in our politics since Franklin has had the same vital relationship with crowds. Franklin would sometimes begin a campaign weary and apathetic. But in the course of campaigning he would draw strength and vitality from his audiences and would end in better shape than he started. I feel that Senator Kennedy is much the same—that his intelligence and courage elicit emotions from his crowds which flow back to him and sustain and strengthen him.[117]

In like manner, James MacGregor Burns, who had expressed misgivings about Kennedy in his admirable campaign biography, wrote an election eve piece for the *New Republic*, in which Kennedy held his own and more when compared to Roosevelt. "As in the case of FDR," Burns wrote, the men around Kennedy were "of two basic types—men of thought who advise him on policy and men of action who conduct the practical work of vote-getting. Also as in the case of Roosevelt, the men of thought have the decisive impact on policies." Burns went further: "The fact that Kennedy demanded and received an emphatically liberal platform . . . is proof that he considers liberalism both politically wise and morally essential. It is instructive to compare, in this regard, the enormous concessions that Franklin Roosevelt made to conservatism when campaigning during the depression of 1932."

Why, then, Burns asked, were some liberals still holding out? "The trouble with Kennedy," he answered, "is that he lacks liberalism's tragic quality. By liberalism's tragic quality I mean that so many of its finest and most passionate causes, like Spain, have been lost causes; that so many liberal heroes have had their tragic denouements, as in Lincoln's assassination, Wilson's defeat on the League, and Roosevelt's death in office." He explained:

> It would be easy to say that Kennedy in office will develop the passionate, evocative qualities that this brand of liberalism demands, just as Franklin Roosevelt did in the White House. For the Presidential office does work its magic on a man. But in Kennedy's case such a prediction might not come true. For he is a different type of liberal from any we have known. He is in love not with lost causes, not with passionate evocations, not with insuperable difficulties; he is in love with political effectiveness.

Given the vital need for action, Burns hoped that "the hold-out liberals" would surrender their reservations about Kennedy and accept "a liberalism without tears."[118]

Not a few of the Roosevelt liberals, however, found Burns's biography more persuasive. In that book Burns made a fair-minded effort to strike a balance but there remained a large unanswered question. In some ways he thought Kennedy and Roosevelt were similar. He observed:

> Like Roosevelt, Kennedy forged his own liberalism out of day-to-day experience rather than abstract dogmas; was caught between different classes and traditions and lingered between different worlds; became a pragmatist, a realist, a hardheaded political tactician willing to compromise—sometimes to the despair of his supporters—in order to gain some progress. . . . Like Roosevelt, he can be courageous, acutely intelligent, quick, responsive. Kennedy, like Roosevelt, is a moderate in his behavior

[96]

as well as in ideas. He has a gentleman's distaste for lack of self-discipline, and self-restraint, for displays of emotion, for personal brawls and scenes.

Yet he saw differences as well. Missing were some of FDR's leadership qualities. "Kennedy lacks Roosevelt's humor and joyousness, his superb acting ability, his magnetism with crowds, his power of oral expression," Burns noted. "He lacks also Roosevelt's blarney and deviousness." Even more, if Kennedy hoped to measure up to the demands of the 1960s, he would need FDR's "imagination and daring." Burns had no doubt that Kennedy could bring "bravery and wisdom" to the struggle ahead; "whether he would bring passion and power would depend on his making a commitment not only of mind, but of heart, that until now he has never been required to make."[119]

VI

If there is one occasion when a president should be able to count on having the limelight all to himself, it is when he steps to the dais to deliver his first State of the Union address; but not John Kennedy. On that January day in 1961, as he began his remarks to Congress and the nation in the great chamber of the House of Representatives, he looked out on a remarkable scene—a sea of white carnations; for his cabinet officers and most of the members, even some Republicans, wore flowers in honor of FDR on the seventy-ninth anniversary of his birth. Kennedy concluded his first State of the Union Message by saying, "In the words of a great President, whose birthday we honor today, closing his final State of the Union Message sixteen years ago, 'We pray that we may be worthy of the unlimited opportunities that God has given us.'"[120]

In other respects, too, Kennedy conveyed the sense of being FDR's successor. As president he showed an abiding interest in the style and performance of Franklin Roosevelt. "Kennedy freely acknowledged their affinities," Schlesinger has noted. "He was endlessly curious about Roosevelt and often demanded Roosevelt quotations for his speeches." It was almost as though Kennedy, for whom Roosevelt had literally been a household word, was just discovering him.[121]

Roosevelt appealed to Kennedy and his circle in no small part because he, like them, appeared to be problem-oriented, unsentimental, liberated from the compulsion to fabricate overarching idea systems. In a book published during his brother's presidency, Robert F. Kennedy wrote: "One of the great creative statesmen of our age was Franklin

[97]

Roosevelt. He was creative precisely because he preferred experiment to ideology. He and the men of his time insisted that the resources of the democratic system were greater than many believed—that it was possible to work for economic security within a framework of freedom."[122]

John Kennedy paid the keenest attention to Roosevelt's administrative style. In the final days of the 1960 campaign, with the issue still very much in doubt, the Columbia political scientist Richard Neustadt gave Kennedy a memorandum, "Staffing the President-Elect," which stated, "If you follow my advice you will commit yourself not to each detail of Rooseveltian practice—but to the *spirit* of his presidential operation; whereby *you* would oversee, coordinate, and interfere with virtually everything your staff was doing." There were "heavy burdens" to running a staff in the FDR manner, Neustadt conceded; "Eisenhower, clearly could not have endured them for a moment." But if "the burdens are heavy the rewards are great. No one has yet improved on Roosevelt's relative success at getting information in his mind and key decisions in his hands reliably enough and soon enough to give him room for maneuver. That, after all, is (or ought to be) the aim of presidential staff work." Hence Neustadt included with his memorandum an appendix on how Roosevelt approached both White House staffing and the budget. After a quick reading Kennedy told Neustadt, "That Roosevelt stuff is fascinating." He was not supposed to read it yet, Neustadt replied. "Fascinating," Kennedy said again.[123]

As chief executive Kennedy conducted the White House in a manner similar enough to FDR's, especially with regard to recruitment of personnel, to remind observers of his predecessor. "Theodore Sorensen, as Special Counsel, is a Rosenman-writ-large," Neustadt observed, and "McGeorge Bundy is a sort of pinned-down Harry Hopkins." So many of the people who joined Kennedy's White House staff were in the New Deal mode that a Republican, casting his eyes on a cadre of presidential assistants on Capitol Hill, said, "All they need now is Eleanor Roosevelt to be den mother." Theodore White has concluded, "Under Kennedy, the kind of men whom Roosevelt had fathered to guide the New Deal's economics and devise arms for the war were subtly but irrevocably brought together in a phantom corps of mandarins."[124]

Even Kennedy's White House study revealed Roosevelt's mark. Kennedy got rid of Eisenhower's desk and put in its place a desk that had last seen service when Roosevelt gave a fireside chat. Like FDR's study, too, Kennedy's had a nautical motif, including ship models and naval pictures. The connection was more than coincidental. It was at Kennedy's suggestion that the National Archives mounted an exhibition of

FDR's collection of naval prints; Kennedy opened the show and even wrote, or put his name to, an article in *Life* on it. (Schlesinger appears to have written the piece, just as he submitted apt quotations for Kennedy's remarks at the opening of the exhibit early in the summer of 1962.)[125]

In fact, Schlesinger provided the most important reminder of the Roosevelt tradition in the Kennedy White House. From his earliest days on the Harvard faculty, Schlesinger had been a political activist, and long before Kennedy became president a close association had developed between the Massachusetts legislator and his Cambridge constituent. When Schlesinger was appointed special assistant to the president, he frequently looked at the events unfolding before him from the perspective of the 1930s—understandably, since the third volume of his *Age of Roosevelt* had just been published in 1960. Thus in September 1961 he wrote a friend: "I hope you have seen Jimmy Wechsler's interviews with the President in the Thursday and Friday *New York Post*. They are an accurate reflection of his present mood. This appears to be the spring of 1934 and the honeymoon is coming to an end." Schlesinger repeatedly furnished Kennedy with bits of Roosevelt lore. When Vaughn Meader attracted notice by his adroit impersonations of Kennedy, Schlesinger fired off a memo, "Imitation of the Presidential Voice: FDR's Experience." The president, for his part, relied on Schlesinger for historical perspective, as when he asked him to look up how other presidents had behaved in midterm elections. (Schlesinger warned him against becoming involved in congressional races because FDR's intervention in the 1938 purge had turned out so badly.)[126] Kennedy was well acquainted with *The Age of Roosevelt*, from which he gleaned an intimate knowledge of the workings of the New Deal and its dramatis personae. He once asked Felix Frankfurter, "Who is the Raymond Moley of this administration?"[127] Moreover, in Kennedy's first days in office, his aide Fred Dutton twice sent him long passages from Schlesinger's work on Roosevelt as highly suggestive for the problems the new chief executive faced.[128]

In part as the result of Schlesinger's memos, in part on his own initiative, Kennedy in less than three years in office mentioned Franklin D. Roosevelt on no fewer than 107 public occasions, and for every conceivable purpose. In the spring of 1962 he paraphrased FDR's Fala speech to say, "'These Republican leaders have not been content with attacks on me, on my wife, or my brothers. No, not content with that, they now include my little girl's pony Macaroni.' Well, I don't resent such attacks, but Macaroni does." That same season Kennedy told a Jefferson-Jackson Dinner in Milwaukee that the assaults that were being made on his programs had earlier been leveled at FDR's. And what were these controversial projects? One was linked to social security. "I thought that matter was settled in the administration of Franklin Roosevelt," he said. Furthermore, every homeowner, builder, and construction worker owed thanks for "the guarantees which were given by earlier programs in the administration of Franklin Roosevelt."[129] Kennedy found, too, that a particular episode of the Roosevelt years continued to loom big. When he attempted to end the stalemate in Congress by enlarging the House Rules Committee, conservative opponents accused him of imitating Roosevelt's effort to pack the Supreme Court, and Kennedy himself alluded to this analogy in a nationally televised discussion.[130]

Kennedy even found the New Deal experience relevant to the civil rights struggle, though in an oblique manner. In May 1963, a week after the terrible bombings in Birmingham, the president went to Muscle Shoals, Alabama, to pay pointed tribute to the Tennessee Valley Authority on its thirtieth anniversary. On the platform with him was Governor George Wallace of Alabama, who had been fiercely resisting every effort to end segregation in his state as an act of tyranny by an alien federal government. Without ever discussing the civil rights issue, Kennedy left no doubt about what he meant when he said that the TVA was not "an outsider, an intruder, an adversary," but an intervention in the South by men such as Roosevelt of New York, "who were not afraid to direct the power and purpose of the Nation toward a solution of the Nation's problems."[131]

In myriad ways Kennedy borrowed from the Roosevelt years and cited FDR in order to legitimate the changes he advocated. His farm program was hailed as a return to the Roosevelt emphases, and his approach to conservation and public power owed much to the New Deal. In his introduction to Stewart Udall's *The Quiet Crisis,* the president wrote, "We must do in our own day what Theodore Roosevelt did sixty years ago and Franklin Roosevelt thirty years ago . . . to make sure that the national estate we pass on to our multiplying descendants is green and flourishing."[132] Kennedy reinstituted a food stamp plan that had originated in the 1930s, and the Accelerated Public Works Act derived from the PWA of the Roosevelt era, though the Kennedy operation was not nearly so wide-ranging. His indebtedness to the Roosevelt period was most conspicuous in the poverty measures he was starting to put together in his final year. The Youth Corps bill was characterized as a "new version of the New Deal's CCC." Even in some of the less spectacular phases of his administration this heritage was noticeable. Asked if he was concentrating his attention on mental retardation just as Roosevelt had on polio, he replied, "Exactly, exactly."[133]

To administer one phase of his welfare program, Kennedy turned to a longtime companion, Franklin D. Roosevelt, Jr. The president initially sought to find a high-level position for him, but Secretary of Defense Robert McNamara would not tolerate FDR, Jr., as secretary of the Navy, and he was ruled unacceptable for other proposed assignments, such as secretary of labor. He was regarded as a playboy, and his associations with the Dominican dictator Rafael Trujillo were embarrassing. Kennedy had to settle for appointing him undersecretary of commerce and chairman of a committee to supervise federal programs in Appalachia, where he could repay his debt to West Virginia.

If his rank was not so high as either of them would have liked, Roosevelt nonetheless found acceptance within the inner social circle at the White House. FDR, Jr., thought of the executive mansion as his home, one that well might have been his a second time if fortune had only been kinder, and the Kennedys took pleasure in the stories he told them of earlier days there. He even accompanied Jacqueline on a voyage on Aristotle Onassis' yacht, a junket that brought criticism on the first lady as a jet setter and on the undersecretary of commerce for associating with a shipping tycoon. According to one unlikely account, Kennedy seriously considered FDR, Jr., for the vice-presidential nomination in 1964, but when, after her return from the Aegean cruise, Jackie asked her husband who his running mate would be, he is said to have replied, "It was going to be Franklin, until you and Onassis fixed that."[134]

Kennedy had a considerably more important relationship with Eleanor Roosevelt, who took it upon herself to serve as roving ambassador for him, as she once had done for her husband. In particular, she pressed the cause of neglected elements in society and aligned herself with the forces for peace. She asked Kennedy to give greater attention to the plight of migratory workers, agitated for more appointments of women to high federal offices, and communicated with Attorney General Robert Kennedy on behalf of civil rights. She visited the White House with a delegation that urged Kennedy to disentangle the country from its growing involvement in Vietnam, and she told him to push ahead on a treaty to end nuclear testing despite the objections of the Pentagon.

Sometimes she offered advice of a personal nature. "I wish you could get someone like my old teacher (probably her daughter) to help you deepen and strengthen your voice on radio and TV," she wrote him early in his term. "It would give you more warmth and personality in your voice." Four days later she wrote him: "I listened to your speech last night with great interest and I found it moving and exciting. I felt that you conveyed the intensity of your own concern, but I still feel there is too much strain on your throat which should be completely free. Please try to take some lessons in breathing and projection because in the long run it will be useful in saving you time and effort." Kennedy, who might well have thought that he was a considerably more accomplished speaker, with better pitch, than the person from whom he was receiving advice, replied, "The problem of my voice is an old one and during the last campaign I attempted to improve it with voice instructions, but I have relaxed my efforts since then. It is difficult to change nature. But I will attempt to nudge it."[135]

Her suggestions about his voice arose from the conviction that he had a problem in communication. She began the letter in which she first counseled him about his voice by saying:

> I hope you will forgive me if I seem presumptuous, but I am concerned because I feel that there is not as yet established a real feeling among the people that you are consulting them and that they must react and carry on a dialogue with you on such subjects as you choose to bring before them. . . . I listened during a rather long drive which I took, to your last press conference and decided that it did not take the place of fireside chats.

Having told him, by implication, that he was not nearly as effective as FDR had been, she explained that, instead of fielding questions that were "much too sophisticated for the average person to understand," he should be talking to the American people more simply. By the fall of 1961, though, she was writing to him, "I want to tell you how courageous and excellent I thought your speech was today. You minced no words, but I thought you made friends for us by that very fact. I was much impressed by your delivery and your depth of sincerity."[136]

If Eleanor Roosevelt was free with her advice, she also tried to maintain a proper relationship with the president. She appeared to understand that her syndicated column could embarrass him, because it was a visible manifestation of the shadow cast by FDR on the White House. When she wrote a piece expressing doubt about Kennedy's faith in air raid shelters and expressing hope that such people as Stevenson and Bowles would be asked to offer new solutions to the Berlin crisis, she courteously sent him a copy, saying, "The column which I have written today will, I hope, not offend you because I have a great sense of admiration for your willingness to shoulder the responsibilities you have to accept, and certainly no one should understand better than I do what a lonely business these decisions are." Nor would Mrs. Roosevelt accept deference from Kennedy. At one point he held a door open for her. "No, you must go first," she told him. "You are the President." With a laugh, he answered, "I keep forgetting." She replied quietly, "But you must never forget."[137]

Mrs. Roosevelt also understood that she posed a bit of a problem for Jacqueline Kennedy. She was a hard act to follow for every subsequent first lady, but especially for the wife of Jack Kennedy. "A Frances Perkins or an Eleanor Roosevelt would not have been on his wave length at all," commented one writer. "After all, he chose a wife who had her own special kind of intelligence, but in the feminine, intuitional sense. As his brother, Robert Kennedy, once described her, she'd never greet him at night by asking, 'What's new in Laos?'" Nonetheless, critics persisted in saying that she should be more like Mrs. Roosevelt, an improbable notion, and in December 1961, when Gallup conducted a poll on the most admired women, Jacqueline Kennedy placed second; ahead of her stood Eleanor Roosevelt.[138]

Mrs. Kennedy herself appears not to have taken the comparison too seriously. She was happy to show the former first lady around the White House, but she did not feel compelled to exert herself to prove that she was a worthy successor to a gadabout preoccupied with social legislation. Attracted to cultural pursuits that gave her a different sphere from Mrs. Roosevelt's, she once told August Heckscher, the president's special consultant on the arts, "I will do anything for the arts you want—except read bills." She added, however, "Of course, I can't be away too much from the children and I can't be present at too many cultural events. After all, I'm *not* Mrs. Roosevelt." Still, in the spring of 1962 she wrote Eleanor Roosevelt, "Jack and I were so touched by your generosity and thoughtfulness in the column you did about me. You are something that is so rare—and so good for all women my age to have to emulate—a great lady."[139]

Eleanor Roosevelt's gestures toward the Kennedys owed no little to the fact that the president was doing all in his power to win her over. Early in his administration, he named her a member of the American delegation to the Special Session of the General Assembly of the United Nations, an appointment that pleased her. She expressed gratitude, too, on learning that he had nominated her for the Nobel Peace Prize, and when he showed his friendship in smaller ways, such as appearing on television programs under her aegis. Mrs. Roosevelt in turn accepted Kennedy's invitations to head the President's Commission on the Status of Women, to serve on the Advisory Council of the Peace Corps, and to be a member of the Tractors for Freedom Committee after the Bay of Pigs disaster.[140]

Mrs. Roosevelt's experience with Kennedy as president completed the metamorphosis of her views that had begun during the 1960 campaign. As early as the spring of 1961, Lawrence Fuchs has written, "the relationship between the President and the Lady was blooming." He went on:

> Impressed and delighted with the way Jacqueline Kennedy was redecorating the White House, she said something like "Franklin would turn over in his grave if he saw it, but I love it. He would never have let me do anything like that." (Not that she would have thought of it herself in those days.) The zest of the Kennedys impressed her, and she told happily of their tearing down walls in the White House, rearranging rooms, and putting in new colors. Kennedy was her young man now.

Fuchs added: "I remember how she used to say that the most important thing Franklin Roosevelt did was to give people hope. I think that was what she liked—the zesty, problem-solving, hope-giving approach to life that Kennedy's personality and convictions exuded. He was a life-affirming person who knew tragedy and felt irony but still cared." By Kennedy's second year in office, no smoldering ember remained of the old Kennedy–Roosevelt family animosity.

Mrs. Roosevelt had only one remaining concern. On a car trip to Brandeis, she asked Fuchs somewhat edgily, "Do you believe the stories they tell about Kennedy having mistresses in New York?" Fuchs said he did not. "Well, good, I don't either," she said with feeling. "People used to tell stories about Franklin, too." She continued, "With all those Secret Service following you around, it's a little ridiculous anyway, isn't it?"[141] In this respect alone did Eleanor Roosevelt underrate John Kennedy.

When on November 7, 1962, Eleanor Roosevelt died, President Kennedy attended the funeral and invited the Roosevelt sons to the White House afterward. (Subsequently, he asked seventeen citizens to serve on a committee to devise a fitting memorial to her and had the report of the President's Commission on the Status of Women unveiled on her birth date.) On returning from the services on that somber November day, Adolf Berle, who had worked under both FDR and Kennedy, recorded in his diary: "This funeral was distinctly the end of an era. . . . In the pew with us, Henry Wallace; behind him, Jim Farley; across, Senator Lehman; the great and lesser great figures of the New Deal. Now old and white-haired they were—and perhaps I with them—visibly going over the horizon line which divided politics and history."[142]

VII

In foreign affairs as in domestic policy, Kennedy drew on the Roosevelt legacy. "In the entire first Roosevelt campaign, foreign affairs were mentioned only once, and then in one paragraph of a speech on the last day of the campaign," Kennedy would point out, a comment that indicates what close attention he paid to details of the Roosevelt era. Yet on the eve of office Kennedy bore in mind FDR's example. "In the final analysis, our foreign policy, our relations with other countries, will be most affected by what we do here in the United States," he said. "It was Franklin Roosevelt's compassionate actions here at home that built his great reputation abroad. What we are speaks much louder than what we say."[143]

Throughout Kennedy's administration the Kremlin gave him pointed reminders of what they expected of a successor to FDR. In a postelection message Khrushchev wired: "Esteemed Mr. Kennedy, allow me to congratulate you. We hope that while you are at this post the relations between our countries would again follow the line along which they were developing in Franklin Roosevelt's time." Two months later, in assessing Kennedy's State of the Union address, *Pravda* wrote:

> It is pointed out in many international commentaries on Kennedy's message that the new administration of the U.S.A. now faces problems as acute and complex as those the administration of Franklin Delano Roosevelt faced 28 years ago. This analogy is by no means accidental. No matter how different the conditions of the 1930s may be from those of our time, there are nevertheless many similarities in the situation of the U.S.A. . . . Franklin Roosevelt had the courage and vision to steer the U.S. ship of state on a new course.

Just as Roosevelt broke new ground with the recognition of the Soviet Union, Kennedy had the opportunity, *Pravda* said, to jettison "the outworn dogmas of the 'cold war.'"[144]

At a dangerous stage of the Cold War, Khrushchev employed memories of FDR as a weapon of argumentation. At Vienna he reminded the president of FDR's pledge at Yalta to remove troops from Germany, and in an interview during the Berlin crisis, he told a *New York Times* correspondent:

> Franklin Roosevelt would have agreed to our solution in Kennedy's place. He would have said it is foolish to fight over this. Many people would have opposed Roosevelt, but the population would have supported him.

Kennedy is too young. He lacks the authority and prestige to settle this issue correctly. He is afraid to take up that position and that is why he has induced these mobilization measures. But he doesn't want to fight. Only an idiot wants war. . . .

The U.S. is the leader in the West. If Roosevelt were in power he would by now have appealed to the people. If Kennedy appealed to the people— if he voiced his real inner thoughts and stated that there was no use fighting over Berlin, no use losing a drop of blood—the situation would be settled quickly.

Even words of approval for Kennedy conveyed his recollections of the leader of the struggle against fascism. The American University address, Khrushchev said, was the best by any American head of state since Roosevelt.[145]

President Roosevelt served as a model for Kennedy especially in relations with Latin America. During the 1960 campaign Kennedy promised to return to FDR's Good Neighbor policy, and before taking office he informed an interviewer, "A new Democratic administration, as the legatee of Franklin Roosevelt, would have a great opportunity to rebuild close relations with Latin America."[146] He instructed his advisers to look for a catch phrase like "Good Neighbor" that he could call his own, and he was given one in "the Alliance for Progress." One of its chief architects described the program as "a New Deal for Latin America."[147] During the Cuban missiles crisis, Kennedy appropriated the word "quarantine" from Roosevelt, and in drafting the portentous address to the nation for the president, Ted Sorensen reread Roosevelt's words on the declaration of World War II.[148]

When Kennedy toured South America in December 1961, he invoked FDR's name again and again, as though he knew it was an open sesame for him. At a resettlement project near Caracas he declared: "I come in the footsteps of a distinguished predecessor, Franklin Roosevelt, who in his own time and generation attempted to bring to fruition the work which Simón Bolívar had so well begun." He gave the same message to the people of Colombia at a dinner at the San Carlos palace in Bogotá. The president said:

In 1934, one of the greatest of my predecessors, President Franklin Roosevelt, was the first President of the United States to visit this country. He came in pursuit of a new policy—the policy of the Good Neighbor. This policy—based on the ideas of Bolívar and San Martín and Santander— recognized the common interests of the American states—denied that any nation in this hemisphere had the right to impose its will on any other nation—and called for a great cooperative effort to strengthen the spirit of human liberty here in the Americas.

I am here today—the second American President to visit Colombia—in that same spirit. For our generation also has a new policy—la Alianza para el Progreso . . . going beyond the Good Neighbor policy to a great unified attack on the problems of our age.[149]

It was on yet another trip to Latin America that Kennedy, in the final year of his life, delivered an address that appeared to encapsulate all of his growing understanding of the significance of the New Deal. To the students and faculty of the University of Costa Rica in March 1963, Kennedy stated:

I can remember my own country when it was quite different from our country today. It was not so many years ago that I was a university student as you are now, and at that time, only 1 in every 10 American farms was electrified, half the farmers in our Southland were tenant farmers and sharecroppers, thousands of families in the Tennessee Valley had cash incomes of less than $100 a year, and all this in addition to a great depression which threw 12 million men and women out of work and had 20 million Americans on relief—that in the time that I was at the university.

Then under the leadership of Franklin Roosevelt, we carried through a great New Deal for the United States. One program after another brought an end to tenant farming in the United States, electrified nearly every farm in our country, transformed the poverty ridden Tennessee Valley into one of the richest agricultural and industrial areas in the United States. It demonstrated in those great years the immense power of affirmative, free government.[150]

VIII

Yet despite the many times he cited FDR, for all of his efforts to cultivate the Roosevelt family, for all of his indebtedness to the earlier period, Kennedy never wholly embraced the Roosevelt tradition and at times he deliberately severed himself from it. After winning election in a campaign in which he profited by identifying himself with Roosevelt, Kennedy, when asked shortly after taking office about the similarity people saw between him and FDR, replied coolly, "There is no validity to the comparison." Shortly after the president's death, the journalist William S. White would reflect, "Kennedy had been for some, although it offended his own great sense of realism, a sentimentalized and idealized reincarnation of Roosevelt—a man he never was and never wanted to be."[151]

Neither Kennedy nor many of the men around him thought that the Roosevelt legacy would be of much use in the 1960s. Kennedy, James MacGregor Burns wrote in 1960, "believes that much of the liberalism of the New Deal and the Fair Deal either has become properly entrenched in our way of life, and hence no longer a disputed political issue, or in a few cases has become outmoded or irrelevant." Even Schlesinger, though he repeatedly reminded Kennedy of ways in which FDR's experience was pertinent, had been arguing since Eisenhower's first term that liberals must move beyond the "quantitative" concerns that had been appropriate to the Great Depression to develop a "qualitative liberalism" befitting an era of prosperity. In 1962, in a new introduction to *The Vital Center,* Schlesinger wrote: "The problems of the New Deal were essentially quantitative problems—problems of meeting stark human needs for food, clothing, shelter, and employment. Most of these needs are now effectively met for most Americans." In the following year, Walter Lippmann, commenting on the "suction toward the center" in the Western world, observed, "President Kennedy, we must remember, is himself a man of the center. He is far removed from the social struggles of the New Deal."[152]

Over and over, as he had in the late 1950s, Kennedy stressed the need to move beyond FDR. In May 1962 he asserted, "All the great revolutionary movements of the Franklin Roosevelt administration in the thirties we now take for granted. But I refuse to see us live on the accomplishments of another generation." He added, "Anyone who says that Woodrow Wilson, as great a President as he was, and Franklin Roosevelt and Harry Truman, that they did it all and we have nothing left to do now, is wrong." Two days later, in an address to a conference for Democratic women, he reemphasized this theme by saying, "I do not take the view that everything that had to be done was done by those who went before us, that Franklin Roosevelt, however extraordinary his record was, and Harry Truman and the others, that they did the job, and ours is now merely to pass through our political period and occupy positions of public significance and not do anything."[153]

Kennedy's separation from Roosevelt went beyond the not unreasonable premise that new problems require new solutions, for he began his administration determined to approach business in a spirit different from FDR's, at least different from that of the FDR who had denounced economic royalists.[154] As Charles Spalding later remarked: "He wasn't antagonistic as Roosevelt was, or appeared to be; he didn't intend to bait business; he didn't intend to chide them or make his antagonism to them an issue of support, which it often seemed to me that Mr. Roosevelt would do. You know, he would turn his scorn on them, and, in turn, would get a reward from a broader number. But Kennedy never proposed to do that." In February 1961, *Time* reported that at a luncheon of the National Industrial Conference Board at which Kennedy called for "a full-fledged alliance" with business, members of his cabinet "tossed in some plums of their own in an outburst of pro-business sentiment that would have stunned an old New Dealer."[155]

Despite entreaties from some of his advisers and scolding from liberal and radical economists, Kennedy persisted in this cautious policy. He had been in office less than two months when Walter Heller sent him a memorandum on behalf of the Council of Economic Advisers stating that he would run no greater political risk with a large deficit than with a small one, and some deficit was inevitable. "Once fiscal virginity is lost, the size of the deficit matters very little to the critics," Heller contended. He added: *"Historical note:* This was FDR's experience. His deficits were small. They worked, but the recovery was slow. The modesty of his fiscal sin never appeased conservative critics, and the slowness of the recovery enabled them to say that it took a war to bail him out. FDR's experience also was that the electorate contains more voters who like recovery and dislike unemployment than people who care about budget balance." Hence, Heller said, Kennedy should seriously consider an aggressive economic program. The president, however, was too committed to cooperation with business to heed advice that he profit from Roosevelt's example.[156]

Kennedy's ultimate disillusionment with collaboration came not because he was persuaded of the worth of FDR's attitude but out of hard experience, similar to Roosevelt's. Not only did he meet business resistance to his proposals, but such publications as the *Magazine of Wall Street* traced the evil heresies of the Kennedy era to the New Deal and especially to John Maynard Keynes, who, it was noted darkly, had married a Russian. Anti–White House sentiment in business circles, James Reston reported in June 1962, had not been so virulent since financiers raged against That Man in the White House in the 1930s. As a result, Kennedy came to sympathize more than he had in the past with FDR's critical view of organized business.[157]

Yet even in 1962 and 1963 Kennedy turned away from the New Deal. When in 1962 he built his legislative program around the Trade Expansion Act, he did so by deciding not to renew the Reciprocal Trade Agreements Act of 1934, an innovation of the Roosevelt era. He refused to endorse a public works bill in the style of the New Deal until it was sharply modified, and he sided with the Budget Bureau in eviscerating a Youth Conservation Corps measure because FDR's Civilian Conservation Corps was regarded as an inappropriate model.[158]

In his administrative style, too, Kennedy departed from the Roosevelt mode in certain respects. Even Richard Neustadt, who had noted perceptively the similarities between the two administrations, cautioned, "The Kennedy White House is not simply Roosevelt's reproduced."[159] Kennedy did not conduct press conferences in the same manner, partly because of the drastic change in communications from FDR's day to his.[160] Nor did he calculatedly pit his administrators against one another. That, Ted Sorensen has observed, was "contrary to [the] Roosevelt fashion."[161]

Furthermore, Kennedy's appointees, it was widely said, differed from FDR's, to a degree in ideology, even more in personality. The *American Banker* was relieved that the views of Kennedy's cabinet were more orthodox than those of Roosevelt's administrators, and a man who had served under Roosevelt objected that Kennedy's people seemed "like good organization men—modern men. They are not a very colorful group." This was the big contrast that a columnist saw at the time of the inauguration. He wrote:

> But no, 1961 isn't 1933! The New Dealers who poured into Washington to take over the government were as gaudy a bunch of amateurs, intellectuals and crackpots as this experienced capital has ever seen—men whom FDR set against each other with sometimes unkind virtuosity, catching the sparks in a net.
> What a gang!—Hopkins, Wallace, Ickes, Fanny Perkins, Tommy the Cork, Henry the Morgue, Ben Cohen, Adlai Stevenson, General Johnson, Ray Moley, Abe Fortas, Alger Hiss—the list goes on and on.
> The Kennedy Cabinet is competent—enormously, reassuringly competent, but nothing like this.[162]

Kennedy found much of the Roosevelt legacy unusable because he was sure that he held office in a very different time. When Nathan Pusey, the president of Harvard, met with him in June 1961, he said, "Nate, when Franklin had this job, it was a cinch. He didn't have all these world problems. He had only to cope with poverty in the United States, but look what I've got."[163] Furthermore, he was aware that he lacked the kind of mandate for bold economic programs that Roosevelt had enjoyed in the Great Depression. He had been in office less than a month when the New Deal economist Robert R. Nathan, on behalf of Americans for Democratic Action, presented a plan for government spending that would result in a $50 billion deficit. "Well, the difficulty with your proposal," Kennedy responded, "is that 93 per cent of the people in this country are employed. That other 7 per cent isn't going to get enough political support to do it. The difference between me and Roosevelt is that he could get these things done. I don't believe that, right or wrong, there's any possibility of doing the kind of all-out economic operation that you want."[164]

No sooner had the 1960 returns been counted than political analysts were predicting that Kennedy would usher in a new "Hundred Days," like FDR's in 1933,[165] but that was not to be. As Senator William Proxmire would remark, "He just didn't have the majority really that Roosevelt had when he was moving so fast and covering so much ground." In the words of a contemporary writer, "Roosevelt was thwarted by nine old men. Kennedy must deal with a Congress full of them."[166] Kennedy himself, though he had written Eleanor Roosevelt about his plans for a first hundred days, appears never to have been as sanguine as some of his supporters, for he comprehended that the legislative tradition he inherited from Roosevelt was not the scintillating Hundred Days but the stalemate in Congress that had begun in 1938.

Nonetheless, the notion did not die easily. As the hundredth day approached, Walt Rostow proposed that Kennedy give a major address on that day to claim credit for achievements and outline future plans, and Sorensen actually put together a document pointing out how Kennedy stacked up against his three predecessors, including Roosevelt, in such categories as the number of bills signed. But it was painfully clear that April 28, 1961, bore no resemblance to the hundredth day of FDR's first administration. Nor, though Kennedy could claim credit for a spate of legislation, did his record ever bear comparison to Roosevelt's. Early in 1963 a Democratic senator, described as "a long-time friend of John F. Kennedy" (quite possibly George Smathers of Florida), stated that while Kennedy wanted to be as successful as Roosevelt in his relations with Congress, there was not the feeling of urgency that had made FDR's success possible.[167]

Kennedy thought, too, that it was much more difficult for him than it had been for Roosevelt to communicate with the American people. That was the main theme of a conversation in the summer of 1962 when the president took the unusual step of paying a call on the ailing justice Felix Frankfurter. A memorandum on that meeting recorded:

He said that he felt that what the Federal Government had to do today was far different, more complicated, and less understandable to the people than it was at the time even as recent as that of F.D.R. He said that F.D.R.'s legislation directly affected various groups of citizens, or perhaps all citizens together, sometimes to their benefit; sometimes, they thought, to their detriment. But he was dealing with the farm problem in a way which was easy to understand, or with housing, or with public works, or with education, or with the right of labor to organize, or with the level of wages, and so on. Today, the President felt, his problems were more in the nature of complicated administrative measures, which people found it difficult to understand. His farm bill, for instance, is not simple and direct in its incidence and effect, as was that of F.D.R. The same was true of the complicated matters of trade, finance, depression, prosperity, etc. The only matter with which he had to deal which resembled earlier problems was medical care. This F.D.R. had not tackled. H.S.T. had tackled it and failed, and the President had now met with a reverse.[168]

Consequently, Kennedy sometimes became annoyed when FDR's devotees badgered him to follow in the footsteps of his predecessor. Holding up a memo from Schlesinger, he said to a caller on one occasion, "Look at that, will you? Seven single-spaced pages. And what a lot of blankety-blank. I dearly love this man. He has a fine mind and some fine ideas, but in this case . . ." He paused, then said with the trace of a smile, "He is proposing that I conduct myself as Franklin Roosevelt did in 1933, but this fellow can't get through his head that first, I'm not FDR and this is 1963, not 1933; that what was fine for Roosevelt simply would not work today for a simple reason—in 1933, Roosevelt faced one central problem, the depression, and he could take more liberties with domestic matters than I could possibly enjoy today. Also, in 1933, there were no nuclear bombs or missiles or jet aircraft or cold war."[169]

It appears never to have occurred to Kennedy that Roosevelt inherited troubles easily as formidable. Far from being free of foreign concerns, he took office one day before Hitler assumed absolute power in Germany and less than eighteen months after Japan occupied Manchuria. In addition, he confronted difficulties in making economic policies explicable to the nation infinitely greater than those Kennedy inherited because he was leading so many forays into unmapped territories. Hardly "simple," his first farm legislation ran 104 pages of small print and introduced American farmers to a forest of regulations with which they were altogether unfamiliar. It was an aspect of FDR's genius that he could take a complex matter like banking and make it seem accessible, and that was the challenge Kennedy had to meet.

Two reporters who covered the White House thought Kennedy's griping unbecoming. When in a colloquy some time after his death

Peter Lisagor remarked on the president's tendency to "whine" about the treatment he received, George Herman replied:

> But, Pete, it went wider than that. I remember one weekend when he came up to New York to speak at housing centers and various odd other things in New York when he said, I think three times in three or four days, that the reason he's not getting this great groundswell of American public opinion support that Franklin D. Roosevelt had was because the issues were clear and simple in Roosevelt's day and today in his own day the issues were so complicated that people couldn't understand them and that that was the only reason he wasn't getting a great groundswell of support. In other words he was saying, "I'm just as great, but you don't understand me."[170]

Critics charged that Kennedy did not elicit the backing FDR had received not because times had changed but because he failed to adopt Roosevelt's techniques, and his counsellors encouraged him to copy his predecessor's methods. Kennedy had been in office only two months when Schlesinger sent him a memorandum stating that such correspondents as Joseph Alsop were complaining that the administration was doing an inadequate job of informing the public. "The Roosevelt Administration was a tremendous success in the field of public education," Schlesinger noted, and though the president could not "just open up the government to make Joe Alsop happy," he would be well advised to consider FDR's pattern.[171]

Kennedy found himself under constant pressure to emulate Roosevelt by giving fireside chats. Even before he took office, his press secretary, Pierre Salinger, told him that he should follow FDR's example, and in late December, after weeks of discussion, Kennedy agreed. But that did not end the matter. When Congress dragged its feet on Kennedy's legislative program, the president was repeatedly admonished to mobilize opinion by speaking to the nation. In March 1961, Lester Markel of the *New York Times* raised this complaint with Kennedy, leading him to ask Schlesinger to check on how many fireside chats Roosevelt had given. "Lester has been in here saying that I ought to go to the people more often," Kennedy explained. "He seems to think that Roosevelt gave a fireside chat once a week." Kennedy was greatly relieved to learn that Roosevelt had delivered far fewer fireside chats than people remembered, an average of only 2.5 a year, and indeed that Kennedy had actually addressed the nation more often than Roosevelt.[172]

Two years later Schlesinger passed on to the president a letter from the Harvard political scientist Samuel Beer, former national chairman of Americans for Democratic Action, which said:

> I certainly do not agree, let alone sympathize, with my liberal friends who say that it is all the fault of the President; that if he would only resort to the magic of the "fire-side chat" he would create great waves of public opinion which would wash away Congressional obstruction. They simply don't remember the way FDR actually worked—e.g. the prolonged and tortured operation by which he got the Wage-Hour bill—and totally forget the political situation that gave him leverage.[173]

Similarly, Lincoln Gordon, ambassador to Brazil under Kennedy, later reflected:

> It was quite clear that among my Harvard friends . . . a lot of people were distressed with the political Kennedy, or the pragmatic Kennedy. They wanted him to be more consistently idealist. It's odd because some of these . . . consider themselves great worshipers of Franklin Roosevelt, but then of course they never knew the living Roosevelt. They only knew Roosevelt as a history and legend, and the living Roosevelt as a person was a great deal less idealistic and much more pragmatic politician than Kennedy, and certainly a very much more difficult man to work for.[174]

Yet, fairly or unfairly, FDR's shadow continued to envelop Kennedy, and Roosevelt provided the measure for Kennedy's performance as he had for Truman's. In summarizing a group of letters the president received early in 1963, the White House reported that the writers were asking Kennedy "to adopt a mood either of sympathy for the poor (like Eleanor Roosevelt) or of vigorous demands for action (like FDR.)" Neither as a communicator of ideas nor as a speaker, his detractors declared, did he match his predecessor. He lacked Roosevelt's "kind of colorful exaggeration," and he could not "make a phrase give off hot sparks as FDR did." Above all, it was asserted, Kennedy could not equal Roosevelt as a legislative leader. After his agricultural measure went down to defeat, a Democrat observed disdainfully, "The next morning, FDR would have had a new ball into the air. Maybe even a brand-new farm bill." A political scientist summed up the prevailing view: "President Kennedy has been bold in word and cautious in deed. In terms of accomplishment, the New Frontier is no New Deal. The one falls thirty years later than the other, and thirty Acts behind it."[175]

For Kennedy it was a bit much. He had never shared in the adulation of FDR, certainly not when he was young, only to a degree in later years, and now he was being called upon to equal a man who was remembered as having been always successful, never in doubt. Unable to meet such demands, he fell back on questioning the legend. At a televised interview, "After Two Years—A Conversation with the President," in December 1962, he was asked by Sander Vanocur of NBC what he planned to do to move Congress to act. "This is a struggle which every President who has tried to get a program through has had to deal with," Kennedy replied. "After all, Franklin Roosevelt was elected by the largest majority in history in 1936, and he got his worst defeat a few months afterwards in the Supreme Court bill." Earlier that year, at a time when he was low in spirits as he contemplated the stalemate of his legislative program and the stress of the forthcoming midterm elections, he was less defensive, more ruminative. "Think of Franklin Roosevelt," he said. "We always imagine him as being a man at the summit of energy and confidence." He paused a moment, obviously reflecting on his own situation, then said wistfully, "But there must have been times in between."[176]

IX

If Roosevelt never cast as large a shadow over Kennedy as over Truman, the last previous Democratic president, or Johnson, his successor, Kennedy nonetheless found it hard to escape the presence of Franklin Roosevelt, in death as in life.[177]

Kennedy had a favorite poem, Alan Seeger's "I Have a Rendezvous with Death," and in one curious respect his own rendezvous with death linked him to Roosevelt. In 1959 an article appeared that pointed out that since 1840 no man elected president in a year ending in zero had left office alive. The skein included William Henry Harrison, Abraham Lincoln, James Garfield, William McKinley, and Warren Harding. The last to carry on the sequence was Franklin Roosevelt. It is not clear what Kennedy thought of the article, which was sent to all of the presidential hopefuls for 1960. According to some accounts, Kennedy scoffed at it. If every prospective candidate took the proposition seriously, he said, 1600 Pennsylvania Avenue might have a "For Rent" sign. In any event, this was one tradition, he declared, that he planned to break. But his personal physician, Janet Travell, has offered a different version. She has recalled that on a November afternoon in 1960, as they sunned themselves by a Florida pool, Kennedy asked her, "What do you think of the rule that for the last hundred years every President of the United States elected in a year divisible by twenty died in office?" He then reeled off the names of the six presidents, ending with Franklin

D. Roosevelt, whose death he could remember. "You don't really believe such a coincidence can continue," she replied. "The odds against it
are too great, and you are not superstitious." Kennedy, she writes,
looked at her "quizzically, silently."[178]

The procedures for Kennedy's impressive state funeral drew upon the
records of the ceremonies of the last president to die in office, Franklin
Roosevelt, and in other respects, too, the events seemed similar.[179] In
both instances there was shock and deep mourning, as well as refusal to
believe that the president was dead. "The memory of Franklin D. Roosevelt's death, in 1945, is still fresh in the minds of most Americans over
25, and . . . many of the reactions at that time were much like those of
November 1963," one scholar noted, while a careful survey reported,
"The death of President Roosevelt brought forth reactions of nearly the
breadth and intensity of those brought forth by the Kennedy assassination."[180]

In certain critical respects, however, the two episodes were not at all
the same. As one writer noted, "John Kennedy was a life and immortality symbol; the destruction of that symbol by violence was all the
more shocking. Violence was missing from the story of Roosevelt's
demise; as it must to all men, death came to him. But John Kennedy
was jerked away from health, from a young family, from leadership, by
a senseless act of violence." The American people, though many noted
the similarities to FDR's death, were considerably more conscious of
the difference. Of those who alluded to any experience similar to that
evoked by the death of Kennedy, one-fourth mentioned the death of
Roosevelt. Yet most people thought the episode was unique; they
"could not recall any other time in their lives when they had the same
sort of feelings as when they heard of President Kennedy's assassination."[181]

In Vance Bourjaily's novel *The Man Who Knew Kennedy,* the protagonist, who narrates the story in the first person, reflects on another
death after hearing the bulletin from Dallas. "Sometime on the long
flight home, . . . I found myself remembering that I was in the air
when the news came that Roosevelt died," he relates. In April 1945, he
had learned what had happened when he landed his Mustang at an
airport. He goes on:

> I sat in the plane, overwhelmed. Roosevelt had always been President—
> except, long before, when I was a child in grammar school. . . .
> That Roosevelt should die was like losing an august, infuriating, immor-
> tal relative, on whom we grudgingly relied. . . . Roosevelt's death . . .
> brought an hour of sadness for an old hero, gone to rest. We were ready

for it, even if we didn't know we were. But I am no more ready for Jack Kennedy's death, I thought, than I am for my own.[182]

David Lilienthal entered in his diary on the evening of November 22, 1963:

The television pictures that are coming through: the casket being lowered from the plane, the new President leaving by helicopter for the White House; how different from the sad hours when F.D.R. came home. How I still remember that cortege through the streets of Washington, the services I attended in the East Room.

But F.D.R. was old and exhausted in the service; this President was *young*, full of vitality and eagerness and joy; shot down without mercy for him and his family, or for his country.

This day ends in anguish.[183]

No sooner had Kennedy died than historians and publicists felt compelled to assign him a place in history, and once more comparison to Roosevelt was inevitable, at the outset not infrequently to Kennedy's advantage. In the aftermath of Kennedy's death, a number of observers rated the late president higher than Roosevelt. Senator Paul Douglas thought that Kennedy "probably had a much better mind than Roosevelt," and a former senator, William L. Benton, stated that his public addresses "transcend in quality Franklin Roosevelt's."[184] Similarly, David Riesman contended that Kennedy was not the heir "of Franklin D. Roosevelt (to whom he was superior in intelligence, knowledge, historical sense, and seriousness)." The president of the AFL-CIO, George Meany, claimed that the labor movement enjoyed "a much closer relationship . . . with the White House . . . than we ever had back in the days of Franklin Roosevelt and, of course, I was here during the Roosevelt Administration and I knew President Roosevelt before I came here."[185] It was left to the president of Senegal to sum up this attitude. Leopold Senghor told an interviewer, "I think that President Kennedy will measure up to one of his Democratic predecessors, to the author of the 'New Deal,' President Roosevelt, only with more youth, perhaps more dynamism, more idealism."[186]

Yet even in the first days after Kennedy's death, most commentators reached quite a different assessment, and as the years went by it was clear that history would not be kind to so brief a tenure. In the issue after the murder, *Time* concluded, "He had asked to be judged by the highest standards, and he died before achieving them. . . . He was a subject of boundless fascination to his countrymen; yet he aroused no such passions of either love or hatred as did Franklin Roosevelt." The most that could be claimed for Kennedy was that the two years and ten months he was allowed were not long enough to establish his greatness. "He had so little time," wrote Schlesinger; it was as though FDR had been killed at the end of 1935. Still, Roosevelt had accomplished much in that period, and other writers emphasized how thin Kennedy's record was. Little more than a month after the assassination, David Bazelon was saying that "it turned out that he was concentrating on getting elected, not on making history as Roosevelt did. . . . Once elected, his hundred days were about as much like Roosevelt's as his civil rights speech was like Lincoln's Proclamation." At the time of his death, it was noted, Washington correspondents had been emphasizing how vexed were Kennedy's relations with Congress, how much resistance he was meeting on getting either civil rights legislation or a tax cut. Kennedy himself, reflecting on the frustrations of the presidency, liked to quote a favorite observation of FDR's: "Lincoln was a sad man because he couldn't get it all at once. And nobody can."[187]

Neither observation of Kennedy's presidency nor the passage of time resolved the doubts James MacGregor Burns had expressed in his campaign biography. Interviewed for the JFK Library some while after the assassination, Burns spoke in admiration of Roosevelt's "very courageous" deeds. "We can say about FDR that in 1940 he was deeply enough committed to stopping Nazi aggression or deeply enough committed to helping the British that he was willing to take pretty risky action in the summer of 1940, in the Destroyer Deal, with an election coming up in the fall," Burns declared. "Whether Kennedy had that kind of ultimate moral commitment is something that I still don't know. . . . After all, he was not a Churchill, he was not a Roosevelt."[188]

But while this historic assessment was going on, something more important was happening—Kennedy was becoming part not of history but of myth, a myth that much of the public embraced and historians could not altogether escape. As Theodore White has observed:

More than any other President since Lincoln, John F. Kennedy has become myth. The greatest President in the stretch between them was, of course, Franklin D. Roosevelt; but it was difficult to make myth of Franklin Roosevelt, the country squire, the friendly judge, the approachable politician, the father figure. Roosevelt was a great man because he understood his times, and because almost always, at the historic intersections, he took the fork in the road that proved to be correct. He was right and so strong, it was sport to challenge him. But Kennedy was cut off at the promise, not after the performance, and so it was left to television and his widow, Jacqueline, to frame the man as legend.[189]

The legend did not take long to evolve. "What remains as the loss . . . is a certain feeling of possibilities, of an élan, and—why not say it?—of an impression of beauty," wrote *Le Figaro* at the time of his death. "These are not political qualities, but surely they are enduring legendary and mythological qualities." Within a month such observations had become commonplace. "In the early weeks of the Johnson Administration the newspapers were beginning to use the words 'the Kennedy legend,' and the phrase was entirely appropriate," Eric Goldman has written. "Alone among American Chief Executives President Kennedy was passing from life to apotheosis with no interval of critical evaluation." By the time of the first anniversary of his death, *Newsweek* was remarking, "In the bare space of a year, . . . Mr. Kennedy had been transfigured from man into myth—an enshrinement that would have pained him to see," and James Reston concluded, "Deprived of the place he sought in history, he has been given in compensation a place in legend," adding, "The heart of the Kennedy legend is what might have been."[190]

The mythmakers focused on Kennedy as romantic hero. Gerald Johnson maintained:

> Logical analysis will certainly be applied to Kennedy's career, and will have about as much effect on his position in history as Mrs. Partington's mop had upon the Atlantic tide. . . . Already it has happened to two of the 35 men who have held the Presidency, rendering them incapable of analysis by the instruments of scholarship; and now Washington, the god-like, and Lincoln, the saintly, have been joined by Kennedy, the Young Chevalier. Historians may protest, logicians may rave, but they cannot alter the fact that any kind of man, once touched by romance, is removed from all categories and is comparable only with the legendary.

William Carleton, too, noted that Kennedy belonged to "the romantic tradition, the tradition of Achilles, David, Alcibiades . . . , Arthur, Roland, Abélard, Richard the Lion Hearted, St. Francis, Bayard, Raleigh, Henry of Navarre, Gustavus Adolphus, Byron." He was, according to one posthumous record album, "The Gallant Warrior of the Thousand Days."[191]

Like the fair youth on Keats's Grecian urn, Kennedy would be forever in pursuit, forever unfulfilled, but also "for ever young," oblivious of Time. Had he lived, Kennedy could not have escaped comparison to Roosevelt, and he would almost certainly have been judged never to have measured up to him. But by passing into myth, Kennedy was at last outside the shadow cast by FDR, a shadow that had first been cast when he was Joe Kennedy's young son. This is an irony that John Kennedy, who never altogether lost his sense of ironic detachment from FDR and from his legacy, would have been the first to appreciate.

[4]

Lyndon B. Johnson

I

On the evening of April 12, 1945, "in a gloomy Capitol corridor," a Washington correspondent came upon Congressman Lyndon Johnson, tears in his eyes, altogether disconsolate about the dreadful news he had just heard. At the end of that day's session, shortly after Harry Truman had left Sam Rayburn's office, Johnson had wandered in. The phone had rung, and Johnson had seen the Speaker pick up the receiver, listen silently, swallow, then look over at him and relay what he had just been told: Franklin D. Roosevelt was dead. Johnson was devastated. Though some minutes passed before the newspaperman encountered him, the thirty-six-year-old Texan still had difficulty putting words together as he sought to explain what FDR meant to him. For, as the correspondent observed, this "leading member of the Roosevelt 'Young Guard'" typified "a hundred formerly obscure young men whose leap into national prominence had been immeasurably aided by President Roosevelt's paternal coaching."[1]

Johnson "clamped a shaking jaw over a white cigarette holder," then said of FDR:

He was just like a daddy to me always; he always talked to me just that way. He was the one person I ever knew—anywhere—who was never afraid. Whatever you talked to him about, whatever you asked him for, like projects for your district, there was just one way to figure it with him. I know some of them called it demagoguery; they can call it anything they want, but you can be damn sure that the only test he had was this: Was it good for the folks?

Johnson went on: "I don't know that I'd ever have come to Congress if it hadn't been for him. But I do know I got my first great desire for public office because of him—and so did thousands of other young men all over the country." He skimmed a eulogy Rayburn had scrawled for the press, then added, "God, God, how he could take it for us all."[2]

Johnson acquired surrogate fathers so often that some writers have been skeptical of how profoundly he felt about this particular daddy, but there is no mistaking his anguish on learning that Roosevelt was gone. "His grief was just unreal," a secretary has recalled. "He just literally wasn't taking telephone calls and he just literally shut himself up. His grief was vast and deep and he was crying tears. Manly tears, but he actually felt like and expressed this in these terms, that it was just like losing his father." Nor was the sorrow short-lived. Johnson's brother has written, "We all knew that Roosevelt's death had deeply affected him. He lost some of his drive, periodically pausing in the middle of his still-crowded work day to stare out the window with a troubled look in his eyes. He might spend a half hour that way."[3]

FDR had greater meaning for Johnson than for any other of his successors. If Roosevelt cast a darker shadow over Truman, it was only because Truman took office immediately after the great man died, and memories were still green. FDR never served as a model for Truman to anywhere near the same extent that he did for Johnson. Nor did any other chief executive associate himself so intimately with Roosevelt's point of view. To Turner Catledge, the managing editor of the *New York Times,* Johnson "was really a good sincere New Dealer—much more sincere a New Dealer for instance than John Kennedy." Similarly, John Kenneth Galbraith has written:

> [Johnson] was less detached, less cerebral, more anxious to show himself involved and successful. Roosevelt was a generation removed from J.F.K., and after Joseph P. Kennedy's break with him, F.D.R. was no household saint in the Kennedy family. Johnson, on the other hand, was truly a Roosevelt man; F.D.R. was ever in his mind as a model of what a good President should be. As with many of our generation when young, Johnson knew his political position only when the President had stated it.[4]

Yet praise and grief were not the only feelings Johnson revealed on learning of FDR's death. Even at that special moment, he said defensively:

> They called the President a dictator and some of us they called "yes men." Sure, I yessed him plenty of times—because I thought he was right—and

I'm not sorry for a single "yes" I ever gave. I have seen the President in all kinds of moods—at breakfast, at lunch, at dinner—and never once in my five terms here did he ever ask me to vote a certain way, or even suggest it. And when I voted against him—as I have plenty of times—he never said a word.[5]

This declaration indicated the attitudes that were to characterize Johnson's behavior for the rest of his days—fealty to FDR's memory combined with a determination to get out from under Roosevelt's shadow. To the very last he remained a Roosevelt man, committed to social reform and a bold foreign policy. Yet he also wanted to put his own brand on the history of his times, indeed to achieve so much that he would outrank even FDR. In the end his ambition not merely to match his master but to surpass him had fateful consequences, for the nation and for his own place in history.

II

Lyndon Johnson had first come to FDR's attention in a significant way at a critical moment in Roosevelt's life. On February 5, 1937, the president had announced a daring scheme to add as many as six justices to the United States Supreme Court, ostensibly to improve the efficiency of the judiciary but in fact, critics charged, in order to pack the Court with judges of the New Deal persuasion. Opponents claimed that the country was overwhelmingly against the plan, while the Roosevelt circle insisted that the nation was with him, as it had been a few months earlier when he had swept all but two of the forty-eight states. No one knew for sure. But in late February a Texas congressman died, and the ensuing election provided the first meaningful test at the polls of how the people felt.

Even before the campaign began, Texas had become one of the main battlefields of the Court fight. On February 9 the Texas Senate had astounded the country by voting 22–3 to instruct the Texas congressional delegation to reject the proposal. In no other state did so large a bloc of Democratic legislators turn against the president. The opposition in Texas stirred up a hornet's nest. In New York, Republicans in both houses of the legislature introduced a measure adopted word for word from the Texas resolution, and in Washington an irate congressman accused the head of the American Bar Association of prompting the resolution and called for a House investigation of that "band of rapacious corporation-controlled lawyers." As the candidates in the special election took to the field, the civil war among the Democrats became more acrimonious. On March 2 Senator Tom Connally, long counted an administration regular, spoke out against the bill in an address to the Texas legislature and received a standing ovation; even the pro-Roosevelt governor, it was said, had been spied clapping his hands under the table. Roosevelt in turn sent first Harold Ickes, then Jim Farley, to Austin to deliver rousing addresses to the Texas legislature. With so much national attention focused on Texas, the White House followed with lively interest developments in the Tenth Congressional District, where two of the nine candidates were outspoken opponents of Court-packing.[6]

Almost no one thought much of the chances in that contest of a twenty-eight-year-old outsider who owed what little claim to recognition he had almost wholly to FDR. An admirer of Roosevelt from the day that he saw him nominate Al Smith at the 1928 Democratic convention in Houston, he had made himself over in his hero's image. When he was chosen Speaker of the Little Congress of congressional aides, he pledged a "New Deal" for his constituents and promised to watch out for the "forgotten man" on Capitol Hill. The president loomed still larger in Johnson's life when in 1935 Roosevelt appointed him to head the National Youth Administration in Texas, the biggest state in the union. Not yet twenty-seven, Johnson was the youngest state director of the NYA.[7]

In a manner that would soon be legendary, Johnson seized upon this opportunity. Driving himself and those around him mercilessly, he put thousands of destitute young men to work on a number of imaginative projects, notably a series of roadside parks that attracted the attention of the White House. On a trip to Texas in 1936, Eleanor Roosevelt made a point of stopping at the NYA office in Austin, explaining to reporters that she wanted to see this young administrator about whom she had heard so much, and a generation later the NYA director for the state of Washington reminded Johnson of a June day in 1936 at Hyde Park: "You were called up to sit near the President and Mrs. Roosevelt and to tell them and the group about your projects in Texas, particularly the roadside parks. I have wondered whether that may have been the time when you were marked for greater things." When the president visited the Texas Centennial exposition in 1936, he was delighted by the tribute Johnson arranged for him: a battalion of NYA workers standing at attention along the highway between Dallas and Fort Worth, their shovels at present arms, Johnson at their head, his hand raised in a military salute. No less important, the NYA provided the nucleus of the political organization that would have its first test under fire in the 1937 primary.[8]

In a race against much better-known candidates, that organization would not have begun to be enough had Johnson not shrewdly exploited FDR's popularity in the Tenth District as his route to a seat in Congress. To the consternation of some of his opponents, Johnson managed to create the impression that he was the only one of the nine candidates who supported FDR's Court-packing plan, a claim that was palpably false. Sure, some others might say they backed Roosevelt, Johnson asserted, but he alone did so unreservedly. "I didn't have to hang back like a steer on the way to the dipping vat," he said. "I'm for the President. When he calls on me for help I'll be where I can give him a quick lift, not out in the woodshed practicing a quick way to duck." If you want to aid the president, he told voters, then cast your ballot for me. "A vote for me will show the President's enemies that the people are behind him," Johnson declared. "Mr. Roosevelt is in trouble now. When we needed help, he helped us. Now *he* needs help. Are we going to give it to him? Are *you* going to give it to him? Are you going to help Mr. Roosevelt? That's what this election is all about."[9]

Johnson reminded the voters that the eyes not only of Texas but of the country were upon them, for they were making a choice that could determine the whole future of the Roosevelt presidency. He leafleted the district with fliers carrying an excerpt from Ray Tucker's "National Whirligig" column: "Major plebiscite on the supreme court will take place in Texas April 10. . . . Young Lyndon Johnson, former national youth administrator, carries FDR's judicial colors. . . . Several senators now lukewarm towards the White House scheme may suddenly shift if Mr. Roosevelt wins out there by proxy."[10]

It did not take long for Roosevelt's circle to buy the idea that Johnson was FDR's "proxy." Elliott Roosevelt announced publicly for Johnson because, as he explained in a telegram to Jim Farley, "Congressional race to pick successor is coming to a head down here as straight out fight between Lyndon Johnson who is backing father wholeheartedly on his whole program including the court issue and two other candidates who have refused to support father on that question." Farley himself deviated from his usual posture of strict neutrality in primary bouts. On a tour of Texas, ostensibly to dedicate some post offices, the Democratic national chairman referred to Johnson as FDR's "champion."[11]

By identifying himself with FDR, Johnson won a stunning victory that was widely interpreted as a vote of confidence for Roosevelt and

Court-packing. The Associated Press ticker announced: "Youthful Lyndon B. Johnson, who shouted his advocacy of President Roosevelt's court reorganization all over the Tenth Texas District, was elected today," while a Texas newspaper headlined the results:

JOHNSON ELECTED TO
CONGRESS BY BIG VOTE
———
FDR'S COURT PROPOSAL
OKAYED BY 10TH
DISTRICT

That was just the way Johnson wanted his success to be perceived. "This is not a personal triumph," he maintained. "This is but approval of the president's program. . . . The people of the 10th district are sending to Washington the message that they are . . . as strong as horse radish for Roosevelt."[12]

The president, gratified by Johnson's victory at a time when the Court struggle was not going at all well, saw to it that his supporter's role was properly acknowledged. When Roosevelt's yacht docked in Galveston at the end of a fishing cruise in the Gulf of Mexico, the newly elected congressman was invited to take part in wharfside ceremonies, where, sporting a huge, garish oleander blossom, he was photographed with FDR and the governor of Texas. (Johnson subsequently had the governor effaced from the photograph to make it appear that he was alone with the president.) Johnson had the further honor of riding in the Roosevelt motorcade through the streets of Galveston, lined with thousands upon thousands of cheering Texans, and of accompanying FDR on the presidential train all the way to Fort Worth.[13]

Johnson did not let this good fortune slip away from him. Though still in pain from an appendectomy and looking so gaunt that a reporter thought he was near death, Johnson overwhelmed the president with questions about how the tarpon were biting and how his family was doing and expressed a keen interest in the welfare of the U.S. Navy, a matter close to Roosevelt's heart. "I can always use a good man to help out with naval matters in Congress," the president responded. As the train pulled into Fort Worth, he scrawled a telephone number on a piece of paper and told Johnson that as soon as he got to Washington he should dial that number and ask to speak to Tom. It was in such fashion, as FDR's protégé, with instant access to Tommy Corcoran, one of Roosevelt's chief White House aides, that Johnson began his congressional career.[14]

III

Lyndon Johnson became Franklin Roosevelt's pet Congressman. Not until 1940 would he go in and out of the White House almost at will, but from the very beginning there were indications that he was the president's favorite. "By the time Lyndon arrived in Washington the word had gone out: 'Be nice to this boy,'" Tommy Corcoran has recalled. Roosevelt saw to it that the new congressman got a coveted spot on the House Naval Affairs Committee. Beyond that, intimates could discern that he was fond of Johnson; he "was kind of tickled to get a liberal from Texas and liked his sort of gung ho qualities," Roosevelt's associates remembered. The president became his tutor, "interested in say, educating him but interesting him in oh, things like water power and forestry; housing; oh, just everything." Roosevelt told one junior cabinet officer, "Keep an eye on that young Texan. He's going places." He even predicted that Johnson would one day be president. Roosevelt was heard to remark, "That's the kind of man I could have been if I hadn't had a Harvard education."[15]

Roosevelt thought so well of Johnson that he offered him the post of administrator of the Rural Electrification Administration, and when Johnson turned him down in order to remain in Congress, the president sent an effusive reply:

> I was very sorry that you did not feel that you wanted to accept the proffer of the Administrator of the Rural Electrification Administration, but I do think I ought to tell you that very rarely have I known a proposed candidate for any position receive such unanimous recommendations from all sources as was the case with you.
>
> But I do understand the reasons why you felt that you should stay as a representative of your district. I congratulate the Tenth District of Texas.[16]

The Tenth District had good reason to receive congratulations, for Johnson made use of his standing with FDR and the New Dealers to obtain millions of dollars in WPA and PWA construction, Federal Housing Project Number One in Austin, and, above all, the Pedernales River Electric Cooperative, which Johnson boasted was "the biggest co-op in the world both in area and power." It took all of Johnson's resourcefulness to get the large REA loan. The first time he secured a fifteen-minute interview at the White House, the president kept him at bay by lecturing him on multiple-arch dams until his time was exhausted. The next time Johnson was determined not to be filibustered. He strode into the Oval Office armed with charts, maps, and statistics, and before Roosevelt had a chance to get a word in he cried, "Water, water everywhere and not a drop to drink; public power everywhere and not a drop for my poor people." For the next ten minutes, a torrent of words, accompanied by photographs of the region, descended on the president. Beguiled by Johnson's histrionics, Roosevelt gave in, though the district was so sparsely settled that it did not qualify for a loan. When that objection was raised, the president retorted, "Those people down there breed pretty fast, you know."[17]

Johnson gave the president full value for what he and his constituents received. He became such a committed agent of FDR both on the Hill and in Texas that in 1940 the president insisted that he be treated as Sam Rayburn's equal in negotiations over the division of the Texas delegation to the Democratic convention. That same year Johnson performed an even more valuable service in running the national campaign to elect Democrats to the House. His astuteness, his energy, and his talent for fundraising impressed everyone, not least Franklin Roosevelt, for Johnson was not shy about keeping him informed about all he was accomplishing. After the election, in which Democratic candidates for the House did better than expected, Johnson wrote the president: "I know some of our Democratic brethren would have been utterly out in the cold except for your good offices. You made it possible for me to get down where I could whiff a bit of the powder, and this note is to say 'Thank you.' It was grand. The victory is perfect." He ended "with assurances of my very great esteem, my pride in your leadership, my confidence in the future under that leadership, and my affection."[18]

In 1941 Roosevelt reciprocated the favor. When Johnson decided to enter the race for the Democratic senatorial nomination, the president arranged for him to make his announcement from the steps of the White House just as reporters were arriving for a scheduled press conference. Asked by a correspondent whether he was endorsing Johnson, Roosevelt replied, "Now it is up to the State of Texas to elect their own Senator, that is number one. Number two, I can't take part in a Texas primary. Number three, if you ask me about Lyndon himself, I can't take part in his election. I can only say what is perfectly true,—you all know he is a very old and close friend of mine. Now that's about all. Now don't try to tie those things together!" As the transcript of the conference noted, "The President brought the house down with laughter," and Roosevelt joined in the merriment.[19]

FDR's attitude permitted the candidate to identify himself in his campaign literature as "Lyndon B. Johnson, upon whom President Roosevelt and the Democratic Party have leaned heavily." Leaflets carried newspaper quotations such as the *Abilene Reporter-News*'s "He stands ace-high with the President," and bumper stickers from Amarillo to Corpus Christi read "FRANKLIN D AND LYNDON B!" From miles away motorists could see billboards with a giant picture of Johnson and FDR shaking hands. If he were elected, Johnson promised, he would be "an all-out Roosevelt Senator."[20]

While professing neutrality, Roosevelt did everything he could to improve Johnson's chances, especially by choreographing an elaborate *pas de deux*. Again and again Johnson sent a wire to the president and got back a telegram, drafted by Johnson or one of his aides, which the candidate would read to Texas voters as yet another sign of FDR's partiality. On one occasion when Johnson was seeking to ingratiate himself with rural voters, Roosevelt wired him, "I am very glad to tell you that I am approving the parity loan bill which you have so ardently supported," a sentence that followed almost word for word Johnson's draft. When Johnson wired the president, "IF MY COMMANDER-IN-CHIEF NEEDS ME DURING THE NEXT FOUR WEEKS IN MY CONGRESS SEAT WILL YOU PLEASE COMMAND ME AND I SHALL COME AT ONCE," Roosevelt obligingly answered, "I SUGGEST THAT YOU STAY IN TEXAS DURING THE CAMPAIGN UNLESS CONDITIONS CHANGE SO RADICALLY THAT YOUR PRESENCE IN WASHINGTON IS NECESSARY. IF THAT HAPPENS I WILL SEND FOR YOU. PLEASE RETURN IMMEDIATELY AFTER THE ELECTION."[21]

Roosevelt all but campaigned for Johnson among the older voters of Texas. On June 5, he wrote "Dear Lyndon":

> I have your letter favoring further help for our senior citizens over sixty years of age. As you remember, you and I discussed this problem before the Chicago Convention of the Democratic Party last year. Our ideas were incorporated in the Party platform which called for the "early realization of a minimum pension for all who have reached the age of retirement and are not gainfully employed."
>
> I agree with you that the implementation of this pledge is the best solution of the problem.
>
> I hope you will come in and talk to me about it when you return.

Two weeks later he told the president of the Social Security League of Texas, "I do not mind reiterating to you that Congressman Lyndon Johnson is an old and trusted friend of mine." Of course, it would be unconscionable for the White House to intervene in a local primary, "but I do not think my Texas friends will misunderstand my position in the Senatorial race." He wanted him to know that "Lyndon, while in Congress, has given me excellent support in the measures I have advocated to provide social security for our people."[22]

Despite FDR's efforts, Johnson fell short. Two days after the election, with the issue still in doubt, the *Dallas News* reported: "Only Miracle Can Keep FDR's Anointed LBJ Out." The final returns, however, showed him a loser, by 1,300 votes out of 600,000. When Johnson got back to Washington, Roosevelt teased him; he had learned in New York, he said, to sit on the ballot boxes during the count. In fact, though, the president was not lighthearted. During the campaign, he had told the son of the mayor of San Antonio not to be downcast about his father's defeat because his ideas would prevail. "The same thing is true about Lyndon Johnson," he added. "I hope he will win but even if he does not the things for which he stands will eventually win."23

Denied a place in the Senate, Johnson retained his seat in the House, where for the most part he continued to serve FDR loyally. Just three days after Pearl Harbor, he became the first member of Congress to go into uniform. He waited only long enough to vote to declare war against Germany. Not content with desk duty, Johnson persuaded the president to send him to the Southwest Pacific, where he flew one mission that won him a Silver Star. On July 1, 1942, Roosevelt ordered all members of Congress in the armed services to return to Washington, and on the day that the president announced that Dr. New Deal had given way to Dr. Win the War, his luncheon guest was the young Texas representative. There was no other Texan Roosevelt relied on with such confidence. In December 1943 Johnson even sided with the president against his own state's oil interests in opposing a bill to raise petroleum prices, the kind of proof of devotion that Roosevelt appreciated. When in 1944 Johnson's first daughter was born, a White House car rolled up to the congressman's residence with a gift, a book about FDR's Scottie, Fala, inscribed "From the master—to the pup." A year later, the master was dead, leaving Johnson bereaved but comforted by the thought that he had been from first to last what one of FDR's closest aides called him, "a perfect Roosevelt man."24

IV

With Roosevelt gone, Johnson felt freer to accommodate himself to the increasing conservatism of his Texan constituents, though never to the point of repudiating FDR directly. Even while Roosevelt was alive, Johnson had deprecated "these old domestic museum pieces, the PWA, FHA and WPA," which "have now outlived their usefulness," and Roosevelt, who understood that Johnson could not go along with him on every question and hope to rise in Texas politics, had tolerated his deviations. Nonetheless, FDR's death made it easier for Johnson to distance himself from the New Deal. When he won election to the Senate in 1948, he insisted that no one should mistake him for a liberal, and after taking over as majority leader in 1955, he behaved not as a latter-day New Dealer but as a man of the center. Still, he continued to think of himself as an FDR follower, one who was adapting Roosevelt's ideas to the age of the cold war.[25]

In the postwar era, and especially during the Eisenhower presidency, both Johnson and his supporters acknowledged that he had shifted to the right. One critic later noted:

> After World War II had ended and the nation was a bit hung-over from its Rooseveltian orgy, Johnson seemed amazed and disturbed when taken for a New Dealer. Him a New Dealer? Pshaw! Oh, he might have mentioned FDR's name once or twice in getting elected in 1937, and he might even have been heard to say that Roosevelt "was like a daddy to me," but that certainly should not be construed to mean that he believed in the Roosevelt philosophy. He told the Associated Press on April 23, 1947, that "the term 'New Dealer' is a misnomer. I believed then and I still believe in many of the causes Roosevelt backed. That includes development of water power and other natural resources. I believe in the REA and think all-weather roads should be built to every farmhouse. But I believe in free enterprise and I don't believe in the government doing anything that the people can do privately."

In 1956 Texas Democrats distributed a column lauding Johnson as "the tall traveler [who] came to Congress as a follower of Franklin Roosevelt but a number of years later . . . was riding in the first-class coach of arch-Republicanism," and the following year Johnson said, "I have to admit, I am perhaps more conservative than I once was."[26]

Johnson's transformation created considerable friction between the majority leader and FDR loyalists. In 1956 Sam Rosenman warned that "Lyndon Johnson and the conservatives of the South will try to capture the Party and change its character for the next decade, unless the New Deal–Fair Deal elements of the Party can overcome this effort." Roosevelt, the FDR faithful told the majority leader, would be heartsick if he knew that his favorite congressman had deserted his liberal colleagues. Richard Rovere has written:

> Once, at a small stag dinner of men who had worked with Roosevelt, this proposition was put in the form of a toast, and Johnson was reduced to tears and to replying that it was all too true but that his old friends simply

could not know his loneliness and the difficulties of his position as a majority leader trying to hold the party together against the day when Eisenhower could no longer cast his magic spells over the country. A day would come, he said, when they would see that he was loyal to his past.

On another occasion, though, when Abe Fortas and others from the Roosevelt era were trying to get Johnson to advance their legislation, Johnson said angrily, "You New Dealers make me sick, because where would you be if you could not get people like me elected to Congress?"[27]

Eleanor Roosevelt constituted a particularly thorny problem for Johnson, as she had for Truman and Kennedy. As majority leader, he did all he could to win her favor. He gave a party for her, and in the midst of a struggle over civil rights legislation, he talked to her about his tribulations. "I'm here every night all night, day and night, but where are all the liberals?" he asked. His entreaties got him nowhere. In August 1957, after the Senate approved a civil rights measure that liberals found inadequate, Johnson wrote Mrs. Roosevelt, "I was very much disappointed by your column last Saturday. I had always thought of you as a fair-minded person who would always insist on knowing all the facts before coming to a conclusion on the motives of men." He added, "If I am 'trying to fool the people,' I have a large company with me," and he named such co-workers as Ben Cohen and Jim Rowe, who had served under FDR.[28]

As these comments indicated, Johnson still wanted to be regarded as one of the Roosevelt circle, and he took particular pains to associate himself with Roosevelt as the 1960 election drew nearer. At the end of a stormy night session of the Senate in August 1958, he corraled Hubert Humphrey and Anthony Lewis of the *New York Times,* gave a bravura performance in instructing Humphrey on how to behave on the Senate floor, then wheeled abruptly and, pointing to FDR's portrait behind his desk, cried, "Look. Look at that chin!" The big Democratic victory in the 1958 midterm elections led him to remind a columnist of "back in Roosevelt's day," when "we used to have Tom Corcoran and Ben Cohen charting policy," and in his campaign for the Democratic presidential nomination in 1960, he let out all the stops. If elected, he told a group of New Yorkers, he would be "more liberal than Eleanor Roosevelt."[29]

Johnson's relationship to FDR helped him rebut the most persistent charge in 1960—that he was too conservative to win the nomination. "Liberal Democrats," the radio commentator Morgan Beatty stated, "should remember that Lyndon was Mr. Roosevelt's leading edge of power in the House of Representatives." When Walter Cronkite inquired whether Johnson was more conservative than when he had been "a protégé, in a sense, of Franklin Delano Roosevelt," Johnson replied somewhat evasively, "I am a great admirer of President Roosevelt now, just as I was then. He hasn't changed in my viewpoint any." Asked by another journalist if he had not shifted position in coming out for public housing, Johnson answered, "Not in the slightest. The first slum-clearance project in the United States, President Roosevelt allocated to my district, Austin, . . . so this is not any new venture for me." When FDR's name came up in an interview with Chet Huntley and David Brinkley, Johnson said, "I think he preserved the Republic. I think except for his great hold on the people and their willingness to follow him, we might well have lost our form of government early in the thirties. He was my hero."[30]

Yet if Johnson ran as a Roosevelt man in 1960, he did so circumspectly. He believed that the Republicans had decided that they could damage him most by appealing to fears that he was a profligate spender and that he was power-hungry, the same tactics they had employed against Roosevelt. The majority leader thought he knew how to outwit them. He told Arthur Schlesinger, Jr., that the more militant Senate liberals had left the impression that they were "wasters, spenders and wild men. . . . The country doesn't want this. The country wants to be comfortable. It doesn't want to be stirred up. Have a revolution, all right, but don't say anything about it until you are entrenched in office. That's the way Roosevelt did it."[31]

His identification with FDR did not suffice to win Johnson the nomination, and he had to be content with the second spot on the ticket. Kennedy chose him as his running mate though Johnson had derided him as the son of the man who had undercut Roosevelt's foreign policy. "I never thought Hitler was right," he cried. "I was never any Chamberlain umbrella man." In the ensuing campaign Johnson's association with FDR helped to attract voters in closely contested southern states, and some people credited the majority leader with an indispensable contribution to Kennedy's narrow victory. But Johnson was determined that as vice-president he would ask nothing of Kennedy, for he did not want to make a nuisance of himself as his fellow Texan John Nance Garner had plagued Roosevelt. Nor did he expect much recognition from Kennedy, for he anticipated that the new chief executive would follow FDR's pattern. He told Franklin D. Roosevelt, Jr., "Your daddy never let his Vice-Presidents put their heads above water."[32] For Lyndon Johnson, Franklin Roosevelt remained in 1960 what he had been for decades past—the ultimate authority, president without peer, the one man who set the course that each of his successors would be expected to follow.

v

When Lyndon Johnson succeeded to the presidency in November 1963, he declared openly that FDR was his model. "In both pride and humility," Johnson said on the occasion of the eighty-second anniversary of the birth of Franklin Roosevelt, "I readily admit that my own course in life has been influenced by none so much as this great man." Johnson relied upon advisers who had been FDR's counsellors—Abe Fortas, Jim Rowe, Anna Rosenberg, Tommy Corcoran, Ben Cohen— and he borrowed freely from the New Deal experience. A White House secretary recalled, "The first winter that he was President, January, it seemed to me that every time I turned around, every time I took a breath, the President was having some kind of a ceremony with relation to FDR."[33] If as president Lyndon Johnson was in Roosevelt's shadow, he gave every indication of purposefully stepping into the shade.

Johnson presented himself to the world as the designated heir of Franklin Roosevelt. He was forever reminding people of the laying on of hands in his own version of apostolic succession and Petrine supremacy. In the spring of 1964 he told a White House audience, "FDR brought me into this house and this room when I was only 27." He boasted of how often in the war years he had partaken of Sunday lunches with Roosevelt, and again and again he would announce that FDR was his beau ideal. He behaved toward him as one should toward paragons. It has been said that "every time he met a young person, Johnson lectured him on the greatness of Roosevelt."[34]

From the outset Johnson surrounded himself with icons of FDR. On his very first day in the White House, he moved into his office a desk that Roosevelt had used. A year later, he said, "Whenever I feel I've done a good day's work, whenever I feel I've really accomplished something, I look at that desk. And then I go back to work, because I know I've only begun." As soon as he took over, he began a search for an appropriate portrait of his idol, and he insisted that it be the very best. At the end of a party on December 23, the day that the black crepe of mourning gave way to Christmas decorations, he led four women reporters to the Cabinet Room to show them where he would mount the painting of Roosevelt, "the ablest man we ever had in this town." It took him longer than he anticipated to find a suitable picture, but when he finally did, he hung it on a wall directly across from where he sat, so

[134]

that FDR's face looked at him through every cabinet meeting of his tenure.[35]

Johnson made a point of associating himself with the younger generation of Roosevelts. He named James Roosevelt as representative to the Economic and Social Council of the United Nations, while Franklin D. Roosevelt, Jr., served under him as chairman of the Appalachian Regional Commission and of the Equal Employment Opportunity Commission. In the 1964 campaign Johnson referred to FDR, Jr., as "a man who rightly wears and proudly wears a great name in American history," and in the following year he opened a White House Conference on Equal Employment Opportunities by stating, "I always feel stimulated and inspired a little bit just to repeat that name—Franklin D. Roosevelt, Jr."[36]

Even when he faced the delicate question of what attitude he should take toward FDR, Jr.'s ambition to be mayor of New York City, he phrased his response in a way that left the impression that he was walking on eggs to give no offense to his patron's son. In reply to an inquiry at a press conference about whether he would agree to speak to Roosevelt about the mayoralty race, the president said:

I have not seen him. I have not talked to him. I will be happy to talk to him. I like him. He performed a very valuable service to this administration but I am not in the business of selecting mayors for any cities. I would, of course, be happy to talk to any prominent citizen, and I include Mr. Roosevelt in that group, who desire to talk to me about his future or any others. As a matter of fact, I talked to Franklin Roosevelt, Sr., about my future a good many times and I would feel very bad if I refused.[37]

Eleanor Roosevelt, never a Johnson fan, served Johnson better in death than in life, for he took advantage of memorial tributes to her to identify himself with her memory. On one occasion he described her as "that very great, grand, and lovely lady." That was not enough, though; he wanted to make clear that he had long been intimately associated with her. "I remember following her on the dusty roads of Texas, in the slums of our cities," he claimed.[38]

Washington observers soon discerned resemblances to Franklin Roosevelt in almost everything Johnson did. It was noted that the LBJ rubric copied the FDR insignia; that Johnson's cabinet sat around a table given to Roosevelt by Jesse Jones; even that the president favored the same kind of soft felt hat that his mentor had worn. The State of the Union message of January 1964 gave Johnson his first opportunity to make a distinctive mark, but correspondents viewed the address as an awkward effort to imitate FDR's style. "Johnson was very much influenced by Roosevelt in every kind of way, even in his manner of speaking when he became President," said an associate who had first met him in the 1930s. "It was very clear to people who had known him over a period of time. I don't think he was consciously mimicking. I think he just had absorbed so much of Roosevelt." So close did the identification become that by the spring of 1964, Eric Goldman has written, "curiously enough, the face of the rough-and-ready Texas President was taking on some of the lines of his hero, the New York patrician FDR."[39]

The president's special assistant, Bill Moyers, remarked that to Johnson, "Roosevelt is a book to be studied, restudied and reread." In an interview at the White House in the fall of 1965, Moyers said:

> Johnson . . . was Roosevelt's pupil. Roosevelt may not have known this but Johnson was always studying him. Roosevelt dominated this town as Johnson does today. Johnson could not help but be affected by Roosevelt. The influence of Roosevelt on Johnson is like the mark a prehistoric river leaves in a cavern. If you go to some place like the Luray Caverns, you may not see the old river but you sense its presence everywhere.[40]

Much of the time Johnson appeared to dwell not in the 1960s but in the 1930s. "Not even the Presidency is more stirring to him" than the age of FDR, observed the correspondent William S. White, who knew him well. He added, "The old years, the New Deal, the Depression, the War, made ineradicable marks upon him at a more impressionable age. And, as with many men of his generation, these old battles stir up the greatest nostalgia of all." Even at a reception in honor of the president of Upper Volta in May 1965, Johnson referred to the period thirty years before, "when as a young man I was crusading for our young people . . . in that great effort [of] many people . . . assembled under the leadership of President Roosevelt."[41]

Johnson had a huge storehouse of tales about the glory days when FDR ruled the land, and he used these anecdotes not just to entertain but as parables to instruct his subordinates. He was particularly fond of telling about the swell-headed Congressman who boasted to his colleagues one day in the thirties of how he had marched into the White House and chewed out the president; Speaker Rayburn is said to have replied, "I am not interested in what you told Roosevelt, but I am damn sure interested in what Roosevelt told you!" A quarter of a century later, whenever a bureaucrat or a member of the White House staff ran on about how he had pressed his ideas on some notable,

Johnson would interrupt him with "Now, that's all very good, but I sure am interested in what Roosevelt told you."[42]

Quite apart from the lasting influence Roosevelt exerted, Johnson found it politically advantageous to link himself to FDR. Many liberals had deep misgivings about a man they remembered as a southern conservative of the Eisenhower era, and Johnson made full use of his association with the age of Roosevelt to reassure them. One of Johnson's aides, Harry McPherson, has recalled:

Memories of the Depression lingered on in the minds of most Democrats, and the mention of FDR's name was enough to arouse the faithful at Democratic dinners. (Indeed, it was sometimes the only thing that did. More than once I heard Johnson, trying to shake a groggy audience out of its torpor, rush to that part of his speech where the names "Franklin D. Roosevelt!" and "Harry S. Truman!" produced a pounding torrent of applause.)[43]

At a time of anxiety about what policies the new president would pursue, Johnson emphasized his fidelity to the FDR legacy. On the day after the assassination, he told Walter Heller that he wanted to go full speed ahead on the poverty program. As Heller started out of the office at the end of their conference, the president beckoned him back and added:

Now I wanted to say something about all this talk that I'm a conservative who is likely to go back to the Eisenhower ways or give in to the economy bloc in Congress. It's not so, and I want you to tell your friends—Arthur Schlesinger, Galbraith and other liberals—that it is not so. I'm no budget slasher. . . . If you looked at my record, you would know that I am a Roosevelt New Dealer. As a matter of fact, to tell the truth, John F. Kennedy was a little too conservative to suit my taste.[44]

Johnson's last sentence is suggestive, for one of the most important benefits he derived from identification with Roosevelt was help in eluding the never-ceasing comparisons to his immediate predecessor. There was no way to come out ahead in a contest with an immortal, and the Roosevelt association diverted attention from that matchup and placed Johnson in a different frame of reference. One study found that after the Kennedy assassination, doubts about Johnson quickly faded. A college student said, "Getting to Johnson, this strikes me again, the fact that we immediately began to think of Johnson in slightly better terms than we have before. . . . I at least began to think things like, well, he was . . . a Roosevelt New Dealer, and so forth." (Johnson, though, never fully escaped the demand that he be John F. Kennedy's legatee. In 1968 he told Robert Kennedy that "he thought that as President Kennedy looked down at him every day from then until now, he would agree that he had kept the faith.")[45]

Johnson also found the Roosevelt heritage useful in devising a program distinguishable from Kennedy's New Frontier, for FDR's New Deal served as midwife at the birth of Johnson's Great Society. The phrase "Great Society" first appeared in the draft of a speech prepared by Richard Goodwin for the president to deliver at an Eleanor Roosevelt Memorial meeting. Johnson decided not to use the talk on that occasion but to save it for later. He liked the draft and became increasingly fond of the phrase, for he was seeking a slogan like "New Deal," and "the Great Society" improved upon the expression he had been toying with, "the Better Deal."[46] When he did unveil his program, commentators had no doubt about its pedigree. One called it a "Second New Deal," a continuation of the later New Deal that had been interrupted by the Court-packing defeat and World War II. Another wrote flatly, "The Great Society is an attempt to codify the New Deal's vision of a good society."[47]

No feature of the Great Society attracted more attention than the War on Poverty, and that, too, was a direct descendant of the New Deal. In January 1964 Johnson declared: "The meek and the humble and the lowly share this life and this earth with us all. We must never forget them. President Roosevelt never did." When Johnson and his aides put together the poverty legislation, they were acutely aware of the experience of the 1930s. The Job Corps provision drew its inspiration from the Civilian Conservation Corps and the college work-study program owed even more to the NYA. "One of the most satisfying jobs of my life was when I was at the age of 27, when President Roosevelt asked me to head the National Youth Administration in Texas," Johnson said in the spring of 1964. "A hundred years from now when historians look back on the Johnson administration, I hope very much that they will be able to say: There, once again, was an era when the young men and the young women of America and their Government really belonged to each other."[48]

In explaining the War on Poverty to the nation, Johnson incorporated essentially the same passage into at least eight separate addresses. The speech took its quintessential form at Franklin D. Roosevelt Square in Gainesville, Georgia, where on May 8, 1964, on the same courthouse steps from which Roosevelt had once spoken, Johnson asserted:

This administration believes in doing the greatest good for the greatest number of people. So today, with Franklin Roosevelt's youngest son, Franklin Roosevelt, Jr., by my side, I have come back to Gainesville to say that his work and ours is not finished; his dreams and ours are not yet realized; his hopes and ours are not yet fulfilled.

As President Franklin Roosevelt did in March 1938, I ask you to give me your heart, to work for the good of the whole people.[49]

If Johnson made much of Roosevelt in his first months in office, he became all but obsessed with him in the 1964 campaign. During the summer of 1964, he asked Eric Goldman to put together a series of memos on the history of Democratic conventions. Goldman has recalled: "As always, the LBJ eye was fixed on FDR. Typically, the memo on acceptance speeches came back with a notation instructing, 'Give me more on R in '32.'" At the president's request Goldman prepared a painstaking dissection of FDR's 1932 presentation, which gave vogue to the phrase "the New Deal." Johnson studied it assiduously in the hope of producing the same kind of effect, and he wound up modeling his own acceptance address on FDR's speech.[50]

As Johnson toured the country in 1964, he made the most of his association with Franklin Roosevelt. To a crowd gathered in the municipal park in South Gate, California, in October, he stated:

I remember the first President I ever saw, and the greatest President I ever knew. I saw him stand up one day in his braces, with pain in his legs, and anguish in his face, but vision in his head and hope in his eyes. I saw him talk to almost this many people, maybe more. It was a rainy, cold day in March 1933. The banks were popping in the country just like popcorn, just like firecrackers going off at Christmastime. They were closing.

The railroad men had come running down to Washington and the insurance companies and all these captains of finance, all these smart conservatives, and the roof had caved in. People were burning their corn. Cotton was selling for 5 cents. You couldn't find a job and relief lines were longer than from here to that airport I landed at, and that is 15 miles away.

But this man stood up in that time when things weren't near as good as they are today, with the braces on his legs, out of his wheelchair, and he grabbed that microphone, and he stuck his chin up, and his jaw out, and he . . . electrified a nation, and he saved a republic.

I say to you today, in the presence of his wonderful son Jimmy Roosevelt, who sits on this platform, that we must cast away the shadows of doubt and these harassing fears that frustrate some of our citizens. . . .The only thing that America has to fear is fear itself.[51]

A little over two weeks later, on the steps of the Los Angeles City Hall, he once more referred to Jimmy Roosevelt and again conjured up the memory of FDR. "Jimmy Roosevelt brought me to Washington," said Johnson, who was never fastidious about the need for accuracy in relating a past event. He then went on to say that the people who were attacking him were the same crowd who had maligned President Roosevelt. "I remember when we had the minimum wage up," he continued. "We had a minimum wage in 1938 for 25 cents an hour. My daddy was on his death bed and he died that night, and I was sitting there listening to the radio with him when President Roosevelt went on the radio and appealed to us to come back to Congress so that widow women wouldn't have to work in pecan-shelling plants for 7 cents an hour."[52]

Johnson had the good fortune to be opposed in 1964 by a man who appeared to place in jeopardy many of the gains of the Roosevelt years and who harbored grievances against FDR more than three decades old. "If I hadn't been a registered Republican, my dissatisfaction with President Roosevelt would have caused me to change my registration," Barry Goldwater later commented. "As a merchant I deeply resented the provisions in the National Recovery Act which gave the federal government the power to impose its will on private business. I think the foundations of my political philosophy were rooted in my resentment against the New Deal."[53]

Johnson's landslide victory in 1964 owed much to the determination of voters to preserve benefits won in the 1930s from Goldwater's assault and to the strength of the Roosevelt coalition. In Florida, a retired auto worker from Detroit interrupted his fishing long enough to tell a reporter: "First, the Democrats gave us the Wagner Act, then Social Security, then they guaranteed deposits in the bank. Lots of people were saved from starvation by the W.P.A. I'm voting for Johnson." An elderly man sunning himself in a waterfront park explained why he, too, would pull down the Johnson lever: "Everything I got, I got under a Democratic administration. You name it—unemployment compensation, Social Security. Goldwater seems to want to tear down a lot of these laws that were made 25 years ago."[54] Blessed by a challenger who permitted him to draw political lines precisely as he wanted to—between those who were faithful to FDR and those who were hostile—Johnson easily won election to a second term.

Returned to office with the biggest Democratic margin in Congress since the 1930s, when he had entered the House as FDR's protégé, Johnson moved quickly to drive through Congress a series of bills that he frankly acknowledged were in the Roosevelt tradition. "The Johnson program was his own, but its roots were in the Roosevelt Administration; in the Roosevelt second term," a writer commented on one Johnson message. "Clearly, the President was picking up where the New Deal left off in 1938." In submitting a report of the Housing and Home Finance Agency in 1965, Johnson observed, "The great Franklin D. Roosevelt first pleaded with Congress to approve housing measures for the good of all Americans." After Congress enacted one of his own housing bills, he remarked, "I have waited for this moment for 35 years." Even when he broke new ground, he looked back toward FDR. On signing the bill appropriating money for the Elementary and Secondary Education Act, Johnson stated, "Twenty-one years ago, President Franklin Roosevelt issued an urgent call to Congress for Federal assistance to education in this country. . . . Today we are helping to write the answer to that historic challenge."[55]

When Lyndon Johnson, with former president Truman by his side, signed the Medicare bill into law in a ceremony at Independence, Missouri, in the summer of 1965, he said:

> In 1935 when the man that both of us loved so much, Franklin Delano Roosevelt, signed the Social Security Act, he said it was, and I quote him, "a cornerstone in a structure which is being built but . . . is by no means complete."
>
> Well, perhaps no single act in the entire administration of the beloved Franklin D. Roosevelt really did more to win him the illustrious place in history that he has as did the laying of that cornerstone. And I am so happy that his oldest son Jimmy could be here to share with us the joy that is ours today. And those who share this day will also be remembered for making the most important addition to that structure.[56]

In the spring of 1965, at a time when the 89th Congress was swiftly advancing his own claim to a place in history, Johnson summed up his public attitude toward FDR. On April 12, 1965, on the twentieth anniversary of FDR's death, Johnson released a statement declaring:

> Twenty years ago—wearied by war, strained by the cares and triumphs of many years—the great heart of Franklin Roosevelt came to a stop.
>
> Most of us here shared the darkness of that day, as we had shared the difficult and shining days which had gone before. And wherever we were, when the unbelievable word came, for a moment the light seemed to waver and dim.
>
> But we were wrong about that. For he had worked too well. What he had set aflame was far beyond the poor and futile power of death to put out. . . .

Therefore, I come here to perform a task which is already done. This entire Nation is at once his grave and monument. Millions of men at work and healthy children are his monument. Freedom here, and in many distant lands, is his monument. And we—his friends, his colleagues, and his followers—are also his monument. . . .

Truly today's America is his America more than it is the work of any man.

But those of us who were lucky enough to know him, also know there was something beyond the long list of accomplishments. He had the gardener's touch. In some mysterious way he could reach out, and where there was fear, came hope; where there was resignation, came excitement; where there was indifference, came compassion.

And perhaps we can remember him most, not for what he did, but for what he wanted to do. We are trying to do it still. And I suppose we always will; as will many others to whom he is just a name and a picture in a book.[57]

Such was the message that Lyndon Johnson conveyed to the world—that he revered Franklin Roosevelt; hoped, as best he could, to carry on his ideas; and was fully content to remain in his shadow.

VI

In fact, Johnson wanted a great deal more than that. He was not satisfied to go down in the history books merely as a successful president in the Roosevelt tradition. He aimed instead to be "the greatest of them all, the whole bunch of them." And to be the greatest president in history, he needed not just to match Roosevelt's performance but to surpass it. As two Washington writers observed, "He didn't want to equal his mentor, Franklin Roosevelt; he wanted to eclipse him."[58]

Johnson had gargantuan aspirations. "Down there inside of Johnson somewhere was an image of a great popular leader something like Franklin Roosevelt, except more so, striding over the land and cupping the people in his hands and molding a national unity that every President dreams about but none is ever able to achieve," a White House correspondent has written. "Johnson's ambitions, of course, were bigger than any other President's." And FDR stood, like a huge thermometer in the town square at the start of a community chest drive, as the gauge of whether Johnson would go over the top. By the summer of 1965, Johnson said later, "I could see and almost touch my youthful dream of improving life for more people and in more ways than any other political leader, including FDR." At the same moment he was expanding the war in Vietnam, for he was determined, in the words of one of his biographers, to "out-Roosevelt Roosevelt" by imposing an American solution overseas at the same time that he achieved unprecedented social reforms in the United States. In the end, he anticipated, the American people, dazzled by his achievement in "pulling off both that war in Vietnam and the Great Society at home," would acclaim him the greatest president of all time.[59]

Though Johnson's desire to go down in history as a greater president than FDR derived in large part from early experiences that shaped his outsized personality, it owed something, too, to resentments built up in the years when he was so much in Roosevelt's shadow. For if there were advantages to being FDR's pet congressman, there was also a price to pay. In the 1941 senatorial contest, Representative Martin Dies dismissed Johnson as a "water carrier," a taunt that led Johnson to write an exceptionally obsequious letter to President Roosevelt:

> In the heat of Texas the last week, I said I was glad to be called a water-carrier—that I would be glad to carry a bucket of water to the Commander-in-Chief any time his thirsty throat or his thirsty soul needed support, for you certainly gave me support nonpareil.
> One who cannot arise to your leadership shall find the fault in himself and not in you!

When Johnson turned up at the Texas Democratic convention in 1944, conservatives cried, "Throw Roosevelt's pin-up boy out of there." In sum, the role diminished him. As the authors of one account have observed, the early Johnson "is but a dim memory to many of the congressmen he served with then. He was known as Roosevelt's man, a man who ran private political errands for the President. . . . His own powerful personality was sublimated to that of his powerful 'chief.' The LBJ of colorful Washington legend would come later; then in the Roosevelt era, Lyndon lived more in the shadows than on the center stage." If history would accord him a higher place than FDR, he would gain a measure of revenge for the humiliation of being Roosevelt's errand boy.[60]

Eleanor Roosevelt's attitude also grated. When he was majority leader, she thought of him as a clever tactician without strong convictions. Told by a friend that Johnson was a "secret liberal," she replied, "You're crazy." In 1959 he agreed to speak at a Memorial Day service in the Rose Garden at Hyde Park. "Mrs. Roosevelt, there's no suggestion that could ever be made to me by any Roosevelt that I wouldn't want to comply with," he told her. In fact, he resented having been asked as a substitute only after Truman could not come, and not until he had left repeated phone messages from Mrs. Roosevelt unanswered did he accept the invitation, just forty-eight hours before the event. When he did appear, Mrs. Roosevelt was conspicuously absent. Nothing daunted, Johnson busied himself saying things that would impress her when his words got back to her. By early 1960 she was beginning to speak publicly of his good points, but she never took him into her fold.[61]

No more than her husband could Mrs. Johnson escape comparison with her counterpart. So admirably did she fulfill her difficult assignment that a few who knew them both came to rate Lady Bird Johnson more highly than Mrs. Roosevelt. Averell Harriman thought her the greatest first lady he had ever encountered, more impressive even than Eleanor Roosevelt because she was much closer to her husband, and David Lilienthal, reporting on a conversation at the White House with Mrs. Johnson, wrote in his diary:

> Out of the corner of my eye I saw a portrait of Mrs. Roosevelt. That portrait, of an older woman, seemed bemused and tolerant, not the crusader. But as great a woman as Eleanor Roosevelt *became,* there was a time, when she lived in that great House, when she was much, much less well organized, focussed, and realistic than this dark-haired intense young woman with the strong Southern accent, sitting there beside me.

These comments were exceptional, however, and Mrs. Johnson could not help knowing that, no matter how well she did, any competition with a personage widely characterized as the greatest woman of the century was a mismatch from the start.[62]

Johnson's rivalry with Roosevelt, though, cannot be accounted for simply by recourse to rational explanations. One senses an obsessive quality that is altogether missing in the attitude of a Truman or a Kennedy. Alone of Roosevelt's successors Johnson was disposed to relate FDR to members of his own family and perhaps to confuse Roosevelt with his own "daddy." Asked in 1964 to comment on presidents he had known, he replied, according to one of his assistants, that "Roosevelt had a heart as compassionate as that of his own mother, and a mind as strategic as that of his father. He recalled that Roosevelt, like his father, 'had a touch of the populist.' "[63]

This comment suggests that Johnson held his father and FDR in very high esteem, but in fact his sentiments were more ambivalent. Toward each man he appears to have felt both affection and resentment. Johnson's lifelong quest for surrogate fathers may have indicated nothing more than a desire to find patrons who would ease his advancement, but it is likely that it also reflected some dissatisfaction with a father he thought to be an unsuitable role model. Furthermore, Johnson's "inner need to both emulate and surpass his father," in Doris Kearns's words, resonated later in his determination to acknowledge the Roosevelt legend but also to outperform the man he called "daddy." Throughout his career, Johnson had cannibalized the fathers he had adopted. As Kearns has written, "he became the invaluable helper, the deferential subordinate willing and able to perform a dazzling range of services for his master, until, step by step, the apprentice accumulated the resources that enabled him to secure the master's role." It would be extravagant to say that in determining to outdo Roosevelt, Johnson was committing a form of symbolic patricide, for in a number of ways he continued to be an admiring son, but at the very least he sought to show that he was a stronger man than his "daddy."[64]

Johnson revealed his feelings nakedly on Election Night, 1964, when the television screen in his hotel suite in Austin showed him rolling up a huge victory over Goldwater. The happy tidings might have been expected to create an enormous sense of contentment, but when he left his suite at 10 P.M., a reporter was startled to have the president snap at him when he asked a question. Johnson was cranky because he did not yet have the answer to the only question that interested him: How was he doing compared to Roosevelt in 1936? For Johnson was not running against Goldwater; he was running against FDR. He phoned Eric Goldman in Washington to ask him whether he was outpointing Roosevelt, and when Goldman warned him against making any premature claims to all-time records, he became peevish. Not until the next day was it fully clear that Johnson's percentage of the popular vote had, in fact, exceeded FDR's in 1936, and that his plurality had broken Roosevelt's record, though his proportion of the two-party vote was not so great, nor was his tally in the Electoral College so impressive.[65]

Johnson could take added satisfaction in the way that others analyzed his victory. Averell Harriman informed him: "For the first time in history, you carried all of the 62 counties in New York State, and all by a comfortable majority. In 1936, FDR failed to carry most of the upstate counties, not even his own—Dutchess County." It was noted, too, that in Maine and Vermont, the two states Roosevelt had lost, Johnson ran up better than 65 percent of the vote. In a postelection commentary, Richard Rovere, remarking that Johnson did not have to depend on southern states to the degree that FDR had, concluded, "Johnson's power base is far more secure than Roosevelt's ever was."[66]

President Johnson continued to vie with FDR when the new Congress convened. Conscious of Roosevelt's achievement in the Hundred

Days of 1933, Johnson harried his congressional leaders to enact as much legislation as possible before the hundredth day of the 1965 session, as though he were in a race with FDR; and when the hundredth day came, he stated that in this period he had compiled "a record of major accomplishments without equal or close parallel in the present era." A week earlier he had told newsmen, "The Senate has already passed 15 substantial measures in this program. I think you will find that they have passed more measures already than were passed the first 100 days of the Roosevelt administration, about which you have been writing for 30-odd years."[67]

These comments indicate that Johnson believed that less than two years after he took office he already overshadowed FDR, and his remarks at the end of the first session of "the fabulous Eighty-ninth Congress" confirm this inference. He called the session "the greatest in American history," and in a White House interview he said of Roosevelt: "He did get things done. There was regulation of business, but that was unimportant. Social security and the Wagner act were all that really amounted to much, and none of it compares to my education act of 1965."[68]

Many of those around him shared that view. "This Congress is a lot more impressive than the Hundred Days Congress," said Johnson's legislative liaison officer for the House of Representatives in 1965. "It's not meeting in a crisis." Such was the attitude, too, of his chief legislative assistant, Lawrence F. O'Brien, who has concluded:

> It has sometimes been said that the record of the Eighty-ninth Congress was the greatest since the New Deal legislation of 1933–34. I'm not sure that goes far enough. You can't really compare the two, of course—one an emergency program passed in the midst of economic depression, the other a burst of national self-improvement passed in a time of prosperity. Yet I tend to think, granting my deep personal involvement, that the break-throughs of the Eighty-ninth Congress—in education, in medical care, in civil rights, in housing—exceeded the New Deal achievements in their impact on American society.[69]

Others besides the White House staff gave Johnson and the 89th Congress the same high marks. In midsummer, at a time when the first session still had more than two months left, Tom Wicker wrote in the *New York Times,* "The list of achievements is so long that it reads better than the legislative achievements of most two-term Presidents, and some of the bills—on medical care, education, voting rights, and Presidential disability, to pick a handful—are of such weight as to cause one to go all the way back to Woodrow Wilson's first year to find a congressional session of equal importance." On Capitol Hill leaders of both parties were prepared to go even further. The Republican Charles Halleck, who had entered the House in 1935, said, when asked about relative political effectiveness, "I thought Roosevelt was pretty good," but Johnson was "the best I ever saw." Even more forthright was the Senate majority leader, Mike Mansfield of Montana. "Johnson has outstripped Roosevelt, no doubt about that," he declared in the fall of 1965. "He has done more than FDR ever did, or ever thought of doing."[70]

VII

Johnson refused to remain in Roosevelt's shadow not only because of his vaulting ambition but because in more than one respect he regarded FDR not as a model but as a bad example. If Johnson sought to emulate Roosevelt, he also attempted to avoid his predecessor's mistakes. "I never wanted to demagogue against business, Wall Street, or the power companies," he once said. "I thought FDR was wrong." In the fall of 1965 Johnson stated:

> If you have great power, you mustn't use it; that was one of the troubles with FDR. The President has terrible power. People are fearful of the President's power. That fear brought this republic into being. When people did not like what Roosevelt was doing, he called them economic royalists and moneychangers. He said they had met their match and would meet their master. It was like people fighting and spitting at one another.

Johnson, who fancied himself the magistrate of a consensus presidency, made a point of claiming in 1965, perhaps the last time he could still do so, "We have cut down the fear that destroyed Roosevelt."[71]

Once the first session of the 89th Congress had concluded its labors, Johnson turned his thoughts less to new programs than to administering what had already been enacted, in part because of lessons he drew from the FDR experience. The outbreak of World War II had prevented Roosevelt from making the final New Deal laws work satisfactorily, Johnson believed, and he did not want that to be said of the Great Society. In a White House interview Bill Moyers declared: "Johnson's approach is to attack and consolidate. The consolidation period may take longer than the advance. Roosevelt advanced too far without consolidation." Moreover, Johnson was determined that the laws would be enforced in a spirit different from that of the New

Dealers. Moyers explained: "This administration has been relatively free of the Ickes-Hopkins kind of feuding. Johnson learned from watching Roosevelt that this did not work. Roosevelt seemed to find enjoyment in watching his own gladiators fighting. Johnson does not like this."[72]

In relations between Congress and the executive, too, Johnson thought FDR had set a bad example. He remembered in particular an episode in 1941 when Sam Rayburn was humiliated by a message from the president about which he had been given no prior warning. "I never know when the damned messages are coming," Rayburn told Johnson at the time. "This last one surprised me as much as it did all of them." Then, Johnson recalled, "he shook his head sadly and walked slowly away." Years later, Johnson reflected, "I could see that his pride was hurt. So was the President's prestige and the administration's program. I never forgot that lesson."[73]

All of the Roosevelt errors that Johnson brought to mind paled beside one vivid episode: the Court-packing fracas of 1937. "I was the only Member of Congress to be elected on President Roosevelt's Supreme Court plan," he pointed out in 1964, and that remained the single most important memory of his earlier years.[74] He had seen a president win an awesome victory at the polls, and then have his expectations for the New Deal explode only a few months later when the Court-packing bill was interred. Johnson, too, had just won overwhelmingly. He was determined that he would not repeat FDR's mistake in judgment.

Again and again, Johnson referred to this ordeal of a president which he had witnessed when he first entered Congress. "Johnson cites the Roosevelt experience all the time," one of the president's White House aides reported in September 1965. "As Congressman, he saw what could go wrong with as big a mandate as that of 1936. He is deeply aware that one major miscalculation and a president has had it. He knows that in the ferocious environment in which a president lives, he may never be careless." On that same day, Johnson himself went out of his way to say, "In 1936, Roosevelt won by a landslide. But he was like the fellow who cut cordwood and sold it all at Christmas, and then spent it all on firecrackers. It all went up with a bang." Two months later at the White House, Bill Moyers recounted a sentence Johnson had once delivered to him: "When Roosevelt reached the summit of his power, he took on the gods of Olympus and got rolled back, and he never reached those heights again."[75]

In the immediate aftermath of his enormous victory in 1964, Johnson let everyone know that his recollection of 1937 led him to be cautious.

He remembered that when he took his seat in the House in April 1937 he found his new colleagues up in arms against the president; FDR, he concluded, had moved too quickly, with too little forethought. He told both White House aides and newspapermen that he planned to "avoid another 1937," that he would not overdraw his account by asking Congress to enact all of the Great Society at once. So rife were these reports that Robert Kennedy said, "It worries me a little when I read these stories about how much the President is thinking about Roosevelt and how he lost his popularity in 1936, because he did too much. But you can lose popularity by doing something, or you lose it by doing nothing. You lose it anyway. It's there to be spent."[76]

Kennedy need not have fretted, for Johnson soon reached precisely the same conclusion. It was imperative, Johnson decided, to seize the hour, not to waste the advantage of his great triumph as he thought FDR had done after his impressive win in 1936. "I have watched the Congress from either the inside or the outside, man and boy, for more than forty years, and I've never seen a Congress that didn't eventually take the measure of the President it was dealing with," he told a gathering of government lobbyists meeting in the Fish Room of the White House in January 1965. He reminded them of FDR's humiliation in 1937. "Here was a man who had just been elected by the biggest landslide in history and had the Congress slap him down," he said. "That poor man sat there in his wheelchair in the White House and just couldn't get around to all the congressional offices." Johnson compared that situation to the one he now confronted:

> I was just elected President by the biggest popular margin in the history of the country, fifteen million votes. Just by the natural way people think and because Barry Goldwater scared hell out of them, I have already lost about two of these fifteen and am probably getting down to thirteen. If I get in any fight with Congress, I will lose another couple of million, and if I have to send any more of our boys into Vietnam, I may be down to eight million by the end of the summer.

Consequently, he had to ram the Great Society program through immediately, while there was still time, by compelling Congress to perform as it had done in FDR's First Hundred Days.[77]

Johnson spoke more prophetically than he knew. For at the very moment when he was carrying out a domestic program that might earn him a higher place in history than Franklin Roosevelt's, he was setting out to send "more of our boys into Vietnam," a course that would gravely imperil his ambition to be regarded as the greatest of American presidents. A correspondent who observed this chain of events later recalled that over lunch in 1964 Johnson told reporters that he would not squander success as Roosevelt had done after 1936 on a single policy error. Tom Wicker wrote:

> Lyndon Johnson would not forget the limits of power; he would not carelessly throw away the fruits of his great victory for some unattainable goal, as Roosevelt had done in trying to pack the Supreme Court.
> But he did.
> . . . He had gone a long way, from the dust of the hill country to the loneliest peak of American political power and opportunity. And then, like Roosevelt before him, he . . . reached too far, believed too much, scaled the heights, only—in the blindness of his pride—to stumble and fall.[78]

VIII

The stumble and fall came in foreign affairs where, at least as much as in domestic policy, Franklin Roosevelt served as Johnson's model. If Johnson sought to outdo FDR, it would not be by departing from his program but by doing more of it, as well as by avoiding the single big error. Though he competed with Roosevelt, he did not reject FDR's ideas. Indeed, it was in the age of Roosevelt that he had absorbed a lesson in foreign policy that he never forgot. World War II, he discerned, had resulted from the appeasement of the fascist powers, which had been emboldened by America's disregard of FDR's warnings. In the Cold War era, Johnson bore Roosevelt's experience constantly in mind. Mechanically substituting Soviet Russia for Nazi Germany, he summed up what he believed to be the appropriate response to Communist aggression in a single phrase: "No more Munichs."[79]

In an interview with the historian Henry Graff in 1965, the president returned frequently to memories of the 1930s and 1940s. Johnson emphasized that his first serious thinking about diplomatic questions had begun as Hitler was rising to power, and he claimed that Roosevelt had wanted him on the Naval Affairs Committee because the Navy had been permitted to deteriorate and the president counted on Johnson to help see to it that the country had adequate force. He took pride in the fact that in 1941 he had persuaded Secretary of State Cordell Hull to write a letter that he liked to think had provided the margin of difference when the House approved by only one vote an extension of the draft less than four months before Pearl Harbor. As Johnson spoke, Graff noted, "he mentioned 'the Nyes, the Borahs, and La Follettes and

Chamberlain'—as if the whole panorama of the isolationist years had come alive for him again."[80]

It had been not just Roosevelt the New Dealer but Roosevelt the Big Navy Man who had first attracted Lyndon Johnson. It was as champion of FDR's rearmament program that Johnson had ingratiated himself with the White House circle, and when in World War II he toned down his enthusiasm for social measures to appease right-wingers in Texas, he retained his value to the administration by clamoring for increased arms spending. The portrait of Roosevelt that Johnson hung in the White House was not that of the champion of the New Deal but that of the World War II commander in chief. And when he stepped up American involvement in Southeast Asia in 1965, he was sure that he was being faithful to FDR's precepts.[81]

Johnson looked at the situation in Vietnam through spectacles ground in the 1930s. He frequently analogized the challenge in Southeast Asia to that posed by Hitler at Munich. When Kennedy sent him to Saigon in 1961, Johnson had likened Ngo Dinh Diem to Roosevelt, and as president he said cheerily that Premier Ky "sounded like Rex Tugwell." He even proposed to establish a TVA in a Vietnamese river basin. "I want to leave the footprints of America in Vietnam," he declared in 1966. "I want them to say when the Americans come, this is what they leave—schools, not long cigars. We're going to turn the Mekong into a Tennessee valley."[82]

In his notorious "Nervous Nellies" speech in Chicago in the spring of 1966, Johnson insisted that "our policy in Vietnam . . . springs from every lesson that we have learned in this century." It was in this same city of Chicago, he emphasized, that Franklin D. Roosevelt in 1937 had called for a quarantine of the aggressors. "The country heard him, but did not listen," he went on. "The country failed to back him in that trying hour. And then we saw what happened when the aggressors felt confident that they could win while we sat by."[83]

Three months later, he again offered FDR as his model in a talk at Campobello Island, New Brunswick, "The Roosevelt Legacy: Facing the Realities of Our Time." Johnson noted that he had first come to Washington just before Roosevelt assumed the presidency, and that by the time FDR's reign was over he was to "help change forever America's course in the affairs of the world" and "leave on a very young Congressman an enduring awareness of both the limits as well as the obligations of power." He added, trusting his audience to draw the parallel to his own predicament in Vietnam: "No man loved peace more than Franklin D. Roosevelt. It was in the marrow of his soul and I never saw him more grieved than when reports came from the War Department of American casualties in a major battle. But he led my nation and he led it courageously in conflict."[84]

In the spring of 1967, the columnist Roscoe Drummond compared Johnson's situation in Vietnam with FDR's on the eve of World War II. Just as bitter words were directed at Johnson from college campuses, so had Roosevelt been required to endure intellectual gadflies who told him to ignore the Axis threat. "President Roosevelt did not take their advice when he concluded that America had to join in resisting aggression in Europe and President Johnson is not following their advice today in his conviction that America must arrest the tide of aggression in Southeast Asia," Drummond stated. "FDR had his critics on resisting aggression but he proved to be right. Mr. Johnson has his critics on resisting aggression but, I believe, he, too, will prove to be right."[85]

That was a line of argument Johnson frequently employed himself. When at a press conference in November 1967 Johnson was asked why there was "so much confusion, frustration and difference of opinion about the war in Vietnam," he replied, "You know what President Roosevelt went through," and others had endured a similar response. "Now, when you look back upon it, there are very few people who would think that Wilson, Roosevelt, or Truman were in error." Such, too, he implied, would be the judgment of history on his own actions.[86]

Some observers agreed that the president had much in common with FDR, but not in the way Johnson intended. When Johnson, having won election on a peace appeal in 1964, soon afterward expanded the Vietnam struggle, it was remembered that Franklin Roosevelt had pledged in 1940 that he would send no boys into foreign wars and then had led the nation step by step toward involvement in World War II. Similarly, Roosevelt's guile and deceit during 1941 suggested Johnson's misrepresentation of such episodes as the Tonkin Gulf affair. One writer later stated: "Roosevelt could be said to have taught his successors, the most worshipful of whom was Lyndon Johnson, that lying succeeded and could be for the 'public good.'"[87]

In Johnson's second term, critics likened his government to the welfare-warfare state that had flourished under Franklin Roosevelt. "For Johnson, as for Wilson and the two Roosevelts before him, as for Bismarck, who created the welfare state, and Lloyd George, who adapted it for assimilation into Anglo-Saxon society, the welfare state evolved as a compound of militarism and reform," one commentator noted. Another charged that Johnson had deliberately chosen war as "the best way to pay off campaign backers" and "to keep a nation working and prosperous and content with his administration." He explained:

It was the natural thing for him to do. If you were a cactus-patch politician who had moved into the Washington stream during the days when FDR was proving the invincibility of a combined welfare-war program; if you were the shrewd kind of mechanic who quickly caught on to the gimmick-ry of the Roosevelt program without picking up the philosophy behind it; if you, furthermore, were convinced, and wisely so, that this nation would put up with anything but joblessness; if your long experience in office had convinced you that the easiest way to prime the pump was through defense spending; and if coupled to that was a basic disposition to "shove it down the throats" of your selected victim—wouldn't you probably hunt up a nicely-paced drawn-out war as just the ticket to prosperity?

. . . But first, the election. He had learned the method from Roosevelt: the promise not to send troops before the election, the plunge after.[88]

Such a view, though far from uncommon, commanded the support of only a minority. The majority rejected it not primarily because the analysis was so simplistic, ignoring as it did that Johnson heated up the Vietnam intervention precisely when the economy was flourishing and when the spectacular success of the tax cut had given every reason to suppose that the nation could prosper without war. More significantly, the conflict in Southeast Asia, however much it owed to such earlier presidents as FDR, had by 1968 unmistakably become "Johnson's war." In particular, there was a quality of grandiosity to the conflict, as there was to the Great Society, which had become LBJ's hallmark. As Doris Kearns has written:

Lyndon Johnson had wanted to surpass Franklin Roosevelt; and Roose-velt, after all, had not only won the reforms Johnson envied; he had also waged a war. But there was a critical difference: Roosevelt did not attempt the New Deal and World War II at the same time. Only Johnson among the Presidents sought to be simultaneously first in peace and first in war; and even Johnson was bound to fail.[89]

With each passing month, critics drummed home the same message: that Johnson had, after all, made the one big mistake; and when it came time to decide what course he should follow in 1968, his most vivid memory of the Roosevelt years returned to him. "He recalled coming in as a Congressman and seeing FDR immobilized domestically over the Supreme Court issue," Walt Rostow has said. "He felt that he could beat Nixon, but wouldn't be able to accomplish anything in his second term. He had too many 'tin cans' tied to him. He had used up his capital on civil rights and on the war." Like Roosevelt, he had miscalculated, and the consequences would be far more costly for him than they had been for FDR. Roosevelt could claim that the Court-packing gamble had ended in victory, for the Supreme Court never again struck down a New Deal law. Moreover, he was returned to office for an unprecedented third term and then elected for a fourth term. For Johnson, though, the string had run out. On March 31, 1968, no longer able to sustain the burdens of an unpopular war and domestic disorder, he shocked the nation by announcing that he would not be a candidate for another term. His strenuous effort to win recognition as "the greatest of them all, the whole bunch of them," had come to an end.[90]

IX

Even as he prepared to take the step that would terminate his political career, Johnson continued to inquire how he stacked up against Roosevelt. On the evening of March 26, 1968, he delivered what was, in effect, a valedictory in a long talk at the White House with the political writer Theodore White and with an adviser, Jim Rowe, who had also been an aide to FDR. His visitors did not know that before the week was out Johnson would reveal his intention not to run for another term, but his conversation was manifestly an attempt to present himself as he hoped history would see him. One feature of his remarks impressed White particularly: "A poor painting of Roosevelt hung in the place of honor in the room where we talked, but Roosevelt, for Johnson, was alive, the master. Roosevelt's name threaded all through the conversation as he went on to review what he had accomplished. Even in recollection, there is a thrill to the memory of this President measuring himself." Johnson listed all the things he had done, all the things he had tried to do, then asked, "How much time did a President have anyway?" White has recorded what came next: "A President has only four years' run from the Congress, he answered. Even Roosevelt—Roosevelt did all he was going to do in his first four years, except for that minimum-wage bill he got through in 1938. The best anybody could hope for was a run of four years, and he himself had had a good four-year run. They'd never repealed any of Roosevelt's legislation, and they weren't going to repeal any of Lyndon Johnson's legislation." He could take pride in a lot of things, he said, but he concluded the interview on a melancholy note: "I guess not many Presidents have been understood in their own time."[91]

The tone of resignation may have indicated that Johnson recognized that he had not outdone FDR after all. He still boasted of his achievements, but not even a man of his colossal ego could continue to think that history would place Roosevelt in his shadow. That was something that he had been compelled to realize in countless ways, large and small. If there was one activity above all others in which Johnson could claim that he was carving out a place in history distinct from Roosevelt's, it was in civil rights. But when the civil rights bill came to the floor of the House in 1964, a California congressman made no mention of Johnson but stressed that the bill was arriving there on FDR's birthday, a day on which, once again, he and his colleagues wore white carnations in memory of the departed leader. When Johnson appointed Thurgood Marshall to the Supreme Court, he expected to see thousands of children named after the new justice, but birth records in Boston and New York showed not one Thurgood but seven Martins, ten Luthers, eleven George Washingtons, and, nearly a quarter of a century after his death, fifteen Franklin Delanos.[92]

The Washington correspondent for *The New Yorker*, Richard Rovere, had noted a curious fact: that "one aspect of Johnson's Presidency . . . presents a direct and somewhat baffling contrast to Roosevelt's." He explained:

> Roosevelt generated vast amounts of political excitement and intellectual stimulation, but Johnson's Washington, on the eve of what promises to be an extended period of extensive innovation, is almost barren of excitement. No State of the Union Message has ever promised larger undertakings than those the President proposed here a week ago tonight. His program is broad, adventurous, and controversial. Yet today, in this great pre-Inaugural tangle of bunting and television cables, the sense of adventure is altogether absent.[93]

Still worse, Johnson found himself to be an object of loathing such as even That Man in the White House had not known. No one had asked FDR how many kids he had killed that day or had likened him to Macbeth, who achieved power by murder. "People *hated* F.D.R. aplenty," David Lilienthal commented in his diary toward the end of 1966. "But contempt, distrust, and scorn—is this something new, reserved for President Johnson?" That obloquy fell particularly hard on a man whose need for affection was so plain. "Lyndon's great desire . . . was to walk in the steps of FDR and to be known as the man of the people who served the common good," William O. Douglas has written. "There was the basic yearning of the man—he had to be loved. It never became so apparent to me as it did the day he took me on a tour of his ancestral home in Johnson City, Texas. The main emphasis was his mother and her love of him. This developed, in his life, to a desire to be loved by everyone, in the manner he imagined FDR was loved by people. . . . Yet it was not possible for him."[94]

Johnson never understood what had happened to him. Through the Great Society he had done the same kinds of things that FDR had achieved and, he was certain, even more, but he could not win the kind of devotion that Roosevelt had received. He had been far more adventurous than FDR in civil rights, yet the best Hubert Humphrey could say was: "President Johnson's firm leadership on civil rights appears to have surprised those who had forgotten his record. They failed to remember that his idol and mentor was Franklin Roosevelt." It bewildered him that FDR had been hailed as champion of the free world for pursuing policies that, to Johnson, seemed identical to his. His advisers and the American people had run out on him in the Vietnam war, Johnson grumbled, though no one had ever jumped ship on Roosevelt in World War II.[95]

Called upon to explain his mounting unpopularity, Johnson frequently alluded to FDR's experience. "Hoover and Roosevelt were more abused than I am," he told a *Time* correspondent. "The things said about Roosevelt were more vicious." Too much should not be made of his party's losses in the 1966 midterm elections, he said; after all, the Democrats had won in a landslide in 1936, then suffered severe losses two years later. When at the end of 1967 a newspaperman asked Johnson to account for the race riots of the previous summer, the president replied that violence was not new in America. "We had a riot in Detroit during President Roosevelt's administration where he had to send out troops that compared very much to the same one we had there this year," he reminded him.[96]

Johnson even attempted to make light of the abuse he was receiving. In comments delivered by telephone to a gathering of Democrats in West Virginia in December 1967, he remarked that Vice-President Humphrey had "been going around the country lately, keeping his finger on the political pulse. And I don't mind telling you that some of his reports make pretty grim reading." Johnson continued:

Just the other day he showed me a letter to a newspaper editor. This particular critic . . . said that 7 years of a Democratic administration had "deluded the American people into believing that a government . . . is an inexhaustible giver-out of jobs, doles, and pensions."

Doesn't that sound familiar? I doubt if there has ever been a Democratic administration that didn't get that kind of criticism. The letter I just read to you, the letter that the Vice President was showing me, in fact, was written on June 17, 1940—not about Lyndon Johnson and the Great Society, but about Franklin D. Roosevelt and the New Deal.[97]

No amount of levity, however, could disguise the fact that Johnson would never achieve his goal of outdoing FDR, a reality that became inescapable with each passing month in 1968. Roosevelt had led the country to victory in World War II, while Johnson was commander in chief of a failing cause. FDR had died while serving a fourth term in the White House, but Johnson was driven from office. The candidate Johnson chose to be his successor remained a fundamentalist New Dealer, but Hubert Humphrey could never recover from being identified with Johnson's one big mistake, and he made matters worse by saying, "I'm Lyndon Johnson's Eleanor Roosevelt."[98] The result was the election of Richard Nixon and the end of any prospect of an Age of Johnson.

x

In the aftermath of Johnson's March 31 announcement, which appeared to signal the demise of the age of Roosevelt, such commentators as Eric Goldman, who had served on the White House staff, offered a compelling explanation for the president's difficulties: he had remained an FDR man in an era altogether different from the Great Depression.[99] "America had been rampaging between the 1930's and the 1960's," Goldman wrote. "The alterations were so swift and so deep that the country was changing right out from under President Lyndon Johnson." Goldman went on to say that "like a good 1930's man, he expressed his authentic thinking during the campaign of 1964 when he would shout, 'Remember Molly and the children,' or 'We Americans don't want much. We want decent food, housing and clothing.'" But in the 1960s, though "there were still plenty of Mollys with plenty of troubles," the main problem had shifted from subsistence to "how to live with a weirdly uneasy general affluence—one that was marked by a maldistribution no longer accepted by a significant section of the population and by a race revolt that was only in part economic." Johnson continued to address himself to the needs and aspirations of the FDR coalition, but "now much of labor sounded like threatened burghers"; white workers had less concern about social reform than status trauma;

black militants were distrustful even of such well-intentioned whites as Johnson; and the young, with no memory of the Roosevelt era, "were inclined to think of bread-and-butter liberalism as quaint if not downright camp." Throughout all of society, the values that had sustained America in the age of Roosevelt and for generations before were being questioned. In such a situation, Goldman concluded, "President Johnson, acting upon the kind of consensus domestic policy that would merely codify and expand the 1930's, was about as contemporary as padded shoulders, a night at the radio and Clark Gable."[100]

Theodore White has made a similar point about the political situation in 1968. "In an age of affluence and education the blind urges that had once created atavistic Democratic votes in slums, factories, ghettos, universities were no longer blind," he has observed. The Roosevelt coalition had been based on the assumption that the working class would be satisfied by the activities of the government in doling out federal benefits. But by 1968 white workers no longer depended on Washington as they had done in the 1930s, and Johnson was asking them to do something Roosevelt had not demanded of them—to accede to the aspirations of blacks for a fair share of power and perquisites that they were reluctant to surrender. "All through 1968," White noted, "the working-class base of the Democratic coalition was to be torn almost as if by civil war, as white workingmen questioned the risk and the pace imposed on them in the adventure."[101]

The reasoning of Goldman and White goes far toward explaining the disappointment Johnson experienced in workers' response to the Great Society. In 1966 he flew to Detroit to speak at a Labor Day rally in that Democratic stronghold. In a city where thousands upon thousands of auto workers had once massed in Cadillac Square to cheer FDR, Johnson attracted only a small turnout. Afterward the president of the United Auto Workers, Walter Reuther, explained that many UAW members were at their lakeside cottages or out boating, while others were joyriding through the countryside. They had no intention of coming into a smoggy city to listen to a politician tell them of his devotion to organized labor.[102]

Two Washington correspondents amplified the argument. Johnson had problems, they wrote, that transcended his own personality. "His hero, Franklin Roosevelt, had come to power in the 1930s when certain fundamental ideas about the nature of government and society and America's role in the world were approaching full time," they explain. One notion was the optimistic one that rational people could, by government fiat and with relatively minor changes in the system, create a just society within a capitalist structure. The other was that America had a mission to safeguard the free world against totalitarian aggression. Unhappily, "it was one of the ironies that marked his life that the intellectual foundations of the New Deal (which he accepted) and the intellectual foundations of America's postwar foreign policy (which he also accepted) were being eroded and discredited even as he took office." As president, Johnson, oblivious of the fact that the political universe was no longer what it had been, applied the Rooseveltian precepts in Vietnam and would be satisfied with nothing short of a Great Society. This meant that he was carrying "the philosophy and ideals of the New Dealers to their logical limits at the very time that the tide was running out on all their premises and assumptions."[103]

Though all of these observations contain important insights, they fall short of fully explaining Johnson's troubles, especially in the realm of foreign affairs. Clearly, there are resemblances between FDR's foreign policy and Johnson's. But there are also critical differences. As Goldman acknowledges, Johnson had "laid hold of an attic doctrine which included even apostrophes to the flag and international deeds of derring-do," an approach that suggests not Roosevelt's measured attitude but an earlier era of forays against banana republics. Johnson's behavior toward the Dominican Republic, in particular, contravened the spirit of FDR's Good Neighbor Policy. Nor is Johnson's persistence in the Southeast Asian disaster readily traceable to Roosevelt. So sympathetic was FDR to the aspirations of the Vietnamese that one student of the Vietnam disaster has concluded, "If Roosevelt had lived, the history of Southeast Asia might have been different." That is probably an overstatement, for by the time of his death FDR had been compelled to beat a retreat in the face of French and British resistance and Chinese weakness. Nonetheless, when Ho Chi Minh appealed to American correspondents for understanding after World War II, he cited the outlook of Franklin Roosevelt as testimony to the rightness of his cause.[104]

It has not been convincingly demonstrated, either, that Johnson came to grief with the Great Society because the FDR legacy was outmoded in the 1960s. In many respects the Roosevelt tradition was a source of strength for Johnson. It provided him with an identity, the core of an electoral coalition, a cadre of advisers, and a storehouse of ideas, especially those for the War on Poverty. To be sure, the problems of the sixties differed from those of the thirties, and Johnson needed to adapt to the imperatives of a new age. But he ran into trouble not so much because he adhered to Roosevelt's programs as because he grafted onto them feckless innovations.

Johnson foundered less because the FDR legacy was faulty than because of his own misconceptions of it and, even more, because of his egregious behavior. When he imitated Roosevelt, he did so with such frenzy that the Johnson White House, one of his aides has written, emerged as a "caricature" of FDR's, "a grotesque and very unattractive scene which, at best, resembled the dances in the Hall of the Mountain King in *Peer Gynt*."[105] In his determination to outdo Roosevelt, he carried everything to excess—the overladen apparatus of the Great Society; the insistence on having both guns and butter, which had calamitous inflationary repercussions; and, most of all, the body counts and the napalm and the saturation bombing.

Johnson had high hopes of history, but those hopes were to be blighted. He would tell visitors to the LBJ Ranch: "This is the tree I expect to be buried under and when my grandchildren see this tree I want them to think of me as the man who saved Asia and . . . who did something for the Negroes in this country." He had thought, too, that his child, the Great Society, would "grow into a beautiful woman" and that the American people would "want to keep her around forever, making her a permanent part of American life, more permanent even than the New Deal." But he lived long enough to see that at the 1972 Democratic National Convention, FDR's picture was displayed along with those of other party leaders but his own portrait was nowhere to be seen. Not many months later, Senator Vance Hartke, peering at his coffin, reflected, "On balance, Lyndon Johnson will be remembered as a sincere humanitarian in the Franklin Roosevelt mold, but with this caveat: the Vietnam War will be hanging over that judgment. Some of the living will forgive him—the dead, never."[106]

Yet if Johnson failed in his effort to put FDR in his shadow, he did not leave the Roosevelt tradition unaltered. A month before Johnson died, the Harris poll released findings that may have been one of the last things he ever read. Asked which recent president "most inspired confidence," respondents chose FDR 393 to 28 over Johnson. (By February 1976 the ratio had risen to 508–14.)[107] The results suggested that the FDR appeal had not faded away in 1968. But, as a result of Johnson's behavior, the Roosevelt emphases were more than ever perceived to contain ingredients of evil as well as good. Johnson's successors would eye the Roosevelt legacy warily, conscious of the malign consequences that could follow from it. It was in this unintended and perverse fashion that Lyndon Johnson, who claimed to want nothing more than to exalt the hero of his youth, did in the end achieve his covert ambition—to cast a shadow on FDR.

[5]

Second Republican Interlude: Richard Nixon and Gerald Ford

On January 20, 1973, Richard M. Nixon took the oath of office, and two days later Lyndon Johnson dropped dead. Less than a month earlier Harry Truman had died. Thus within two months of Nixon's enormous victory over George McGovern, a triumph likened to Franklin Roosevelt's in 1936, the two men who had lived most under FDR's shadow were gone and the country appeared to be entering a new era. A book published in Nixon's second term summed up that line of thinking: "The deaths of Truman and Johnson symbolized the passing of the long legacy left from FDR's reign in the White House," and "seemed to add a solemn, funereal note to McGovern's defeat, which itself was being interpreted as a final and definitive repudiation of the Roosevelt-Democratic approach to governmental action."[1]

The new era, it was said, would take its character from a president altogether disconnected from the age of Roosevelt. In his sparkling biography *Nixon Agonistes,* Garry Wills wrote:

> Nixon is a postwar man. Politically, he does not preexist the year 1946. . . . He lived through the Depression, studying, working, going to school. He was then at a formative age. Yet neither the Depression nor the New Deal, neither cause nor cure, had any discernible effect upon him. . . . History ended in 1924, with the death of his boyhood hero Wilson, and did not start up again until 1946.[2]

One can understand how such an interpretation could arise. Nixon never laid eyes on FDR, and not until 1946 did he know that the president was crippled. Roosevelt's first election in 1932 does not seem to have meant much to him, and he appears never to have voted for FDR, though his father probably did.[3] Years later, when asked whether Roosevelt had affected his political thinking, Nixon replied, "I would say probably not," then added as if this clarified matters, "You understand that in the thirties, of course, I was still in school, in law school."[4]

In fact, though, Nixon did preexist 1946. As an undergraduate at Whittier, he studied the New Deal assiduously and, in response to the growth of the leviathan state under Roosevelt, debated such topics as whether the national government was overreaching. An NYA job helped him work his way through Duke Law School, and he was in his final term there when FDR's Court-packing plan stirred a national controversy. Five years later he went to Washington to seek a position with the Office of Price Administration, one of the most liberal of the wartime agencies, and from January to August 1942 he served with the OPA.[5]

Furthermore, FDR cast a dark shadow over Richard Nixon, one of a very different sort from that projected upon Lyndon Johnson. Indeed, one commentator has gone so far as to suggest that Nixon was as ghost-ridden as the people of Norway in Ibsen's overwrought drama. "When each new president moves into the White House, he finds that he shares it with the ghosts of his predecessors," a Nixon speechwriter has said, and "the ghost that did most to shape his presidency was that of Franklin Delano Roosevelt. . . . It was the Roosevelt pattern in domestic policy that Nixon sought to reverse, the Roosevelt coalition he sought to replace, the Roosevelt legacy he sought to supplant."[6]

Theodore White has offered the same perspective. "Nixon considered his greatest rival to be Franklin D. Roosevelt, Harvard '04," White asserted. The tremendous victory in 1972, he observed, gratified Nixon but left him with an oppressive sense of burden. White explained:

> It meant that if he were to make his mark on history permanent, he would have to do it with greater individual boldness, with greater personal exercise of authority, than any victorious President before him. And that, in turn, meant that he would still be running, as really he always had been running, against the personality and work of Franklin Roosevelt. . . . Anyone who has talked to Richard Nixon, over a period of years and privately, knows that, without ever avowing it, he has been running against Franklin D. Roosevelt since he began campaigning for office. He speaks of Roosevelt not with bitterness or disrespect or anger—but in a way that makes clear in all conversation that his own measure of himself is a measure against Franklin Roosevelt.[7]

On this, as on so many other matters, Nixon's own testimony is not always reliable. He has recently stated:

I never ran against Roosevelt. I mean, some of my friends on the Republican side did. Because I admired him. Perhaps it goes back to my earlier background, the fact that my father thought that he was doing something about the Depression, although he was unable to do anything about . . . really solving it, the war did that. And also in the foreign policy area, I felt that Roosevelt spoke for the country. And consequently, I would say that I was more pro Roosevelt than against.[8]

The evidence is to the contrary. Nixon made his political debut in the 1940 campaign by assailing Roosevelt, doing the rounds of service clubs in southern California with attacks on the 1937 Court-packing plan, though that issue was less than burning in 1940. His memoirs shrug these activities off. "As the 1940 elections approached, I strongly supported Wendell Willkie because, while I favored some of Roosevelt's domestic programs, particularly Social Security, I opposed his attempt to break the two-term tradition," he wrote. "I even made a couple of speeches for Willkie before small local groups in Whittier." A college girl friend, though, has indicated a longstanding animus. "I thought Roosevelt was wonderful," she has recollected, "and he detested him." His brief government service further alienated him. He was not at ease with the fast-moving OPA lawyers, and his assignment on tire rationing was dreary. He came out of the experience with a distrust of government regulation and resentment against what he subsequently called "the old, violent New Deal crowd" who wanted to skewer Big Business. Not for many years afterward would he even directly acknowledge that he had been on the OPA staff.[9]

In 1946 Nixon won election to Congress for the first time as an avowed foe of FDR's policies. When Republican leaders were looking him over to see if he would be an acceptable candidate, Nixon told them that there were two attitudes toward the American system: "One advocated by the New Deal is government control to regulate our lives. The other calls for individual freedom and all that initiative can produce. I hold with the latter viewpoint." Reflecting on the 1946 race, a California Democrat has said, "I am sure that Roosevelt, in addition to the many fine things that he did, for good or bad, certainly changed the whole future of this country. Possibly many of the things which he instituted were needed, but from the standpoint of what I think and possibly what others who were backing Dick Nixon would have said, we went too far too fast. At that time, it was the one thing that helped elect Dick."[10]

During the ensuing years, Nixon, while commending Roosevelt as "very effective" as a war president and "dynamic" in foreign affairs, had more ambivalent feelings about his performance in the Great Depression. Noting that Roosevelt had run on a pledge to slash government spending, "a conservative economic platform if you ever read one," Nixon commented:

> Roosevelt probably honestly thought he was going to put it into effect. But he could no more have done that than fly to the moon because the times called for something else. The times called for spending, for government action to stop the depression. So when Roosevelt took office he became, in effect, a captive of circumstances. Since he couldn't turn the tide backwards, he had to go with it. By the force of his personality he directed the course it took. He turned it into the channels of the great social reforms of the 1930's, some of which were very admirable and others of which proved to be unworkable and undesirable.

Yet whatever his reservations about the soundness of FDR's economic policies, Nixon had a keen sense of the political rewards the Democrats had reaped from the New Deal. The GOP badly needed a social welfare position, he wrote Charles Percy. "As you know, since 1933 the Democrats have used programs in this field to their great advantage and to our marked disadvantage."[11]

In addition, while continuing to align himself with those who deplored the changes Roosevelt had helped bring about, Nixon looked toward FDR to clue him on how to operate, to provide leads that he could exploit, like one power broker eying another. It was in such fashion that Nixon's cocker spaniel found a place in history hitherto monopolized by FDR's Scottie, Fala.

In 1952, when the revelation that he had been the beneficiary of a secret fund threatened to drive him off the national Republican ticket, Nixon summoned Roosevelt to the rescue. On a plane from Portland, Oregon, where a crowd had hurled pennies at his car and men with canes and dark glasses shook tin cups marked "Nickels for poor Nixon," to Los Angeles, where he was to address the nation on television, Nixon took out some postcards and scribbled down random thoughts. He later wrote:

> I . . . thought about the stunning success FDR had in his speech during the 1944 campaign, when he had ridiculed his critics by saying they were even attacking his little dog Fala, and I knew it would infuriate my critics if I could turn this particular table on them. I made a note: "They will be charging that I have taken gifts. I must report that I did receive one gift after the nomination—a cocker spaniel dog, Checkers, and whatever they say, we are going to keep her."[12]

The Checkers speech served to lower still further Nixon's repute among the Roosevelt liberals, who had singled him out as a particularly treacherous enemy as early as 1946. In each of his political endeavors, he had the Roosevelt family arrayed against him, with Eleanor Roosevelt in particular voicing her contempt. In 1956 Mrs. Roosevelt announced that she had "no respect" for the way Nixon had gone after Helen Gahagan Douglas in the 1950 senatorial race in California. "I have always felt that anyone who wanted an election so much that they would use those means did not have the character that I really admire in public life."[13]

Nixon's election to the presidency in 1968 gave him an opportunity to get even with the Roosevelt Democrats at the same time that he freely borrowed from the FDR legacy for rhetoric, ideas, and procedures. As Nixon contemplated his first inaugural, Roosevelt served both as a model and, much more markedly, as a point of departure. In preparation for his great day, he read every previous inaugural address. FDR's 1933 effort was one he especially esteemed, but also one he rejected. He told his aides at Key Biscayne as he worked over a draft that the theme of FDR's discourse was "to kick hell out of someone else and tell the American people they're great," and he added, "We've got to write the section about the spirit of America, about confronting ourselves, in a way that we don't condemn everybody. We mustn't appear to be scolding the people." Nixon's presentation, too, could define the goals of his administration. His chief speechwriter has explained:

One of those goals was summed up in a theme we developed during the campaign: to break the pattern of the century's middle third at the start of its final third. In a neat bit of historical symmetry, the administrations from Franklin Roosevelt's through Lyndon Johnson's precisely spanned the middle third of the twentieth century. FDR was inaugurated in March 1933. He was the architect of the modern presidency, and of the vast expansion of federal powers that continued from his administration onward, reaching its zenith under Johnson, who came to Washington in the 1930s as a Roosevelt protégé.[14]

On January 20, 1969, his presentation having been whipped into shape, Nixon both acknowledged FDR's role at the outset of the second third of the century and delineated his own different conception. He stated:

Standing in this same place a third of a century ago, Franklin Delano Roosevelt addressed a nation ravaged by depression and gripped in fear.

[165]

He could say in surveying the Nation's troubles: "They concern, thank God, only material things."

Our crisis today is in reverse.

We find ourselves rich in goods, but ragged in spirit; reaching with magnificent precision for the moon, but falling into raucous discord on earth.[15]

Nixon drew upon Roosevelt on several occasions in his first term, as he had during the campaign, not always in a manner that would have pleased FDR. The president's speechwriter William Safire went more than once to volumes of Roosevelt's public papers for inspiration, and on transmitting a reorganization plan to Congress in March 1970 Nixon referred to FDR's 1939 reorganization as having laid the basis for the modern presidency.[16] When Nixon signed a bill amending the Social Security Act in 1971, he quoted from Roosevelt not to celebrate the welfare state but to exalt the work ethic. "Over the last four decades," he said, "we have learned, at inestimable social cost, the truth of Franklin Roosevelt's words: 'Continued dependence upon relief induces a spiritual and moral disintegration fundamentally destructive to the national fibre. To dole out relief in this way is to administer a narcotic, a subtle destroyer of the human spirit.'"[17]

Like other Republican leaders of his generation, Nixon was critical of FDR's performance at Yalta, but that did not stop him from making use of the association between Roosevelt and Stalin. When at the Kremlin in 1972 Brezhnev stressed the need to cultivate a personal relationship, saying, as Nixon has recorded it, "that the name of Franklin D. Roosevelt was warmly cherished in the memory of the Soviet people," Nixon replied that the relationship between Roosevelt and Stalin (and Stalin and Churchill) taught the importance of achieving an agreement between the two leaders that would circumvent disputes among subordinates. Two years later, Nixon again emphasized the broad perspective in talking to Brezhnev. He noted in his diary:

I had used this argument with him in pointing out how Roosevelt, Churchill, and Stalin had gotten along well, particularly emphasizing the Roosevelt-Stalin relationship in fighting the war, because they did not allow differences on what the peace was going to be like to deter them from their main goal of defeating the Nazis.

Of course, historically, my own view is that this was a mistake—that Churchill was right in insisting that there be more discussion at that point and that we should have made some kind of a deal that would have avoided the division of Europe on the basis that it finally came out.[18]

Nixon also found the memory of FDR helpful in exculpating his behavior in Vietnam. Called upon to explain the "credibility gap"— early in 1971 seven out of ten Americans said they did not believe what the administration was saying about Vietnam—Nixon summoned Roosevelt to his side. After reminding his interviewer, Howard K. Smith, that Wilson had pledged to keep the country out of war on the eve of American intervention in World War I, the president added:

> And you remember Franklin D. Roosevelt once made the statement in a speech before World War II: I will not send your sons to fight on foreign shores. I think both Wilson and Franklin D. Roosevelt meant exactly what they said. They were not lying to the American people.
> On the other hand, the great events made it necessary for them each to take the Nation into war. . . .
> It is the events that cause the credibility gap, not the fact that a President deliberately lies or misleads the people.[19]

The president's defenders, too, used the FDR legacy to justify his foreign policy. Nixon's decision to give military aid to autocratic governments, said William Buckley, amounted "to nothing more than the continuation of broad policies originated by Franklin Delano Roosevelt (who kissed the devil's nose by giving aid to Stalin)." Incensed at Americans for Democratic Action for adopting a resolution in 1971 to impeach President Nixon for "high crimes" in Vietnam, Buckley wrote of the ADA leaders:

> What do they have in common? Above all, their early devotion to Franklin Delano Roosevelt. Out of that devotion developed an ultramontanism not known outside the Roman Curia. Anything Roosevelt did was all right, and any challenge to Roosevelt's executive prerogatives was reactionary, nihilistic, and anarchistic. Roosevelt used to make secret commitments in behalf of the United States every couple of weeks, with extras on Halloween—armies to Iceland, fleets to the Mediterranean, marines to Singapore. Never mind, what now we are taught to call the military-industrial complex, in those days we called the arsenal for democracy—you couldn't do business with Hitler—we had to shoulder the responsibilities of a great power—had to have a strong President. Impeach Roosevelt? As well impeach the Statue of Liberty.[20]

Other observers who were drawn to the Roosevelt comparison, however, regretted that Nixon was much less accessible to the press than FDR and not nearly so accountable to the American people. Milton

Eisenhower complained that whereas FDR averaged eighty news conferences a year, Nixon scheduled only four in all of 1970, and in the fall
of that year a columnist observed: "At this point in his first term of
office Franklin Roosevelt had held 150 Washington press conferences.
President Nixon has held 12. It has changed the whole tone here. It has
made the presidency once removed. . . . The bold, direct press conference, 'How about it, Mr. President?' has turned into the timid news
leak, and news ooze."[21]

Even when Nixon cited FDR, he did so not to perpetuate the Roosevelt tradition but with the altogether contrary purpose of destroying
the FDR coalition. The *New Republic*'s veteran commentator Richard
L. Strout wrote, "As to politics we have little doubt which way Mr.
Nixon will go; he will try to demolish the old FDR Democratic coalition and create one of his own. His wrecking ball in 1968 shook the
FDR coalition but knocked out only one segment, the South." In 1972
he would see to it that the FDR coalition gave way to a "New American
Majority."[22]

One morning near the close of the 1972 campaign, Nixon told three
of his aides, as they chatted in the Oval Office, how his "New American
Majority" differed from FDR's coalition. He explained:

> The Roosevelt coalition was just that—a coalition. He played one against
> another—big city bosses, intellectuals, South, North. By contrast, our
> New American Majority appeals across the board—to Italians, Poles,
> Southerners, to the Midwest and New York—for the same reasons, and
> because of the same basic values. These are people who care about a strong
> United States, about patriotism, about moral and spiritual values.

The great healer who nurtured spiritual values then went on to explain
that he got support for such decisions as saturation bombing not from
college presidents, for "they have no guts, no character," but rather
"from those areas the elitists look down their noses at. . . . Square
America is coming back."[23]

In order to make an impressive showing for the New American
Majority, the White House put almost all its campaign chest into re-
electing Nixon rather than helping Republican candidates generally. As
Safire explained:

> What amounted to the "Schorenstein Rationale" was put forth. Hymie
> Schorenstein was a Brooklyn district leader in the Twenties who refused
> to spend a nickel on local campaigns, sending his collections instead to the
> campaign of Franklin Roosevelt for Governor. "You ever watch the ferries

come in from Staten Island?" he asked his pleading candidates. "When that big ferry sails into the ferry slip, it never comes in strictly alone. It drags in all the crap from the harbor behind it." After a dramatic pause, Schorenstein would conclude, "FDR is our Staten Island Ferry."

So Nixon was supposed to be the Staten Island Ferry; the money spent on the presidential campaign, Clark MacGregor was told to argue, would build up a landslide so huge that weak candidates would be swept in.[24]

It did not take long for evidence of a landslide to mount, and once again Nixon revealed his intimate knowledge of the Roosevelt years. In September he discounted polls that showed him with a 34-point lead by saying, "No President except Washington ever won by two to one. The best was 63/37 for Roosevelt." After he did, in fact, nearly match FDR's figures, he responded to the suggestion that his big victory might raise unreasonable expectations by remarking that he was well aware of FDR's experience in 1937.[25] Nonetheless, to those assigned to draft his second inaugural address, Nixon sent only two previous efforts, one of them FDR's 1937 speech.

Observers of all political stripes never wearied of matching Nixon's totals in 1972 with FDR's a generation before. Nixon's supporters exulted in the fact that in winning forty-nine of fifty states, though not the District of Columbia, he surpassed FDR's mark of forty-six out of forty-eight, long thought to be unbeatable. Unimpressed, however, was one Democratic partisan who wrote sourly, "Franklin Roosevelt carried all but two states by telling the people they had nothing to fear but fear itself. Richard Nixon carried all but one state by making them fear everything, especially each other." More dispassionate analysts concluded that Nixon diverged markedly from FDR in failing to carry his party through to control of Congress. Even in victory he was a loner.[26]

Nixon, though, scored his performance much as he did the exploits of his gridiron heroes. He was quick to point out that he and Roosevelt were the only chief executives in the history of the country who had run for the offices of president and vice-president five times, each with the same record: four wins, one loss. This tally, critics objected, conveniently obscured the fact that FDR had won the presidency each of the four times he ran while Nixon had prevailed twice, failed once. Still, as Theodore White commented, "Between them, these two men go down as the most enduring American politicians of the twentieth century, and they span a period of fifty years of continuing American revolution."[27]

Richard Nixon's ambitions did not stop with replacing the FDR coalition, for he fully intended to use his mandate to turn the country away from the New Deal tradition. Two days before the 1972 election

Nixon told an interviewer for the *Washington Star* that he expected his administration to bring about the most significant change since Franklin Roosevelt had been elected in 1932, but his program would be the reverse of FDR's. "Roosevelt's reforms led to bigger and bigger power in Washington," he said. "It was perhaps needed then. . . . The reforms that we are instituting are ones which will . . . diffuse the power throughout the country." Nixon, as he explained in his memoirs, would launch a frontal assault on "the ideas and ideology of the traditional Eastern liberal establishment that had come down to 1973 through the New Deal" and its successors.[28]

One of Nixon's chief aides carried this hostility to the point of recommending that the new administration refuse to be gauged by the criterion fixed by FDR in 1933. An in-house memo counseled:

> For a third of a century, the fashionable critics have been measuring progress according to the standard established by Roosevelt in his first 100 days. If we're going to change the pattern of government, we've got to change the standards of measurement. . . .
>
> The fact of the matter is that the nation still is suffering from the first 100 days of Johnson, from the first 100 days of Kennedy, and even, lingeringly, from the first 100 days of Roosevelt. It should be neither our plan nor our style to repeat those 100 day stunts—and we should present this not defensively, but as a positive virtue.[29]

Nixon's desire to dismantle the apparatus of the New Deal and its progeny never got very far because even as the pollsters were forecasting a landslide, Washington was beginning to reverberate to an ill-omened catchword: Watergate, a development that once again echoed the FDR White House. To each of the charges raised, the president and his appointees responded that Roosevelt had done everything Nixon did, and worse. By far the most important aspect of the relationship between FDR and Nixon was the allegation that in all that "Watergate" implied, Nixon was the true heir of FDR, for if this argument could be developed persuasively, Nixon's historical reputation might yet be redeemed. In June 1975 Safire wrote, *"Nixon never lied to the people about his health just before an election.* We have known for about a year that F.D.R. knew he was dying in 1944 and concealed that fact from the voting public with the connivance of his doctors."[30] The Nixon circle was delighted when a memo arrived from a disgruntled former FBI official asserting that Roosevelt, among others, had manipulated the agency, and were disappointed when they were not able to make much use of it.[31]

The president's supporters charged that it was Roosevelt who first installed a hidden recording device in the Oval Office, tapped the wires of his foreign policy critics and had their tax returns examined, and used the FBI for his own ends. They noted that when J. Edgar Hoover reported to Roosevelt that an FBI agent had been caught trying to tap the phone of a radical labor leader, Roosevelt, in the words of his biographer James MacGregor Burns, had "roared with laughter, slapped Hoover on the back, and shouted gleefully, 'By God, Edgar, that's the first time you've been caught with your pants down!'" Defenders of Nixon could make use of another passage in Burns about FDR's pressing Attorney General Francis Biddle to prosecute wartime dissenters: "When Biddle pleaded that it was hard to get convictions, Roosevelt answered that when Lincoln's Attorney General would not proceed against Vallandigham [the antiwar Copperhead], Lincoln declared martial law in that county and then had Vallandigham tried by a drumhead court-martial. Earlier he had treated Biddle's earnest support of civil liberties as a joking matter." Nor, asserted the Nixon camp, could any breach of freedom by Nixon begin to match FDR's internment of thousands of Japanese-Americans.[32]

To his champions Watergate represented nothing more than the application to Nixon of codes that FDR had violated with impunity. "Nixon did not lie as much as FDR; it's just that we look differently upon his purposes," said one of his friends, while his speechwriter Raymond Price has reported that in a phone call to San Clemente Jimmy Roosevelt cried, "Everything they're accusing him of my father did twice as much of!" On another occasion, Price has reported, Tommy Corcoran came up to him at a Washington party and, with a roguish smile and a twinkle in his eyes, said, "The trouble with your people is that they're always writing memos. When we did that sort of thing, we never put it on paper!" In sum, Price has concluded, "It was the old double standard, with a vengeance; what was acceptable for FDR and his successors to do was unacceptable for Nixon even to think about doing."[33] So deeply held was this conviction that it was impervious to the substantial body of evidence of the many ways, in degree and in kind, in which FDR's open presidency had differed from Nixon's furtive one.[34]

At times, though, even Nixon and those close to him recognized that Roosevelt and Nixon were not at all the same. "What Presidents are remembered?" Nixon once asked. It was about midnight near the end of 1970, and he was shooting the breeze with a speechwriter while they worked over an economic talk. Nixon, in a reflective mood, ticked off those chief executives, such as FDR, who had made their mark. Like

[171]

them, he observed, he lived in a time of controversy, and he did not fear controversy. One had to understand, too, he went on, the mystique of leadership, as de Gaulle did. The speechwriter William Safire, who heard all of this, has recorded his response:

> I said I thought he was carrying the aloof, mysterious leader bit a little too far. FDR was mysterious, but he was human. Anecdotes about Roosevelt abounded, and Americans who loved him or hated him at least thought they knew him as a person, not as a remote resident of the fenced-in White House. But with Nixon, I suggested, the danger was he would become totally depersonalized—the plastic, hollow man that his critics always maintained he was.

Nixon, who often talked about himself as though he were altogether detached from the subject of discussion, replied, "We don't disagree about that."[35]

Unable to convince Congress of the legitimacy of the FDR parallel, Nixon surrendered his office in disgrace, still believing, as he made clear years later, that he and Roosevelt, who were being assigned such different places in history, were brothers under the skin. He thought of FDR not as the builder of the welfare state or the architect of a global foreign policy but as a potentate manipulating the levers of power in order to act out his aggressions.

In an extraordinary interview with David Brinkley, Nixon revealed more about his own projections than about Roosevelt. Popular though FDR was, "a lot of people hated him," Brinkley remarked. "I suppose that's common to all public figures." Nixon replied, "Oh yes, I would perhaps be a pretty good witness to that effect." But he added, "I would say that in Roosevelt's case, he somewhat asked for it." John Connally, Nixon noted, "used to say that Roosevelt's political philosophy was [that] it was always necessary to have an enemy." Nixon continued:

> Roosevelt of course attacked the princes of privilege who set class against class, and so forth. A man like that who chooses enemies therefore is going to have friends to balance them. So you will generally find that as far as presidents, leaders, generally are concerned, that in order to have strong friends, they also have to have strong enemies. And Roosevelt welcomed it, he fought his enemies, and therefore had his friends. So there was a love-hate relationship as far as Roosevelt was concerned.

Having unburdened himself in this fashion, Nixon permitted Brinkley to lead him to a more conventional observation, though one that still bristled with indicators of disapproval. "If you were to set up a pantheon of presidents, as in the pantheon in Rome, where would you put Roosevelt?" Brinkley asked him. Nixon answered:

Oh, I'd put him very high. . . . I'm sure that many of my good conservative and Republican friends would disagree, but at his best he was really a great leader. He was a great leader during the Depression, although I disagreed with many of the things that he did. . . . I would say that Roosevelt would have to rate very high, and very high as a war leader. However, at the last, unfortunately, I don't think he was effective, after he of course had had his stroke. And then went to Yalta and thereafter. I think then it was downhill. But in his prime, he has to be among the very top 4 or 5.

Shortly after saying this, though, Nixon, in a murky passage that reads like a dream sequence, came as close as he ever would to saying what he really thought about FDR. He told Brinkley:

As I look back on FDR, he, uh, he was, he got across the impression that he was simply an idealist, and that was his manner, his speeches, uh, which were very, very effective, he, he would, he talked always in idealistic terms, but he was an operator, he was a pragmatist, he punished us politically, he punished his enemies, and he rewarded his friends. He did that to the press, . . . he punished them and he rewarded them if they were nice to him in their columns. . . . He handled the Congress the same way, uh, he he dealt that way with his Allies until very late in his life, when uh, after he was not at his [best] in my opinion, the last few months, uh, when he went to Yalta. And so, one of the reasons for the success of Roosevelt's policies to the extent they were successful, he could lift people, he could inspire them.[36]

When the clamor over Watergate became too loud, Nixon gave way to his personal choice, Gerald Ford, a man situated quite differently with respect to the shadow of FDR.[37] To be sure, like Nixon, Ford was a dyed-in-the-wool Republican who viewed Roosevelt as the most successful commander of the enemy forces, disapproved of much of the New Deal, and looked mournful whenever anyone mentioned the sick man at Yalta. But Ford's view of FDR had none of the obsessive quality of Nixon's. Indeed, save in the most obvious ways in which he affected any American of Ford's generation, and more particularly any GOP congressman, Roosevelt influenced Ford hardly at all. It has been said that the shortest book in the world is the collection of Irish haute cuisine. A volume on the impact of Franklin Roosevelt on Gerald Ford would be even briefer.

Ford, who cast his first ballot in 1936, never voted for Roosevelt, and, like Nixon, never saw him. "None of my own family was the beneficiary of any of the New Deal programs at all," he said recently.[38] When at the Presidential Suite at the Waldorf in New York City in late December 1981 the historian David McCullough interviewed Ford about Roosevelt, the former president spoke listlessly and picked out his words as though he were protecting himself at a press conference. Asked how he had responded to the news of FDR's death, Ford answered, "Refresh my memory on the day that he died."[39]

The limited relationship Ford did have to Roosevelt differed little from that of other small-town midwesterners. In 1940 he got his first exposure to politics when he worked actively to deny Roosevelt a third term. That spring he took weekends off from Yale Law School to go to Manhattan to take part in Wendell Willkie's campaign, and that summer he went home to Grand Rapids determined to help Willkie in Michigan. He came out of the experience a confirmed anti-FDR Republican, and he would remain one through all his years in Congress, the vice-presidency, and the White House.[40]

At a Lincoln's Birthday gathering in Detroit in 1950, Congressman Ford alluded to "one of the blackest Tuesdays in the history of this country, November 2, 1948," the occasion for a Democratic victory that left him feeling "that the United States was on the brink of disaster, with little or no hope of recovery." He further remarked:

> As a young man, or at least relatively so, I am one of those who became of voting age after the New Deal came into power, and as a result have had no opportunity to point to the White House and say "A Republican, a man who believes in our American way of life, now occupies the highest and most respected office in the world." All of my contemporaries are in the same category and as a result have never had the opportunity to appraise the difference between sound administration and maladministration. . . . There has been no concrete opportunity to contrast good and evil.

Not only had the Democrats sinned at Yalta, Ford said, but they had "a seeming fiendish allegiance to the Wagner Act."[41]

As president, Ford consciously developed a different approach from Roosevelt's. True, he did direct his speechwriters to read FDR's State of the Union addresses for 1942, 1943, and 1944 because as the time for his own first State of the Union message neared, the grim economic forecasts reminded him of the somber days of World War II. But as he prepared his message with the help of Robert Hartmann, Ford deliberately distinguished his downbeat approach from FDR's method. In his memoirs Ford recalled: "I told Bob to insert a line saying that I didn't expect much, if any, applause. Ever since Roosevelt, I knew, American Presidents had responded to economic challenges by trying to come up with crash programs that carried short-term benefits. My programs were designed to foster a long-term recovery even at the cost of short-term suffering. Such proposals aren't likely to elicit cheers."[42]

So much the opposite of FDR did Ford seem that his critics compared him to Roosevelt's most conspicuous antagonist. When in the summer of 1976 the president vetoed a public works bill, Speaker Carl Albert read a quotation to his colleagues on the floor of the House, then revealed that the familiar words were not Ford's, but came from a 1932 veto message by Herbert Hoover. Albert declared: "On the eve of the greatest depression this Nation has ever known, President Hoover vetoed a progressive, job-creating public works bill sponsored by a Democratic Congress. Now, some 44 years later, almost to the day, an equally conservative Republican President has again demonstrated the lack of economic understanding and human sensitivity which has enshackled the Republican Party." Like Hoover, the Speaker said, Ford denied that public works legislation generated jobs, "not withstanding all of the experience to the contrary of the 1930's with the WPA, TVA, and other agencies."[43]

Yet what is more striking than Ford's rejection of FDR is how little Roosevelt mattered to him. One of Ford's most important aides could recall no occasion when he ever spoke of Roosevelt at the White House. Nor did he appear to have read much of the FDR literature. In contrast to Nixon, who frequently mentioned Roosevelt, however perfunctorily, Ford, as president, only once referred to FDR in a public address. On October 8, 1974, wearing a freshly minted WIN (Whip Inflation Now) button on his lapel, Ford told Congress, "In his first inaugural address, President Franklin D. Roosevelt said, and I quote: 'The people of the United States have not failed. . . . They want direct, vigorous action, and they have asked for discipline and direction under our leadership.' . . . We must whip inflation right now." Symptomatically, on this lone occasion when he cited Roosevelt, Ford did so in a manner characteristic of the Hoover era, long on public relations and short on substance. Ford himself admitted to a *Washington Post* reporter that he could not offer "that kind of electrifying leadership that FDR gave."[44]

With so few cues from Ford, observers rarely thought to match him with FDR. Journalists did make the inevitable comparisons of Ford's first hundred days to Roosevelt's, and it was said of Betty Ford, as it had been and would be routinely said of others in her spot, that she "invested the First Lady position with a sense of purpose not seen since Eleanor Roosevelt." Right-wing critics charged that in signing the Act of Helsinki Ford had endorsed FDR's capitulation to Stalin at Yalta, and one of the president's speechwriters, who deplored the paucity of new thoughts in the Ford White House, remarked, "Some people may not like Harry Hopkins, but he gave Roosevelt an idea an hour." These few items, however, make up virtually the entire corpus of associations of Ford with FDR.[45]

For his own part, Ford saw only one way in which he could be likened to FDR, and even this observation had to be drawn out of him. On the centennial of Roosevelt's birth David Brinkley remarked that both Ford and FDR had come to office at a time of widespread distrust and faced the need to restore confidence in government. "If you have the capability of . . . engendering public trust by being yourself, the public then begins to feel that you're honest, that you're being straight-forward, and that you're not trying to fool them," Ford responded. "I happen to believe that is what Mr. Roosevelt did in those very difficult times. And that's what I tried to do in those very tough times in 1974 and '75."

In retrospect, Roosevelt got higher marks from the Gerald Ford who had known what it was to hold the responsibilities of the Oval Office than he had received from the zealous Republican congressman. Asked whether FDR's resort to deficit spending had been good or bad, Ford answered, "In 1933, '34 and '35, during the depths of the Depression, it was an absolutely essential policy. We needed whatever Federal budget stimulant we had in order to revive the economic circumstances in this country." Brinkley persisted. Might not "a wiser President" have kept Joe Stalin out of Eastern Europe and avoided the cold war? "I wouldn't put it quite that way," Ford returned. He did indicate that he thought the imperial presidency had begun with FDR, but instead of following this up, Brinkley said, "Well, I gather that in general you admired him." Ford, perhaps more positive than he would have been without prompt-ing, replied, "I did, although I had vast philosophical differences with him. He intrigued me as a politician; I was impressed with him as a persuader; I admired the strong stance that he took, even though I differed with him; so, yes, the bottom line is you couldn't help but think he was a good President for the country at that time."[46]

Ford's true sentiments came out in a more freewheeling interview a month later. After trying with difficulty to arouse some spark of interest in FDR, David McCullough posed a final question to Gerald Ford. If he were ranking FDR alongside Truman, his immediate successor, whom would he put first? Ford, who had once thought that Truman's election spelled the death of the republic, answered unhesitatingly: "I'm prejudiced. I think Harry Truman was more my kind of guy."[47]

[6]

Jimmy Carter

I

Dawn had not yet broken when the long caravan of cars, their head-lights piercing the dark of a Georgia night, set out upon the highway. By the time the procession reached its destination, the sun had risen on a lovely Labor Day morning and people had begun to stir in anticipa-tion of holiday pleasures. As the automobiles rolled through the streets of the village, thousands cheered and waved banners and a drum-and-bugle corps sounded its welcome. Up through a tree-lined avenue the ten-car motorcade made its way until it came to a halt before a hand-some white edifice, and out of one of the limousines stepped the former governor of the state, James Earl Carter, Jr. As they caught sight of him, the crowd let out another cheer, for never before had one of their own been nominated for the highest office in the land, and the towns-folk gathered there understood that they were present at a singular occasion. For years past Detroit's Cadillac Square had been the starting place for every Democratic presidential candidate, but with deliberate forethought Jimmy Carter had chosen to launch his 1976 presidential campaign not in Detroit but here in Warm Springs, at the Little White House, where on so many occasions Franklin D. Roosevelt had carried out the functions of his office, and where, thirty-one years before, he had died.

Carter did all he could on this special day to identify himself with the former president. He was introduced to the throng, including patients in wheelchairs from the spa that was FDR's favorite retreat, by Jimmy Roosevelt, with Franklin D. Roosevelt, Jr., seated conspicuously on the portico of the Little White House. He spoke from a lectern displaying the Yalta portrait of Roosevelt, and when he concluded his remarks,

Graham Jackson, the black Navy veteran whose weeping countenance was the subject of the best-remembered photograph of the mourning at FDR's death, played "Happy Days Are Here Again" on the accordion. All that was missing, said one correspondent, was Jim Farley and Fala.[1]

In his formal remarks Carter discussed Roosevelt and Hoover in a manner that intimated that he was drawing an analogy to his own contest with Gerald Ford. "Although he was born into a family with wealth and prominence, Franklin Roosevelt yet understood and served well the millions of American families who were left hopeless and hungry and jobless and despairing by the Great Depression," he said. He added:

> His opponent in 1932 was an incumbent President, a decent and well-intentioned man, who felt that the government could not and should not with bold action try to correct the economic ills and the problems of a great nation. He led the Republican Party which lacked the strength to bring us out of those dark days. But Roosevelt knew that our country could do better; and with bold and forceful action he restored confidence to our economic system, he put our nation back to work, and he unified our people. And that changed our lives. . . . This year, as in 1932, our nation is divided, our people are out of work, and our national leaders do not lead.[2]

But anyone who thought that all Carter had in mind was to associate himself with Roosevelt and the New Deal was not paying close enough attention to the tableau at Warm Springs. If Carter praised the economic policies of the 1930s, he also made clear that he did not approve of large-scale government spending and that he wished to "decentralize power" and rely on "private responsibility." The Washington correspondent for the *Atlanta Constitution* went so far as to say:

> The Warm Springs speech offered yet another sign that Carter's liberal-courting phase is at an end. "They have nowhere else to go," a Carter aide noted.
> There was a call for work instead of welfare. There was a call for a "muscular" military and for the prospect of a peaceful "struggle" with the Soviet Union.
> One section of the Carter kickoff speech could easily have been mistaken for a President Ford text.[3]

Even the selection of Warm Springs reflected something besides homage to FDR. Carter's advisers doubted that he could draw a huge crowd to Cadillac Square, and they feared that television cameras would be panning over empty spaces. Furthermore, street gangs had been mugging pedestrians in downtown Detroit, and his aides did not want the opening of the campaign marred by some ugly incident or the display of a small army of police to protect the candidate. Michigan, too, was Gerald Ford's state. It seemed more advisable to start in Georgia, which was Carter country, and in a small town, where a huge turnout would not be necessary for effective TV coverage.[4]

In truth, the episode revealed an ambiguity in Carter's attitude toward Roosevelt. He was careful not to seem too zealous a New Dealer, and his references to FDR were expressed without ardor. Yet in picking Warm Springs for his campaign debut, he undoubtedly hoped to reassure liberal Democrats, who were suspicious of him as an outsider, that he, too, revered their patron saint. In particular, he understood that it was essential for him to reconstruct the Roosevelt coalition. So he regarded Roosevelt in 1976 as he had throughout his life—as someone at a great distance who never had moved him very deeply but was expected to receive ritualistic obeisance.

The shadow of FDR that at times for Lyndon Johnson had all but obscured the sun cast only the haziest of impressions on Carter, which was not at all what one might have expected. For Carter was raised in what Roosevelt, because of his association with Warm Springs, had regarded as his "second state," even, on occasion, his first state. "He always claimed to be from Georgia," the agrarian reformer Will Alexander remembered; Roosevelt would say to him, referring to a southerner, "It's somebody from down our way."[5] Warm Springs was less than eighty miles from Plains, where Carter grew up, and if FDR was a formidable figure to most Americans of Carter's youth, he was an especially vivid presence to the people of Georgia. Beyond this Carter sought office as candidate of a party that idolized Roosevelt. Only rarely, though, did Carter indicate that he shared these enthusiasms or could even relate to them. In the end, his detachment from a sentiment that so many in his party and in the nation shared would contribute no little to foreshortening his public career and to consigning him to his place in history.

II

In October 1976, on the eve of a debate with Gerald Ford that could determine the outcome of the presidential contest, Jimmy Carter chatted with a young assistant who sought to put his mind at ease by talking not about the present but about the past. In discussing presidents of bygone years, his aide said, "I just don't think that reverence is felt anymore." He did not idolize General Eisenhower, the first chief executive he remembered, the young man remarked, and "I certainly didn't feel a special reverence for any of the more recent presidents." Carter interrupted him: "I felt it for Roosevelt."[6]

It was the closest Carter would ever come to expressing so strong an emotion about FDR during the campaign, even in private, but after he left the White House he sometimes claimed to hold such sentiments. "I always felt he was our special President," he would say then. He was only eight when FDR was first elected, he pointed out, "and he was just my President. I never even thought about— when folks said 'The President,' you didn't say which President." Carter recalled that he "helped to make concrete blocks and construct buildings under the WPA programs" when he was in high school and remembered that people in Georgia looked on FDR as a "fellow Georgian almost. Every time he came to Georgia, that was *the* story." As a consequence of the state's law permitting eighteen-year-olds to vote, he cast his first vote for Roosevelt in 1944. When the news came over the loudspeaker in Bancroft Hall in Annapolis of the president's death, he was "heartbroken with grief."[7]

Though Carter gave no evidence of such feelings in 1976, he did at various times during the campaign acknowledge an awareness of what FDR signified. In his acceptance speech at the Democratic convention in 1976, he recalled that as a country boy he and his family had congregated outside on a summer night in Georgia to listen to convention proceedings in some distant northern city reported on a radio wired to a car battery. "Ours is the party," he said, "of the man who was nominated by those distant conventions and who inspired and restored this nation in its darkest hours—Franklin D. Roosevelt."

One of Carter's earliest biographers has given a slightly different and more graphic description of this episode. James Wooten has written:

He often remembered . . . a deliciously warm summer's night in rural Georgia in the early 1930s when his parents had allowed him to postpone his regular bedtime so that he could hear one of Franklin Roosevelt's fireside chats on their battery-powered radio, and although the precise date was always vague in his mind, he saw himself as no older than nine or ten—a slightly built, almost fragile, child with hair the color of straw and a sunburned face full of Huck Finn freckles—and he recalled that for years after that hot, heavily humid evening, even after his stern and stolidly conservative father had summarily dismissed the talk as so much New Deal twaddle, the resonant tones of the President of the United States, slicing crisply through the static from faraway Washington, would remain and endure for him as an oral symbol of authority and strength and leadership and hope, a force in his life that somehow he would never quite escape or outgrow.[8]

On more than one occasion, Carter has mentioned that the New Deal had quickened his interest in politics. "During the Depression years, political decisions in Washington had immediate and direct effect on our lives," he wrote in his memoir, *Why Not the Best?* "Farm programs, Rural Electrification, Works Progress Administration, Civilian Conservation Corps, and others were of immense personal importance." At a Democratic party dinner in New York during the 1976 campaign, he illustrated the theme of national innovation by saying, "I think of the Civilian Conservation Corps that I knew about when I was a child on the farm. I was too young to participate, but my first cousins did. I think about the REA when it turned on the electric lights in my house when I was fourteen years old."[9]

Carter particularly stressed the contribution of the Rural Electrification Administration. "Those who dispute the ability of men and women to improve the lot of mankind have never seen the impact of the REA on the life of a small boy in the rural South," he said. As he walked across a South Dakota farm in the autumn of 1976, he told his listeners, "I think the best day of my life was when they turned the lights on in our house about 1937, when Roosevelt was President." Earlier, he had explained, "My father was a natural leader in our community and with the advent of the Rural Electrification Program, when I was about thirteen years old, my father became one of the first directors of our local REA organization. He then began to learn the importance of political involvement on a state and national basis to protect the program that meant so much in changing our farm life-style."[10]

A week after his pilgrimage to Warm Springs, Carter carried the theme he had enunciated there even further in a talk to an AFL-CIO convention in Dearborn, Michigan. On the September day that Gerald Ford opened his campaign, Carter asserted that the contest had begun long before Ford's initial address. "This campaign was under way in 1932, when his party nominated Herbert Hoover and ours nominated Franklin Roosevelt," he said. Carter made a point of emphasizing that he had chosen Warm Springs to launch his campaign, and he remarked upon FDR's struggle there against polio. He went on to speak of the earlier political confrontation in a way that unmistakably implied that Ford, widely thought to be a good-natured president, was another Hoover. Roosevelt, Carter reminded the union delegates, had run in 1932 against Hoover, "a decent man, a well-intentioned man perhaps, but who didn't see that his responsibility was to try to ease the handicap of people who were without jobs and were without hope and were discouraged." He continued:

> Roosevelt moved forward in the tradition of the Democratic Party. He had confidence in us and he helped us. He proposed a twenty-five-cent-an-hour minimum wage. Twenty-five cents. The Democratic Congress finally passed it, but ninety-five percent of the Republicans in Congress voted against it.
>
> He gave Rural Electrification to farm homes like mine. He thought people ought to have security in their old age and he put forward Social Security. There were ninety-five Republican House members, and ninety-four voted against Social Security. That draws a distinct difference between this good man, Franklin Roosevelt, in the tradition of the Democratic Party, and Herbert Hoover, in the tradition of the Republican Party.
>
> That's when this campaign began.[11]

Carter's references to FDR continued throughout the fall of 1976. "Today Carter is running as, and with, a liberal in the New Deal mold," wrote George Will in July. "He is a budding architect, anxious to add new wings to FDR's mansion." In the ensuing weeks Carter remarked upon the CCC work camps as a solution for the problem of idle urban youth, and in one of his televised debates with Ford he scored well on rheostat devices when he pledged to renew FDR's fireside chats. Subsequently, Ford's press secretary would observe sardonically, "He did everything to invoke the memory of the founder of the Democratic coalition except roll out in a wheelchair puffing on a cigarette through a long holder."[12]

These allusions to the age of Roosevelt prompted a variety of observers to suggest that Carter was another FDR. Mike Mansfield thought that Carter could unify the Democratic party much as Roosevelt had done, and his speechwriter James Fallows, impressed in the summer of 1976 by the way Carter, with his gubernatorial experience, grappled with problems, has written, "The last governor to become President was Franklin Roosevelt, and I told my friends that summer that Carter had at least the potential to leave the government forever changed by his presence." In a television commercial for Carter, E. G. Marshall said, "I've always felt that when Franklin Roosevelt died that was the end of the good and great presidents," that he had come to feel the same way about Truman and Kennedy, and that he would vote for Jimmy Carter, who was "in the tradition of the best Democratic presidents."[13]

Campaign correspondents filled in the appropriate biographical data. As a boy in Plains, they reported, Jimmy Carter encountered a teacher who was one of the three greatest influences in his life. Julia Coleman was an ardent admirer of FDR, like him a victim of polio who had made a success of herself. Miss Julia, it was said, had served with Eleanor Roosevelt on a committee that picked textbooks for high schools, and she had once spent a night at the White House. When she returned to Georgia, she had excited Jimmy and her other pupils by her tales of her visit, especially her account of Franklin Roosevelt with his dog, Fala, on his lap.[14]

With such details sketched in, journalists obligingly drew the appropriate parallel. "What Carter shares with Roosevelt is the self-image which allowed FDR to work love and aggression into a political style of unmatched grandeur—combative, resourceful, disruptive," wrote William Greider in a well-regarded series in the *Washington Post*. Like Carter, Roosevelt was "the righteous outsider ready to shake up the temple, eager to challenge the established order, impatient with the consensual atmosphere of regular politics, yet cunning and relentless in his own tactics." Carter, said the columnist Max Lerner, was one of a number of presidential candidates, including FDR, who "took the city of the politicians by surprise, if not by storm." He added, "In his political instincts, Carter may be closest to Roosevelt, with perhaps an even more ravenous power hunger than the squire of Hyde Park had. . . . There seems to be the same combination of strength and guile." Another veteran columnist made a different kind of comparison that required a greater stretch of the imagination. Carter, observed Richard L. Strout, had "a homely face of the most attractive sort that reminds one of Eleanor Roosevelt."[15]

The most frequent analogy centered on the notion that each man in his first bid for office had been perceived to be a dissembler who equivocated on the leading questions of the day. "The comparison seems far-fetched because FDR is now a mythological giant of history," Greider noted, "but the real Roosevelt who entered office in 1933 was described in much the same terms as are now applied to Carter: charming but insincere, shallow and inconstant on the issues, occasionally slippery, sometimes deceitful." Another writer noted that what people said of Carter in 1976 was precisely what the *Brooklyn Eagle* had stated about FDR in 1932: "He can smile more than any man in American politics without being insipid."[16]

When Carter squeaked through in November, analysts once again looked toward FDR. The pollster Louis Harris stated, "Jimmy Carter's victory was not a personal victory: He won because of the revival of the old coalition that first sent Franklin D. Roosevelt to the White House in 1932." Carter attracted a number of the elements of that alignment—

blacks, white ethnic workingmen, Catholics, Jews, and liberal professionals. He also came close to restoring one component of the FDR coalition that had been missing in recent years—the Solid South. As in the Roosevelt years, too, the Democratic candidate took less than 11 percent of *Fortune*'s panel of business executives; in fact, the chairman of Seagram specifically compared the likely impact of a Carter win to the consequences of Roosevelt's in 1932. (A question arises, however: if Carter's alliance so closely resembled FDR's, why did Carter succeed so narrowly when Roosevelt prevailed by huge margins? Pat Caddell suggested the answer: both men had the same base, but in 1976 the base had shrunk, for as early as the 1950s white-collar employees outnumbered blue-collar workers.)[17]

As the day of Carter's inauguration approached, Washington heard the same kinds of comparisons to FDR that had marked the campaign. A month after the election, the Baltimore essayist Gerald Johnson stated that his perspective was that of a "minority of Americans whose memory of politics reaches back 43 years, when we were watching another President-elect in a fairly similar situation. In us it produces a sensation comparable to what psychologists call the phenomenon of *déjà vu,* that is, a sensation of familiarity although we are certain that we have never seen the like before."[18]

III

In truth, writers should have been more cautious in their analogies, for by neither background nor disposition was Jimmy Carter an FDR.[19] Some have stressed that Carter's maternal grandfather, Jim Jack Gordy, had been a follower of the Populist Tom Watson and a man who, though he was in the camp of Roosevelt's enemy Eugene Talmadge, "the Wild Man from Sugar Creek," had admired FDR. But Carter was raised in a household with a decidedly different complexion. Carter's father could not forgive Roosevelt for the slaughter of the little pigs and the plowing up of cotton, and after 1932 he never voted for him. Billy Carter has recalled that James Earl Carter's denunciations of Roosevelt provoked heated quarrels with Gordy, and an old friend, once an FDR partisan but subsequently a critic, has remembered that Jimmy's father was so outspokenly hostile to Roosevelt in the 1930s that he "gave conservatives a bad name." He felt even greater animosity toward Mrs. Roosevelt. "I just really think that Earl's hatred for Roosevelt grew out of his dislike for his wife," Lillian Carter has said. "He couldn't stand to see her picture in the magazines or the newspapers. It wasn't really very nice, but that's the way he felt." Jimmy's mother may not have differed much. She and her husband had postponed having another child after the Wall Street crash, "and when I finally got pregnant with Billy, we joked about naming him for FDR, since we both thought he was the man who had helped us out of the Depression." Early in 1980, however, when Miz Lillian ranked the seven best presidents, Franklin Roosevelt failed to make the list (though her son did). But then, neither did George Washington.[20]

Though there is evidence of Roosevelt's presence in Carter's early years, the shards are remarkably few. Raised in a family steeped in politics, Carter showed little interest in public affairs throughout the age of Roosevelt and even beyond, and one does not sense very much awareness of FDR's activities despite the proximity of Warm Springs. Insofar as the New Deal did lodge itself in Carter's mind, it was less the effort to create a more humane social order that captivated him than the technological marvel of rural electrification.

Carter's teacher may have imbued him with a sense of the majesty of FDR after sleeping at the White House, observing Fala, and becoming an intimate of Eleanor Roosevelt, but the only record of the association in Mrs. Roosevelt's papers fails to sustain such a conclusion. Early in 1934 a touching ten-page handwritten letter to the first lady from Miss Julia began, "I am an obscure teacher in South Georgia." She explained that she was superintendent of a rural consolidated school in the village of Plains ("We have a splendid class of graduates, twenty two this year"), and she implored Mrs. Roosevelt to deliver the commencement address. She wrote: "The problem of education in Georgia is a great one. It is with heroic sacrifice that we have kept our school open. . . . With your great heart, you must know something of the struggle of the masses of humanity. . . . You have ideals. I know you have. Catch this beautiful vision of service. Come to our obscure rural school." Some days later Miss Julia received a reply: a routine turndown from Mrs. Roosevelt's secretary.[21]

If Carter did hear much that was positive about FDR when he was young, it did not penetrate very deeply. As governor, Carter only rarely alluded to Roosevelt, and when he did once speak of "a powerful and great and kind and compassionate and humane man—Franklin Roosevelt," it was in the context of ceremonies at the Warm Springs Foundation.[22] Unlike Truman, Kennedy, and Johnson, he had never met Roosevelt, and, uniquely, he took office as president without having made the acquaintance of any of his Democratic predecessors. To a very large extent, Carter lived outside the history of the party, beyond the shadow cast by FDR.[23]

When Carter made his bid for the Democratic presidential nomination in 1976, he ran against a field of candidates who fought strenuously with one another over who would be regarded as FDR's heir while Carter was railing against the concentration of power in Washington, a legacy of the Roosevelt era. After winning the Massachusetts primary, Henry Jackson told his followers, "The essence of our victory is the fact that we put together once again the grand coalition that elected Franklin D. Roosevelt, Harry Truman, John F. Kennedy, and Lyndon Johnson." Hubert Humphrey continued to speak in the authentic voice of FDR; Morris Udall and Fred Harris advanced Roosevelt-style reforms; and the crippled George Wallace, to whom Nixon had sent a print of the movie *Sunrise at Campobello,* told a North Carolina crowd, "Franklin Roosevelt was elected President of the United States four times in a wheelchair. Maybe you've forgotten that." But neither Udall nor Harris could build a majority, and as Elizabeth Drew observed, "Jackson is trying to reconstruct a coalition that will not coalesce. He is not Franklin Roosevelt, and the year is not 1932." Wallace himself conceded, "You just can't get in a wheelchair and go out in crowds. Roosevelt was in a wheelchair but that was before television. A lot of people didn't know he was in a wheelchair." In the end, the stop-Carter forces tried to unite around Humphrey and failed.[24]

The Carter nomination, Democrats said, marked the close of an era, a transition symbolized by the death of Jim Farley, FDR's campaign manager, a month before the convention. At Madison Square Garden, Jimmy Roosevelt approached unrecognized, while Jim Rowe, after hearing Hubert Humphrey's uncharacteristically brief remarks, said, "It's his last hurrah," then added, "It is the last hurrah for all of us." A historian who has written authoritatively on the relation of the national government to the cities in the modern era concluded: "Carter's populist attacks on the 'Washington establishment' . . . in effect denounced the political apparatus that the New Deal had built. . . . Since the Democrats went on to nominate this outsider who repudiated the New Deal promise of an ever-expanding federal pie, a political epoch had seemingly ended."[25]

In the ensuing campaign against President Ford, Carter, for all of his citations of FDR, continued to repudiate the Roosevelt heritage of big government. Some months after he took office, the *New York Times,* commenting on the conservative character of his administration, reflected: "It was only infrequently and not too convincingly . . . that Mr. Carter in his campaign donned the economic mantle of F.D.R. or the social cloak of L.B.J. He said far more often and more passionately that he intended to cut waste, run things efficiently and balance the budget. If he now seems even more zealously dedicated to those propositions than some of us might have expected, no one can fairly say he wasn't warned."[26]

So conservative were some of his statements that key elements in the Roosevelt coalition wondered what to make of him. One Jewish leader, Carter has related, told him that Jews were anxious about his attitude toward Israel and his religious beliefs, but "they were also concerned about the degree to which I was committed to the Great Society and New Deal programs. Because if there was social unrest . . . intersocietal conflict, quite often the Jewish people were the ones who suffered." A Washington figure, puzzled by how to chart Carter's ideology, said, "I don't know if he's Franklin Roosevelt or Richard Nixon." In like manner the *New York Times* observed: "One of the most intriguing questions of the Carter campaign is whether the Georgian is correct in so often comparing himself with Presidents Roosevelt, Truman, Kennedy and Johnson. With his stress on morality and seeming naivete about undertaking major restructuring of the Federal Government, Mr. Carter strikes a chord more reminiscent of Woodrow Wilson."[27]

Carter's performance as a twice-born FDR did not play well, and eventually he had to admit it. The experience of the New Deal years did not seem to have much meaning for him (at one point in his debate with Ford he referred to the "Great Depression of the 1940s"), and his allusions to the Democratic tradition were mechanical. "He memorized lines extolling the virtues of Harry Truman and FDR, which he rattled off machine-gun-style," remarked a reporter who covered the 1976 campaign. In the last phase of the campaign Carter changed course when he recognized that the notion that he was an FDR Democrat was credible neither to the country nor to those around him. "We didn't use it subtly," one of Carter's lieutenants conceded. "Saying 'Vote for me because I belong to the same party as Roosevelt' was unsalable." As Ford gained rapidly on Carter, Rosalynn Carter thought she knew what had gone wrong—among other things, "too much Truman and FDR." A Carter aide agreed. He told a reporter that Carter "started sounding like Hubert Humphrey, talking about the great traditions of FDR. On the DNC whistlestop train trip I went to Jody [Powell] and said, 'For God's sake, get him off that. He is not in the tradition of FDR. People like him because they think he's different.' He finally went back to the old primary theme that he was good at, but it may be too late."[28]

At the end of a campaign in which it remained unclear what Carter stood for, not every commentator agreed that his victory demonstrated the durability of the FDR political alliance. Richard Rovere conceded that "the conventional wisdom . . . that Jimmy Carter succeeded this year because he reassembled the Democratic coalition that Franklin Roosevelt mobilized . . . works reasonably well." But he pointed out that if the Democrats had really wanted a candidate in the Roosevelt lineage, they would have nominated "someone like Morris Udall or Fred Harris or Henry Jackson, all of them more in the New Deal mold than Carter." Furthermore, he noted that though both FDR and Carter had carried the South, this congruence concealed a sharp divergence, for, at a time of widespread black disfranchisement, Roosevelt's ballots had come from whites, whereas Carter had relied on black voters; Ford actually had a small edge in the white South, FDR's old stronghold. From a different perspective, one of the country's foremost political scientists was skeptical that the 1976 contest resembled the earlier Roosevelt–Hoover match. "I would say that the last truly critical election came in 1932, when Franklin Roosevelt came in with his 'New Deal,'" observed Walter Dean Burnham. Though Carter had won by "gathering just enough fragments of the New Deal coalition," the political terrain was not the same as in the 1930s.[29]

The ill-defined character of the 1976 campaign left seasoned president watchers puzzled about how much Carter was likely to resemble FDR after he took office. The sense of *déjà vu* Gerald Johnson noted in his postelection commentary derived in part from the fact that at the outset of his quest for the White House, Carter had assembled a "Brain Trust" so that he would be able to move on appointments as soon as he won. "You can estimate this as supreme confidence or colossal gall, but in either case it is very Rooseveltian," Johnson said. Nonetheless, he added, one still could not be sure whether Carter "has enough, or indeed any, of his predecessor's uncanny power to see in a particular man a special ability to deal with a particular crisis," to light upon a Harry Hopkins or a Harold Ickes. "What is doubtful," he thought, "is Carter's possession of Roosevelt's ability . . . to pick them out and put them on the particular kind of job that they can handle."

Despite these reservations, Johnson viewed the prospect of a Carter presidency with greater equanimity than did those who looked back longingly toward the FDR years. "This is certainly no occasion for bedecking ourselves with garlands and dancing in the streets, but it is no occasion for dragging out the sackcloth and ashes, either, or weeping over the obvious fact that Carter isn't a Roosevelt," he wrote. "Roosevelt's work is done, and it was so well done that practically everything built during the Hundred Days still stands, stronger than ever after 43 years." Carter was a man of enormous energy and indomitable courage. "In the name of common sense, what more have we the nerve to ask?"[30]

IV

Carter had been president of the United States less than a month when he stirred up memories of Franklin Roosevelt by appropriating one of FDR's best-known trademarks: the fireside chat. Carter even went Roosevelt one better by delivering his nationally televised address beside a real fire—a crackling, three-log blaze in the hearth of the White House library. Garbed in a cardigan sweater, he reminded no one of Franklin Roosevelt, but the telecast, which attracted 80 million viewers, provided the occasion for numerous accounts associating Carter in the public mind with FDR.[31]

Though Carter rarely compared himself directly to FDR, this would not be the only occasion when he linked himself to his predecessor. At a White House dinner for the National Governors' Association he pointed out, "I'm the first President who was a Governor since Franklin Delano Roosevelt," and in response to those who questioned his credentials, Carter told a writer, "I know ministers, teachers, blacks, Jews. I have consulted the best minds on every subject. I am as well prepared as anyone has been, including Roosevelt back in the '30s." Nor did he think that his record paled in comparison to FDR's. At a Democratic fundraiser in New Jersey in the fall of 1979, Carter said, "You remember the mess that Franklin Roosevelt inherited in the early thirties. He put America back to work. Since I've been in office, in the last 3—almost 3 years, we have added a net increase of 8-1/2 million new jobs in this country, because we believe in work."[32]

During the 1976 campaign, Carter, asked to explain what role his wife would play in his administration, had replied, "She'll be more like Eleanor Roosevelt." He continued, "She'll be active in both her domestic and foreign programs, and she'll help me to carry out mine, both in this country and abroad." (This may have been the first time that anyone conceived of a first lady's having "domestic and foreign programs.") On election night, a journalist spoke to a high-ranking politician who thought the Carters were carbon copies of each other, save that "he has the Eleanor Roosevelt teeth and she has the Eleanor Roosevelt brain." "It can't be all bad to have a first lady traveling around the country shaking hands and identifying social problems that need attention," he went on. "She has studied Eleanor Roosevelt—that's her heroine—and I think she'll be just like her." Like Eleanor Roosevelt, too, it was said, Rosalynn Carter had to make clear that she, not her mother-in-law, was first lady, and again like Mrs. Roosevelt, who had descended coal shafts to be her husband's eyes and ears, Rosalynn Carter surveyed the flood areas of Georgia for her husband.[33]

Carter adopted a number of programs that could trace their ancestry to the New Deal. Soon after he took office he announced a $1.8 billion proposal to give work to young people and teach them skills, a project that stirred memories of the CCC and the NYA. Under the Comprehensive Employment Training Act, new opportunities opened up for public service jobs, notably in the field of the arts, where the Roosevelt administration had pioneered. By the fall of 1978 CETA's payroll had reached 725,000, and the assistant secretary of labor said of the art project: "All in all, it constitutes the largest federal investment in the arts since the Great Depression and in many ways has outpaced the earlier commitment." When in the fall of 1977 Carter signed a bill raising the minimum wage, he remarked that there were several people at the ceremony who had been at the White House thirty-nine years before when Franklin Roosevelt had signed the first such law, and in his statement to the Democratic national convention on the 1980 platform he boasted of his achievement in sponsoring such New Deal–style programs as food stamps. "On the eve of the forty-fifth anniversary of the Social Security Act, proposed by President Roosevelt," Carter added, "I am pleased that the platform has reaffirmed our strong support for the Social Security system."[34]

President Carter also markedly altered the nature of the Tennessee Valley Authority. When he came to office, he found that the TVA had become little more than a huge electric power company, and, shockingly, that it led the nation's utilities in fighting against clean-air laws. Carter changed this situation by naming S. David Freeman chairman of the board and instructing him to effect a turnabout in policy. Freeman attempted to do just that. As one correspondent observed on the forty-sixth anniversary of the project, Freeman had busied himself "reconnecting T.V.A. to its roots as a New Deal social and economic experiment." After the first chairman of the Authority, David E. Lilienthal, toured the valley with him, Freeman stated, "Now, we're beginning to come back to what Lilienthal called the seamless web."[35]

In drawing upon the age of Roosevelt, though, Carter found the FDR who was Dr. Win-the-War more pertinent than Dr. New Deal. The Second World War had greater salience for Carter than the Great Depression, and in coping with the major domestic problems of his administration—the energy crisis and inflation—he and his advisers looked at World War II gasoline rationing and explored the instrumentalities of the war mobilization. Late in June 1979, Carter's domestic affairs adviser, Stuart E. Eizenstat, sent the president a memorandum recommending creation of a National Energy Mobilization Board that would draw upon the experience of World War II, and in a major energy speech in July 1979 Carter adopted this suggestion in calling for a new agency modeled on the War Production Board of the 1940s.[36]

Carter's "malaise" address, with its imagery of war, stirred up memories of the earlier period. It moved one citizen to write an op-ed piece for the *New York Times* in which she said:

> Jimmy Carter bridged the generation gap in a few intensely felt moments in my household the other night. . . . As Mr. Carter spoke, I heard Franklin D. Roosevelt's voice again and smelled my father's cigar and saw our family of six sitting up straight around the radio in a dim room listening intently to our leader in a time of fear and hardship. I remembered how it was when the blackout sirens sounded in New York City and how we saved every scrap of paper for the paper drive and how the subways were too dark to read in. Gas rationing? That was a problem only for the rich. Sugar rationing, shoe rationing—we could cope with that. It was a good way of easing anxiety about our family members overseas in wartime. We had the certain knowledge that each of us had a contribution to make.
>
> That feeling, as I say, bound my son and me in tight attention as we heard the new-old Jimmy Carter sternly tell us that the crisis was real, that we have been enslaved by OPEC, but that he would lead us to freedom.

The *Times* ran the essay under an arresting title: "Listening to Carter, But Hearing F.D.R."[37]

v

On March 4, 1977, six weeks after Carter took office, 900 survivors of the age of Roosevelt gathered at Washington's Mayflower Hotel to commemorate the forty-fourth anniversary of FDR's first inauguration. Here were Rex Tugwell and Grace Tully, Tommy Corcoran and Ben Cohen, and, younger than they but afflicted by the cancer that would soon claim his life, Hubert Humphrey, conspicuously bald from radiation treatments but still bouncy, loquacious, beaming, speaking confidently of the future. Cohen, once one of Roosevelt's bright-faced young men but now a stooped, frail octogenarian, gave the featured address, "The New Deal Looks Forward." Writing in *Time,* Hugh Sidey observed, "It was as if Franklin Roosevelt were still in the White House and his staff members were rolling up their sleeves for another job. . . . Cohen, 82, one of FDR's ubiquitous counselors and troubleshooters, struck the chord of marching on. Indeed, the New Deal in flesh and emotion and philosophy does seem to go on forever."[38] That was a truth, though, that not everyone was prepared to recognize, least of all the new Democratic incumbent.

None of the distinguished guests at the Mayflower dinner attracted so much notice as one man who was invited but did not come: Jimmy Carter. He not only failed to show up at an occasion just six blocks from 1600 Pennsylvania Avenue, but did not even send a message. Fritz Mondale was supposed to appear in Carter's place, and since he was expected to arrive late, the banquet committee substituted fruit cup for hot soup. No use. The vice-president, though he accepted the invitation, chose to go ice fishing in Minnesota instead.[39]

As the aging veterans struggled out of their seats at the end of a long evening, the folk singer Joe Glazer signed off on his guitar with "Happy Days Are Here Again," played not as a joyous fanfare but as a dirge, a fitting finale to an occasion that left the FDR loyalists lamenting the steep descent from Roosevelt to Carter. In ignoring the event, Carter appeared to be suggesting that the New Dealers were irrelevant, and their comments that evening and those by journalists afterward paid him back in kind. When he introduced Cohen, Tommy Corcoran drew knowing laughs by saying that the problems a president faced in 1977 were "peanuts" compared to the difficulties Roosevelt confronted, and the master of ceremonies, Marquis Childs, observing that there were no Carter people in the room, said, "This is a clean break between the past and the present." The press commentary was biting. Why, asked David Broder, could not Jimmy Carter, who had risen before dawn to be sure his campaign was launched in Warm Springs, have spared a half hour to stop by? And why did none of Carter's White House staff care to meet their counterparts from the FDR era? "You would have thought that just in human terms, they might like to establish that link. But no."[40]

Carter's behavior toward the New Deal reunion characterized most of his presidency. In striking contrast to his Democratic predecessors, he rarely referred to FDR in his public statements, and then usually in the most perfunctory manner. Through all of 1978, he found not one occasion to mention him. When after many years of dispute the Fine Arts Commission approved a brilliant design by a West Coast landscape architect for a memorial park in Washington honoring Roosevelt, Carter's secretary of the interior turned it down as too expensive, though in fact it was not exceptionally costly. Nor was this regarded as merely a temporary setback. The secretary believed that the question of whether to create such a memorial to FDR should be left to "a future generation of Americans."[41]

Jimmy Carter had won office by capitalizing on distrust of the government leviathan that had emerged in the Roosevelt era, and as chief executive he self-consciously acted out the role of a man with a different perception of power from FDR's. He eschewed a capacious limousine in order to stroll down Pennsylvania Avenue on Inauguration Day, and he let it be known that he was restricting the playing of "Hail to the Chief." "The imperial presidency of Franklin Delano Roosevelt and his successors was no more," wrote one commentator. "Or so it was advertised." Furthermore, his principal domestic policy official stated that "we realize Washington does not have all the answers or possess all the resources or have the power to solve every problem plaguing society."[42]

Carter's chief aides rejected the best-remembered touchstone of Roosevelt's first year. "The country doesn't want another 100 Days," Pat Caddell announced barely a week after the president took office. When the hundredth day arrived, the same note was struck. "Since the beginning of Franklin Roosevelt's term, the first one hundred days of an administration have been closely watched as a sign of what can be expected over the course of the entire administration," Stuart Eizenstat wrote in April 1977 in a memo to the president that the White House leaked to the press. Though claiming credit for "major initiatives" and "significant achievements" since the inauguration, Eizenstat observed, "As you know, we have consciously tried *not* to emphasize the administration's first one hundred days out of a desire to avoid seeking hurried changes when more deliberate ones are needed." In truth, the memo was self-serving, for it occurred to no one that Carter's modest accomplishments held a candle to FDR's.[43]

Nor did the Carter circle bring to mind Roosevelt's Brain Trust or Felix Frankfurter's prodigies. Eizenstat could have found a home in the FDR White House, but he was an exception. One Washington columnist observed:

> It is questionable whether Roosevelt could have put over the New Deal with a staff as inexperienced and provincial as Carter's. Some of them seem to regard Congress as a kind of Georgia legislature. FDR's gnome-like secretary, Louis Howe, was born in Indianapolis, Marvin McIntyre in Kentucky, Steve Early in Virginia, Bill Hassett in Northfield, Vermont, Rex Tugwell in New York. By contrast the Carter staff is extraordinarily homogeneous, with a relatively narrow viewpoint.[44]

When Tugwell sent some ideas to Carter, his letter was referred to a staffer, and when the New Dealers convened at the Mayflower, he was still awaiting a reply.

Tommy Corcoran drew on his service in FDR's government to reprimand Carter and his aides for not making good use of the available talent in the country. He told a reporter:

I remember that my chief, Mr. Roosevelt—a convinced Democrat whose imagination could encompass the whole universe and yet close in on the last six inches—was willing in his crises to accept the participation and advice of all men, no matter what their fathers' parties.

The Carter group is an impenetrable circle. They won't let the people through who want to help them. Ben Cohen, who was in charge of domestic inflation under Roosevelt, has been trying desperately to get through to the White House to explain how to deal with the problem. They won't let him in. It's a frozen situation.[45]

Throughout his administration Carter rejected the New Deal as a model, save in the most limited respects. In formulating a reindustrialization plan he turned down recommendations for a public corporation patterned on the RFC, and he was appalled by Senator Adlai Stevenson III's proposal for an oil and gas corporation fashioned after the TVA which would provide a yardstick to determine the fairness of prices charged by private industry. Whereas in the Roosevelt years government regulation of business had been extended to new sectors, Carter persuaded Congress to deregulate transportation and banking. He also wanted to trim social security benefits and cut back on urban, health, and welfare programs. As the *New York Times* observed, "Instead of satisfying the coalition that has sustained Democratic Presidents since Franklin Roosevelt, he proposes to tame that hungry beast as Republican Presidents since Eisenhower never could." When Carter looked back on his presidency, he would say: "My main political problem was with the so-called liberal wing of the Democratic party. I went into office demanding deregulation of the private enterprise system, and balancing budgets and . . . cutting back on some of the excessive social programs that I thought were overly costly. This was the biggest political problem when I was in office."[46]

No one did more to steer the president away from the liberals than his wife—who was no Eleanor Roosevelt, however often the parallel was drawn. Under the headline, "Mrs. Carter's Model Is Very Much Her Own: Mrs. F.D.R.," a *New York Times* writer noted that Jimmy had called Rosalynn his "political partner," a term that could well be applied to Eleanor Roosevelt. She added, however, "Mrs. Roosevelt ultimately evolved a separate identity in a way that Mrs. Carter has indicated she has no wish to do. Mrs. Carter appears content to see herself as an extension of her husband, without feeling submerged." When Rosalynn Carter herself was asked whether she was a second Mrs. R., she retorted, "That's press speculation. I've never considered trying to be another Eleanor."[47]

If Rosalynn Carter brought to mind Eleanor Roosevelt, the resemblance lay in the power that both wielded, not from a congruence of viewpoints. Whereas Mrs. Roosevelt was an ardent reformer, Mrs. Carter served as a force for restraint. One correspondent noted, "It is Rosalynn Carter who is the fiscal conservative; Rosalynn who warned him in his postconvention slide to stop scaring off voters by trying to solve the social problems of the world, and to remember 'why we won the primaries—because people say Jimmy Carter does not believe in wasting money, does not believe in massive federal spending programs, that he is not going to spend money the government does not have.'"[48]

With the first lady's active encouragement, the Carter strategists calculatedly moved away from the Roosevelt coalition while hoping not to alienate its components. Gerald Rafshoon prepared a long memorandum stating, according to one account, "that the liberal base is illusory," that the public was "pro-military," and that Carter should cater to the suburban middle class, which disliked bureaucracy and government spending. Others were not prepared to go that far, though they agreed that it was essential to halt spiraling prices even if that meant adopting policies that antagonized such traditional Democratic allies as union labor. "Carter can't put together the Roosevelt coalition, but he can't afford to lose it," said one aide midway through the president's term. "He could say to the old Roosevelt coalition, 'You're not going to like what I'm doing, but it's important to get in the mainstream of American thinking. Bear with me. We have to get inflation under control; then we can get on with some of the things you care about.'" Another White House assistant added, "We're in a period of no happy choices, and this makes it increasingly difficult to put together the traditional coalition. Carter had certain elements of the old coalition—blacks, the U.A.W., and so on—and you can't hope to get re-elected without substantial portions of that coalition backing you. But if we don't get inflation under control we're out of the ballgame with everybody." Still, he acknowledged, "There is going to be very little good news for our constituencies."[49]

FDR's influence on Carter's foreign policy is more uncertain. Nearly a year after his term expired he informed one interviewer, "I went back and studied Roosevelt's relationship with the Soviet Union," and he told another that he had followed FDR's precept of being a good neighbor toward Latin America. "The only presidents that I knew about whose policies I could emulate were Roosevelt's and Kennedy's," he explained. "And I've looked on myself as carrying on that legacy." Perhaps. But he had not mentioned Roosevelt in these connections at the time, and even after he left office he was critical of FDR in the one area where he claimed to have studied him. "I think we gave away too much at Yalta," he said to David Brinkley. "The granting to Stalin of an almost undisputed control over Eastern Europe was a very serious historical mistake." Carter wondered whether if FDR had been firmer he could not have forced the Russians to give in, as Truman had managed to do in Iran.[50]

Long before then Carter had revealed that if he had an idol it was not Roosevelt but Truman. On the eve of the 1976 debates a national magazine, in an exclusive interview, asked Carter, "Which of our previous Presidents would you call yourself most akin to in philosophy?" The governor replied, "My own personal favorite is Harry Truman." On entering the White House, he faced the choice of which portrait of a predecessor to hang in the place of honor, and bypassed Roosevelt in favor of Truman. In his 1978 State of the Union Address, Carter said that the situation he faced was not like those confronting Franklin Roosevelt in depression and war but like the one that Harry Truman had been required to cope with—a time "when there is no single overwhelming crisis, yet profound national interests are at stake." It was not surprising, then, that he would tell Brinkley, "I think that there was a much greater parallel between Truman's administration and my own than there was between Roosevelt's and my own."[51]

Some of those close to Carter expressed skepticism, not without reason, about how great his attachment to Truman was, but Truman did have some influence on him and undoubtedly served his purposes. As Jody Powell has pointed out, Truman was the first president Carter ever saw, and it was no small matter in 1948, in the midst of the Dixiecrat rebellion, for a Georgian to speak out for him. Though there is no evidence that Carter was stirred by any of FDR's campaigns, he was "just very, very interested" in Truman's race, Rosalynn has recalled. "I remember Jimmy was the only one in the sub school who was for him." Carter's political maturation may well have taken place not in the Roosevelt years, despite the intensely political environment of his family, but in 1948. Moreover, Carter must have recognized that as an outsider in 1976 he could profit by identifying with the gritty Truman, whose cause had been deemed hopeless but who had surprised them all in the end. It is less clear what Carter meant when he said that his problems were closer to Truman's than to FDR's, but his remark suggests that he thought his task to be neither the achievement of social advances nor the awakening of the nation to foreign peril, but the more inchoate assignment of managing an economy in a twilight world between war and peace.[52]

During all of his White House years Carter was called upon to demonstrate that his presidency was something more than Gerald Ford's second term, and when it came time to sum up his thinking about Roosevelt on the centennial of FDR's birth, he sounded like no one so much as Ford. In the rank order of American presidents he would place Roosevelt "near the top," he said. Yet, in addition to criticizing FDR on Yalta, Carter pointed to "some of the mistakes he made like trying to pack the United States Supreme Court," and said that Roosevelt had "hurt himself" when he "misjudged his popularity" and tried to purge Senator Walter George of Georgia. Carter implied that what he claimed was his "75 percent batting average with the Congress" was better than that compiled by FDR, who, he asserted, "never got a major bill through Congress in his last seven years in office," a palpable misstatement. When, finally, Carter was asked, "Do you feel, as many do, that he is the most important president since Lincoln?" there was a long pause that spoke volumes before he gave a grudging "Yes" barren of emotion. Quickly he added, "He is not my favorite—I don't want to mislead you." Who, then, was his favorite? Like Gerald Ford, he had no hesitation about his answer: "Truman."[53]

VI

When in Carter's first spring in office the novelist Francine du Plessix Gray was given three wishes, she used one of them for a whimsical response: "To continue to believe that Jimmy Carter will be another F.D.R." Four months earlier, at the time of Carter's inauguration, John Osborne, one of the most perceptive of Washington writers, had observed: "No comparison with Franklin Roosevelt will wash. It is, of course, precisely that comparison which Carter tried to evoke in launching the fall campaign from Warm Springs. But, as one Washington wag put it, that's where FDR died, not where he and the experiments he fostered came alive." In 1979 one of Carter's biographers acknowledged, "Certainly he is no leader of Franklin Roosevelt's stature," and that same year a cartoonist in the *Charlotte Observer* drew a savage sketch on the president's malaise address. A gruff, cigar-wielding Winston Churchill rumbles "Blood, Sweat, and Tears," a confident Franklin Roosevelt, his cigarette holder at a rakish tilt, declares, "We Have Nothing to Fear but Fear Itself," while an obtuse Carter, an idiotic smile button on his lapel, gestures with his index finger as he admonishes, "Say Something Nice About America!" Throughout his four years in office Carter heard the same lament: "Why can't he be more like FDR?"[54]

Commentators on the Carter presidency never tired of using FDR's performance as a benchmark. Many months before Carter took office, Mo Udall confided, "I told him, politely, of course, he could jack around waiting to get his feet on the ground or he can strike before the congressional honeymoon's over—like in FDR's first hundred days," and when the magic date on the calendar came around in the spring of 1977, Hedrick Smith commented, "Mr. Carter has gotten some pieces of legislation through Congress. Yet, he has . . . fallen well short of the legislative blitz achieved by Franklin D. Roosevelt during the first 100 days of the New Deal." Even when he prepared to visit Mark Twain's old hometown in Missouri, the press listed the 70,000 turnout for Roosevelt in 1936 as the mark Carter would have to beat when he arrived in Hannibal.[55]

Any number of observers spelled out the ways in which Carter was no FDR. Those who acknowledged that Roosevelt had been less than a paragon as an administrator faulted Carter for being as contradictory as his predecessor but lacking the master's touch. "Not since the gaudier years of Franklin Roosevelt has so much confusion over authority been so visible in Washington," wrote the *New York Times* in an editorial leader. "The confusion is Rooseveltian; the orchestration is not." One of Carter's detractors, a prominent Capitol Hill Democrat, regretted that the president lacked FDR's legislative skills, while another was saddened by his "inability to establish emotional rapport with enough constituencies so he has a political bank account." In contrast, Roosevelt, though "a very cynical man in some ways and a horse trader," could always count on fervent support from a large segment of the public.[56]

Again and again, critics complained that Carter lacked Franklin Roosevelt's magnetism and his capacity to arouse the people by offering a vision of a better America. "I like Mr. Carter, I respect him," said the executive director of the NAACP. "But, in all honesty, when he walks into a room, it doesn't light up." Carter's Democratic predecessors had offered catching slogans—New Freedom, New Deal, New Frontier, Great Society; "alone of all Democrats to occupy the White House since Wilson," noted one observer, "the thirty-ninth President has felt no need to raise any such plain standard." Carter, it was said, had fixed the direction for his whole administration when he stated, "I have no new dream to set forth today."[57]

Carter's one feeble effort to find a slogan for his administration was a flop. The president's speechwriters all agreed that their rubric should copy FDR's by being two words long and start with "new," but the best anyone could come up with was "New Foundation." Nobody believed it was really satisfactory, though it is indicative of the limited range of the Carter circle that the president's advisers pondered such substitutes as "groundwork" and "building blocks," and even considered using "improved" instead of "new." The real difficulty was that Carter himself had no conceptual design to provide guidance for his aides. Asked by Bill Moyers what "single theme" would characterize his administration, Carter could offer none, and instead muttered something about Kierkegaard. When it came time to draft his State of the Union message in January 1979, his speechwriters dusted off "New Foundation," then some two months old, for want of anything better. The phrase was stillborn, and no one ever mentioned it again, save as a painful example of Carter's inability to capture the magic of his predecessors.[58]

Nor when he spoke did Jimmy Carter bring to mind the silver-tongued Roosevelt. While he was preparing his malaise address at Camp David (FDR's "Shangri-la") in the summer of 1979, the *New York Times* reported: "Oratorically, the Presidential entourage concedes, Mr. Carter has had problems with uninspiring speech delivery. The President himself concedes that he is not Winston Churchill or Franklin Delano Roosevelt." Similarly, a commentator stated that Carter's fireside chat was "hardly memorable," in part because the energy crisis "did not compare with the immediate, numbing paralysis of the closing of the banks in F.D.R.'s day." Yet just as important was Carter's own failure to rise to the occasion; "the studied informality of the Carter 'Fireside Chat' gave it a certain stiffness." "Fireside chats . . . delivered with Roosevelt's verve," concluded a Washington correspondent, were "an impossibility for Jimmy Carter."[59]

To Arthur Schlesinger, Jr., who as the most prominent chronicler of the age of Roosevelt performed a sacerdotal function, Carter's claim to be an apostle of FDR seemed almost blasphemous. In March 1978 Schlesinger contrasted Carter to Roosevelt and found the incumbent woefully lacking. The *Washington Post* printed this address alongside a cartoon in which, as one writer has described it, "a worried, drawn Carter is shown overshadowed by the jaunty silhouette of the squire from Hyde Park." Two years later, Schlesinger, who found Carter's political success despite his shortcomings exasperating, wrote:

Let him speak for himself: "Government cannot solve our problems. It

can't set the goals. It cannot define our vision. Government cannot eliminate poverty, or provide a bountiful economy, or reduce inflation, or save
our cities, or cure illiteracy, or provide energy." No, children, this is not
from a first draft of Ronald Reagan's inaugural address. It is from Jimmy
Carter's second annual message to Congress. Can anyone imagine Franklin
D. Roosevelt talking this way? If he had taken Carter's view of government, we still would be in the Great Depression.[60]

Those who sought to account for Carter's failure to profit from
FDR's experience offered one explanation more than any other—that
he was a technocrat with little awareness of history. One prominent
Democrat who was regarded as a presidential aspirant said that, unlike
such men as Roosevelt, Carter was "an engineer without deep philo-
sophic roots and hence without an instinctive way of orienting himself
on issues." Not at all like FDR's, his speeches were almost barren of
historical content. Eisenhower's speechwriter, Emmet Hughes, found
it odd that a man who came from the nation's most history-conscious
section showed "no very lively sense of history at all," while James
Fallows, who resigned as Carter's speechwriter in dismay, wrote that
the first clue to his "Passionless Presidency" was "Carter's cast of mind:
his view of problems as technical, not historical, his lack of curiosity
about how the story turned out before." Fallows added: "In two years,
the only historical allusions I heard Carter use with any frequency were
Harry Truman's rise from the depths of the polls and the effect of
Roosevelt's New Deal on the southern farm. The rest of Roosevelt's
record . . . was uncharted territory."[61]

The most compelling testimony on this point comes from the president's senior adviser, Hedley Donovan. Carter, he has said, did like to
talk about the early years of the White House, but about the structural
details of the edifice, not the people who lived there. Not once did
Donovan hear Carter refer to FDR. But then neither did he ever hear
him mention Jefferson or, curiously given his Georgian antecedents,
Wilson. Nor, again strangely for a southerner, did he ever allude to the
Civil War. During Donovan's months in the White House, Carter was
embroiled in problems of economic mobilization, but at no time did he
say anything to his senior adviser about the two world wars or the
policy implications of the age of Roosevelt.[62]

Consequently, when those who observed Carter closely sought an
analogy, they were inclined to compare him not to FDR but to that
other engineer in the White House, Roosevelt's *bête noire,* Herbert
Hoover. It became commonplace to say that Carter was "Jimmy Hoov-

er."[63] Emmet Hughes, noting that Hoover had been the only other chief executive with a technological background, has concluded:

> For this or whatever case, there has been no President since Hoover so absorbed and fascinated as Carter by the "machinery" of his government and the monitoring of all its details. There has been no President since Hoover so devoted to "run a desk" with an industry decreed by a presidential work-ethic of exhaustive briefings and exhausting hours.
>
> In a private interview last month in the Oval Office, Jimmy Carter commented upon his own presidency in terms that would have been appreciated by few other chief executives so much as by Herbert Hoover. Not surprisingly, he ventured no notions in economic philosophy to which the earlier President could have taken serious exception—nor any regretful longing for a social program abandoned for the sake of the battles against inflation, deficit, waste, and bureaucracy.[64]

At midterm it remained to be seen whether the fact that Carter did not even feel "any regretful longing" would have political consequences. Toward the end of his second year in office, a writer in the *Washington Post* observed:

> He did not promise to excite us or entertain us or even "lead" us in the public fashion of a Franklin D. Roosevelt, John F. Kennedy or Lyndon B. Johnson. He promised only to manage our affairs sensibly and with a degree of charity. We in turn responded, and so elected the country's first national city manager.
>
> Is that enough? Along with all the other variables that go into such a close election, it certainly was enough in 1976. But times, and the temper of the American electorate, change. And Carter, having failed to establish much of an emotional bond with the American people these last two years, seems particularly vulnerable to a change in the national temper.[65]

VII

When President Carter concluded his address to the Democratic midterm convention in Memphis, the band struck up "Happy Days Are Here Again" and almost nobody clapped. Throughout the meeting Carter's people had trouble with critics who used praise for "the party of Franklin Roosevelt" as a way of criticizing the president, and afterward one of the delegates wrote, "The Democratic Party's real strength lies in its progressive tradition and its commitment to Franklin Roosevelt's Economic Bill of Rights," and he deplored "President Carter's failure to give any indication of more than lip-service to that commitment." Though Carter held a majority of the delegates, he failed to inspire the zealotry aroused by the senator from Massachusetts, Edward Kennedy, the favorite of those who hoped for a new age of Roosevelt. Kennedy's challenge and the spirit of the Memphis meeting spelled out an inescapable message—that before Carter could turn his thoughts toward winning reelection he had to worry about gaining renomination. "The party will sit in judgment on him first," observed *Newsweek,* "and his estrangement from the old liberal-labor minority coalition forged by F.D.R. could haunt him then."[66]

Ted Kennedy presented himself in 1980 as a latter-day New Dealer only after having taken a quite different approach. When he first announced his candidacy, he assumed a more moderate stance, for it had seemed likely that he would wrest the nomination from Carter and that his main task would be to capture the center from his Republican rival. In a biography published in 1980, Kennedy was advised to shift away from liberalism, since "the constituency that traditionally supports the party of FDR, the lower middle class, is now attracted to conservative populism." In keeping with that view, Kennedy told a group of New York businessmen: "We are making a clean break with the New Deal and even the 1960's. We reject the idea that government knows best across the board, that public planning is inherently superior or more effective than private action. There is now a growing consensus, which I share, that government intervention in the economy should come as only a last resort." When Carter climbed in the polls and took the Iowa caucuses, however, Senator Kennedy quickly reminded himself that his greatest strength lay in the blue-collar FDR coalition and among voters who still cherished Roosevelt's memory. As one representative response to a direct mail campaign put it, "I would like to see a president take charge of our nation like Franklin D. Roosevelt, and I think that Teddy Kennedy comes closest to him."[67]

Once he had oriented himself, Kennedy campaigned unflaggingly as Franklin Roosevelt's legatee, the rightful heir to the party's New Deal heritage who was seeking to depose the pretender in the White House. The problem of economic reconstruction, he told voters, was "Lincolnesque or Rooseveltian in dimension," and only a "real Democrat" like himself could meet such a challenge. "Surely the nation that came back from the Depression half a century ago can roll back inflation," Kennedy declared. His statement, "The only thing that paralyzes us today is the myth that we cannot move," was, as Anthony Lewis remarked, "an echo, surely deliberate, of Franklin Roosevelt's pithier 'the only thing we have to fear is fear itself.'" The leading publicist for Kennedy, Arthur Schlesinger, Jr., provided a visible link to the Roosevelt tradition, while another of FDR's biographers, James MacGregor Burns, counseled him to cultivate the sort of "activist followership" that had congregated about Roosevelt in 1936.[68]

Kennedy and his supporters took full advantage of the cry that the president was "Jimmy Hoover." "In the hurried effort of the Democratic incumbent to flee with the political wind, he has left behind the best traditions of the Democratic Party," Kennedy told the American Society of Newspaper Editors. "We are instructed that the New Deal is old hat and that our best hope is no deal at all." Kennedy's followers sounded the same theme. In a television campaign advertisement, Carroll O'Connor, TV's Archie Bunker, said, "I've seen some oddities offstage as well as on, but never anything odder than Jimmy Carter in a Democratic primary. He may be the most Republican president since Herbert Hoover." And in an appeal to Alaska's Democrats, the senator's nephew Joseph Kennedy stated, "Carter is taking the same steps Herbert Hoover took in the 1930s. It was a miserable failure then and it will be a miserable failure now."[69]

Senator Kennedy's address to an Irish cultural center in San Francisco encapsulated all of these arguments. He declared:

> We have a President now that doesn't really believe that a President of the United States or an individual can make a difference. . . . And I say to you that a President of the United States can make a difference. . . . We can read the history of this country and see it so clearly. Franklin Roosevelt made a difference when he pulled this country up by its bootstraps when it was facing the Depression in the period of the nineteen-thirties.[70]

In meeting this challenge Carter had three formidable advantages. One was that Kennedy could not articulate until too late what it meant to be a Roosevelt man in the 1980s. It was all very well for Kennedy to state that one must meet the needs of the poor, but he did not really say what he would do about inflation, noted Elizabeth Drew. "There is no question that he is rousing this audience," she wrote from Memphis, "but where is he taking it?" One logical destination might have been to a controlled economy, but as Garry Wills wrote, "controls were the love that dare[d] not speak its name." Second, Carter had the better of Kennedy in being able to act "presidential." When on May 29, 1980, he finally left the White House to open his first acknowledged political tour, he did so by telling a noontime rally in a sunstruck plaza in

Columbus, Ohio, that his effort was like FDR's in 1944, when Roosevelt said that he would not campaign for reelection but would feel at liberty from time to time to correct any misstatements made by his opponents. Finally, Carter was able to appeal to a mood of retrenchment by heeding the advice of those who counseled him to attack Kennedy in the same fashion in which Hoover had castigated Roosevelt—as a profligate spender, "a New Dealer of the 1960s who would bankrupt the country with grandiose schemes."[71]

Furthermore, Carter refused to concede to Kennedy the FDR legacy, and his domestic policy adviser even developed a rationale for the claim that Carter was being faithful to the Roosevelt tradition. In the most thoughtful address by any of Carter's counselors, Stuart Eizenstat declared that though the president would continue to honor the traditional obligations of the Democrats to the less advantaged, he also had to adapt to "new realities": the huge deficit he had inherited, the "new phenomenon" of stagflation, and the widespread distrust of government. Carter, Eizenstat told a luncheon meeting of the Women's National Democratic Club, was an innovator like his predecessors precisely because he chose not to imitate them but to respond to this unfamiliar situation.

Though Carter was diverging from some well-worn paths, he was also carrying out "the Democratic Party's historic mission," Eizenstat insisted, and the Carter presidency should be judged in this light. He maintained:

> Emerson once said that mankind was divided between the Party of Conservatism and the Party of Innovation, between the Past and the Future, between Memory and Hope. There can be no doubt in modern times where the Democratic Party has stood in this great division. We have been for decades and remain the majority party in this country precisely because the American people see in our Party and in the Presidential Administrations which have embodied it during our lifetimes—Roosevelt, Truman, Kennedy, Johnson, and Carter—their own commitment to the future—not the past—to hope, not memory, to innovation, not the status quo.[72]

Such language had considerably greater appeal to most of the delegates than did Kennedy's rhetoric. Many Democrats, particularly those of an older generation, continued to regard themselves as FDR loyalists and quickened to Kennedy's reminder that their party should not neglect the downtrodden. But they worried about how to justify New Deal–style spending in an age of limits, when there was a new awareness that resources are finite.[73] Well before the delegates gathered in

New York it was clear that the nomination would go not to Kennedy but to Carter. Yet there remained a large residue of Kennedy followers as well as many others who, though they voted for Carter, were put off by the way he distanced himself from the New Deal and would jump to their feet cheering the moment they heard the magic words "Franklin Delano Roosevelt."

When it came time for him to address the delegates in New York, Ted Kennedy showed a sure understanding of this nostalgia for the Roosevelt years in one of the most electrifying speeches ever made at a national convention. With a commanding presence and speaking with a power he had not shown in the primaries, Kennedy detonated a thunderous response by firing away at the Republicans:

> We heard the orators at their convention all trying to talk like Democrats. They proved even Republican nominees can quote Franklin Roosevelt to their own purpose. The Grand Old Party thinks it has found a great new trick. But 40 years ago, an earlier generation of Republicans attempted that same trick. And Franklin Roosevelt himself replied: "Most Republican leaders have bitterly fought and blocked the forward surge of average men and women in their pursuit of happiness. Let us not be deluded that overnight those leaders have suddenly become friends of the average men and women. You know, very few of us are that gullible."
>
> And four years later, when the Republicans tried that trick again, Franklin Roosevelt asked: "Can the Old Guard pass itself off as the New Deal? I think not. We have all seen many marvelous stunts in the circus, but no performing elephant could turn a handspring without falling flat on its back."

Kennedy's speech transformed the listless convention into a chanting, shouting revival meeting and altogether redid the 1980 Democratic platform. Richard Strout wrote that he would rank Kennedy's address with Roosevelt's Fala speech, adding, "He used excoriating humor, as FDR did," while a Connecticut Democrat who had attended every convention of his party since 1928 said, "I heard tham all back to Al Smith and Kennedy's speech ranks with F.D.R. back in '32. Carter could never produce one like it." He had achieved such success, wrote a columnist for the *Washington Post,* "by conjuring up FDR, and by taking Democrats back to their roots. It is Ted Kennedy who seats you by an old radio and makes you hear the voice of Franklin Roosevelt." When he told the delegates that the Republicans should not be permitted to snatch FDR away from them by quoting him for their own ends, the hall erupted and the demonstration that followed his talk was longer than the address itself. Carter's agents took one look at the scene and surrendered. On behalf of the president, they accepted a series of planks that Carter had been sternly opposing, including a $12 billion economic stimulus, which were characterized as an "updating of New Deal proposals."[74]

Despite his capitulation on the platform, Carter had the satisfaction of delivering the acceptance address, a presentation that also looked back to the age of FDR, but in a different fashion. He started by declaring, "We will win because we are the party of the great president who knew how to get reelected—Franklin D. Roosevelt." In reciting this litany, though, he was lauding not the architect of the welfare state but the champion campaigner. He went on to remind the delegates, "Forty years ago, President Franklin Roosevelt said that there are times in our history when concerns over our personal lives are overshadowed by our concern for 'what will happen to the country we have known.' This is such a time." Later in his speech, he boasted, "We have slashed government regulation and put free enterprise back into the airline, trucking and financial systems of our country, and we are doing the same for the railroads. This is the greatest change in the relationship between business and government since the New Deal."

Only near the end of his talk did Carter take note of the opposition's attempt to capture Roosevelt for the Republicans. He responded:

What have the Republicans proposed? Just an attack on almost every achievement in social justice and decency we have won in the last 50 years—since Franklin Roosevelt's first term. They would make Social Security voluntary. They would reverse our progress on the minimum wage, full employment laws, safety in the work place, and a healthy environment.

Lately the Republicans have been quoting Democratic Presidents—but who can blame them? Whom would you rather quote—Herbert Hoover or F.D.R.?

If Carter cited Roosevelt, however, he also spoke of other Democratic presidents, and the press thought he was less concerned with evoking Roosevelt than with calling up the image of the underdog Harry Truman.[75]

Carter entered the ensuing campaign against Ronald Reagan with formidable liabilities, quite apart from such specific difficulties as the Iranian captivity. He headed a divided party many of whose members identified not with him but with Teddy Kennedy and his New Dealish aspirations, and he could not, or would not, reach out to them. After the election, one of Carter's cabinet officers reflected, "We lost sight of the fact that what really united the Roosevelt coalition was the commitment to providing people opportunities for productive work." It was frequently remarked, too, that he lacked FDR's deftness as a campaigner. In scolding Carter for cutting such a poor figure against Reagan, Anthony Lewis wrote:

> What fun a Franklin Roosevelt would have with that Reagan picture of a pitiful America. He would tell the voters that the men in the Kremlin have much more reason for nervousness—in Poland, in Afghanistan, in their own economic muddle. We have problems, he would say, but we have the will and the ingenuity to solve them. He would give people dreams. He would inspire.
>
> But there is no fun in Jimmy Carter, and very little of the self-confidence that Roosevelt communicated.[76]

Fittingly enough, Carter's defeat marked the first time that an elected incumbent chief executive had lost a reelection contest since Hoover was ousted by FDR in 1932.

After the election, a number of analysts pointed out that whatever else the Reagan–Carter duel may have been, it surely was not a referendum on the New Deal. In nearly four years in office, Carter had hardly ever been able to bring himself to mention Franklin Roosevelt's name, and both his policies and his rhetoric departed repeatedly from the New Deal tradition. Indeed, much of Carter's difficulty on Election Day came from being so little in the image of FDR that millions in the Roosevelt coalition—union members, big-city dwellers, Catholics, Jews—did not go to the polls, and many others were so uninspired that they did nothing to keep him in office save cast a dutiful vote.[77] Though by no means the only cause of his defeat, Carter's inability to understand how strong a shadow FDR still cast contributed no little to the fact that he would leave Washington a one-term president with no prospect of ever being revered as Roosevelt was.

To be sure, the many comparisons that were made between Carter and FDR were often unfair. Carter operated within a much narrower range of options than Roosevelt had in 1933. If he had sought to institute a modern version of the New Deal, he would have been circumscribed both by budgetary imperatives and by stiff resistance from a sizable sector of opinion that had come to distrust the national government. Carter, for his part, had no grandiose notion of his place in history and felt no compulsion to outperform FDR. He had his own agenda, and he left a not inconsiderable record of accomplishment—from Camp David to Panama, from his appointments of blacks and women to his achievements with respect to the environment. Furthermore, to ask Carter to be another FDR is to ignore how he got to the White House in the first place—by campaigning as an outsider who proposed to curb the excesses of the imperial presidency, a pledge he largely fulfilled.

Carter's single term had a melancholy ending because that promise was not enough. Once the memory of Watergate faded, numbers of Americans began to recall wistfully the dynamic leadership they associated with FDR. Unlike Roosevelt though, Carter, for all his good intentions, could not offer a standard around which his partisans could rally. As a Washington correspondent said, his greatest shortcoming was not any specific error in policy but an incapacity to present an "overall vision that would distinguish his Administration, as the New Deal, the New Frontier and the Great Society distinguished past Democratic Presidencies." Moreover, even those prepared to concede that Carter had to jettison much of the Roosevelt legacy because of the harsh imperatives of a changed economic environment could not understand why he did it with so few misgivings. *Time* concluded: "In a sense, Carter was an irrelevance to his own party. He was never a Democratic leader by either blood or inclination—not really. He never sought, like Franklin Roosevelt or Lyndon Johnson, to preside as paterfamilias over the great brawling Democratic coalition."[78]

Even before the returns were counted, a historian suggested that Carter was doomed from the beginning. "Since FDR, the presidency has been prototypically defined as activist," observed Frank Annunziata, and "so captivating" was the strong presidency model "that Jimmy Carter became, from the very outset of his presidency, a predictable 'failure.'" It was thus inevitable that Arthur Schlesinger, Jr., would call him the most conservative Democratic president since Cleveland, and that Leonard Silk, financial editor of the *New York Times,* would write that Carter in 1980 had come "to New York not to praise Mr. Roosevelt's policies but to bury them." He concluded:

Jimmy Carter will not be remembered for a New Freedom, a New Deal, or a New Frontier, or for winning the "hearts" of his fellow Democrats. He will, however, be remembered as the first Democrat who reoriented the party away from its fixation with the New Deal into a new, if unwelcome, recognition of the constraints imposed by a maturing welfare state. . . . Even if subsequent historical judgments assess this role as having been "necessary," Jimmy Carter will never escape the verdict of being the first Democratic president to violate the spirit and substance of New Deal liberalism.[79]

[7]

Ronald Reagan

I

The Republican delegates arrayed row on row at the 1980 national convention in Detroit could not believe what they were hearing. This was supposed to be the finest hour for American conservatives in half a century. In nominating Ronald Reagan they had chosen an uncompromising right-wing ideologue, and one who, unlike Barry Goldwater sixteen years before, had a good chance of winning. They had come to the great arena that night to take part in a secular rite at which their candidate would pay homage to the totems of their party, and here he was quoting not Lincoln, not Coolidge, but—would you believe it?— Franklin D. Roosevelt. Up to that point, they had been cheering lustily, but when they heard those words, they fell into a chilled silence. Still worse, when Reagan reached the peroration of his acceptance address, he once more quoted Roosevelt, paragraph after paragraph, and wound up by calling upon the delegates to fulfill FDR's promise. When the *New York Times* appeared on the streets the next morning, its editorial leader had an eye-catching title: "Franklin Delano Reagan."[1]

Nothing appeared more preposterous than Reagan's claim of kinship with FDR. Reagan had, after all, first come to national political attention in 1964 as a Goldwater partisan delivering "the Speech," a diatribe against the New Deal and all its offspring, and ever since he had been the lodestar of the anti-Roosevelt right. Well before 1964, Reagan had been an outspoken foe of the showpiece of the age of Roosevelt, the Tennessee Valley Authority. So it was understandable that *Time* thought that Reagan's reliance on Roosevelt in his acceptance address was "an awkward reach even for a candidate striving for Democratic votes," and that Hugh Sidey remarked, "When Dutch stood there the other night in his Eastern Establishment dark suit, giving a speech that could have been written by a Democrat and invoking the ghost of F.D.R. in the name of the Republican Party, some of us had to pinch ourselves."[2]

Neither the Republican delegates nor the national commentators should have been so surprised. As far back as "the Speech" Reagan had shown his fondness for one of the fruitier of FDR's sentences, "This generation of Americans has a rendezvous with destiny," a line he quoted again in Detroit. Furthermore, he had cited Roosevelt three times on announcing his candidacy for the Republican nomination, and when he opened his presidential campaign in New York City he was to say, "A troubled and afflicted mankind looks to us, pleading for us to keep our rendezvous with destiny."[3]

In its "Franklin Delano Reagan" leader, the *New York Times* expressed not amazement but admiration. Noting that it was customary for presidential nominees to associate themselves with the past heroes of their party, the *Times* thought it "audacious, even brilliant" for Reagan to identify himself with FDR. The political advantages were obvious, for "if Ronald Reagan casts himself as the latter-day equivalent of Franklin Roosevelt, guess which part Jimmy Carter is meant to play." Besides, "by using F.D.R. as a model, Mr. Reagan suggests that he is not content to be the darling of narrow ideology. On the contrary, he suggests that there will be a tidal change, 1932-like, in the way Americans vote, and that he aspires to lead it." To achieve such a shift, Reagan had to move toward the center, and one important step in that direction was "the effort to kidnap Franklin Roosevelt."[4]

The *Times* editorial, though discerning, missed the point. In quoting FDR in Detroit, Reagan had not modified his views but exploited Roosevelt for conservative ends. He had concluded his acceptance address by stating:

> The time is now to redeem promises once made to the American people by another candidate, in another time and another place. He said:
>
> "For three long years I have been going up and down this country preaching that government—Federal, state and local—costs too much. I shall not stop that preaching. As an immediate program of action, we must abolish useless offices. We must eliminate unnecessary functions of government.
>
> "We must consolidate subdivisions of government and, like the private citizen, give up luxuries which we can no longer afford.
>
> "I propose to you my friends, and through you, that government of all kinds, big and little, be made solvent and that the example be set by the President of the United States and his Cabinet."

So said Franklin Delano Roosevelt in his acceptance speech to the Democratic National Convention in July 1932.

The time is now, my fellow Americans, to recapture our destiny, to take it into our own hands. But, to do this will take many of us, working together. I ask you tonight to volunteer your help in this cause so we can carry our message throughout the land.

Yes, isn't now the time that we, the people, carried out these unkept promises? Let us pledge to each other and to all America on this July day 48 years later, we intend to do just that.[5]

Far from reflecting a "new Reagan" seeking an accommodation with liberal thought, the Detroit speech encapsulated what the Republican candidate had been saying for more than two decades: government had become too big, too remote.

The *Times,* in common with other observers, misconstrued the address in yet another respect, for it perceived Reagan primarily as a calculating political animal. Though Reagan must have known how much he would profit by associating himself with Roosevelt, his allusions to FDR came naturally. Roosevelt had been his first political hero, and he never got over that initial adulation. When a historian interviewed Roosevelt's successors as the FDR centenary approached, he found Ford listless, Carter guarded, but Reagan so chockful of enthusiasm that in the midst of a busy White House schedule he went on talking about FDR beyond the allotted time and "with the most obvious fondness." Reagan, David McCullough concluded, "sees Roosevelt as his 'kind of guy'—confident, cheerful, theatrical, larger than life."[6]

If even astute writers found it hard to come to terms with this paradox—that Reagan was a sincere Roosevelt admirer intent on ridding the land of FDR's influence—one should not wonder, for no one did more to spread confusion about his relation to Roosevelt than Reagan himself. He was forever reinventing his past. A dyed-in-the-wool Roosevelt partisan, he implied that he had cast but a single vote for FDR. Committed to Roosevelt liberalism at least as late as 1950, he claimed that he was disaffected from the New Deal almost from the outset. Again and again he dropped pebbles that led searchers astray. Furthermore, it was hard to find coherence in his statements and actions. Though he never ceased to express admiration for Roosevelt, that did not stop him from saying more than once that FDR headed a government that sought to bring fascism to America. In the end he would make the bewildering record complete by running a campaign designed to smash the Roosevelt coalition and then putting his name to legislation that would enshrine FDR, alongside Washington, Lincoln, and Jefferson, among the immortals in the capital of the republic.

II

"I didn't desert my party," Reagan once said in accounting for his defection from the Democrats. "It deserted me." He explained: "I looked up FDR's old platform, and I discovered that it called for a restoration of states' rights and a reduction in the national budget. You know what? I'm still for that." This would turn out to be the most enduring of Reagan's rationales for the transformation of a Roosevelt man into a right-wing Republican. He had been consistent all along, Reagan claimed. True, he had once voted for FDR, but for the FDR of 1932 who "had promised to cut federal spending by 25 percent, had promised to return to the states and local communities authority and autonomy that had been unjustly seized by the Federal Government." When the party abandoned these principles, he remained true to them, and consequently he had no choice but to bolt.[7]

In advancing this notion Reagan told one interviewer that "while he was still Governor of New York, Roosevelt warned of the evils of big government" and said that in such fields as public utilities "Washington must be discouraged from interfering."[8] It hardly needs saying that Reagan was misconstruing FDR's record. To be sure, Roosevelt held orthodox views about budget balancing, as did almost everyone else in the pre-Keynesian era, but he made clear in 1932 that he would not permit fiscal concerns to stand in the way of relief to the unemployed. The distinguishing fact about Roosevelt in 1932 was not that he sometimes spoke of the need for retrenchment but that he stood out among the nation's governors precisely because he was willing to go much further in advocating government regulation of utilities, public power development, and the responsibility of the state to the jobless.

Nonetheless, with an insistence bordering on perversity, Reagan maintained again and again that he was following in Roosevelt's footsteps. When in the 1980 campaign debates Carter said, "I noticed recently that Governor Reagan frequently quotes Democratic Presidents" (symptomatically, Carter did not mention FDR by name), Reagan replied: "The president that I quoted had made a promise—a Democratic promise—and I quoted him because it was never kept. . . . It was a promise for less government and less taxes and more freedom for the people." After nearly a year in office Reagan was still saying to David Brinkley, "When I cast that first vote for him, I cast it for a man who had campaigned on a pledge to reduce the cost of government by twenty-five percent." This latest repetition of Reagan's lines was too much for Brinkley, who replied, "Well, I thought you, Mr. President, in your younger days, earlier days, were something of a New Dealer." Reagan answered, "I was. Yes," then raced through a jumble of words that clarified nothing.[9]

In truth, as Brinkley's remark suggested, Reagan's version of events would not wash, for it misstated his own history even more than Roosevelt's. Far from having supported FDR only in 1932, as his comments implied, Reagan voted for Roosevelt in 1936, 1940, and 1944 as well. Having cast his very first ballot, at the age of twenty-one, for FDR in 1932, he seized every opportunity to vote for him thereafter. Indeed, Reagan's devotion to Roosevelt was greatest not in 1932, when FDR pledged to cut government spending, but after he had put through the precedent-smashing legislation that centralized authority in Washington. Reagan voted for FDR in 1932 not because he was attracted by Roosevelt's desire for a balanced budget but because he was born into a Democratic family. "I was, I guess, a Democrat because my father had been," Reagan has recalled. Moreover, in 1932 he "wasn't particularly excited or anything." But in 1936, when Roosevelt was unmistakably a New Deal candidate, Reagan was thrilled when, for the first and only time, he saw him in a parade that passed by the Des Moines radio station. Did he cheer him? "Oh, of course!" he assured McCullough. "Yes!"[10]

Three years earlier, when Roosevelt delivered his first inaugural address, the radio announcer manning the booth at WHO Des Moines was Ronald Reagan, and he never forgot that day. In 1976 he told a reporter, "I still believe when he was first inaugurated, yes, if he didn't do anything else, he gave back to the people of this country their courage. His line 'We have nothing to fear but fear itself' was one that can be repeated many times in many circumstances." Reagan learned passages of the first inaugural by heart, and he developed a convincing impersonation of FDR, even to the right flourish with an imaginary cigarette holder. From 1933 on he listened to each of Roosevelt's fireside chats, and he subsequently acknowledged that he based his own style on his recollections of those talks. Toward the end of his first year in the White House he remarked, "You know, it's pretty hard for most people to realize . . . at this time the impact of those fireside chats—that they, to this day, still hold the radio record for audience. When he came on, it was *the* biggest radio audience . . . ever." The admiration in his voice was unmistakable.[11]

Far from being a consistent opponent of the welfare state linked to the age of Roosevelt only by his 1932 vote, Reagan had the most intimate connection with the New Deal, for the head of the WPA in

Dixon, Illinois, Ronald Reagan's home town, was his father, Jack. An unemployed shoe salesman, Jack Reagan got back on a payroll by ringing doorbells for FDR in 1932. As reward he received a job in the Roosevelt relief operation, first with FERA, then with WPA. Even in the 1980s Ronald Reagan was capable of forgetting his commitment to limited government long enough to wax eloquent about the WPA, the one agency above all others that FDR's conservative opponents scorned. "Now, a lot of people remember it as boondoggles and . . . raking leaves," he noted. But that was not right, Reagan said. "Maybe in some places it was. Maybe in the big city machines or something. But I can take you to our town and show you things, like a river front that I used to hike through once that was swamp and is now a beautiful park-like place built by WPA." There were other good things that the WPA had done for Dixon, Reagan added, his voice vibrant, such as the improvements in the town's airport. He sounded for all the world like a 1936 Democratic campaigner making a stump speech for FDR and Big Government.[12]

Roosevelt's conduct of foreign affairs gave Reagan yet another reason to think well of his predecessor. At the close of his interview with McCullough early in December 1981, President Reagan's desire to say all that he could in praise of FDR left him momentarily out of control of his thoughts, but he quickly recovered himself to add still more to the record. The president said:

> He gave confidence to the people. He never lost faith in this country for *one minute*. And a—oh, there was just one more that I was going to a—oh dear! Oh, the most famous thing— . . . when the threat of Hitler was obvious to the world, and he was building up the same kind of military monster that the Soviet Union has now built up. He was making a speech at a dedication of a bridge in Chicago, and he called for the entire free world, the rest of the world, to quarantine Nazi Germany. . . . The press literally kicked his brains out for saying such a thing. You look back now and say, "If the free world had done it, would there have been World War II?"[13]

Reagan's respect for FDR's performance in World War II was virtually unbounded. He informed McCullough:

> I must say I think he was a great war leader. I think there were less of the great tragic blunders that have characterized many wars in the past than this one. . . . I remember him when he . . . said that he was going to ask for 50,000 planes a year, and I remember when the American press tore him to ribbons for that. . . . They said that, you know, that this was

impossible. It couldn't happen. But when you look at what this country did starting from the low point of Pearl Harbor in 44 months—something like 350,000 planes and hundreds of thousands of tanks and of trucks and of every kind of weapon, we truly were the arsenal of democracy. . . . I think his leadership in the war was great.

Three weeks later he told David Brinkley: "There's no question about his leadership in that war as commander-in-chief. Our war effort was just absolutely magnificent, and we succeeded literally in saving the . . . world and probably achieved the greatest victory in . . . the history of war, in . . . the total surrender of . . . the principal enemy."[14]

This attachment to Roosevelt and his views did not end in 1945 but carried into the postwar period. In his autobiography *Reagan*, abandoning his claim to have been only a 1932 Democrat, confessed that he had been "a near-hopeless hemophilic liberal," a characterization that embraces his behavior not only in the age of Roosevelt but in the years after the war. He served on the boards of directors of both the United World Federalists and the Hollywood Independent Citizens Committee for the Arts, Sciences, and Professions, and on several occasions the Democratic left tried to get him to run for Congress or the California legislature. Reagan was regarded as so far to the left that when he turned up at a caucus of anticommunists, Olivia de Havilland was astonished because she thought that he was with the Stalinist cadre, though in fact he had never been a fellow traveler but rather, as he would later admit to a journalist, "a very emotional New Dealer."[15]

In 1947 Reagan helped found the California organization of Americans for Democratic Action, the main legatee of Roosevelt liberalism. His participation in a group that was denounced by the Republican right was far from perfunctory. Next to his name, ADA wrote the words "dues paid," and he subsequently served as a member of the national board. When in the fall of 1947 he testified in Washington, James Loeb, Jr., ADA's executive secretary, wrote him a "fan letter" saying that he had heard "from our New York office and from all around this town of Washington, D.C., that your testimony was considered, by all odds, the most honest and forthright from a decent liberal point of view." Loeb added: "It was an encouraging experience to have had a chance to talk to you and to know that there are people in your position who share so completely a liberal point of view. . . . What we liberals need most of all on our side is a bit of genuine liberal fanaticism."[16]

The testimony that elicited such encomiums from ADA came before the House Committee on Un-American Activities, where Reagan gave a good account of himself. While Gary Cooper denounced the "pink mouthings" of Hollywood Communists and Robert Montgomery blustered that he was ready to take up arms against the Reds, Reagan, the "boyish-looking movie hero," stated that the best way to combat communism was "to make democracy work," adding that he shared Jefferson's belief that "if all of the American people know all of the facts, they'll never make a mistake." With regard to the popular proposal to outlaw the Communists, Reagan told the committee, "As a citizen I would hesitate, or not like, to see any political party outlawed on the basis of its political ideology." When the handsome movie star, in a tan gabardine suit set off by a blue knitted tie, walked into the hearing room, "there was a long drawn-out 'ooooh' from the jampacked, predominantly feminine audience," said the *New York Times,* but Reagan was not content to behave as a matinee idol. He not only responded well to the questioning but after the committee chairman dismissed him he still had a thought he wanted to express about the Communists: "Sir, . . . I detest, I abhor their philosophy, . . . but at the same time I never as a citizen want to see our country become urged, by either fear or resentment of this group, that we ever compromise with any of our democratic principles."[17]

A year later Reagan headed the Labor League of Hollywood Voters for Truman and gave a radio address under the sponsorship of the International Ladies Garment Workers Union on behalf of the president and the Democratic senatorial candidate Hubert Humphrey. He praised Humphrey for "fighting for . . . adequate low-cost housing, for civil rights, for prices people can afford to pay and for a labor movement free of the Taft-Hartley law," while Humphrey's opponent, Reagan said derisively, was "the banner carrier for Wall Street." Noting that inflation had eaten into the incomes of ordinary people, he pointed his finger at the fat return reported by Standard Oil. "High prices," Reagan contended, "have not been caused by higher wages, but by bigger and bigger profits." In 1976 California partygoers still played a 1940s tape of Reagan introducing Humphrey that was described as "quintessential left-wing stuff."[18]

In 1950, to his subsequent discomfort, Reagan backed the California ADA Democrat Helen Gahagan Douglas in her campaign against Richard Nixon for a U.S. Senate seat. Reagan later said that he never made any speech for Mrs. Douglas but only supported her in the course of giving a general endorsement to the Democratic slate in 1950. By then, he claimed, he had already reached the conclusion that she was "awfully naive about the subject of Communists," but he did not think it was right to say so publicly. In fact, a Douglas campaign office memo in December 1949 listed "Ronnie Reagan" as one of the Hollywood personalities to be signed up in January, and by March he was in a select group of a dozen actors and actresses, including Myrna Loy, Lena Horne, and Eddie Cantor, who were "sponsors" of the candidacy of Helen Gahagan Douglas. During the campaign he taped a number of three-minute radio spots for her that were widely aired in California. He was even recommended by her campaign manager to be a "State-wide front" for her effort, but, according to one account, her top aides decided to keep Reagan's name off the campaign letterhead because he had too leftist a reputation.[19]

When Reagan did change his views, he gave no evidence of a sudden revulsion against FDR and the Democrats. In 1952 he was a Democrat for Eisenhower, but so were a lot of others that year, and in 1953 he chaired a committee to reelect as mayor of Los Angeles a man strongly backed by liberals and unionists in the city. In the 1960 election he still identified himself as a Democrat, though for Nixon. Not until 1962 did he switch his registration to Republican, and as late as 1966 Nelson Rockefeller, claiming not to know where Reagan stood, said, "Reagan was a Roosevelt New Dealer once, wasn't he?"[20]

Even in these years Roosevelt still provided Reagan with a model for leadership, more particularly with a pattern for communicating. In the 1950s, Theodore White has written, Reagan "learned new rhythms, the hesitation, the toss of the head, the style that he claimed had been inspired by watching Franklin D. Roosevelt." In Sacramento, Reagan released a report on the first hundred days of his administration and adapted FDR's fireside chats to the demands of television. Again and again writers likened his manner of governing to FDR's. His most sagacious biographer has concluded: "Though Reagan's politics ultimately would evolve into opposition to some of the most enduring legacies of the New Deal, his style has remained frankly and fervently Rooseveltian throughout his life. His cadences are Roosevelt's cadences, his metaphors the offspring of FDR's."[21]

III

When Reagan was not attempting to resolve the contradiction between his identification with FDR and his right-wing ideology by denying his past, he did so by insisting that he and Roosevelt shared the same conservative outlook. To this end he kept on hand a cache of FDR quotes to be drawn upon at his pleasure, and often with little regard for the facts. For example, he did not hesitate to claim that Roosevelt "said the federal government had no business trying to regulate banks."[22] By citing isolated sentences from Roosevelt's Albany days or wrenching statements from his White House years out of context, Reagan suggested that there was a continuity between his policies and FDR's because, he contended, both were hostile to the emergence of a powerful national government. One would never guess from the parallels Reagan drew that this was the same Roosevelt who expanded the national state, made Wall Street answerable to Washington, placed a host of industries under federal regulation, and introduced the welfare state.

There is no clearer instance of Reagan's distortion of Roosevelt's record than his frequent citation of a sentence from a presidential message of January 1935 to prove that his attitude toward the unemployed was consistent with FDR's. In 1976 Reagan told a correspondent that Roosevelt "said the federal government should get out of the business of welfare," and he was still maintaining at the end of 1981: "Roosevelt at one time made a statement that the Federal Government had to get out of the business of—we didn't call it 'welfare' then, we called it 'relief.'"[23] One would suppose that Reagan, with a vivid memory of a father who headed a WPA operation, could not help knowing how altogether misleading this allusion is.

Roosevelt did say, "The Federal Government must and shall quit this business of relief," but he said it in a message to Congress in which he called for a massive federal works program to give the able-bodied jobless not "relief" but "employment" through the biggest peacetime appropriation in the history of this or any other nation. In quoting the sentence he was so fond of citing, Reagan neglected to point out what Roosevelt said next:

> The Federal Government is the only governmental agency with sufficient power and credit to meet this situation. We have assumed this task and we shall not shrink from it in the future. It is a duty dictated by every intelligent consideration of national policy to ask you to make it possible for the United States to give employment to all of these three and one half million employable people now on relief.

Congress responded with a multibillion-dollar appropriation that made possible the creation of the WPA and the NYA. To help those who were not employable, Roosevelt submitted an unprecedented social insurance proposal and less than eight months later Congress made good his promise by enacting his plan into law: the landmark Social Security Act of 1935.[24]

When Reagan has admitted to consciousness the fact that Roosevelt did preside over a vast expansion of governmental authority, he has insisted that FDR intended this departure only as a temporary expedient, and that after the war he planned to sound retreat. Typically, Reagan reached this conclusion not by careful study of the data but from hearsay. "I have known his sons for years," he said at the end of 1981. "I know from their own conversations about what he believed. . . . Had he lived, and with the war over, we would have seen him using government the other way." It did not occur to him that what he had heard reflected the latter-day conservatism of two of Roosevelt's sons (FDR, Jr., felt quite differently), or that there was overwhelming contrary evidence. As Arthur Schlesinger, Jr., pointed out in rejoinder, Roosevelt had clearly expressed his intentions for the postwar world in his 1944 State of the Union address. In that message the president outlined an "economic bill of rights," and said:

> After this war is won, we must be prepared to move forward . . . to new goals of human happiness and well-being. . . . Our fighting men abroad— and their families at home—expect such a program and have the right to insist upon it. It is to their demands that the Government should pay heed rather than to the whining demands of selfish pressure groups who seek to feather their nests while young Americans are dying.[25]

Reagan could hardly deny that there had been a transformation in the age of Roosevelt which carried into the postwar era, but he attributed this legacy not to the president but to the men about him, for he never wanted to blame the idol of his youth for anything.[26] Even when he pointed out that FDR had run in 1932 on a promise of retrenchment, he could not bring himself to find fault with him. "I'm not saying that he turned around," Reagan said. "I believe that Franklin Roosevelt believed in our federal system of sovereign states." Nor did he hold FDR responsible for the leviathan in Washington. "President Roosevelt started administering medicine to a sick patient, but those people who then gathered around and became the structure of government had no intention of letting the patient get well and cut him off the medicine," he asserted. "Their goal was supreme centralized authority." After noting the allegedly statist view of such men as Harold Ickes, he added, "Well, I don't believe that that was really in Roosevelt's mind." One gathers that people like Ickes somehow slipped into government offices and assumed positions of power when Roosevelt's back was turned.[27]

In the spring of 1976 Reagan bought himself a pack of trouble by carrying his charges about FDR's statist advisers to the point of absurdity. He told an interviewer: "Fascism was really the basis for the New

Deal. It was Mussolini's success in Italy, with his government-directed economy, that led the early New Dealers to say, 'But Mussolini kept the trains running on time.'"[28] The remarks did not draw much attention when they were made, but in the 1980 campaign they would be taken up by Democrats seeking to forestall Reagan's attempt to "kidnap Franklin Roosevelt."

At the 1980 Democratic convention Teddy Kennedy drew the delegates out of their chairs applauding and yelling when he charged that "the same Republicans who are invoking Franklin Roosevelt have nominated a man who said in 1976, and these are his exact words: 'Fascism was really the basis of the New Deal.' And that nominee, whose name is Ronald Reagan, has no right to quote Franklin Delano Roosevelt." In commenting on Kennedy's address, a *New Republic* editor remarked, "Kennedy . . . eviscerated Ronald Reagan, of course, making the most of some wonderful nuggets of negative research. . . . The Reagan quotation that 'fascism was really the basis of the New Deal' should shut Reagan's mouth forever in attempting to invoke the name of Franklin Roosevelt as a new Republican deity."[29]

Two days later Fritz Mondale, in another rousing speech to the convention, also paid his respects to the Republicans and to Reagan's attempt to appropriate the FDR legend. "They spoke of truth—and said Franklin Roosevelt caused World War II," he said disapprovingly. The vice-president went on:

> All of a sudden we are told the Republican Party is for jobs. The Party that gave us both the Great Depression, and the highest unemployment since then, would have us believe they're now for the working people and are leaving no one behind.
>
> I've been in politics for many years, and I've noticed that the closer Republican oratory moves to Franklin Roosevelt, the closer their policies move to Herbert Hoover.

As for the GOP candidate, "Only if he destroyed the Social Security system and all who depend on it—only then would the job be done." Mondale declared: "It's hard to believe that anyone—even Ronald Reagan—would actually do that. After all, what kind of person would try to wipe out every program since Roosevelt? He'd have to be a person who believes, 'Fascism was really the basis for the New Deal.' Who would ever say something like that? Ronald Reagan."[30]

Reagan would have been well advised to let Mondale's reminder of his earlier misstatement lie, but when newspapermen questioned him about the pounding he had taken at the Democratic convention, he insisted on repeating it. "Anyone who wants to look at the writings of the members of the brain trust of the New Deal will find that President Roosevelt's advisers admired the fascist system," he declared. With an abandon that revealed what he truly thought of the New Dealers, he added, "They coined the expression that Mussolini made the trains run on time. They thought that private ownership with government management and control à la the Italian system was the way to go and that has been evident in all their writings."[31]

In truth, such allegations rested on the flimsiest grounds. Even the most uncritical admirer of the New Deal would acknowledge that the head of the NRA, the idiosyncratic Hugh Johnson, did once sign a "proclamation" with the pseudonym "Muscleinny," and that there are certain resemblances between the NRA and corporatism. But John P. Diggins, the author of the definitive study of the impact of Mussolini on America, has stated flatly, "Hugh Johnson notwithstanding, the published writings of the Brain Trusters reveal no evidence of the influence of Italian Fascism upon the New Deal," and he has denied "that Roosevelt was in any way influenced by Mussolini or that the New Deal was a bastard of the Corporate State." Corporatism, *Fortune* pointed out in the second year of the New Deal, was "probably less well known in America than the geography of Tibet." The claim that Mussolini made the trains run on time was a commonplace long before the New Deal and it was advanced not by liberals but by the right, by the men who would be FDR's fiercest critics. Mussolini himself was disappointed by Roosevelt's refusal to embrace fascism, while Roosevelt was an instinctive democrat who viewed Mussolini's strutting and bombast with contempt.[32]

How can one account for the fact that Reagan blundered so badly? Only by his extraordinary hostility to government and his inability to distinguish between totalitarianism and social democracy. Throughout the world in the 1930s, the pace of government intervention quickened, but the contrast between Italy and Germany on the one hand and such countries as the United States, Great Britain, and Sweden on the other was one not of degree but of kind. No recital of contrary evidence, though, would persuade Reagan to abandon his tale—that FDR was a heroic statesman, much to be admired, who came close to bringing fascism to America.

IV

All of Reagan's declarations served to obfuscate the truth, which is not that Reagan had been a one-time-only FDR supporter, not that

Roosevelt had been a fellow conservative, not that the New Dealers had derived their ideas from Mussolini, but that sometime in the 1950s Reagan radically altered his political colors. To cover up this fact Reagan again sought to rewrite the past. Even when he conceded that he became alienated from the Roosevelt program, he pushed the moment of changeover much earlier in time than is credible and ascribed to himself motivations that do not bear scrutiny.

Reagan, never at a loss for explanations, offered more than one reason for his departure from the Democratic party and its New Deal emphases. Sometimes he traced his estrangement to memories of his father "coming home day after day so frustrated that you wouldn't believe it" because relief agency bureaucrats were more interested in preserving a system of handouts than getting their "clients" back to work. At other times he said that his growing suspicion of centralized government increased during World War II, when civil service regulations restrained him, as base personnel officer at Culver City, from firing civilian employees who he thought should be dismissed. Yet neither of these recollections explained why he voted for Roosevelt all four times and remained a "hemophilic liberal" in the postwar period. He may well have had "some misgivings," as he claimed in his autobiography. More to the point, though, was his frank acknowledgment, "I had followed FDR blindly."[33]

On still other occasions Reagan has said that his encounters with the Stalinists changed his political complexion. When Jimmy Roosevelt asked the board of the Hollywood Independent Citizens Committee of Arts, Sciences, and Professions to adopt an anticommunist resolution, Reagan came to his aid, only to be denounced as "capitalist scum" and "enemy of the proletariat." He later said, "Light was dawning in some obscure region in my head. I was beginning to see the seamy side of liberalism," a curious statement given the fact that Jimmy Roosevelt had provided the leadership and that his colleagues in ADA took a strong stand against communism.[34] Furthermore, not for some time after his ICCASP days did he abandon his liberal associates and join the ranks of the conservatives.

One cannot say with confidence what brought about this shift, save that it seems to have been related to his economic circumstances. A man of considerable wealth from movie contracts and land investment, he came to resent the bite federal taxes took from his income. He felt adversely affected, too, by the Truman administration's antitrust suit against the movie studios, and during the four months he spent in England in 1949 filming *The Hasty Heart* he became irritated at such vexations of the new social order as the restriction on the amount of currency he could take home with him. Furthermore, the switch came at a time when his life was breaking up—his first marriage had ended in divorce, his career was fading.[35]

In this critical period of readjustment Reagan signed up with General Electric, and once he became part of the GE team the outcome could not be in doubt. He contracted not only to introduce the weekly General Electric Theater and appear in some of its presentations but also to tour the country for ten weeks each year on behalf of the firm. As a pitchman for GE he told the business audiences what they wanted to hear, and as a biographer has observed, "Reagan believes in what he says, and he wound up believing what he was saying."[36]

Once converted, Reagan became more Catholic than the pope. On his speaking tour of GE's 135 plants he established a reputation as an unrestrained critic of the New Deal and all its works. "He questioned every social program enacted since 1932," notes one of his biographers. Reagan was especially vehement in his objections to government electrical programs, from the TVA to the REA. "Except among the die-hard right wing, debate had ceased in American life over such accepted plans as social security and the progressive income tax," a writer observed. "Reagan was now intent on reviving that debate."[37]

Reagan's fulminations against the Tennessee Valley Authority proved to be a liability. When it was pointed out that GE was doing a multimillion-dollar business with the TVA, Reagan's employer told him to pipe down, and when he persisted in preaching the conservative gospel, the firm canceled his program. His hostility to the TVA cost him even more dearly in 1976, when he was locked in a close race with Gerald Ford for the Republican presidential nomination. Asked what he thought of the idea of selling the TVA to private industry, Reagan replied, "It would be something to look at." In his memoirs Gerald Ford wrote: "'It would be something to look at'—my campaign aides seized upon that with glee. . . . The TVA 'issue' turned things around for me in Tennessee, which I won by fewer than 2,200 votes. It probably helped me as well in Kentucky."[38]

Through all of this, Reagan continued to draw on his memory of Roosevelt, but selectively. He recalled the FDR who promised budget balancing in 1932, who fashioned a winning political coalition, who forged a strong foreign policy, and who was, as Reagan thought himself to be, a great communicator. He quite forgot the Roosevelt who expressed concern for "one-third of a nation ill-housed, ill-clad, ill-nourished." When he quoted from FDR, he turned his words to markedly dissimilar ends. Where Roosevelt had spoken of "the forgotten man at the bottom of the economic pyramid," Reagan offered himself as the champion of "the forgotten American, the man in the suburbs working sixty hours a week to support his family and being taxed heavily for the benefit of someone else."[39]

In 1964 he got maximum exposure for these ideas when he delivered what to Reagan watchers became known as "the Speech," a calcification of all of the random thoughts he had been experimenting with for the past dozen years. Released from GE's restraints, he felt free to take out after the TVA without reservation, though that was an agency, he acknowledged, that was "considered above criticism, sacred as motherhood." In other segments of "the Speech," he piled abuse on Roosevelt-style programs in areas ranging from agriculture to public housing to social welfare. He concluded, as he would in 1980, with a "rendezvous with destiny" quotation from Franklin Roosevelt, but he gave it a diametrically opposite meaning from the one FDR had given it. Where Roosevelt summoned the nation to set an example to the world by democratic social action, Reagan warned of the slippery slope into statist tyranny.

In the years after 1964 Reagan's attitude hardened. He continued to view Senator Goldwater not as a right-wing extremist but as a man gifted with foresight. "There's no question," he told a reporter, "Goldwater tried to tell us some things that maybe eleven years ago we weren't ready to hear. We still were wrapped in the New Deal syndrome of believing that government could do all these things for us." At the end of 1981, he stated, "I would have to say . . . that . . . the problem of the Great Depression . . . was not solved by any of the so-called New Deal panaceas."[40] By then it was clear that it was not the Democrats who had changed but Reagan, and that Ronald Reagan had come a long way since that autumn day in 1936 when, as a young radio announcer, he had cheered FDR, the protagonist of the New Deal, through the streets of Des Moines.

v

While repudiating the New Deal legacy of the age of Roosevelt, Reagan continued to identify himself with FDR. In campaigning for the presidency in 1980 he made good use of his larder of Roosevelt quotations, not just in his acceptance address but throughout the year. Noting that Carter had cited Roosevelt in a trip to Michigan at the beginning of October, Elizabeth Drew wrote, "Perhaps he and Reagan are competing over who mentions him more often." It was a duel in which Reagan had Carter at a disadvantage. Recalling how Roosevelt had not only saddled Hoover with the blame for hard times but had taught a whole generation of Americans to associate "Republican" with "Depression," Reagan sought to carry out another political revolution by charging that the country was in "a new Depression—the Carter Depression," and by implying that Carter was a Hoover who could not cope. As one of his biographers has written, "Reagan set out in 1980 to achieve a '1932' in reverse." At the victory celebration following the November election, Reagan made remarks that it was said sounded "a subliminal echo of Franklin Delano Roosevelt," and during the inter-regnum and while in the White House, Reagan comported himself in a manner that again and again invited comparison to FDR.[41]

Reagan's identification with Roosevelt served him in several ways. It associated him with the last president historians have placed in the "great" category. It permitted him to leap over comparison to more recent predecessors such as Nixon or to ideologues such as Goldwater which would have been awkward. It suggested that, like FDR, Reagan would inaugurate an era, construct an enduring political coalition, con-tribute an imaginative domestic agenda, and originate a foreign policy that would reshape the world. And it reassured those of his Democratic followers who continued to have warm memories of the Roosevelt of their youth though they had subsequently come to prefer stability to social change.

As Reagan's most recent biographer has written perceptively:

> Culturally, he remained a Democrat who drew his metaphors and inspira-tion from the New Deal. Other Republican politicians spoke to the major-ity of the electorate as outsiders, trying to induce Democrats to come over to their side. Reagan spoke as an insider. Though he had left the party of Franklin Roosevelt, he refused to abandon the words and phrases which provided a shared language and a common bond with his fellow citizens. When Reagan spoke, ordinary Americans did not have to make the mental translation usually required for conservative Republican speakers. He un-dermined the New Deal in its own vernacular. . . . Reagan's speeches were peppered with . . . borrowings from Roosevelt, whose words and memo-ries stoked hidden fires of approval and patriotism among American work-ing men and women.[42]

Reagan presented himself as Rooseveltian, however, not in order to perpetuate FDR's political tradition but for exactly the opposite pur-pose: to dismantle the Roosevelt coalition. "Once an ardent apostle of F.D.R., Reagan had closely studied the ways his former hero had formed the coalition that had produced his unprecedented success in politics," a biographer has written. "After long research and reflection,

Reagan had determined how he would assemble his own coalition to create a Conservative Age." Not only Reagan but the men around him cultivated the impression that the 1980 campaign was destined to bring about a realignment comparable to that effected by Roosevelt in the 1930s. "Reagan is like Roosevelt, the activist who restored hope after Hoover's failure to overcome the Depression," said Congressman Jack F. Kemp. "But Reagan's activism is in the private sector, rather than in spending public funds as F.D.R. did." Like Roosevelt, Kemp declared, Reagan would create a new majority party by adding to the Republican core disaffected independents and blue-collar Democrats.[43]

More than any other prominent Republican, Kemp publicized the idea that Reagan was the architect of a new political era as FDR had been a generation before. "There is a tidal wave coming equivalent to the one that hit in 1932, when an era of Republican dominance gave way to the New Deal," he predicted in 1979. "Is it crazy to suggest this?" he asked, then pointed out that blacks who had once seemed wedded forever to the party of Lincoln had been persuaded by Roosevelt to switch parties because "Hoover offered a balanced budget, and FDR offered buttered bread." He concluded, "Just wait. It will not be long before the Democrats are forced to preach hellfire and damnation against a tidal wave of blacks voting for the GOP and growth." After the 1980 election, the congressman claimed, "Ronald Reagan and a new Republican majority in the U.S. Senate were swept into office in 1980 on the crest of such a wave. Like Roosevelt in 1932, Reagan offered the hope of a better future at a time of crisis."[44]

Across a wide political spectrum, politicians and journalists shared Kemp's view of the significance of the election. "The old coalition that has given the party its strength since the days of Franklin D. Roosevelt completely shattered at Tuesday's election," asserted a writer in the *Washington Post,* while the *Christian Science Monitor* headlined its election feature: "Reagan era begins, New Deal era ebbs." More surprisingly, a number of present and former Democratic senators agreed. Gary Hart thought people were "weary of the old New Deal approach"; Sam Ervin believed the country had "been running on New Deal programs for too many years and the people got tired of them"; and Paul Tsongas said bluntly, "Basically, the New Deal died yesterday."[45]

Some of these same observers, though, anticipated that Reagan, the purported destroyer of the Roosevelt coalition, would follow FDR's style once he took office. The *New York Post* featured Reagan's victory under the banner, "I have a rendezvous with destiny, he told America 16 yrs. ago," a phrase, it explained, he had borrowed from "an early Democratic idol, FDR," and in December Congressman Kemp again predicted, "He's going to be the Franklin Delano Roosevelt of the Republican Party." On the eve of Reagan's inauguration Ronald Steel observed:

> He is not F.D.R. and the times are very different. But Reagan himself has drawn a parallel to F.D.R. The political model of this man of the resurgent right is the hero of the liberal left. The revealing references to Roosevelt in his campaign speeches were not mere genuflections. Name another Republican politician who extols the greatest Democratic vote-getter of all time. Reagan's evocations express the admiration of a man who once glimpsed a leader he could believe in—a leader with vision, and the inner strength to pursue that vision. Like so many men of his generation, indeed like Lyndon B. Johnson, who said he modeled himself on F.D.R., Reagan learned from Roosevelt the possibilities of the Presidency.[46]

Though there were striking contrasts between the America of 1981 and that at the end of the Hoover era, some of the most thoughtful analysts were even more impressed by how alike they were. In the feature article of a national economic survey supplement published by the *New York Times,* Leonard Silk wrote:

> As an unconventional conservative, Mr. Reagan sees the challenge facing him as comparable to that which confronted the liberal Franklin D. Roosevelt in 1933. This year will mark the start of an experiment to resolve a national economic crisis that is comparable to the program begun by the New Deal nearly half a century ago.
>
> Now, as then, a new President senses that the nation is plagued by anxiety over its economic future and knows that a key part of the job of reconstruction will be psychological. Mr. Roosevelt's unforgettable rallying cry was, "We have nothing to fear but fear itself," and Mr. Reagan has not hesitated to quote him. . . .
>
> The present situation is not as grim and urgent as the one which Mr. Roosevelt sought to resolve 50 years ago, when one-fourth of the labor force was jobless. But, for the longer run, stagflation threatens America's economic strength as seriously as did depression in the 1930's.[47]

Much of this preinaugural speculation derived from the brouhaha aroused by a memo written by Kemp and the incoming budget director, David A. Stockman, recommending that Reagan put through an emergency program modeled on FDR's first hundred days immediately upon taking office. Additionally, the president-elect's counselor, Edwin Meese III, stated that though he did not "contemplate at this point anything as drastic as closing the banks, or even the stock exchange," as in 1933, he did foresee "major executive steps." In response a columnist wrote:

> What's going on here? GOP calls for another New Deal? In terms of substance, of programs, certainly not. But in terms of political psychology, exactly that. . . . Ronald Reagan is being urged to follow, or advised not to follow, the FDR example: seize the moment of national discontent, draw at once and heavily on his election mandate, dominate Congress with a flood of specific legislative requests and a flurry of executive actions, push through a comprehensive economic program in those first 100 days of the new administration.[48]

Reagan did not choose to follow the course outlined in the Kemp-Stockman memo in precise detail but that did not dampen the enthusiasm of writers bent on finding congruities. One historian wrote of Reagan's inaugural address: "It is the ghost of Franklin Roosevelt which hovers over this speech; Reagan, today a conservative Republican, was once a liberal, New Deal Democrat. Thus it is not surprising that the new chief executive chose to devote the opening of his speech to the economic crisis presently facing this nation, much in the same manner that F.D.R. delivered his first inaugural address in the shadow of the Great Depression."[49]

That spring, Reagan's hundredth day in office brought on another round of comparisons. In London a writer in *The Observer* found it odd that without fail the media were comparing Reagan's first hundred days to FDR's though Reagan sought to obliterate the Roosevelt record, and in truth American correspondents had become altogether entranced by the similarity they perceived. In a representative piece assessing "the most dramatic first 100 days since FDR," a White House correspondent for the *New York Times* wrote:

> With a gift for political theater, Mr. Reagan has established his goals faster, communicated a greater sense of economic urgency and come forward with more comprehensive proposals than any new President since the first 100 days of Franklin D. Roosevelt, the hero of his youth and the man whose record of achieving social change Mr. Reagan seeks to emulate—albeit at the opposite end of the political spectrum.
>
> In Rooseveltian fashion, Mr. Reagan has commanded the attention of the public, the Congress and America's allies and adversaries.[50]

The press analogized the experiences of the two presidents even when their programs were quite dissimilar. Under the headline "F. D.

Reagan calls America to his side," the *New York Daily News* reported that the new president had delivered an economic message "in a style reminiscent of Franklin Delano Roosevelt's fireside chats," and *Newsweek* featured the same program under the banner "RWR's Own New Deal," though "RWR," patently an imitation of "FDR," never caught on. *Newsweek* reported: "Barely a month into his Presidency, Ronald Wilson Reagan asked America last week to follow him on a decisive right turn in its history—a second New Deal potentially as profound in its import as the first was a half century ago." Even Reagan's courageous behavior after he had been wounded by a would-be assassin was likened to FDR's response to the attempt on his life in Miami in February 1933.[51]

Comparison of Roosevelt and Reagan became particularly commonplace in 1982, the centennial year of FDR's birth, and it sometimes took an unusual form. A compilation by Ross Baker, a Rutgers political science professor, attracted attention in the nation's press. Baker noted that the two presidents were the same height and weight (6 foot 2, 190 pounds); that each reached the White House after serving as governor of the most populous state; that both pledged to balance the budget and failed; that Roosevelt named the first female cabinet member and Reagan the first woman justice. Still, Baker acknowledged, there was one fundamental difference: "When FDR was Reagan's age, he'd been dead for eight years."[52]

By 1982 commentators had become so carried away by matching the two men as to suggest that Reagan's assault on liberal programs actually served to safeguard Roosevelt's policies. "Folks laughed in 1980 when Reagan invoked FDR's name," wrote George F. Will, "but in 1981 he began doing for the welfare state what FDR did for capitalism: saving it by tempering its excesses." His biographer took this idea still further. "Reagan may turn out to be the salvation of the New Deal much as his idol Franklin Roosevelt proved the savior of capitalism," Lou Cannon asserted. "He was a conservative, but one who was conserving the New Deal. Like Roosevelt, he saw himself as a force of history. Like Roosevelt, he was anathema to those whom his policies ultimately benefited most."[53]

Any other right-wing Republican would have bristled at such a suggestion, but Reagan welcomed it. When the National Conference of Christians and Jews voted him its annual gold medal for "courageous leadership in government, civic and humanitarian affairs," a mob of 10,000 protesters, shocked at the granting of an award to a man who had been slashing government funds for social programs, created a monster traffic jam outside the New York hotel where Reagan accepted the honor. At the banquet, the president, responding to the criticism, said:

> Today, I'm accused by some of trying to destroy government's commit-ment to compassion and to the needy.
> Does this bother me? Yes. Like FDR, may I say I'm not trying to destroy what is best in our system of humane, free government—I'm doing everything I can to save it: to slow down the destructive rate of growth in taxes and spending; to prune non-essential programs so that enough re-sources will be left to meet the requirements of the truly needy.[54]

VI

Like the jeering demonstrators outside the New York hotel, a num-ber of scholars denied that Reagan had any right to claim descent from Roosevelt. Yes, said the economist Robert Lekachman, Reagan's pro-gram was just like Roosevelt's New Deal, "with the trifling difference that FDR sought to alleviate poverty and Ronald Reagan enthusi-astically enriches further the already obscenely rich." Another promi-nent economist, Paul Samuelson, declared, "For 40 years since Roose-velt's New Deal America has been seeking a more humane society—a welfare state. . . . Now Ronald Reagan seeks to end that trend." Simi-larly, a historian commented, "More ludicrous than talk of similarities to the Depression are comparisons of Mr. Reagan and Franklin D. Roosevelt. F.D.R.'s supporters rode in freight cars, Mr. Reagan's travel in Lear jets; F.D.R.'s people stood in soup lines, Mr. Reagan's stand at cocktail parties; F.D.R.'s backers sold apples on street corners, Mr. Reagan's are more likely to sell real estate in Orange County, Califor-nia." Reagan, observed another historian, FDR's biographer Frank Freidel, raises "difficult questions when he tries to remodel President Roosevelt into his own image. . . . The Franklin D. Roosevelt of the centennial celebration should not be transformed into a Ronald Roosevelt."[55]

Commentators scoffed at the idea that Reagan's first three months in office resembled FDR's. After describing the scene when Roosevelt entered the White House, "TRB" in the *New Republic* observed, "Peo-ple compare that to Ronald Reagan's 100 Days. How silly can you get?" To be sure, he went on, in 1981 as in 1933 the country had a personable president, and on both occasions nobody was sure what ailed the econ-omy. But there the resemblance ended. With business in the saddle, "what is happening now is a kind of counter-New Deal, an anti-Roosevelt." The columnist David Broder noted yet another distinction. "Franklin D. Roosevelt, who is in so many ways a model for Reagan, took a wholly pragmatic view, experimenting with a variety of programs to cure the Depression that fit no consistent economic theory," he observed, whereas Reagan was placing all his bets on a single doctrine.[56]

Washington writers assigned to cover the president pointed out that far from seeking to perpetuate the New Deal, Reagan sought to end it. On the day of Reagan's inauguration, Hedrick Smith in a feature article in the *New York Times* called the new president "the first missionary conservative to gain the White House with the aim of reversing the liberal New Deal revolution of government activism and Democratic Party dominance established by Franklin D. Roosevelt nearly half a century ago." With "that same jaunty, smiling self-confidence of Mr. Roosevelt," Reagan was "preaching the gospel that 'government is not the solution, government is the problem.'" In the months that followed, reporters observed that whenever Reagan cited FDR, an action contrary to the spirit of the New Deal was sure to ensue. By August a columnist could write, "He is a president who has just completed repealing the New Deal." If this was an exaggeration, it was closer to the line of direction of the Reagan administration than the claim that he was the savior of FDR's policies.[57]

Indeed, not a few critics suggested that Reagan resembled Roosevelt less than FDR's ill-remembered adversary. When in February 1982 Reagan arrived in Minneapolis for the first Republican rally of the new year, he was greeted by a placard proclaiming "Welcome President Hoover" as hundreds of demonstrators turned out in bitter subzero cold, while in Lafayette Park, across from the White House, protesters set up a tent city of homeless people which they named Reaganville to evoke memories of the Hoovervilles of the Great Depression. "If things continue, there is a fair chance that Ronald Reagan will be our second Herbert Hoover—elected in triumph, thrown out in ignominy," wrote Robert Heilbroner. No less scathing was an editorial in the *New York Times* early in 1982. "In one sense, the President has truly become Franklin Delano Reagan," the *Times* asserted. "Knight of the balanced budget, archenemy of Federal borrowing, he is now the premier deficit spender of all time." In another sense, though, it said, "the President has become Ronald Hoover," for he was seeking to turn back the clock to a day when the problems of the nation's economy were not dealt with by the federal government but were Balkanized by being dumped on the states.[58]

A month after the Minneapolis demonstration, an address to the annual convention of Americans for Democratic Action by the Democratic congresswoman from Maryland, Barbara Mikulski, reflected growing resentment at Reagan's claim to be faithful to the memory of Roosevelt. "FDR's life, his administration, and his devotion to a decent life for all Americans are still the standards by which we judge presidents and administrations now," she declared. The "simple human kindness" of Franklin and Eleanor, she continued, pointed up the essential difference between the New Deal and Reagan's New Federalism: "one was warm and human, flawed but bold; the other is cold and mechanical, flawed and unfeeling." "What a far cry," she said, were FDR's humane concerns from "a President who believes in coddling the wealthy and condemning the poor." Noting that the first lady wore "$1000 designer gowns when welfare families are only allowed $1000 for all they have in the world," she etched a caricature of "Mrs. Reagan in her gown, and her china, and her hairdo that never seems to move. . . . The contrast to Eleanor Roosevelt is poignant and sad."[59]

If such comments sounded strident, that was because liberal Democrats were coming to a most unwelcome conclusion: Reagan was getting away with it. It did not matter that there was a wealth of evidence demonstrating that the 1980 election was not a rejection of the New Deal. It did not matter that there was even more proof that Reagan had turned away from Roosevelt's ideas a full generation before. It did not even matter that before the eyes of the entire nation Reagan was approaching modern-day problems in the spirit of FDR's onetime enemies. Despite all of this, Reagan had managed to persuade a significant sector of opinion that in style and even in substance he was a latter-day Franklin Roosevelt. So contrary was this notion to reality that one might register it as the greatest sleight-of-hand of modern American politics, save for one thing. No one believed it more sincerely than Ronald Reagan.

VII

January 20, 1982, marked the centennial of Franklin D. Roosevelt's birth, and it could not have come at a worse time. No one seemed to care, not even the Democrats. Carter never lifted a finger to plan for an occasion that many anticipated would fall early in his second term. Even the veterans of the New Deal were resigned to letting the day pass largely unnoticed. Late in the Carter administration, at a luncheon meeting in the State Department which brought together such notables as Secretary of State Edmund Muskie, Franklin D. Roosevelt, Jr.,

Tommy Corcoran, Averell Harriman, Jim Rowe, and Grace Tully, agreement was universal that it was too late to do anything of significance. And the birthday, it seemed, would arrive altogether unpropitiously with a right-wing Republican in the White House.[60]

The more choleric of Reagan's fellow conservatives left no doubt as to how they felt about the occasion. In the fall of 1981, *Source,* the publication of the Republican National Committee, called a proposed FDR memorial an "eyesore" and denounced Roosevelt as "the great chiseler," and in the very month of the centennial observance Roosevelt was blamed for Poland's distress because of his actions at Yalta and was being flayed for the excesses of the bureaucracy. As one writer said, "It is as if FDR had been holed up all these years at Federal Trade Commission headquarters spinning new regulations to cripple the captains of industry." In a sardonic commentary the *National Review* summed up the conservative attitude:

> Some Chicago lout had to go and notice that we are coming up on the centennial of Franklin D. Roosevelt's birth (January 30, 1982), so now all the gears are grinding toward a year-long, tax-financed celebration of the event. Not inappropriately, the lout picked up a $200,000 federal grant to plan it. If the celebration is truly to be in the FDR mold, it will be bureaucratic, Cabinet-rank, unconstitutional, more expensive than any before, and perpetual so that our children's children can help pay for it a hundred years from now.[61]

In fact, had it not been for the efforts of the "Chicago lout," there would have been no national observance, and even then the recognition was grudging. Unable to believe that no one was doing anything to commemorate Roosevelt's birth, a young Chicagoan, Peter Kovler, took it upon himself to mobilize the country and virtually single-handedly carried it off. Congress, however, stipulated that the cost of a joint session in FDR's honor could not exceed $25,000, though a Democratic-controlled Congress in 1974 had appropriated $7 million for the centenary of Herbert Hoover's birth. From only one official quarter was the response altogether openhearted. Others might be mean-spirited or indifferent, but Ronald Reagan did not intend to let the day go by without paying tribute to FDR in the grand manner.

When the celebrants who had been attending the joint session of Congress arrived at the White House, they found that President Reagan had arranged a joyous fête. As they filed in to lunch to the fox-trot beat of a red-coated Marine band, they walked into a brilliantly lit room where each table was beautifully set with White House china, bright bouquets of tulips gracing every table. Nor had the president stinted on the meal: lobster bisque, supreme of chicken Véronique with wild rice, a praline ice cream mold surmounted by an American eagle, all accompanied by a Château St.-Jean Chardonnay 1980. Gathered there that day were people who had served under the shadow cast by FDR in every administration from Truman through Carter. None, though, showed any more enthusiasm for Roosevelt's natal day than the president of the United States.

Into a room buzzing with talk of earlier times strode the president, handsome, red-cheeked, smiling radiantly in a manner that signaled that here was no chief executive dutifully carrying out a ritual in honor of a leader of a rival sect but a man who altogether shared the sentiments of his guests and was pleased by the opportunity to say so. FDR, Reagan declared, was "one of history's truly monumental figures," "an American giant, a leader who shaped, inspired and led our people in perilous times." The president adroitly linked himself to his predecessor by quoting Walter Lippmann's notorious 1932 sentence about FDR's being a pleasant fellow with no conspicuous qualifications for the office and then saying, "I think I have been hearing an echo," a remark that drew good-natured laughter from the Roosevelt partisans. He went on to repeat the comment of the one member remaining from the Hundred Days Congress of 1933, Jennings Randolph of West Virginia, who had said that FDR made everyone feel "I count."

The president recalled fondly that day in 1936 when he had seen Roosevelt riding through the streets of Des Moines in an open-top car. "What a wave of affection and enthusiasm swept through that crowd," he remembered, "drawing from us a reservoir of affection that we did not know we felt in those hard times." Only obliquely did he lay claim to carrying on FDR's ideas; Americans, he stated, always know "when things have gone too far—when it is time for fundamental change." The theme of his message was of a different sort—that it was from Franklin Roosevelt on that day in Des Moines that he had first gained a sense of the majesty of the office he now held. At the end of his gracious remarks the president raised his glass in a toast, and as everyone in the room rose he said, "Happy days, now, again, and always."[62]

Six months later Reagan brought his allegiance to FDR to a climax, or anticlimax. In July 1982 he signed into law an authorization for a garden wall monument to FDR to be built in the Tidal Basin. Thus the long-frustrated campaign to give Roosevelt a fitting memorial, an effort that had failed under every Democratic president, that the Carter administration had flatly rejected, was carried to fruition by this paladin of the Republican right. On the following day newspapers carried detailed descriptions of how the well-designed memorial park would appear. Only one thing wrong. Not a penny was to be appropriated for the project that year, nor could anyone foresee when the money would come. No expression of the baffling, labyrinthine relationship of Ronald Reagan and Franklin Roosevelt could have been more fitting.

[8]

Waiting for Franklin D.

I

There is an Illinois legend that for an entire year after Lincoln died, in April 1865, no brown thrush sang. FDR's death on an April day eighty years later reminded many people of that earlier event and brought a comparable sense of deprivation. Each president had been taken in the final days of a great war, his work not quite completed. Each had achieved so much that the ensuing generation was left with a sharp awareness of living in a "post-heroic age," in George Forgie's phrase, an era "shaped by the memory of the revolutionary age that preceded it." In the Illinois capital of Springfield legislators have sensed Lincoln's brooding spirit, and for the past generation Americans, looking back toward the age of Roosevelt, have felt "nostalgia for a lost presence." More than a quarter of a century after that April day in 1945, Rexford Tugwell said of FDR, "'What would he have done?' is still a relevant question."[1]

Writing in 1971, nearly four decades after he had first become a member of the Brain Trust, Tugwell declared that the history of the postwar world "was drastically different than it would have been if [FDR] had lived." Roosevelt had died at sixty-three, much too young. If he had been granted twelve more years, "he would have finished out his fourth term and had a fifth and a sixth." Even if he had enjoyed only eight more years, the world would have been spared the disaster of Truman and perhaps Eisenhower, Tugwell said. To be sure, "he survived in people's memory, a standard for his successors; but, much as they might be granted for effort, they failed." Ever since his death the world had gone "off course," Tugwell concluded. "For him, death may have had no sting; for those who were left it did."[2]

Even when commentators were less fanciful and more fair-minded than Tugwell, FDR's successors have never been able to escape unflattering comparisons, though there was no way that they could reasonably have been expected to match Roosevelt's record. No president could ever again introduce the welfare state. None, after the Constitution was amended, could ever again serve as long as FDR. None, in an atomic age, could anticipate fighting a world war through to the kind of victory achieved in 1945. None could be the first to lead the country out of isolation into a United Nations and a dominant role in world affairs. In short, each of the chief executives since Roosevelt's death has been, in Sainte-Beuve's phrase, a "late-comer" who bore the special disadvantage of coming directly after an eminent figure. As Pliny observed, "The burthen of government is increased upon princes by the virtues of their immediate predecessors."[3]

II

Men of letters have been especially attuned to the kinds of disadvantages that successors face, for they have concentrated much of their attention on a single question: How can one find scope for one's talents when so much has already been achieved? Though their focus is on "the burden of the past" for the poet, their comments are no less pertinent in the political sphere.

"When a great poet has lived," T. S. Eliot has said, "certain things have been done once for all, and cannot be achieved again." That lament has been a persistent one among writers and artists. Robert Burton complained that "we can say nothing but what has been said," and Thomas Carew regretted that there were naught but "rifled fields" from which all the "buds of invention" had been taken. The situation, La Bruyère grumbled, left a writer with two choices: resort to "forced conceits" to make one's mark or slavish imitation of predecessors. The latter was the more likely course. Robert Louis Stevenson could speak for many others when he confessed, "I have . . . played the sedulous ape to Hazlitt, to Lamb, to Wordsworth, to Sir Thomas Browne, to Defoe, to Hawthorne, to Montaigne, to Baudelaire and to Obermann."[4]

The realm of music holds many similar examples of composers in awe of a mighty forerunner. Handel all but exhausted the possibilities of the oratorio, and the "passion" form did not long survive Johann Sebastian Bach. In the nineteenth century, composers viewed Beethoven as "a dread idol, a jealous god whose Ninth Symphony stood as the pinnacle of human artistic creation." So dark a shadow was cast by Beethoven's achievement that Brahms could bring himself to write only four symphonies. Even more telling is the behavior of Gustav Mahler and Anton Bruckner, each of whom wrote more than nine symphonies but would not acknowledge what he had done. Mahler left his Tenth Symphony unfinished, while Bruckner would not number two of his early works; his D-minor symphony is called *Die Nullte* (Number Zero). Yet Beethoven himself spent his final days rereading Handel's scores.[5]

Though the sensibility of the statesman is not that of the artist, political leaders, too, have had to live with the "anxiety of influence," and they have often attempted to deal with it by associating themselves with some past figure of enormous potency. Alexander drew strength from his conviction that he descended from Heracles and Achilles, while Ptolemy I moved Alexander's body to Egypt and created a cult of Alexander throughout his kingdom. To identify herself with Peter the Great, who had come to be thought of as possessing godlike qualities, the empress Catherine commissioned a statue of him so mammoth that "a miniature cliff of 1,600 tons of granite was dragged to the bank of the Neva to form a pedestal." In France, Napoleon III calculatedly fostered the legend of the first Napoleon in order to exploit the obsession with the emperor typified by Julien's fixation in Stendhal's *Rouge et Noir*.(It did little good; Victor Hugo continued to refer to him as *Napoleon le petit*.)[6]

In America as well, leaders have sought to bracket themselves with past heroes. In the age of Andrew Jackson party rivals spent an inordinate amount of time debating whether Jefferson, who had opposed Jackson's nomination in 1824, had changed his mind before his death in 1826. During these years, Merrill Peterson has noted, politicians showed "acute sensibility . . . to the value of Jefferson's benediction"; Thomas Hart Benton, in particular, "sprinkled Jefferson's holy water on every issue from slavery to salt." A generation later the martyred Lincoln was regarded as so essential to the plans of both Andrew Johnson and his Radical opponents that the struggle between them degenerated, as David Donald has written, into "a ghoulish tugging at Lincoln's shroud."[7]

Frequently, though, presidents have shared the sentiment of the Irishman who cried, "Get history off our backs!" The weight of having to live up to the reputation of a former resident of the White House has been too heavy to endure. More than once they have seemed much like Holgrove in *The House of the Seven Gables*, who says: "Shall we never, never get rid of this Past? It lies upon the Present like a giant's dead body! In fact, the case is just as if a young giant were compelled to waste all his strength in carrying about the corpse of the old giant. . . . A dead man sits on all our judgment-seats."[8]

In one respect a long line of earlier presidents had a tougher time than FDR's successors, for they were subject to being outclassed by a predecessor who was still around to hog the spotlight. At John Adams's inauguration, George Washington was the center of attention, and in James Madison's presidency, critics often charged that "the long arm of Monticello" still managed the government. They found proof in the revelation that in a brief period Madison had written Jefferson twelve times. (In fact, all of the communications were about the disposition of a lamb.) Martin Van Buren fared no better. When he was inaugurated in 1837, the crowd reserved its greatest cheers for Andrew Jackson. "The rising sun," remarked Thomas Hart Benton, "was eclipsed by the setting sun."[9]

Understandably, these experiences sometimes aroused resentment. In later years Adams claimed that his role of minister plenipotentiary to negotiate peace in 1779 far outranked in significance that of Washington as commander in chief, and he even asked, "Would Washington have ever been commander of the revolutionary army or president of the United States if he had not married the rich widow of Mr. Custis?" He also thought it a bit much to say that God had denied Washington children so that he could be father of the whole country. In like fashion Jefferson was to write, in an introduction for the *Anas*, that in his second term George Washington had approached senility and had permitted himself to be exploited by politicians.[10]

No president has been able to evade a confrontation with his forerunners, not only because they provide a guide to action to be taken (or avoided) but also because they have so palpable an effect on how he will ultimately be measured. Theodore Roosevelt once remarked, "Often when dealing with some puzzling affair I find myself thinking what Lincoln would have done," and toward the end of FDR's first term, Anne O'Hare McCormick, a correspondent for the *New York Times*, observed:

> As soon as a man moves into the White House, even though up to that moment he has been only an ambitious politician, he becomes conscious of himself as a historic figure. The White House is a gallery of dead Presidents, among whom the living occupant lives as a man among his ancestors. . . . Increasingly he is aware of those who stand out from the crowd, still alive in the memory of the nation.[11]

III

Franklin D. Roosevelt proved to be an especially tough act to follow. In his more than three terms in the White House, he had become, as one writer has stated, "the Paul Bunyan of American Presidents: a myth based on vividly remembered reality." So large did he loom in the popular imagination that he even affected the reputations of those who had come before him. As one of Grover Cleveland's biographers has noted perceptively:

> Perhaps the harshest thing that happened to Cleveland was Franklin Roosevelt. . . . FDR's glowing presidential style and achievement cast shadows in all directions—forward to encompass each of his successors, and backward to measure every predecessor. Dexterity, innovation, and public compassion now became the main criteria for comparing presidents. . . . History insured that the linkage between Cleveland and FDR would be defined to Cleveland's disadvantage.

Much the same observation could have been made by the biographers of other presidents, certainly with respect to Herbert Hoover and even, or perhaps especially, to Woodrow Wilson.[12]

Decades after his death, Roosevelt continued to cast a shadow. When Jimmy Carter campaigned in West Virginia in the midterm elections of 1978, pictures of FDR still adorned the walls of miners' shacks. In the 1980s millions of Americans still drew on the accomplishments of the Roosevelt years: old people counted on social security benefits; Southerners electrified their homes with TVA power; big-city residents lived in New Deal housing projects; New Yorkers crossed the Triboro Bridge and Virginians traveled the Skyline Drive. The jobs legislation enacted in 1983 owed an obvious debt to the WPA, and a bill to create a new program modeled on the CCC won wide support in Congress. Five miles from Willow, in southwestern Oklahoma, the first of the more than 200 million trees planted in FDR's pet project of a shelter belt against dust storms on the dry western plains still thrived. Some of the most prominent political figures of the 1980s looked back half a century for guideposts. Teddy Kennedy frequently alluded to FDR, while Fritz Mondale recalled having been raised in a family that regarded Franklin Roosevelt as a household god.[13]

FDR's successors in the White House faced an imposing set of challenges. Their greatest problem was how to solve the question that troubles the artist—"What is there left to do?"[14] Roosevelt had handed down a rich legacy of ideas and institutions to his successors. But by that very token he had also made it much less likely that their achievements would equal or surpass his. They had to cope, too, with a further demand—to remain loyal to FDR, as the Roosevelt idolators expected them to be, and yet to establish their own identity in order to create a record comparable to his. Ironically, the more faithful they were to FDR, the more unlike him they would be, for Roosevelt had made his place in history by diverging from the pattern of his predecessors. They could succeed by greatly enlarging what he had accomplished or by finding new fields of endeavor, neither of which was an easy task, or by departing from his legacy, an action fraught with difficulty, for it seemed a kind of filial disobedience.

It was a staple of the pop psychology of the times to refer to Roosevelt as a father figure, and though only Johnson seems in any significant way to have confused FDR with his own family, other presidents may well have viewed him as a parental preceptor. To the extent that his successors thought of FDR as a father, they became involved in all the complicated emotions that any effort to displace a father entails. "The essence of success," Freud observed, is "to have got further than one's father . . . as though to excel one's father was still something forbidden." In fact, the relationship is deeply ambiguous, for a son may love his father and seek his approval while also wanting to surpass him. The effort of Roosevelt's successors to deal with this dilemma—to prove their fidelity to FDR while distancing themselves from him—has done much to shape the course of events from the spring of 1945 to the present.[15]

At times the injunction to emulate FDR has had mischievous results. Roosevelt has seemed so Promethean a figure that it has too often been forgotten that he, like his trouble-plagued successors, made mistakes and ran into difficulties. Though he greatly improved the economic situation, he did not bring the country out of depression short of war, and, for all of his success as a political tactician, he left his successors the legacy of a stalemate in Congress that began in his second term. Nor is it always remembered that it was in FDR's presidency that Japanese-Americans were herded into internment camps and European Jews were all but abandoned to their fate. Moreover, some of the developments of the postwar era that were to be most deplored, such as the baleful influence of the military-industrial complex, had their origins in the age of Roosevelt. Comparison of his successors not to the historical Roosevelt, warts and all, but to a legendary FDR has inevitably produced not just disappointment but an inordinate sense of depression at the decline in quality of the presidential office.

The requirement that postwar presidents live up not only to the real Franklin Roosevelt with his multifarious accomplishments but to the legendary FDR has carried with it the same unfortunate consequences that attended the canonization of other national leaders, not excepting George Washington. As one historian has commented:

The most fundamental problem with the Washington myth was . . . that it created a heroic abstraction for patriots to emulate which . . . was quite distant from the complex realities of daily existence. It discouraged patriots from dealing on realistic terms with the variously imperfect people and the periodically unstable social conditions that necessarily surrounded their daily lives. The Washington myth made patriots less tolerant of human frailties and diversities (even in themselves).[16]

It was not always sensible, either, to instruct FDR's successors to apply his prescriptions to the solution of contemporary difficulties, for three decades after Roosevelt's death much of the New Deal looked very different than it had in the 1930s. The TVA, once hailed by conservationists, had become one of the nation's worst polluters; some federal housing projects were cancers in the inner city; and the social security system demanded a thorough overhauling. Roosevelt's expansive view of the role of his office seemed less attractive when, especially after the experience with Johnson and Nixon, the country saw a need to deflate the imperial presidency. In bypassing the traditional departments to set up emergency agencies, Roosevelt had resorted to a strategy that proved effective in the 1930s, maintained one writer. "But Roosevelt left his successors a much bigger government, and in due course, the iron law of organization began to transform what had served as brilliant expedients for FDR into dead weight."[17]

Even if FDR's successors did want to follow in his path, they could not always be sure they were doing so. So broad was the trail Roosevelt left that it permitted those who sought an accommodation with the Kremlin to claim FDR as their model and those who insisted on resistance to the Soviet Union to equate their efforts with those of Roosevelt against totalitarianism.[18] It was spacious enough to allow those who wished to embark on new social experiments to quote FDR's utterances and, though with less credibility, those who insisted that there were limits to how much society should be transformed to cite chapter and verse from Roosevelt.

Not even members of the Roosevelt family were always reliable exegetes of the legacy. John Morton Blum has said of Eleanor Roosevelt's impact on FDR's successors that she "seemed to put herself in their way, though her interpretations of FDR's intentions reflected distortions that dated back to her continual impatience with his sense of a practicable pace for change." In 1972, James Roosevelt endorsed Nixon, noting that he had been toughened in spirit and soul by his defeat in the gubernatorial race in 1962 just as FDR had surmounted the ordeal of polio, while his brother Franklin, Jr., came out for McGovern because he was certain that his mother had been right in saying earlier, "I doubt if the country can stand Nixon as President." Twelve years later, when the Reagan White House arranged a commemoration of the centennial of Mrs. Roosevelt's birth, some of the former president's family showed up but FDR, Jr., made a point of staying away, for he thought that Reagan had betrayed the ideals of his father.[19]

However difficult it was to agree on the precise nature of the FDR legacy, none of the post-1945 presidents could doubt that there was a price to be paid for taking office in the aftermath of the age of Roosevelt. Harry Truman could not escape incessant, and often unreasonable, contrasts with his predecessor; Dwight Eisenhower concluded that FDR's historical reputation would determine his own place in history; John Kennedy was faulted for lacking Roosevelt's passion and commitment; and Lyndon Johnson's duel with the spectral presence of Franklin Roosevelt helped bring about his downfall. Both Richard Nixon and Gerald Ford heard that they did not measure up to FDR, while Jimmy Carter learned that even in an age of limits he was expected to be a latter-day Roosevelt.

By reconstructing the past, his own and that of the nation, and by seeking to undo the New Deal tradition, Ronald Reagan alone appeared to elude FDR's shadow, but the appearance was deceiving. His distortion of history brought him savage criticism, and, he, like his forerunners, continued to be measured by the yardstick of FDR's achievements, to his disadvantage. Writing in 1984, nearly four decades after Roosevelt's death, Herbert Stein, who had served as chairman of the President's Council of Economic Advisers under Nixon, observed:

> There was . . . this difference between the Roosevelt revolution and the Reagan would-be revolution. The Roosevelt revolution was incorporated in statutes, programs and agencies that were not subject to annual reconsideration and that developed constituencies—bureaucracies and beneficiaries—that resisted counterrevolution. The Reagan changes were changes in numbers, mainly budget numbers, that are the subject of redetermination every year. They would not have the lasting effect that the Roosevelt changes had.[20]

IV

Yet if FDR still casts a shadow, that shadow has been waning. Though Nixon, Carter, and Reagan have all affirmed the influence of Roosevelt, that acknowledgment has been largely ritualistic. It is not a little like the play-acting at Versailles, where Louis XV maintained the tradition of the *coucher* that had come down from his great-grandfather; when the courtiers had left his bedroom, the king would flee by a back door and spend the night elsewhere.[21]

Memories of the Roosevelt era have receded further with each passing year. A historian wrote in 1979 that "what exists now in literature of a revised Roosevelt is little more than a shadowy figure lurking in the gazebo of Clio's estate," and the following year the chief of *Newsweek*'s Washington bureau remarked that "the days of F.D.R. [seem] for so many of us now . . . pre-history." Mondale, his biographer notes, remembered the "clear, patrician voice" he had heard over the radio as "distant and somewhat disembodied." Even Arthur Schlesinger, Jr., the admiring chronicler of *The Age of Roosevelt*, wrote, "The New Deal is of course over." Each season brought news of the death of another of the Young Turks of the New Deal—Tommy Corcoran, David Lilienthal—and on the prairie bulldozers were leveling trees that had been planted in FDR's shelter belt. In 1981 the organizer of the FDR centennial celebration observed, "While most people over age 45 feel passionately about FDR one way or another, those younger than 30 often cannot distinguish Franklin Roosevelt from Theodore Roosevelt. Young people today see his name on a school and often cannot tell you who he was."[22]

A cleavage of this sort between generations has been an enduring aspect of political culture, especially in America. "To see the Revolution in terms of an uprising of sons against father was natural, given the frequency of intergenerational conflict in colonial American life," Morton Keller has noted. It has even been argued that rival parties—Federalists and Jeffersonians, or Jacksonians and Whigs—had more in common with their antagonists than they did with counterparts in an earlier generation. Similarly, Ortega y Gasset has written, "The reactionary and the revolutionary of the nineteenth century are much nearer to one another than either is to any man of our own age." Observations of that kind may understate the continuities between generations; there were, in truth, significant linkages between the architects of the New Deal and latter-day reformers—from the Fair Deal to the Great Society. It is indisputable, though, that by the end of the Carter era the ligatures connecting the postwar age to Roosevelt's times were no longer as taut as they had once been.[23]

A generational fault line now bifurcated the Democratic delegation on Capitol Hill. The Great Depression shaped the ideas of the congressional leadership, which remained faithful to the ideology of the age of Roosevelt. "I did not become Speaker of the House to dismantle the programs that I've worked all my life for," said Thomas P. O'Neill, Jr. Tip O'Neill had learned in his youth that government was a benefactor while a younger group of House Democrats had been taught in the era of Vietnam and Watergate to distrust government. "Clearly we don't think of ourselves as New Dealers—at all," stated a Michigan representative with no recollection of FDR. "We don't assume that what was enacted in 1939 should set the priorities for 1979."[24]

Many of the younger Democrats continued to think fondly of Roosevelt but they were perplexed about how to make the best use of his legacy. Early in 1982 a Washington commentator wrote:

> The Democrats, willy-nilly, are FDR's true political legatees. They must build a house of their own in which to hang his portrait, and we have no doubt in time they will. But for the moment they are like the listless heirs of some departed magnate, picking sadly over the threadbare furniture in a cobwebby mansion.

Another observer maintained that the nation Roosevelt had inherited on March 4, 1933, bore "scant resemblance to the one in which we live today. Yet Roosevelt's response to the dire conditions he faced upon uttering the oath of office hardened into a rigid ideology that has manacled the Democratic Party to a set of hidebound solutions increasingly untenable in today's world."[25]

With uncommon boldness a cadre of "neoliberals" expressed their dissatisfaction with developments that had made the Democrats the party of memory rather than the party of hope. "This is a different generation," Senator Paul Tsongas of Massachusetts told the stunned delegates to the national convention of Americans for Democratic Action in 1980. "And if we do not speak to this generation in its terms, liberalism will decline, and if we do not meet these needs, liberalism *should* decline." A year later Ed Koch sounded the same theme. "I believe that over the past decade the national Democratic Party lost the sense of where it came from," the mayor of New York declared. He added:

> What happened over the last decade is that we became the party of the status quo, the party of government for government's sake, the party of abstraction. Rather than seeing ourselves as the inheritors of a dynamic, pragmatic, humane tradition, we sought to embalm our past successes—the New Deal, the Fair Deal, the New Frontier, the Great Society.[26]

In the 1984 campaign the most conspicuous of the neoliberals, Senator Gary Hart of Colorado, made a bid for the Democratic presidential nomination by claiming that he offered an alternative to reliance on the age of Roosevelt. Disenchanted by the efforts of what he called the "Eleanor Roosevelt wing" of the party to perpetuate the 1930s and convinced that "American liberalism was near bankruptcy," Hart had run for the Senate in 1974 with a staple speech entitled "The End of the New Deal." He opened the 1984 presidential primary season by telling a New Hampshire audience, "The New Deal, although a brilliant response to the problems of the 1930s, cannot solve our problems today," and throughout the campaign he depicted his chief opponent, Walter Mondale, as the captive of the vested interests of the FDR coalition. Though he insisted that his attempts to address the needs of a post-industrial economy offered "Rooseveltian presidential leadership," he was widely understood to be rejecting the FDR mode. "Underlying Gary Hart's campaign for the Democratic presidential nomination as the candidate of 'new ideas' is a desire by a generation whose connection to the New Deal is faint and remote to get out from under the shadow of Franklin Roosevelt," noted one commentator that spring. "This election may well mark the last national election in which the Roosevelt legacy will serve as a rhetorical stimulant and a metaphor for action."[27]

In contrast to Hart, Fritz Mondale found himself cast as "the last, pale heir of the once mighty New Deal coalition." At the beginning of the 1984 campaign he was accused of "waving the bloody shirt of the New Deal," and six months later, the *New York Times* was still observing: "Despite Mr. Mondale's talk of change, most strategists felt that his nomination marked the playing out of a great cycle of Democratic Party history rather than the start of something new. . . . Most Democrats expect that Mr. Mondale will be the last nominee with personal ties to the definition of the party rooted in the 1932 election." Commentators acknowledged that Mondale's success in overcoming Hart's challenge demonstrated the continuing strength of the FDR elements in the party, but so bleak were his prospects in November that his nomination was characterized as "Franklin Delano Roosevelt's last funeral."[28]

The press billed the ensuing campaign as a contest pitting the custodian of the age of FDR against a president who turned his back on the liberal past, but, in fact, the situation was more ambiguous. Presented with a sluice of quotations from Franklin D. Roosevelt for his acceptance speech at the Democratic national convention in San Francisco, Mondale chose instead one from Harry Truman, "A President has to be able to say yes and no, mostly no," and, as David Broder noted, the address, centrist in focus, "offered no New Deal." The Republicans confused matters further at their own gathering in Dallas, where they played "Happy Days Are Here Again." Gerald Ford quoted FDR approvingly (and accused Mondale of failing to be a proper Roosevelt follower); Elizabeth Dole told the delegates, "I was raised believing in Roosevelt's insistence on equal opportunity," and Howard Baker declared: "The Democrats are doing their best to rebuild the old coalition that elected Franklin Roosevelt so many times. But it's not going to work. *Walter Mondale* is running for president this year and *he ain't no FDR*."[29]

Nonetheless, no one doubted that the future of the FDR tradition lay not with Reagan but with Mondale. Only a year earlier the former vice-president had stated, "As Franklin Roosevelt and the 'New Dealers' recognized, we cannot do without a strong national government if we wish to achieve our shared economic and social objectives." For all of his moderation in San Francisco, he still could not evade the charge the Republicans raised in Dallas: "What he really wants to do is . . . rerun the campaign of 1932." The endeavor of the GOP to kidnap FDR once again in 1984 drew Mondale into a series of efforts to reclaim the party's idol. "What a cynical rewrite of history that is," he said of the behavior in Dallas. "Can you imagine Roosevelt giving tax breaks to millionaires and socking it to working people, as this crowd did?" For a generation, Mondale asserted, Reagan had fought liberal programs, "but now, six weeks before the election, he sprinkles his speeches with Roosevelt quotes." Consequently, when in November Mondale went down to a resounding defeat, almost every postelection autopsy issued the same finding: the FDR coalition was at long last dead.[30]

To be sure, political analysts had been performing last rites on the Roosevelt coalition for a long while. Gerald Pomper had found that from 1944 to 1964 there was "an indication of the decreasing salience of the New Deal ideological division between the two parties," and after the 1966 elections Walter Dean Burnham had announced the approaching "liquidation of the older New Deal alignment and political styles associated with it." The president of Common Cause, David Cohen, recalled that when he was a boy every store in the neighborhood carried a picture of FDR; but in 1980 he reflected on "the fracturing of the Roosevelt coalition—its last hurrah was the 1968 Hubert Humphrey campaign." By 1980, commentators pointed out, voters who had cast their first ballot for FDR in 1932 were in their seventies, and to a younger generation the Great Depression was as remote as Sarajevo.[31]

No previous outcome, however, had seemed quite so categorical as that in 1984. Not only had Reagan won by the widest electoral margin in a contested election in American history, save for Franklin Roosevelt's advantage in 1936, but he had defeated a man who was universally regarded as FDR's legatee. "An apostolic laying-on of hands connected him, through Hubert Humphrey and Lyndon Johnson, back to the patron saint, Franklin Roosevelt," noted a Washington correspondent. "So the repudiation of Mondale was a repudiation of the Democratic Party that had emerged from the old Roosevelt coalition."[32]

After such a debacle, what were the Democrats to do? From every side, they heard the same refrain—that, in the words of *U.S. News & World Report*, "the November 6 presidential wipeout signaled the end of the New Deal coalition that has ruled the party for 50 years." Even true believers conceded that the coroners might well be right. A liberal Democratic congressman from New York City acknowledged that "the tectonic plates of American politics are shifting," and a disgruntled North Carolinian wrote: "The truth is that Republicans and conservatives have never been able to forgive God for letting Franklin Delano Roosevelt be a Democrat. Ever since the end of World War II, their tactic has been devoted to undoing the good that was done by the New Deal. And they are close to succeeding." To many in the party leadership it seemed clear that there was only one course open, and in the aftermath of the disaster the Democratic party chairman of Mississippi put it succinctly: "We must let Franklin Roosevelt rest in peace."[33]

V

Not everyone, though, agreed that the Roosevelt legacy no longer had any meaning or that FDR was a Ghost of the Democratic Past who should be exorcised. True, 43 percent of voting-age citizens in 1984 were born after his death, and he could not be expected to be as vivid a presence to that cohort as he had been to those who had lived through the age of Roosevelt. But he was still remembered, and valued, by a good many Americans, including some with no personal recollection of the grim March day on which he had first taken office. In Arizona in 1983 an aspiring Democrat circulated a tract under the title "What Would FDR Say to the Democrats Today?"[34] and at the Democratic national convention Jesse Jackson, in one of the cruder pieces of image-making, said he would rather have FDR in a wheelchair than Ronald Reagan on a horse.

Nearly forty years after Harry Truman found it difficult to think of anyone but Mr. Roosevelt as "the President," people continued to view FDR as the only genuine article. In a Jules Feiffer cartoon published in the midst of the 1984 campaign a troubled man mutters, "President

Mondale, *President* Mondale, President *Mondale*. It doesn't sound right to me." In the next several panels, he says, "But *President* Reagan sounds just as wrong—and President Carter sounded wrong—and President Ford sounded wrong and President Nixon and President Johnson. And President Kennedy and President Eisenhower and President Truman sounded wrong." Finally, he speaks the words *"President Roosevelt,"* and his face lights up. But he ends disconsolately, "The last time a President sounded right was when I was twelve."[35]

If Americans were waiting for the reappearance of FDR, they were right to wait, declared Wilson Carey McWilliams in an election-year column, for the memory of Roosevelt provided a gauge of the quality of the political culture in one's own day. He explained:

> A people's memory sets the measure of its political freedom. The old times give us models and standards by which to judge our time; what has been suggests what might have been and may yet be. Remembering lifts us out of bondage to the present, and political recollection calls us back from the specialization of everyday existence, allowing us to see ourselves as a people sharing a heritage and a public life.[36]

Nor did everyone concede that the FDR coalition had perished. To be sure, no one could deny that Mondale had been routed or that the Republicans had won four of the past five presidential contests. Yet it was also true that the Democrats held most of the governorships, maintained the majority in the House they had enjoyed for more than three decades, and were in a strong position to recapture the Senate. If the Roosevelt coalition no longer had all of its original vigor, its main components—have-nots and certain ethnic groups—continued to be the most reliably Democratic segments of the electorate. Mondale carried better than seven out of every ten voters making less than $5,000 a year, 89 percent of black voters, and a majority of union households, the unemployed, hourly wage earners, Jews, and big-city residents.

The dissenters suspected that the noisy insistence in the days after the 1984 election that the Roosevelt coalition was defunct and that FDR was no longer with us expressed less a historical judgment than a political conviction. There was something suspect about its very stridency, especially when one recalled how often it had been said before. It was far from clear why if, as Gary Hart claimed, the New Deal was dead in 1974 it was necessary for him to kill it off in 1980 and again in 1984. Not without reason did critics of neoliberalism ask whether the message "We must let Franklin Roosevelt rest in peace" was not code language for sloughing off commitments to the poor, especially blacks. For if the historical Roosevelt sometimes fell short of being the benefactor of one-third of a nation, he also has been all but universally remembered as the architect of the welfare state, and those at the bottom of the economic pyramid could least afford to have the FDR myth vanish from sight.

Roosevelt continued to be esteemed because in contrast to more than one president of the past generation, he had demonstrated a willingness to concern himself about excluded groups and a conviction that intervention by the state, though not always well advised, is often indispensable. It has even been said that he "essentially reinvented the federal government."[37] These emphases continued to be meaningful to at least some members of the rising generation of political leaders. "Franklin D. Roosevelt spoke for more than his generation when he said that the measure of a healthy society is its response to the most vulnerable," stated Congressman (now Senator) Paul Simon in 1982. "A WPA-type project-oriented jobs program could be implemented again today," he added, as he listed nearly two pages of worthwhile ventures such an agency could undertake—from tree planting to building bicycle paths to staffing day-care centers. Even Democrats who were less persuaded by the pertinence of New Deal remedies voiced a yearning for those special qualities that distinguished FDR's stewardship. The governor of Arkansas, Bill Clinton, told the Democratic convention in 1980:

> It seems that everyone in this convention and half the people at the Republican convention quoted Franklin Roosevelt. Everyone can quote him, but his words out of context mean little. And they do very little to illuminate what was really significant about his leadership. When Franklin Roosevelt ran for reelection in 1936, . . . he was returned to office, but not because the depression was over. . . . Far from it. We were still in the teeth of the depression. Why was he returned to office? Because people knew what sort of vision he had for America. They knew what action he was taking to transform the country. And they were willing, most important, to accept hardship for the present, because they believed they were part of a process that would lead them to a better tomorrow.[38]

In retrospect, too, it was evident that if FDR was a burden to his successors, he also benefited them in countless ways. It is improbable that Harry Truman would ever have reached the White House if Roosevelt had not agreed to select him as his running mate, or that Dwight Eisenhower would ever have gotten there if he had not been jumped over so many other officers in World War II. For a much greater stretch of time, Lyndon Johnson was indebted to FDR—his model when he was congressional secretary, the man who appointed him to head the NYA in Texas, the leader with whom he identified in his first race for Congress, and the president who advanced his political career from the moment of their encounter on the Galveston embarcadero.

Roosevelt left those who succeeded him, also, a political legacy of immense value, not just "the FDR coalition" but the record of his own performance as the Great Campaigner. From Truman's whistle-stop appeals to rail depot audiences to safeguard the gains of the New Deal to Kennedy's invocation of FDR in the West Virginia hollows to Johnson's barnstorming as a longtime Roosevelt intimate in courthouse towns that remembered the four-time president to Carter's tableau in Warm Springs, Democratic contenders found that FDR iconography remained compelling. Roosevelt even functioned as a guide to the opposition on how to put together an enduring combination. Only days after Reagan's landslide triumph in 1984, Representative Newt Gingrich of Georgia, a leader of the Republican New Right, asserted, not altogether persuasively, that he and his associates were acting in the spirit of FDR's "successful American revolution" and declared, "We seek to build a majority around a new vision of government with many new ideas, precisely in the 'Brains Trust' tradition of the New Deal."[39]

As that remark suggested, Roosevelt contributed not only to a party realignment but to statecraft. Dr. New Deal left behind a medicine bag that was ransacked by the Fair Deal, the New Frontier, and the Great Society, and Dr. Win-the-War presided over experiments in economic mobilization that were still pertinent in the 1970s. Roosevelt's foreign affairs emphases as well as some of the international institutions he helped to create, including the United Nations, lived on long after him. And the young men FDR brought to Washington in the 1930s were continuing to counsel presidents more than forty years later.

VI

Legacies, though, do have a way of coming undone, and each generation must redefine for itself the significance of the heritage handed down to it. Not even Alexander, in giving his signet ring to Perdiccas, could determine the course of events after his death, and Charlemagne's empire did not long survive him. The test of each president in this regard is how successful he is in maintaining continuity with what is worthwhile in the past and adapting old ideas to new ends. Alfred North Whitehead has observed:

> The art of free society consists in the maintenance of the symbolic code; and secondly in fearlessness of revision, to secure that the code serves those purposes which satisfy an enlightened reason. Those societies which can-

not combine reverence to their symbols with freedom of revision, must ultimately decay either from anarchy, or from the slow atrophy of a life stifled by useless shadows.[40]

In recent times the treatment accorded FDR's legacy has revealed more "fearlessness of revision" than reverence for symbols. The manipulation of the past recalls nothing so much as Lenin's comments in *State and Revolution*:

> During the lifetime of great revolutionaries, the oppressing classes constantly hounded them, received their theories with the most savage malice, the most furious hatred and the most unscrupulous campaigns of lies and slander. After their death, attempts are made to convert them into harmless icons, to canonise them, so to say, and to hallow their *names* to a certain extent for the "consolation" of the oppressed classes and with the object of duping the latter, while at the same time robbing the revolutionary theory of its *substance*, blunting its revolutionary edge and vulgarising it.[41]

Like those who followed him, Roosevelt, too, had been required to conjure with the past. Anne O'Hare McCormick wrote of him in 1936:

> More than most Presidents, he measures himself by his official ancestors. At a first meeting, before he went to Washington, this reporter was struck by his frequent allusions to the Presidents who in his mind have served as instruments of historic change. Once he enumerated the characters in history he most admires, and I was struck again by the fact that all were Americans and three were Presidents—Washington, Jefferson and Theodore Roosevelt.
>
> The reason for his admiration is just that these men led the country from one phase of development into another. He thinks of them as translating into policy and action revolutions already far advanced in the national mind.[42]

For the most part, the memory of his predecessors served Roosevelt well. FDR, as David Donald has remarked, "seemed to rummage through the clothes closet of American history and take his pick of garments. He understood what was meant by 'the usable past.'" In one address in the 1936 campaign he mentioned no fewer than five of his predecessors—Jefferson, Jackson, Lincoln, Theodore Roosevelt, and Wilson. As a Democrat FDR identified most particularly with Andrew Jackson. On Election Day in 1936 he wore Jackson's hefty gold watch chain for good luck, and he stipulated that the reviewing stand for his inauguration in 1937 should be a replica of the Hermitage.[43]

Roosevelt even appropriated the totem of the Republican party. Four years before he entered the White House, he said, "I think it is time for us Democrats to claim Lincoln as one of our own," and as president he made a pilgrimage to Lincoln's birthplace, long the exclusive shrine of the GOP. He employed as his speechwriter the author of *Abe Lincoln in Illinois*, Robert Sherwood, who gave Broadway a Great Emancipator who was an early New Dealer. Frequently he likened his situation to Lincoln's. Asked by young radicals how he could justify rearmament, he replied, "Have you read Carl Sandburg's *Lincoln*?" He even compared the antiwar critic Charles Lindbergh to Clement Vallandigham, the Copperhead leader. When after meeting with Churchill at the Atlantic Conference he was asked to draft his own headline for the ensuing press interview, he answered, "I'd say, 'President Quotes Lincoln—And Draws Parallel.'"[44]

Only Woodrow Wilson caused him some anxiety. Roosevelt often referred to his experience as assistant secretary of the Navy in the Wilson administration, but he said that he had profited more from Wilson's errors than from his successes. In particular, he saw Wilson's unhappy experience in the League of Nations fight as an example of what he must avoid. (After the president viewed the movie *Wilson* in 1944, his blood pressure rose to the worrisome rate of 240 over 130.) In pacing off the path for a postwar United Nations, Roosevelt tried, as Ernest May has written, "step by step to stay out of Woodrow Wilson's footmarks." His insistence on unconditional surrender signified a deliberate departure from Wilson's action in acceding to an armistice that permitted the "stab in the back" legend to build. As Robert Sherwood said, "The ghost of Woodrow Wilson was . . . at his shoulder."[45]

Roosevelt, however, bequeathed his successors a lesson on how to cope with an awesome predecessor, notably in the nimble manner in which he adapted the legacy of an even more formidable forerunner than Wilson: Thomas Jefferson, the party's patron saint. When he first campaigned for the presidency in 1932, it was widely understood that "Jeffersonian" implied faith in limited government. But as early as April 1932 Roosevelt chose the occasion of a Jefferson Day dinner in St. Paul to come out for national economic planning. Five months later, in his Commonwealth Club address in San Francisco, he announced the end of the "long and splendid" day of Jeffersonian individualism, while still claiming the Sage of Monticello as authority for the view that government might be "a refuge and a help."[46]

In his years in the White House Roosevelt so reversed the emphasis on states' rights that his opponents called themselves "Jeffersonian Democrats," but he did so while keeping faith with Jefferson's distrust of single-interest government and while emphasizing the democratic and egalitarian strains in Jefferson's thought. FDR's program, a scholar wrote approvingly in 1935, was "essentially Jeffersonian." He added: "It is merely selecting for emphasis the social rather than the individualistic side of the tradition. One emphasis is as necessary as the other if a working balance between liberty and equality, the basic concepts of democracy, is to be effected."[47]

President Roosevelt also took the greatest pains to make sure that Jefferson received all the honors due him. He frequently quoted Jefferson, put his face on a postage stamp and a nickel, and in 1939 arranged to have a grove of twenty tulip poplars planted on the White House grounds in tribute to the third president. Roosevelt also played a critical role in overcoming opposition to the site and the design for the Jefferson Memorial in the Tidal Basin, even going to the trouble of scrutinizing carefully each of the six plaster models of sculptures that were submitted. In January 1940, he wrote bluntly, "I went to see the statues of Thomas Jefferson and I am sorry to have to tell you in utter frankness that I do not like any of them!" He then delineated the shortcomings of each. The commission supported his aesthetic judgments, and a new search was begun that took more than a year to complete. "I think it vitally important that whatever is chosen should be thoroughly original and completely indicative of Jefferson's part in our history," Roosevelt explained. In 1943, after four years of contention, the temple to Jefferson's memory was completed on the banks of the Potomac.[48]

In this fashion Roosevelt managed to pay homage to Jefferson at the same time that he was supplanting him as the party's most revered figure. In 1934 he took no part in Jefferson Day festivities and even stated that it would be a "fine thing" if as many Republicans as Democrats served on the banquet committee. "Much as we love Thomas Jefferson we should not celebrate him in a partisan way," he told Colonel House. As Merrill Peterson observes, "The partisan symbol was dying in the house of democracy." Peterson adds, "After Roosevelt, there was no 'return to Jefferson,' though there might arise at some future time the wish to return to Roosevelt. The party was furnished with a new tradition." Even the tree planting was symptomatic: Jefferson was identified with the Lombardy poplar, not the tulip poplar, which was FDR's favorite. Never, though, did Roosevelt make explicit what he was doing. On the contrary, he saw to it that a wreath was laid on Jefferson's tomb on each anniversary of his birth. The final wreath was placed there on April 13, 1945, as the funeral train carrying FDR's body from Warm Springs to Washington passed through Virginia.[49]

Sources

Almost nothing has been written about the impact of Franklin Roosevelt on his successors. There is no book on the subject, not even a substantial article. As a consequence I have had to rely on archival sources and on fragmentary references in works designed for other purposes.

Nor has the subject of this book—the influence of a head of state on those who succeeded him—attracted historians of other periods or of other countries. The closest models I have been able to find are Merrill D. Peterson, *The Jefferson Image in the American Mind* (New York: Oxford University Press, 1960); George B. Forgie, *Patricide in the House Divided: A Psychological Interpretation of Lincoln and His Age* (New York: Norton, 1979); and Peter Karsten, *Patriot-Heroes in England and America: Political Symbolism and Changing Values over Three Centuries* (Madison: University of Wisconsin Press, 1978). These books have a focus different from mine, but each has proved useful. In comparing FDR's legacy with that of powerful political figures elsewhere in the world, I have profited from reading Miguel A. Bretos, "From Banishment to Sainthood: A Study of the Image of Bolivar in Colombia, 1826–1883," Ph.D. dissertation, Vanderbilt University, 1976; Jonathan D. Spence, *Emperor of China: Self-portrait of K'ang-hsi* (New York: Knopf, 1974); and Silas H. L. Wu, *Passage to Power: K'ang-hsi and His Heir Apparent, 1661–1772* (Cambridge: Harvard University Press, 1979).

Some writers have shown considerable awareness of FDR's shadow. There is speculation about what would have happened if Roosevelt had lived in Rexford G. Tugwell, *Off Course: From Truman to Nixon* (New York: Praeger, 1971) and Otis L. Graham, Jr., "1945: The United States, Russia and the Cold War—What If Franklin Roosevelt Had Lived?" in *Speculations on American History*, ed. Morton Borden and Otis L.

[255]

Graham (Lexington, Mass.: D. C. Heath, 1977). Michael R. Beschloss, *Kennedy and Roosevelt: The Uneasy Alliance* (New York: Norton, 1980), is excellent on FDR and Joe Kennedy, while Lawrence H. Fuchs, "The Senator and the Lady," *American Heritage* 25 (October 1974), is beguiling on John Kennedy and Eleanor Roosevelt. David K. Adams, "Roosevelt and Kennedy," *Bulletin of the British Association for American Studies* 7 (December 1963), and Frank Freidel, "Roosevelt in Reagan's Eyes, and in History's," *Boston Globe,* January 24, 1982, are brief suggestive accounts. I have also drawn upon such works as Robert A. Caro, *The Years of Lyndon Johnson: The Path to Power* (New York: Knopf, 1982); Eric F. Goldman, *The Tragedy of Lyndon Johnson* (New York: Dell, 1969); Alonzo L. Hamby, *Beyond the New Deal: Harry S. Truman and American Liberalism* (New York: Columbia University Press, 1973); Doris Kearns, *Lyndon Johnson and the American Dream* (New York: Harper & Row, 1976); Joseph P. Lash, *Eleanor: The Years Alone* (New York: Norton, 1972); David E. Lilienthal, *The Journals of David E. Lilienthal,* 6 vols. (New York: Harper & Row, 1964–76); Merle Miller, *Plain Speaking: An Oral Biography of Harry S. Truman* (New York: Berkley, 1973); Arthur M. Schlesinger, Jr., *A Thousand Days: John F. Kennedy in the White House* (Boston: Houghton Mifflin, 1965); James Wechsler, "Did Truman Scuttle Liberalism?" *Commentary* 3 (March 1947); and John Farrington, "A Study of New Deal Thought in the Kennedy and Johnson Administrations," Ph.D. dissertation, University of Colorado, 1973.

In attempting to place FDR's legacy in a larger context, I have found especially stimulating the work of literary critics, notably W. Jackson Bate, *The Burden of the Past and the English Poet* (Cambridge: Belknap Press of Harvard University Press, 1970), and Harold Bloom, *The Anxiety of Influence: A Theory of Poetry* (New York: Oxford University Press, 1973).

ABBREVIATIONS

COHC	Columbia Oral History Collection, New York, New York
DDEL	Dwight D. Eisenhower Library, Abilene, Kansas
ER	Eleanor Roosevelt
FDRL	Franklin D. Roosevelt Library, Hyde Park, New York
HSTL	Harry S. Truman Library, Independence, Missouri
JFKL	John F. Kennedy Library, Boston, Massachusetts
LBJL	Lyndon Baines Johnson Library, Austin, Texas
OF	Official File
OH	Oral History

POF   President's Official File
PPF   President's Personal File
PSF   President's Secretary's File

PAPERS CONSULTED

Joseph W. Alsop, Library of Congress, Washington, D.C.
Americans for Democratic Action, State Historical Society of Wisconsin, Madison, Wisconsin.
Americans for Democratic Action, Southeastern Pennsylvania Chapter, Urban Archives, Temple University, Philadelphia, Pennsylvania.
Charles O. Andrews, University of Florida, Gainesville, Florida.
Thurman Arnold, University of Wyoming, Laramie, Wyoming.
Eben A. Ayers, HSTL.
Newton D. Baker, Library of Congress, Washington, D.C.
Claude A. Barnett, Chicago Historical Society, Chicago, Illinois.
Bernard Baruch, Princeton University, Princeton, New Jersey.
H. R. Baukhage, State Historical Society of Wisconsin, Madison, Wisconsin.
Robert Bendiner, State Historical Society of Wisconsin, Madison, Wisconsin.
Adolf Berle, FDRL.
Alexander M. Bickel, Yale University, New Haven, Connecticut.
Van Bittner, University of West Virginia, Morgantown, West Virginia.
Roy Blough, HSTL.
Richard Bolling, University of Missouri, Columbia, Missouri.
Vance Bourjaily, Bowdoin College, Brunswick, Maine.
Chester Bowles, Yale University, New Haven, Connecticut.
Isaiah Bowman, The Johns Hopkins University, Baltimore, Maryland.
Louis D. Brandeis, University of Louisville Law School, Louisville, Kentucky.
Overton Brooks, Louisiana State University, Baton Rouge, Louisiana.
Walter Brown, Clemson University, Clemson, South Carolina.
Arthur F. Burns, DDEL.
Harry C. Butcher, DDEL.
Arthur Capper, Kansas State Historical Society, Topeka, Kansas.
Frank Carlson, Kansas State Historical Society, Topeka, Kansas.
John Franklin Carter, University of Wyoming, Laramie, Wyoming.
Oscar L. Chapman, HSTL.
Marquis Childs, State Historical Society of Wisconsin, Madison, Wisconsin.
Gordon R. Clapp, HSTL.
Grenville Clark, Dartmouth College, Hanover, New Hampshire.
Joseph S. Clark, Historical Society of Pennsylvania, Philadelphia, Pennsylvania.
Clark Clifford, HSTL.
Tom Connally, Library of Congress, Washington, D.C.
Norris Cotton, University of New Hampshire, Durham, New Hampshire.
Oscar Cox, FDRL.
Homer S. Cummings, University of Virginia, Charlottesville, Virginia.

Sources

Hugh Dalton, London School of Economics and Political Science.
Jonathan Daniels, University of North Carolina, Chapel Hill, North Carolina.
Jo Davidson, Library of Congress, Washington, D.C.
Joseph E. Davies, Library of Congress, Washington, D.C.
William L. Dawson, Chicago Historical Society, Chicago, Illinois.
Democratic National Committee, HSTL.
Joseph M. Dodge, DDEL.
Helen Gahagan Douglas, University of Oklahoma, Norman, Oklahoma.
Lewis W. Douglas, University of Arizona, Tucson, Arizona.
Paul H. Douglas, Chicago Historical Society, Chicago, Illinois.
Ernest G. Draper, Library of Congress, Washington, D.C.
Dwight D. Eisenhower, DDEL.
The Papers of Dwight David Eisenhower, The Johns Hopkins University, Baltimore, Maryland.
Allen J. Ellender, Nicholls State University, Thibodaux, Louisiana.
George Elsey, HSTL.
Roscoe C. Emery, University of Maine, Orono, Maine.
James A. Farley, Library of Congress, Washington, D.C.
Walter Wagner Faw, Tennessee State Library and Archives, Nashville, Tennessee.
Doris Fleeson, University of Kansas, Lawrence, Kansas.
Gerald R. Ford, Gerald R. Ford Library, Ann Arbor, Michigan.
Felix Frankfurter, Library of Congress, Washington, D.C.
Harry W. Frantz, HSTL.
John Kenneth Galbraith, JFKL.
Richard Goodwin, privately held.
Harold Gosnell, HSTL.
James C. Hagerty, DDEL.
Bryce N. Harlow, DDEL.
Harris Polls, University of North Carolina, Chapel Hill, North Carolina.
William H. Harsha, Ohio University, Athens, Ohio.
William D. Hassett, FDRL.
William D. Hathaway, University of Maine, Orono, Maine.
Brooks Hays, JFKL.
Walter Heller, JFKL.
Charter Heslep, HSTL.
Charter Heslep, University of Wyoming, Laramie, Wyoming.
Stephen H. Hess, DDEL.
Ben Hibbs, DDEL.
Stanley High, FDRL.
Charles D. Hilles, Yale University, New Haven, Connecticut.
Oveta Culp Hobby, DDEL.
Richmond P. Hobson, Library of Congress, Washington, D.C.
Spessard L. Holland, University of Florida, Gainesville, Florida.
E. M. House, Yale University, New Haven, Connecticut.
Thomas Lomax Hunter, University of Virginia, Charlottesville, Virginia.

Harold L. Ickes, Library of Congress, Washington, D.C.
Independent Voters of Illinois, Chicago Historical Society, Chicago, Illinois.
Lyndon B. Johnson, LBJL.
Jesse Jones, Library of Congress, Washington, D.C.
John F. Kennedy, JFKL.
Robert F. Kennedy, JFKL.
Frank R. Kent, Maryland Historical Society, Baltimore, Maryland.
Dorothy Kenyon, Smith College, Northampton, Massachusetts.
Harley Kilgore, FDRL.
Horace R. Kornegay, University of North Carolina, Chapel Hill, North Carolina.
James M. Landis, Library of Congress, Washington, D.C.
Donald Richard Larrabee, University of Maine, Orono, Maine.
John H. Lewis, Urban Archives, Temple University, Philadelphia, Pennsylvania.
Breckinridge Long, Library of Congress, Washington, D.C.
Douglas MacArthur, MacArthur Archives, Norfolk, Virginia.
Frank McCallister, University of Illinois at Chicago Circle, Chicago, Illinois.
Margaret McHenry, Historical Society of Pennsylvania, Philadelphia, Pennsylvania.
Clifford G. McIntire, University of Maine, Orono, Maine.
Kenneth McKellar, Memphis/Shelby County Public Library, Memphis, Tennessee.
Frank McNaughton, HSTL.
Henry Roemer McPhee, Jr., DDEL.
I. Jack Martin, DDEL.
Joseph W. Martin, Stonehill College, North Easton, Massachusetts.
Joseph T. Meek, Chicago Historical Society, Chicago, Illinois.
Robert E. Merriam, DDEL.
Victor R. Messall, HSTL.
Eugene Meyer, Library of Congress, Washington, D.C.
Patsy Mink, Smith College, Northampton, Massachusetts.
Gerald D. Morgan, DDEL.
Charles S. Murphy, HSTL.
National Committee against Limiting the Presidency, HSTL.
New York Journal-American, University of Texas, Austin, Texas.
The New York Times, Washington Bureau, DDEL.
Richard Nixon, Duke University Archives, Durham, North Carolina.
Barratt O'Hara, University of Illinois at Chicago Circle, Chicago, Illinois.
Victor A. Olander, University of Illinois at Chicago Circle, Chicago, Illinois.
John Callan O'Laughlin, Hoover Archives, Stanford, California.
Joseph C. O'Mahoney, University of Wyoming, Laramie, Wyoming.
Edward A. O'Neal, State of Alabama Department of Archives and History, Montgomery, Alabama.
Drew Pearson, LBJL.
Mrs. Sidney N. Pelayo, Louisiana State University, Baton Rouge, Louisiana.

Sources

Claude Pepper, privately held.
Charles H. Percy, Chicago Historical Society, Chicago, Illinois.
Joseph Pulitzer, Library of Congress, Washington, D.C.
George Radcliffe, Maryland Historical Society, Baltimore, Maryland.
George Reedy, LBJL.
Republican National Committee, DDEL.
Rice Millers' Association, Southwestern Archives and Manuscripts Collection, Lafayette, Louisiana.
Eleanor Roosevelt, FDRL.
Franklin D. Roosevelt, FDRL.
Samuel I. Rosenman, HSTL.
Charles Ross, HSTL.
Richard Rovere, State Historical Society of Wisconsin, Madison, Wisconsin.
Adolph Sabath, Tulane University, New Orleans, Louisiana.
Dore Schary, State Historical Society of Wisconsin, Madison, Wisconsin.
Arthur Schlesinger, Jr., JFKL.
Frank E. Smith, JFKL.
Harold D. Smith, FDRL.
Bertrand Snell, State University of New York at Potsdam.
Theodore Sorensen, JFKL.
Henry Stimson, Yale University, New Haven, Connecticut.
Harold Phelps Stokes, Yale University, New Haven, Connecticut.
Harlan Fiske Stone, Library of Congress, Washington, D.C.
George Sutherland, Library of Congress, Washington, D.C.
Harry S. Truman, HSTL.
Rexford Tugwell, FDRL.
Hunt Unger, University of Illinois at Chicago Circle, Chicago, Illinois.
Fred M. Vinson, University of Kentucky, Lexington, Kentucky.
John M. Vorys, Ohio Historical Society, Columbus, Ohio.
James P. Warburg, JFKL.
Zebulon Weaver, Western Carolina University, Cullowhee, North Carolina.
Theodore H. White, JFKL.
Ann Whitman, DDEL.
Claude R. Wickard, FDRL.
A. L. M. Wiggins, HSTL.
Edwin E. Willis, Southwestern Archives and Manuscripts Collection, Lafayette, Louisiana.
A. J. Wirtz, LBJL.
Ellen S. Woodward, Mississippi Department of Archives and History, Jackson, Mississippi.

ORAL HISTORY MEMOIRS

George D. Aiken, LBJL.
Will Alexander, COHC.
George E. Allen, HSTL.

John E. Amos, JFKL.
Norman Angell, COHC.
Toinette Bachelder, LBJL.

Roger Baldwin, COHC.
Malcolm Bardwell, LBJL.
William L. Batt, Jr., JFKL.
Jack L. Bell, HSTL.
Jack L. Bell, JFKL.
Robert Benjamin, JFKL.
William L. Benton, JFKL.
Andrew J. Biemiller, HSTL.
Barry Bingham, COHC.
John Blatnik, JFKL.
Hale Boggs, JFKL.
Hyman Bookbinder, JFKL.
Juan Bosch, JFKL.
Chester Bowles, COHC.
Chester Bowles, JFKL.
Mrs. Chester Bowles, COHC.
Spruille Braden, COHC.
Philip W. Buchen, Gerald R. Ford
    Library, Ann Arbor, Michigan.
James MacGregor Burns, JFKL.
Prescott Bush, COHC.
Cass Canfield, COHC.
John Franklin Carter, HSTL.
Joseph Casey, JFKL.
Turner Catledge, recorded at the
    University of Southern Mississippi,
    Mississippi State University, State
    University, Mississippi.
Arthur Chapin, JFKL.
Oscar L. Chapman, LBJL.
Cesar Chavez, JFKL.
Marquis Childs, COHC.
William Chilton III, JFKL.
Sidney Christie, JFKL.
Tom C. Clark, LBJL.
Charles W. Cole, JFKL.
George Hamilton Combs, Jr., COHC.
Council of Economic Advisers, JFKL.
Jonathan Daniels, HSTL.
Willard Deason, LBJL.
Marion Dickerman, COHC.
Michael V. Di Salle, JFKL.
Margaret Dixon, JFKL.
Helen Gahagan Douglas, LBJL.
Lewis W. Douglas, COHC.
Paul Douglas, JFKL.
Eddie Dowling, COHC.
Virginia Durr, COHC.
Frederick Dutton, JFKL.
Charles Earl, JFKL.
Harry Easley, HSTL.
Milton Eisenhower, DDEL.
Allen J. Ellender, LBJL.
Claude Ellis, JFKL.
Oscar R. Ewing, HSTL.
James A. Farley, LBJL.

James A. Fayne, JFKL.
Phil Fine, JFKL.
Frank Fischer, JFKL.
Ray Fitzgerald, JFKL.
Edward T. Folliard, HSTL.
Edward T. Folliard, JFKL.
Felix Frankfurter, JFKL.
Orville L. Freeman, JFKL.
Lawrence Fuchs, JFKL.
Edward Gallagher, JFKL.
George Gallup, COHC.
Charles Garabedian, JFKL.
Warner W. Gardner, HSTL.
Sim Gideon, LBJL.
Roswell L. Gilpatric, JFKL.
Arthur E. Goldschmidt and Elizabeth
    Wickenden, LBJL.
Elizabeth Wickenden Goldschmidt,
    LBJL.
Robert C. Goodwin, JFKL.
Lincoln Gordon, JFKL.
Michael G. Gretchen, JFKL.
Kay Halle, JFKL.
Charles Halleck, JFKL.
Carl Hamilton, COHC.
Fowler Hamilton, JFKL.
John Harllee, JFKL.
Florence J. Harriman, COHC.
Richard Harris, Richard Nixon Oral
    History Project, California State
    Fullerton.
Seymour Harris, JFKL.
Walter Hart, JFKL.
William D. Hassett, HSTL.
Anne Hearst, JFKL.
William R. Hearst, Jr., JFKL.
August Heckscher, JFKL.
John F. Henning, JFKL.
F. W. Henshaw, COHC.
Henry Hirshberg, LBJL.
Luther Hodges, JFKL.
William Bruce Hoff, JFKL.
Jackson J. Holtz, JFKL.
John Jay Hooker, JFKL.
Welly Kenon Hopkins, LBJL.
William J. Hopkins, JFKL.
Andrew Houvouras, JFKL.
Robert H. Jackson, COHC.
Arnold Roosevelt Jones, DDEL.
Marvin Jones, LBJL.
Roger W. Jones, HSTL.
Ira Kapenstein, JFKL.
Robert F. Kennedy, JFKL.
Gerald Kepple, Richard Nixon Oral
    History Project, California State
    Fullerton.

Sources

Arthur Krock, JFKL.
Chester Lane, COHC.
Gene Latimer, LBJL.
William Lawrence, JFKL.
Ray E. Lee, LBJL.
Gould Lincoln, HSTL.
Peter Lisagor, JFKL.
Mary Lord, COHC.
Katie Louchheim, JFKL.
Charles Love, JFKL.
John W. McCormack, LBJL.
Robert F. McDonough, JFKL.
George McGovern, JFKL.
Walter Staunton Mack, Jr., COHC.
Edward D. McKim, HSTL.
John F. Macy, JFKL.
Leonard Mayo, JFKL.
George Meany, JFKL.
A. S. Mike Monroney, LBJL.
Mike Monroney, Jr., COHC.
Edward Morgan, JFKL.
Warren Moscow, COHC.
Robert Nathan, JFKL.
W. Walter Neeley, JFKL.
Robert G. Nixon, HSTL.
Lyle Otterman, Richard Nixon Oral
    History Project, California State
    Fullerton.
Bradley Patterson, JFKL.
Claiborne Pell, JFKL.
Frances Perkins, COHC.
Charles Peters, JFKL.
Esther Peters, JFKL.
Press Panel, JFKL.
William Proxmire, JFKL.
Nathan Pusey, JFKL.
Daniel Quill, LBJL.
Daniel J. Quill, LBJL.
Jennings Randolph, JFKL.
Mary Rather, LBJL.
Joseph Rauh, JFKL.
Emmette S. Redford, LBJL.
Stanley F. Reed, COHC.

George Reedy, LBJL.
Thomas Rees, JFKL.
Cyrus Rice, JFKL.
William Richardson, JFKL.
Robert L. Riggs, HSTL.
Arch Riley, JFKL.
Charles Roberts, JFKL.
A. Willis Robertson, LBJL.
Dorothy Rosenman, COHC.
James H. Rowe, Jr., HSTL.
Dean Rusk, JFKL.
Dore Schary, JFKL.
Leopold Senghor, JFKL.
Theodore C. Sorensen, JFKL.
Charles Spalding, JFKL.
Miles Stanley, JFKL.
Max Starcke with Mrs. Max Starcke and
    Dorothy Palmie Alford, LBJL.
J. S. Stillman, COHC.
Sam V. Stone, LBJL.
Anna Lord Strauss, COHC.
Richard L. Strout, HSTL.
Ludwig Teller, COHC.
Arthur T. Thompson, JFKL.
Frank Thompson, JFKL.
Lawrence E. Tierney, Jr., JFKL.
Bascom Timmons, LBJL.
Walter Trohan, HSTL.
Grace Tully, LBJL.
Harry H. Vaughan, HSTL.
Carl Vickers, JFKL.
H. Jerry Voorhis, LBJL.
Henry A. Wallace, COHC.
James P. Warburg, COHC.
Marshall G. West, JFKL.
Burton K. Wheeler, COHC.
Claude Wheeler, DDEL.
Claude C. Wild, Sr., LBJL.
Donald M. Wilson, JFKL.
M. L. Wilson, COHC.
James Wine, JFKL.
Dick Wright, JFKL.
Albert Zack, JFKL.

Notes

Preface

1. Sir James George Frazer, *The Belief in Immortality and the Worship of the Dead: The Belief among the Micronesians* (London: Macmillan, 1924), 3:243; Roy P. Basler, *The Lincoln Legend* (Boston: Houghton Mifflin, 1935), p. 4 (for Lincoln and the Osiris myth); Elizabeth A. R. Brown, "The Ceremonial of Royal Succession in Capetian France: The Funeral of Philip V," *Speculum* 55 (April 1980): 286–87; Adolf A. Berle, *Navigating the Rapids,* ed. Beatrice Bishop Berle and Travis Beal Jacobs (New York: Harcourt Brace Jovanovich, 1973), p. 535; Ernst H. Kantorowicz, *The King's Two Bodies: A Study in Mediaeval Political Theology* (Princeton, N.J.: Princeton University Press, 1957).

2. Hugh Sidey, *A Very Personal Presidency* (New York: Atheneum, 1968), pp. 242–43; Lady Bird Johnson, *A White House Diary* (New York: Holt, Rinehart and Winston, 1970), p. 485.

3. Theodore H. White, *America in Search of Itself: The Making of the President 1956–1980* (New York: Harper & Row, 1982), p. 47; Peter Karsten, *Patriot-Heroes in England and America: Political Symbolism and Changing Values over Three Centuries* (Madison: University of Wisconsin Press, 1978), pp. 106–8; T. A. Heppenheimer to the editor, *Newsweek,* September 1, 1980, p. 4. He was paraphrasing Richard Scammon and Ben Wattenberg. For the expectation that political attitudes will persist for a lifetime, see Marvin Rintala, "A Generation in Politics: A Definition," *Review of Politics* 25 (1963): 512–16.

4. Henry F. Graff, *The Tuesday Cabinet* (Englewood Cliffs, N.J.: Prentice-Hall, 1970), p. 179.

5. *Durham* (N.C.) *Morning Herald,* July 30, 1981. An earlier proposal that FDR's face be carved on Mount Rushmore was resisted by the sculptor Gutzon Borglum on the grounds that there was not enough granite. Thomas A. Bailey, *Presidential Greatness: The Image and the Man from George Washington to the Present* (New York: Appleton-Century-Crofts, 1966), p. 12. It should be noted, though, that the response to a fundraising drive begun in 1833 to erect the Washington Monument was so feeble that the obelisk did not go up until 1885

(Karsten, *Patriot-Heroes,* p. 92). Not until 1846 did a significant monument to Simón Bolívar appear anywhere in South America, and five years after that statue was unveiled in Bogotá's main square it was riddled with buckshot. Miguel A. Bretos, "From Banishment to Sainthood: A Study of the Image of Bolivar in Colombia, 1826–1883," Ph.D. dissertation, Vanderbilt University, 1976, pp. iii, 112.

6. Silas H. L. Wu, *Passage to Power: K'ang-hsi and His Heir Apparent, 1661–1722* (Cambridge: Harvard University Press, 1979), p. 9. See, too, Jonathan D. Spence, *Emperor of China: Self-Portrait of K'ang-hsi* (New York: Knopf, 1974).

1. Harry Truman

1. Harry S. Truman, *Memoirs by Harry S. Truman,* 2 vols. (Garden City, N.Y.: Doubleday, 1955–56), 1:4–5; Robert H. Ferrell, *Off the Record: The Private Papers of Harry S. Truman* (New York: Harper & Row, 1980), pp. 14–15; John Toland, "The Day a Generation Wept," *Ladies' Home Journal,* June 1966, p. 64; Sam Rayburn, "The Speaker Speaks of Presidents," *New York Times Magazine,* June 4, 1961, p. 37; Joseph E. Davies MS Diary, April 30, 1945; Frances Perkins COHC, pp. 774–75. Accounts of this episode differ in detail, and the matter was further confused by Truman himself in his letter of October 31, 1959, in *Strictly Personal and Confidential: The Letters Harry Truman Never Mailed,* ed. Monte M. Poen (Boston: Little, Brown, 1982), p. 31.

2. William S. White, "A Plain Politician from Missouri," *New Republic,* November 7, 1955, p. 16; J. B. West, *Upstairs at the White House* (New York: Warner, 1974), p. 54. See, too, Roger W. Jones HSTL OH, pp. 17–18.

3. *New York Times,* July 23, 1944, cited in Melvin I. Urofsky, "The Election of 1944," term paper, Columbia University, May 1961. A Washington reporter who did not care much for FDR's policies, when asked later what his response was to Roosevelt's death, replied, "Well, 'Something's wrong with God.' I mean I almost thought that man would live forever" (Jack L. Bell HSTL OH, p. 32). Hubert Humphrey has written, "Possibly 40 per cent of the American population knew no other president" (Humphrey, *The Education of a Public Man: My Life and Politics,* ed. Norman Sherman [Garden City, N.Y.: Doubleday, 1976], p. 66). In 1944 a man explained that he was moved to vote for Dewey by a news story "about a bunch of school children who, when polled, voted 97% for Roosevelt. Of course! They never knew any other President. It's time they did" (Harold Phelps Stokes to Arthur Krock, October 31, 1944, Stokes MSS, Box 2).

4. Jack Bell, *The Splendid Misery: The Story of the Presidency and Power Politics at Close Range* (Garden City, N.Y.: Doubleday, 1960), p. 149; Claude R. Wickard MS Diary, April 12, 1945, Wickard MSS, Box 16. See, too, Jack L. Bell HSTL OH, p. 34.

5. Lela Stiles, "The Day F.D.R. Died," *Saturday Evening Post,* April 16, 1955, pp. 153–54.

6. Rexford Guy Tugwell, *The Stricken Land: The Story of Puerto Rico* (Garden City, N.Y.: Doubleday, 1947), p. x; Merle Miller, *Plain Speaking: An Oral Biography of Harry S. Truman* (New York: Berkley, 1973), p. 209. See, too, Oscar Cox MS Diary, April 13, 1945, Cox MSS, Box 151; "Original Leahy Notes," April 12, 1945, Charter Heslep MSS, University of Wyoming, Box 30. A veteran White House correspondent wrote of the train journey from FDR's burial at Hyde Park: "When I got aboard and settled down in the drawing room in which I had traveled so many thousands of miles with Mr. Roosevelt, I didn't feel at all like I was covering a new President. There just didn't seem to be any President at the moment" (Merriman Smith, *Thank You, Mr. President: A White House Notebook* [New York: Harper, 1946], p. 205). Tugwell later recalled the mood in New York in August 1945 in the week after Hiroshima: "More than one person I heard say, as I had said to myself, 'The President would not have let the military people use it.' I knew who they meant by 'the President.' It was not the present occupant of the White House; it was *their* President, who was now gone" (Tugwell, *A Chronicle of Jeopardy, 1945–55* [Chicago: University of Chicago Press, 1955], p. 27).

7. Truman, *Memoirs*, 1:30.

8. Robert E. Sherwood, *Roosevelt and Hopkins: An Intimate History* (New York: Harper, 1948), p. 881. See, too, D. E. Johannsen, "Reactions to the Death of President Roosevelt," *Journal of Abnormal and Social Psychology* 41 (1946):218–22; D. C. Miller, "A Research Note on Mass Communication: How Our Community Heard about the Death of President Roosevelt," *American Sociological Review* 10 (October 1945):691–94; Jim Bishop, "The Day Roosevelt Died," *American Weekly,* April 13, 1958, pp. 10–15 and April 20, 1958, pp. 18–23, clipping, Dore Schary MSS, Box 59; R. Sterba, "Report on Some Emotional Reactions to President Roosevelt's Death," *Psychoanalytical Review* 33 (October 1946):393–98; "Outline of Script for 'Our Foreign Policy' Broadcast," April 14, 1945, John M. Vorys MSS, Box 85; Thomas F. McAllister to Oscar L. Chapman, April 21, 1945, Chapman MSS, Box 4; Florence J. Harriman COHC, pp. 37–38; Margaret McHenry MS Diary, April 14, 1945; Franklin Delano Roosevelt, "Poems and letters sent in to the Times, Chicago's Picture Newspaper after the death of the President," Chicago Historical Society; Ray Henle, "Excerpt from 'Washington Bureau Reports,'" April 14, 1945, Harley Kilgore MSS, Box 96; F. D. Roosevelt Scrap Book, Van Bittner MSS; Agradecimento do Embaixador Americano, na Cerimonia em Homenagem á Memoria do Presidente Roosevelt, May 12, 1945, Adolf Berle MSS, Box 77. Though Roosevelt's death was a shock, some people claimed that they had expected it. Their statements, however, came after the fact. See, for example, Harlan Fiske Stone to Marshall Stone, April 17, 1945, Stone MSS, Box 2; Stanley F. Reed COHC, p. 310. Particularly illuminating for the refusal to believe that FDR could be dying, despite evidence that he was failing, are Robert L. Riggs HSTL OH, pp. 10–11; Robert G. Nixon HSTL OH, pp. 66–73; Jonathan Daniels HSTL OH, pp. 51–53.

9. Truman, *Memoirs*, 1:29.

10. Samuel I. Rosenman, "Franklin Roosevelt: One Year Later," *New York*

Times Magazine, April 7, 1946, p. 9; James Wechsler, "Did Truman Scuttle Liberalism?" *Commentary* 3 (March 1947):222; Alfred Steinberg, *The Man from Missouri: The Life and Times of Harry S. Truman* (New York: Putnam's, 1962), p. 238. Speaking as chairman of the Independent Citizens Committee of the Arts, Sciences, and Professions, the sculptor Jo Davidson said, "Franklin Roosevelt is not dead. He belongs to the immortals. He is right here with us now" (transcript, n.d., Jo Davidson MSS, Box 10). For the belief in the summer of 1945 that FDR was still alive, see Ernest W. Baughman, "About the Death of President Roosevelt," *Hoosier Folklore* 6 (September 1947):111.

11. Cabell Phillips, *The Truman Presidency: The History of a Triumphant Succession* (New York: Macmillan, 1966), p. 23; Eugene F. Schmidtlein, "Truman the Senator," Ph.D. dissertation, University of Missouri, 1962; memo, "Truman, Harry S.: Biographical Material" folder, Truman MSS, Senatorial File, Box 168; Margaret Truman, *Harry S Truman* (London: Hamish Hamilton, 1973), p. 120. In 1955 Samuel Rosenman, who had assisted both FDR and Truman, commented on a draft of Truman's memoirs: "The statement, 'Though I went along fully with the Roosevelt program,' seems quite unenthusiastic. The fact is that you not only went along but almost a hundred per cent supported it" (Samuel I. Rosenman to HST, June 14, 1955, Rosenman MSS, Box 11). Though Truman claimed, "I was a New Dealer from the start," the leading authority on the subject has shown that he overstated the matter (Truman, *Memoirs,* 1:149; Richard S. Kirkendall, "Truman's Path to Power," *Social Science* 43 [April 1968]:70). In the ten years he served in the Senate, Truman moved in a leftward direction, though not as a result of ideological inclinations. At the beginning of his tenure, he showed by his votes on legislative amendments that he thought there were limits beyond which the government should not go. By the war years, however, he was among the more advanced members of the upper house in defending New Deal gains. Still, he remained a moderate who was not aligned with the insurgent liberals, and he was motivated primarily by loyalty to Roosevelt and to his party (Gary M. Fink and James W. Hilty, "The Senate Voting Record of Harry S. Truman," *Journal of Interdisciplinary History* 4 [Autumn 1973]:211–13).

12. Robert S. Allen and William V. Shannon, *The Truman Merry-Go-Round* (New York: Vanguard, 1950), p. 10; Bert Cochran, *Harry Truman and the Crisis Presidency* (New York: Funk & Wagnalls, 1973), pp. 82–83. Even his friends acknowledged his limitations as a public speaker. When Senator Lewis Schwellenbach went to Missouri in 1940 to help Truman in his bid for reelection, he told a campaign rally that "there has been no more loyal or better friend of President Roosevelt in the United States than Harry Truman," but he added, "I need not tell you that Harry Truman is not an orator. He can demonstrate that for himself" (Cochran, *Harry Truman,* p. 95).

13. Steinberg, *Man from Missouri,* p. 130; Phillips, *Truman Presidency,* pp. 26–27.

14. Steinberg, *Man from Missouri,* pp. 130, 132; HST to Frank McMurray, February 14, 1940, Truman MSS, Senatorial File, Box 166. Burton K. Wheeler, who had become a bitter critic of FDR's, said of Truman, "Privately he

would criticize Roosevelt, I think more often than I did on many things, and criticize the bureaucrats up hill and down hill" (Burton K. Wheeler COHC, p. 48).

15. Miller, *Plain Speaking*, pp. 152, 157; Margaret Truman, *Harry S Truman*, pp. 118–26; James T. Crenshaw, "The 1940 Senatorial Campaign in Missouri," *Whistle Stop: Harry S. Truman Library Institute Newsletter* 8 (Winter 1980):3; Harry Easley HSTL OH, pp. 44–45; Robert Underhill, *The Truman Persuasions* (Ames: Iowa State University Press, 1981), p. 93; Stephen Early to R. H. Wadlow, "Personal and Confidential," July 30, 1940, FDRL PPF 6337.

16. Richard F. Haynes, *The Awesome Power: Harry S. Truman as Commander in Chief* (Baton Rouge: Louisiana State University Press, 1973), p. 22; Richard Tanner Johnson, *Managing the White House: An Intimate Study of the Presidency* (New York: Harper & Row, 1974), p. 53.

17. Miller, *Plain Speaking*, p. 165. See, too, Wilbur D. Sparks OH, pp. 168–69.

18. Phillips, *Truman Presidency*, p. 45; Edwin W. Pauley memo, George E. Allen HSTL OH; Truman, *Memoirs*, 1:192. See, too, Turner Catledge OH, pp. 34–35.

19. Interview with Harry Truman, November 12, 1949, Jonathan Daniels Notebooks, Daniels MSS, Box 45; Daniels, *Man of Independence* (Philadelphia: Lippincott, 1950), p. 259; Robert G. Nixon HSTL OH, p. 128; Charles E. Bohlen, *Witness to History* (New York: Norton, 1973), p. 301; Daniel Yergin, *Shattered Peace: The Origins of the Cold War and the National Security State* (Boston: Houghton Mifflin, 1978), p. 70n; HST to FDR, April 5, 1945, HSTL PSF 333; Harry S. Truman, "My Dear Margie . . . ," *Good Housekeeping*, January 1979, p. 168; personal memo, n.d., HSTL PSF 333. See, too, William D. Hassett HSTL OH, pp. 4–5; Edward T. Folliard HSTL OH, p. 2; Gould Lincoln HSTL OH, p. 7; Allen Drury, *A Senate Journal, 1943–1945* (New York: McGraw-Hill, 1963), p. 410; Mary H. Blewett, "Roosevelt, Truman, and the Attempt to Revive the New Deal," in *Harry S. Truman and the New Deal*, ed. Alonzo L. Hamby (Lexington, Mass.: D. C. Heath, 1974), p. 81. For a contrary view, see Arthur F. McClure and Donna Costigan, "The Truman Vice Presidency: Constructive Apprenticeship or Brief Interlude?" *Missouri Historical Review* 65 (April 1971):341.

20. Tugwell, *Stricken Land*, p. xvii.

21. Miller, *Plain Speaking*, pp. 196–97. For skepticism about Truman's claim from a well-informed source, see Jonathan Daniels HSTL OH, pp. 89–90.

22. Jim Bishop, *FDR's Last Year* (New York: Morrow, 1974), p. 610; interview with Harry Truman, November 12, 1949, Jonathan Daniels Notebooks, Daniels MSS, Box 45; Harold D. Smith MS Diary, May 21, 1945. Not until nearly two weeks after Truman took office did a member of a secret intelligence unit write to him, explaining, "I simply wish at this occasion to spare you the possible embarrassment of being consulted on a matter concerning which only President Roosevelt and myself had full knowledge" (John Franklin Carter, "Secret: Report on Operations of This Unit," April 24, 1945, Carter MSS, Box 10). See, too, Harry H. Vaughan HSTL OH, pp. 82–83.

23. Yergin, *Shattered Peace,* p. 156; James David Barber, *The Presidential Character: Predicting Performance in the White House* (Englewood Cliffs, N.J.: Prentice-Hall, 1972), p. 249; George E. Mowry, "The Uses of History by Recent Presidents," *Journal of American History* 53 (June 1966):11. See, too, HST to Joseph E. Davies, April 19, 1945, Davies MSS, Box 16; Rexford Tugwell MS Diary, August 23, 1945, Tugwell MSS, Box 19; "Conversational Club: Presidents and the Fourth Estate," December 18, 1961, William D. Hassett MSS. For evidence that Truman thought that FDR would die in office and that he would become president, see Robert L. Riggs HSTL OH, pp. 3–4; Edward D. McKim HSTL OH, pp. 105–6; Harry H. Vaughan HSTL OH, pp. 76–77; Walter Trohan HSTL OH, p. 21; Harry Easley HSTL OH, p. 99. See, too, Joseph Pulitzer, Confidential Memo to B. H. R., August 28, 1944, Pulitzer MSS, Box 75.

24. Truman, *Memoirs,* 1:482–83. Though this account has been published as Truman's own, it was actually drafted by Rosenman and taken over by Truman virtually word for word. See Samuel I. Rosenman to HST, July 7, 1954, Rosenman MSS, Box 11.

25. *Public Papers of the Presidents of the United States: Harry S. Truman, 1945* (Washington, D.C.: Government Printing Office, 1961), pp. 263–309. See, too, Richard O. Davies, "Social Welfare Policies," in *The Truman Period as a Research Field,* ed. Richard S. Kirkendall (Columbia: University of Missouri Press, 1967), p. 161. For the use of FDR's words verbatim in the opening lines of the full employment bill, see Stephen Kemp Bailey, *Congress Makes a Law: The Story Behind the Employment Act of 1946* (New York: Columbia University Press, 1950), p. 47.

26. Congressman Jennings in "Executive Session—Confidential, Conference of Republican Members of the House of Representatives," September 14, 1945, House Chamber, Joseph W. Martin MSS; Steinberg, *Man from Missouri,* p. 262; Cochran, *Harry Truman,* pp. 200–201.

27. Samuel I. Rosenman, "Franklin Roosevelt: One Year After," *New York Times Magazine,* April 7, 1946, pp. 57–58; Francis H. Heller, ed., *The Truman White House* (Lawrence: Regents Press of Kansas, 1980), p. 9; Truman, *Memoirs,* 1:72. See, too, C. L. Sulzberger, *The Last of the Giants* (New York: Macmillan, 1970), p. 341.

28. *The Truman Administration: Its Principles and Practice,* ed. Louis W. Koenig (New York: New York University Press, 1956), p. 325; Harry S. Truman, *Truman Speaks* (New York: Columbia University Press, 1960), p. 67; Daniels, *Man of Independence,* pp. 269, 281. Conservatives had no trouble perceiving continuity. In commenting on the foreign aid program, a Louisiana congressman noted in his diary: "European W.P.A. can not keep up forever. We must protect our own country" (Overton Brooks MS Diary, September 1, 1947, Brooks MSS). This entry is reconstructed from Brooks's notes, which are partly in shorthand.

29. Steinberg, *Man from Missouri,* pp. 242–43; Joseph C. Goulden, *The Best Years, 1945–1950* (New York: Atheneum, 1976), p. 214.

30. Joseph and Stewart Alsop, "Candidate Truman's Magic Brew," *Saturday Evening Post,* December 31, 1949, p. 12; ER to HST, May 14, 1945, HSTL PSF 322.

31. Truman, *Memoirs,* 1:438; Eben A. Ayers MS Diary, August 15, 1945; James F. Byrnes, *All In One Lifetime* (New York: Harper, 1958), p. 373; Joseph P. Lash, *Eleanor Roosevelt: A Friend's Memoir* (Garden City, N.Y.: Doubleday, 1964), pp. 297, 312. Four days after Truman took office, a prominent black editor urged him to put Eleanor Roosevelt in his cabinet (Associated Negro Press release, April 16, 1945, Claude Barnett MSS, Box 42). See, too, *Drew Pearson Diaries, 1949–1959,* ed. Tyler Abell (New York: Holt, Rinehart & Winston, 1974), p. 49.

32. West, *Upstairs at the White House,* pp. 51, 77, 87. See, too, Goulden, *Best Years,* pp. 211–12; Harold F. Gosnell, *Truman's Crises: A Political Biography of Harry S. Truman* (Westport, Conn.: Greenwood, 1980), p. 64; Mrs. Chester Bowles COHC, p. 18; Dorothy Rosenman COHC, p. 59; Anna Lord Strauss COHC, p. 364; Helen Bradford to Don Bermingham, April 13, 1945, Frank McNaughton MSS, Box 17.

33. Henry Wallace MS Diary, March 14, 1946, Wallace COHC, p. 4626; Steinberg, *Man from Missouri,* p. 294; Joseph P. Lash, *Eleanor: The Years Alone* (New York: Norton, 1972), pp. 78–79; Harold D. Smith MS Diary, May 29, 1946.

34. William Hillman, *Mr. President: The First Publication from the Personal Diaries, Private Letters, Papers, and Revealing Interviews of Harry S. Truman* (New York: Farrar, Straus & Young, 1952), p. 51; *St. Louis Star-Times,* February 17, 1948, Democratic National Committee Clipping File.

35. Truman, *Memoirs,* 1:9–13.

36. Claude Pepper MS Diary, April 24, 1945. I am indebted to Mr. Pepper for permitting me to read his diary in his congressional office. Pepper may well have been to the left of Roosevelt, too. For FDR's irritation at Pepper for pushing the poll-tax issue in wartime, see Virginia Durr COHC, p. 137.

37. West, *Upstairs at the White House,* pp. 60–62, 71. Structural changes were made, too; when they were completed, one feature of the White House of the Roosevelt era was gone—FDR's wheelchair ramp.

38. Eben A. Ayers MS Diary, May 24, 1945.

39. David E. Lilienthal, *The Journals of David E. Lilienthal,* 6 vols. (New York: Harper & Row, 1964–76), 2:564; Clinton P. Anderson with Milton Viorst, *Outsider in the Senate: Senator Clinton Anderson's Memoirs* (New York: World, 1970), p. 65; R. Gordon Hoxie, *Command Decision and the Presidency* (New York: Reader's Digest, Crowell, 1977), p. 118.

40. Jonathan Daniels, *White House Witness: 1942–1945* (Garden City, N.Y.: Doubleday, 1975), p. 287; Heller, *Truman White House,* p. 229; Miller, *Plain Speaking,* p. 400; Adolf A. Berle, *Navigating the Rapids,* ed. Beatrice Bishop Berle and Travis Beal Jacobs (New York: Harcourt Brace Jovanovich, 1973), p. 573. See, too, Mary H. Blewett, "Roosevelt, Truman, and the Attempt to Revive the New Deal," in *Harry S. Truman and the Fair Deal,* ed. Alonzo L. Hamby (Lexington, Mass.: D. C. Heath, 1974), p. 82. Truman's secretary of

state, Dean Acheson, had broken with FDR. At the end of 1933, Tommy Corcoran reported, "Dean says he knows the President didn't like Dean the very minute they met. Dean thoroughly despised the president as a political trimmer, a skimper of problems, and an arrogant bully" (Thomas G. Corcoran to Felix Frankfurter, December 30, [1933], Frankfurter MSS, Box 49). Remembered grievances also played an important part in Truman's attitude toward the vice-president in his second term. Truman, who never forgot that the secret of the atomic bomb had been kept from him, saw to it that Alben Barkley was made a member of the National Security Council (Leonard Baker, *The Johnson Eclipse: A President's Vice Presidency* [New York: Macmillan, 1966], pp. 97–98). The National Security Council had been created with powers carefully defined to avoid "Rooseveltian free-wheeling" (Richard E. Neustadt, "Approaches to Staffing the Presidency: Notes on FDR and JFK," *American Political Science Review* 57 [December 1963]:860).

41. Ferrell, *Off the Record*, p. 174; Jonathan Daniels Notebooks, November 12, 1949, Daniels MSS, Box 45.

42. W. S. White, *Citadel: The Story of the U.S. Senate* (New York: Harper, 1957), p. 174; Lilienthal, *Journals*, 2:434; Alonzo L. Hamby, *Beyond the New Deal: Harry S. Truman and American Liberalism* (New York: Columbia University Press, 1973), p. 83.

43. Claude Pepper MS Diary, June 28, 1945; Warner W. Gardner HSTL OH, pp. 18–19; Eben A. Ayers MS Diary, May 28, 1945; Morgenthau to HST, July 5, 1945, Roy Blough MSS, Box 6; *Drew Pearson Diaries*, p. 381; Richard J. Walton, *Henry Wallace, Harry Truman, and the Cold War* (New York: Viking, 1976), p. 50. See, too, Richard Wilson, "What's Become of the New Dealers?" *Look*, April 27, 1948, p. 26; Clifton Brock, *Americans for Democratic Action: Its Role in National Politics* (Washington, D.C.: Public Affairs Press, 1962), pp. 43, 87; memo, Frank McNaughton to Don Bermingham, April 15, 1945, McNaughton MSS, Box 7.

44. Harold Brayman, ed., *The President Speaks Off-the-Record: From Grover Cleveland to Gerald Ford . . . ; Historic Evenings with America's Leaders, the Press, and Other Men of Power, at Washington's Exclusive Gridiron Club* (Princeton: Dow Jones, 1976), p. 405.

45. Henry Wallace MS Diary, June 8, 1945, Wallace COHC, p. 3891.

46. Ibid., April 14–15, 1945, p. 3694.

47. Interview with Harry Truman, November 12, 1949, Jonathan Daniels Notebooks, Daniels MSS, Box 45; Goulden, *Best Years*, pp. 216–17. See, too, Charles Ross MS Diary, February 16, 1948; Eben A. Ayers MS Diary, May 28, 1945, March 20, 1946; Warner W. Gardner HSTL OH, pp. 24–25; Rexford Tugwell MS Diary, July 21, 1945; Henry A. Wallace MS Diary, February 14, 1946, Wallace COHC, p. 4544.

48. HST, memo, January 14, 1952, HSTL PSF 333; *Nashville Tennesseean*, February 14, 1946, clipping, Walter Wagner Faw MSS, Box 197.

49. Walton, *Henry Wallace*, pp. 70, 105–6, 113; Goulden, *Best Years*, p. 221. See, too, Turner Catledge OH, p. 47; Eben A. Ayers MS Diary, September 5,

1946. For Secretary Byrnes's early determination to curb Roosevelt holdovers, see Walter Brown MS Diary, August 10, 1945. The New Dealers were to get another jolt when, early in 1948, the White House notified Marriner Eccles, architect of FDR's banking legislation, that he would not be reappointed as chairman of the Federal Reserve Board. See Ernest Draper MS Diary, "Stirring Times," February 2, 1948, pp. 217–22, Draper MSS, Box 3; Marriner S. Eccles, *Beckoning Frontiers: Public and Personal Recollections* (New York: Knopf, 1966), pp. 434–56; A. L. M. Wiggins MS Diary, February 9, 1948, Wiggins MSS, Box 1.

50. That was an expression I heard guffawed over many times when I worked in the national office of Americans for Democratic Action in Washington. For the Andrew Johnson analogy, see Daniels, *Man of Independence*, p. 289.

51. Susan M. Hartmann, *Truman and the 80th Congress* (Columbia: University of Missouri Press, 1971), p. 6; Steinberg, *Man from Missouri*, p. 13.

52. Goulden, *Best Years*, pp. 209, 211. See, too, *Wichita Eagle*, April 14, 1945, clipping, Victor R. Messall MSS, Box 12; Harry W. Frantz, "Washington Relaxes in First Spring after World War," April 10, 1946, Frantz MSS, Box 1. Truman the haberdasher was a staple of news accounts about the president; see *Baton Rouge State Times*, April 12, 1945, clipping, Mrs. Sidney N. Pelayo Papers.

53. Lilienthal, *Journals*, 1:690, 697. Throttlebottom was a bumbling officeholder in the 1932 musical hit *Of Thee I Sing*.

54. Samuel and Dorothy Rosenman, *Presidential Style: Some Giants and a Pygmy in the White House* (New York: Harper & Row, 1976), p. 439; C. B. Baldwin, quoted in Curtis D. MacDougall, *Gideon's Army*, 3 vols. (New York: Marzani & Munsell, 1965), 1:22. See, too, Harold D. Smith MS Diary, April 18, 1945.

55. Lilienthal, *Journals*, 2:5.

56. Steinberg, *Man from Missouri*, p. 352; Cochran, *Harry Truman*, p. 135. See, too, James E. Pollard, *The Presidents and the Press: Truman to Johnson* (Washington, D.C.: Public Affairs Press, 1964), p. 41. For contrary views, see A. Merriman Smith, *Thank You, Mr. President*, pp. 14, 25, 26; Sarah McClendon, *My Eight Presidents* (New York: Wyden Books, 1978), pp. 24–25. The press hovered over Truman, watching for the smallest signs of departure from FDR's policies. See *Washington News*, May 3, 1945, clipping, Scrapbook R, Joseph C. O'Mahoney MSS.

57. Allen and Shannon, *Truman Merry-Go-Round*, p. 55; James H. Rowe, Jr., HSTL OH, p. 37.

58. Claude Pepper MS Diary, April 13, 16, 22, May 21, 1945.

59. Allen and Shannon, *Truman Merry-Go-Round*, p. 47; Cochran, *Harry Truman*, p. 125; Hamby, *Beyond the New Deal*, p. 142. Some also thought that in naming Fred Vinson chief justice of the United States, Truman had failed to carry out FDR's intent to appoint Robert Jackson to that post (Eugene C. Gerhart, *America's Advocate: Robert H. Jackson* [Indianapolis: Bobbs-Merrill, 1958], p. 287).

60. I. F. Stone, *The Truman Era* (New York: Monthly Review Press, 1953),

p. xv. For the view of a conservative columnist that Truman's appointees were superior to "the pretentious humbugs and frauds by whom the late Roosevelt was surrounded," see Frank R. Kent to Frederic Nelson, May 2, 1949, Kent MSS, Box 7. For the idea that, in general, Truman was a welcome change from FDR, see Charter Heslep MS Diary, HSTL, May 14, 1945; Drury, *Senate Journal*, pp. 414–15; Dewey Short, quoted in Frank McNaughton to Don Bermingham, April 16, 1945, McNaughton MSS, Box 7; Richard H. Hunt to Charles O. Andrews, April 17, 1945, Andrews MSS, Box 52; Brooks Hays to "Dear Managers," May 5, 1945, Hays MSS, Box 36; Ernest Draper MS Diary, "Stirring Times," pp. 89–90, Draper MSS, Box 3; Richard Wilson, "Five Ways F.D.R. Changed Your Life," clipping, Hunt Unger Papers.

61. Lisle A. Rose, *Dubious Victory: The United States and the End of World War II* (Kent, O.: Kent State University Press, 1973), pp. 274–75; MacDougall, *Gideon's Army*, 1:36. See, too, Charles L. Mee, Jr., *Meeting at Potsdam* (New York: M. Evans, 1975), pp. 75, 99; Chester Bowles to Mrs. Kaye de Bermingham, April 2, 1947, Bowles MSS, ser. I, Box 38. It has been suggested that the need to prove that American resolve had not been weakened by the death of FDR may have given Truman an added shove in a "get tough" direction (Yergin, *Shattered Peace*, p. 86). For a stimulating discussion, see Otis L. Graham, Jr., "1945: The United States, Russia and the Cold War—What if Franklin Roosevelt Had Lived?" in *Speculations on American History*, ed. Morton Borden and Graham (Lexington, Mass.: D. C. Heath, 1977), pp. 139–61.

62. Harold J. Laski, "If Roosevelt Had Lived," *Nation*, April 13, 1946, pp. 419–20.

63. Chester Bowles, *Promises to Keep: My Years in Public Life, 1941–1969* (New York: Harper & Row, 1971), p. 172; Hamby, *Beyond the New Deal*, p. 67.

64. Barton J. Bernstein, "Economic Policies," in Kirkendall, *Truman Period*, p. 101. For the extent to which farm leaders wanted to curb labor, see the Edward A. O'Neal Scrapbook, 1946/1947, O'Neal MSS.

65. Goulden, *Best Years*, pp. 229–30. See, too, Oscar R. Ewing HSTL OH, p. 119.

66. Hamby, *Beyond the New Deal*, p. 138. Adolf Berle, a member of FDR's original Brain Trust, noted in his diary, "The election returns are in, which merely confirm what anybody could see coming. The New Deal dissolved with Roosevelt" (Berle, *Navigating the Rapids*, p. 574). For the view that Truman led his party in 1946 to a disaster that Roosevelt would have avoided, see Norman D. Markowitz, *The Rise and Fall of the People's Century: Henry A. Wallace and American Liberalism, 1941–1948* (New York: Free Press, 1973), p. 148.

67. Brock, *Americans for Democratic Action*, p. 40; Jack Redding, *Inside the Democratic Party* (Indianapolis: Bobbs-Merrill, 1958), pp. 50–51.

68. James Wechsler, "Did Truman Scuttle Liberalism?" *Commentary* 3 (March 1947):222–23. I have changed the final term in the text from "1944," which is clearly a misprint.

69. *New York Daily News*, quoted in Max Lerner, *Actions and Passions: Notes on the Multiple Revolution of Our Time* (New York: Simon & Schuster, 1949),

p. 209; *Congressional Record,* 79th Cong., 1st sess., p. A2556; "The Eleanor Roosevelt Memorial Scholarships," Frank McCallister MSS, Box 306; First Annual Roosevelt Day Dinner, January 28, 1949, Palmer House, Chicago, Hunt Unger Papers, Folder 10; Jerome W. Sidel to Marquis Childs, January 9, 1953, Childs MSS, Box 2; Hamby, *Beyond the New Deal,* p. 141. See, too, Betty Glad, *Jimmy Carter: In Search of the Great White House* (New York: Norton, 1980), p. 366; Robert H. Jackson COHC, pp. 1523–24; "Roosevelt Anniversary Address for The President," Samuel I. Rosenman MSS, Box 7; "Baukhage Talking," Hyde Park, N.Y., January 30, 1947, H. R. Baukhage MSS, Box 1; Dean Acheson, Memorandum for the President, April 8, 1947, Clark Clifford MSS, Box 29; Meyer Berger, "They Speak As If He Still Lives On," *New York Times Magazine,* April 13, 1947, p. 8.

70. Elmo Roper, *You and Your Leaders: Their Actions and Reactions* (New York: Morrow, 1957), p. 22; John M. Fenton, *In Your Opinion . . . : The Managing Editor of the Gallup Poll Looks at Polls, Politics, and the People from 1945 to 1960* (Boston: Little, Brown, 1960), p. 68. See, too, Chester Bowles to Franklin D. Roosevelt, Jr., August 9, 1948, Bowles MSS, ser. I, Box 45; Address Given by Congressman William L. Dawson, Democratic National Convention, July 14, 1948, Dawson MSS, Box 1.

71. Memo, n.d. [1948], Drew Pearson MSS F169; Fenton, *In Your Opinion,* p. 62.

72. Richard M. Dalfiume, *Desegregation of the U.S. Armed Forces: Fighting on Two Fronts* (Columbia: University of Missouri Press, 1969), pp. 141–42; Truman, *Memoirs,* 1:30

73. Andrew J. Biemiller HSTL OH, p. 53; Humphrey, *Education of a Public Man,* p. 112; Steinberg, *Man from Missouri,* p. 315. For FDR's final action on civil rights, see Adolph Sabath Memoirs, Sabath MSS, Box 1, Folder 6.

74. Albert Eisele, *Almost to the Presidency: A Biography of Two American Politicians* (Blue Earth, Minn.: Piper, 1972), p. 61; Walton, *Henry Wallace, Harry Truman, and the Cold War,* pp. 34, 85, 119, 149; MacDougall, *Gideon's Army,* 1:98, 229; Daniels, *Man of Independence,* p. 309. See, too, Claude Pepper MS Diary, May 14, 1945, and the account of the Philadelphia rally of March 9, 1947, in John H. Lewis MSS, Box 1.

75. Wechsler, "Did Truman Scuttle Liberalism?" pp. 22–23. See, too, J. S. Stillman COHC, p. 38.

76. Elliott Roosevelt, *As He Saw It* (New York: Duell, Sloan & Pearce, 1946); Eleanor Roosevelt to Joseph W. Alsop, December 5, 1946, and Alsop to Roosevelt, December 17, 1946, Alsop MSS, Box 2. For conflicting assessments of the controversy, see Norman Angell COHC, p. 228; Marion Dickerman COHC, p. 222; Richard Rovere MS Diary, February 23, 1948, Rovere MSS, Box 3. After an interview with Elliott Roosevelt, Rovere wrote in his diary, "I cannot exaggerate the heaviness, the thickness, the dullness of the man's speech and presence." For Elliott Roosevelt's continuing criticism of Truman, see Abraham L. Pomerantz to Jo Davidson, December 22, 1947, Davidson MSS, Box 6; MacDougall, *Gideon's Army,* 1:179–80.

77. Joseph Alsop and Arthur M. Schlesinger, Jr., to The Editor, *The Times,* London, England, April 15, 1947, Alsop MSS, Box 2.

78. Theodore H. White, *In Search of History: A Personal Adventure* (New York: Warner, 1979), p. 256; Henry Wallace COHC, p. 3669. See, too, F. W. Henshaw COHC, p. 160; John Morton Blum, ed., *The Price of Vision: The Diary of Henry A. Wallace, 1942–1946* (Boston: Houghton Mifflin, 1973), p. 372.

79. MacDougall, *Gideon's Army,* 2:517–18; *New York Times,* July 25, 1948.

80. Humphrey, *Education of a Public Man,* p. 110; Bowles to James P. Warburg, March 18, 1948, Warburg MSS, Box 13; Claude Pepper MS Diary, April 2, 1948; MacDougall, *Gideon's Army,* 1:472; Finlay Lewis, *Mondale: Portrait of an American Politician* (New York: Harper & Row, 1980), p. 57. See, too, Chester Bowles to Samuel Rosenman, March 31, 1948, Bowles MSS, ser. I, Box 45; Minutes, Board of Directors, April 20, 1948, Independent Voters of Illinois MSS, Box 2.

81. Hartmann, *Truman and the 80th Congress,* pp. 32–35; Statement by the President (*not used*) regarding fight on Mr. David Lilienthal (March 1947), HSTL PSF 322. When he resolved to renominate Lilienthal to head the TVA, he told Jonathan Daniels, "McKellar will have a shit hemorrhage" (Daniels, *White House Witness,* p. 287). See, too, HST to Kenneth McKellar, March 11, 1947, McKellar MSS, Political Correspondence, Box 58.

82. Lilienthal, *Journals,* 2:378–79.

83. Steinberg, *Man from Missouri,* p. 329; Cochran, *Harry Truman and the Crisis Presidency,* p. 237.

84. Markowitz, *Rise and Fall of the People's Century,* p. 259; "An Appeal to the Liberals of America," ADA MSS, Administrative File, Box 94; Allen Yarnell, *Democrats and Progressives: The 1948 Presidential Election as a Test of Postwar Liberalism* (Berkeley: University of California Press, 1974), pp. 104–5. See, too, Norman Mackenzie, "Dilemma for Liberals," *New Statesman and Nation* 12 (March 6, 1948):187–88.

85. "Henry A. Wallace: The First Three Months," n.d. [1948], Americans for Democratic Action, Southeastern Pennsylvania Chapter MSS, Box 17.

86. Clark Clifford, Memorandum to the President, November 19, 1947, Clifford MSS, Box 21; "The Politics of 1948," Confidential Memo, James H. Rowe, Jr., HSTL OH; *Public Papers of the Presidents of the United States: Harry S. Truman, 1948* (Washington, D.C.: Government Printing Office, 1964), pp. 407, 410. "Truman will, in all probability, be beaten," wrote a columnist, "but Democratic progressivism is not dead. Its aliveness is underlined by the fact that in this hour of its great crisis its candidate knows he must assume the mantle and militancy of FDR if he is to stand even a chance of winning" (Lerner, *Actions and Passions,* p. 234). See, too, Roper, *You and Your Leaders,* p. 139; George Gallup COHC, p. 33; John Frederick Martin, *Civil Rights and the Crisis of Liberalism: The Democratic Party, 1945–1976* (Boulder, Colo.: Westview, 1979), pp. 79–80; George Radcliffe, address as chairman of the Democratic State Convention of Maryland, n.d., Radcliffe MSS, Box 45.

87. Richard O. Davies, *Housing Reform during the Truman Administration*

(Columbia: University of Missouri Press, 1966), p. 89; *Public Papers of the Presidents, 1948,* p. 850.

88. ER to HST, March 22, 1948, HSTL PSF 321; Walton, *Henry Wallace, Harry Truman, and the Cold War,* p. 190; ER to HST, October 4, 1948, Eleanor Roosevelt MSS, Box 4560; Lash, *Eleanor Roosevelt,* pp. 307–8; Lash, *Eleanor: The Years Alone,* p. 146. See, too, Eben A. Ayers MS Diary, July 1, 1948.

89. Redding, *Inside the Democratic Party,* pp. 226–29. There are contradictory accounts in Margaret Truman, *Harry S Truman,* p. 38, and James Roosevelt with Bill Libby, *My Parents: A Differing View* (Chicago: Playboy Press, 1976), p. 329. Despite her effort, Truman lost New York.

90. Spessard L. Holland to M. Lewis Hall, November 5, 1948, Holland MSS, Box 41. See, too, Warren Moscow COHC, p. 15. Some writers thought Truman's campaign speeches "were consistently more aggressive and more radical than any Franklin Delano Roosevelt ever uttered," and that in such areas as health insurance he was "well to the left of the Roosevelt New Deal" (Joseph and Stewart Alsop, quoted in Irwin Ross, *The Loneliest Campaign: The Truman Victory of 1948* [New York: New American Library, 1968], p. 265; Richard L. Strout, *TRB* [New York: Macmillan, 1979], p. 71).

91. John Hersey, "Profiles: Mr. President, II. Ten O'Clock Meeting," *New Yorker,* April 14, 1951, p. 38; Allen and Shannon, *Truman Merry-Go-Round,* p. 3; "What I Miss Most about Franklin D. Roosevelt," *Look,* April 22, 1952, p. 100. Nor did tributes to FDR diminish. See, for example, Labor League for Political Education, Cook County Branch, First Annual Dinner, September 5, 1949, Victor A. Olander MSS, Folder 238.

92. Robert A. Divine, *Since 1945: Politics and Diplomacy in Recent American History* (New York: Wiley, 1945), p. 24; MacDougall, *Gideon's Army,* 3:769; Allen and Shannon, *Truman Merry-Go-Round,* p. 41; Robert J. Donovan, *Conflict and Crisis: The Presidency of Harry S. Truman, 1945–1948* (New York: Norton, 1977), p. 438. See, too, Brock, *Americans for Democratic Action,* p. 101; Ross, *Loneliest Campaign,* p. 263; Fenton, *In Your Opinion,* pp. 62–64; Benjamin V. Cohen to Felix Frankfurter, November 6, 1948, Frankfurter MSS, Box 45; Arthur Schlesinger, Jr., to Chester Bowles, November 5, 1948, Bowles MSS, ser. I, Box 45.

93. Truman, *Memoirs,* 2:171; Miller, *Plain Speaking,* p. 249; Samuel I. Rosenman HSTL OH, pp. 55–56. This is a point that has been made to me very forcefully by Averell Harriman. See, too, Pollard, *Presidents and the Press,* p. 27; John Franklin Carter HSTL OH, p. 62; Alonzo L. Hamby, "Introduction," in *Harry S. Truman and the Fair Deal,* ed. Hamby (Lexington, Mass.: D. C. Heath, 1974), p. vii. One historian has noted, "The election returns, according to his most intimate friends, gave Truman a feeling of being out from under the shadow of Roosevelt at last, although the domestic program he was to propose in his second term was essentially a continuance of the New Deal. When Representative Sam Rayburn, Democrat, of Texas, who would become Speaker of the House in the newly elected Congress, visited Truman at Key West

after the election, he found the President's mood transformed from the humility of 1945 and 1946" (Robert J. Donovan, *Tumultuous Years: The Presidency of Harry S Truman, 1949–1953* [New York: Norton, 1982], p. 17).

94. Fenton, *In Your Opinion*, p. 46.

95. *Drew Pearson Diaries*, p. 13. On another occasion, Pearson noted: "March 15: Income tax day. Harry Truman today lost the battle of the filibuster—in my opinion one of the most important battles in his political career and in the recent history of the country. It was handled with inexcusably poor strategy. Truman scolded Congressmen instead of soft-soaping them as did Roosevelt" (ibid., p. 30).

96. Thomas Sancton, "Second Chance for the New Deal?" *Nation*, January 15, 1949, pp. 61–62. Many historians agree that the Fair Deal was merely an extension of the New Deal. For example, Richard O. Davies states, "The reforms that Truman advocated were, for the most part, New Deal retreads— programs that had originated in the Roosevelt administration" (Davies, "Social Welfare Policies," in Kirkendall, *Truman Period*, p. 152). See, too, Louis W. Koenig, "Truman's Global Leadership," *Current History* 38 (October 1960):227. Others, however, claim that the Fair Deal had a distinctive identity, for in contrast to the focus of the New Deal on poverty, the Fair Deal looked toward a more equitable sharing of abundance. See, for example, Phillips, *Truman Presidency*, pp. 162–63.

97. Joseph and Stewart Alsop, "Candidate Truman's Magic Brew," *Saturday Evening Post*, December 31, 1949, p. 12.

98. *Drew Pearson Diaries*, p. 120. For the linkage of McCarthy to the Roosevelt era, see Samuel Lubell, *Revolt of the Moderates* (New York: Harper, 1956), p. 71; Robert Griffith, *The Politics of Fear: Joseph R. McCarthy and the Senate* (Lexington: University Press of Kentucky, 1970), p. 6; Herbert S. Parmet, *Eisenhower and the American Crusades* (New York: Macmillan, 1972), pp. 301–2; Bates Macgowan to Edwin E. Willis, January 22, 1959, Willis MSS, Box 171.

99. Telegram received by Herbert Lehman and Robert Sherwood, quoted on January 24, 1949, Americans for Democratic Action, Southeastern Pennsylvania Chapter MSS, Box 6; Eben Ayers MS Diary, November 8, 1952. See, too, HST to Jesse Jones, May 12, 1951, Jones MSS, LC, Box 32; Margaret Chase Smith to Roscoe C. Emery, April 8, 1949, Emery MSS, Box 537; Maeva Marcus, *Truman and the Steel Seizure Case: The Limits of Presidential Power* (New York: Columbia University Press, 1977), pp. 139, 155–57; Norris Cotton, "Your Congressman Reports," May 1, 1952, Cotton MSS.

100. Truman, *Truman Speaks*, p. 81. The interviewer was Henry Graff.

101. Joseph and Stewart Alsop, "Candidate Truman's Magic Brew," p. 12. After Truman left office, Averell Harriman implied that the Fair Deal was more advanced than FDR's program in saying, "Stevenson has at long last accepted the New Deal. Now we've got to see that he accepts the Fair Deal and moves on from there" (Averell Harriman to HST, August 31, 1956, Samuel I. Rosenman MSS, Box 11). See, too, Raymond H. Fosdick, "'We Must Not Be Afraid of Change,'" *New York Times Magazine*, April 3, 1949, p. 58.

102. HST, memo, September 20, 1945, HSTL PSF 333; Poen, ed., *Strictly Personal*, pp. 31, 153.

103. Walter Trohan HSTL OH, p. 38.

104. Ferrell, *Off the Record*, pp. 134, 144.

105. Interview with Harry Truman, November 12, 1949, Jonathan Daniels Notebooks, Daniels MSS, Box 45. Truman's attitude was far from idiosyncratic. For the widespread hostility to the Roosevelt boys, see Henry A. Wallace COHC, p. 2543; Marquis Childs COHC, pp. 106–7; Carl Hamilton COHC, p. 294; Spruille Braden COHC, p. 2972; Ludwig Teller COHC, pp. 73–74; George Hamilton Combs, Jr., COHC, pp. 142–45; Walter Staunton Mack, Jr., COHC, p. 74. As early as June 1945 Truman wrote in his diary, "My great predecessor had a lot of trouble with his family. Most all of 'em sold him down the river and when they weren't selling him they 'sold' the country" (Ferrell, *Off the Record*, p. 40).

106. Miller, *Plain Speaking*, pp. 254–55. See, too, James Roosevelt with Bill Libby, *My Parents*, p. 327.

107. Margaret Truman, *Harry S Truman*, p. 8.

108. Ibid.

109. Lash, *Eleanor: The Years Alone*, pp. 172, 250–51; Lash, *Eleanor Roosevelt*, p. 326. For Mrs. Roosevelt's prominence at the United Nations and as the gray eminence of the Democratic party, see press release 1325, December 1, 1951, John M. Vorys MSS, Box 69; W. A. Harriman, Memorandum for the President, March 24, 1952, George Elsey MSS, Box 4; Chester Bowles COHC, pp. 435, 681–82.

110. HST, memo, April 16, 1950, HSTL PSF 333. See, too, Bill Lawrence, *Six Presidents, Too Many Wars* (New York: Saturday Review Press, 1972), pp. 183–87.

111. Lilienthal, *Journals*, 2:431; Wechsler, "Did Truman Scuttle Liberalism?" p. 222. See, too, "Article—New Republic, June 20, 1946," Thurman Arnold MSS, Box 38; Richard L. Strout HSTL OH, p. 59.

112. Miller, *Plain Speaking*, pp. 408–9.

2. First Republican Interlude: Dwight D. Eisenhower

1. Henry L. Stimson and McGeorge Bundy, *On Active Service in Peace and War* (New York: Harper, 1948), pp. 442–43; Stephen E. Ambrose, *The Supreme Commander: The War Years of General Dwight D. Eisenhower* (Garden City, N.Y.: Doubleday, 1970), p. 308. For surprise at the choice of Eisenhower, see Fleet Admiral William D. Leahy, *I Was There* (New York: McGraw-Hill, 1950), pp. 214–15; Captain Harry C. Butcher, USNR, *My Three Years with Eisenhower* (New York: Simon & Schuster, 1946), p. 454. Shortly before the decision was made, Butcher noted in his diary, after a conference with Hopkins, "Harry said it was definite that Marshall would be Supreme Commander" (p. 448). See, too, Forrest C. Pogue, *George C. Marshall, Organizer of Victory,*

1943–1945 (New York: Viking, 1973), pp. 319–22; Winston S. Churchill, *Closing the Ring* (Boston: Houghton Mifflin, 1951), p. 418; Arthur Bryant, *Triumph in the West: A History of the War Years Based on the Diaries of Field-Marshal Lord Alanbrooke, Chief of the Imperial General Staff* (Westport, Conn.: Greenwood, 1959), pp. 73–74; "For: The EYES of General Eisenhower or General Smith ONLY for delivery to the Prime Minister, To: Personal and Secret to the Former Naval Person, No. 424, From: The President," December 23, 1943, FDRL PPF 8912. "Former Naval Person" was, of course, Winston Churchill, who had served as first lord of the Admiralty. In his characteristically thoughtful fashion, Marshall troubled to get hold of the original draft of Roosevelt's message from the code room and sent it to Eisenhower as a memento (G.C.M. memo, December 8, 1943, FDRL PPF 8912). Roosevelt decided on Eisenhower because Marshall was indispensable as chief of staff and invaluable at sessions of the Combined Chiefs of Staff (Stephen E. Ambrose, "How Ike Was Chosen," *American History Illustrated* 3 (November 1968):28–29).

2. Kay Summersby, *Eisenhower Was My Boss* (New York: Prentice-Hall, 1948), p. 88.

3. Forrest C. Pogue, *George C. Marshall: Ordeal and Hope* (New York: Viking, 1966), pp. 162–63; James F. Byrnes, *All in One Lifetime* (New York: Harper, 1958), p. 114; Kenneth S. Davis, *Soldier of Democracy: A Biography of Dwight Eisenhower* (Garden City, N.Y.: Doubleday, 1946), pp. 299, 300, 309.

4. Memos in FDRL PPF 8912; Robert E. Sherwood, *Roosevelt and Hopkins: An Intimate History* (New York: Harper, 1948), p. 689; E. K. G. Sixsmith, *Eisenhower as Military Commander* (New York: Stein & Day, 1972), p. 115.

5. Dwight D. Eisenhower, *At Ease: Stories I Tell My Friends* (Garden City, N.Y.: Doubleday, 1967), p. 268; Dwight D. Eisenhower, *The White House Years: Waging Peace, 1956–1961* (Garden City, N.Y.: Doubleday, 1965), p. 104; Dwight D. Eisenhower, *Crusade in Europe* (Garden City, N.Y.: Doubleday, 1948), p. 195; Relman Morin, *Dwight D. Eisenhower: A Gauge of Greatness* (New York: Simon & Schuster, 1969), p. 97; Ambrose, *Supreme Commander*, pp. 301, 303. See, too, Butcher, *My Three Years*, p. 452.

6. Sherwood, *Roosevelt and Hopkins*, p. 701; *The State of the Union Messages of the Presidents of the United States, 1790–1966*, ed. Fred L. Israel (New York: Chelsea, 1966), 3:2883. The president sent Eisenhower a message through his aide: "Tell Ike that not only I, but the whole country is proud of the job he has done. We have every confidence in his success" (Butcher, *My Three Years*, p. 280).

7. DDE to FDR, January 17, 1943, DDE MSS, Pre-Presidential, Box 92; Peter Lyon, *Eisenhower: Portrait of the Hero* (Boston: Little, Brown, 1974), p. 111; Virgil Pinkley with James F. Scheer, *Eisenhower Declassified* (Old Tappan, N.J.: Fleming H. Revell, 1979), p. 127; DDE to Major General Watson, December 5, 1943, FDRL PPF 8912.

8. Theodore H. White, *In Search of History: A Personal Adventure* (New York: Warner, 1979), pp. 349, 406; Eisenhower, *Crusade in Europe*, p. 138.

9. Typescript of article, Ben Hibbs MSS, Box 2. The article subsequently

appeared as "Some Thoughts on the Presidency," *Reader's Digest,* November 1968, pp. 49–55.

10. DDE to Mamie Eisenhower, April 15, 1945, in Dwight D. Eisenhower, *Letters to Mamie,* ed. John S. D. Eisenhower (Garden City, N.Y.: Doubleday, 1978), p. 248; Davis, *Soldier of Democracy,* p. 546; Eisenhower, *Crusade in Europe,* p. 409. See, too, Robert Murphy, *Diplomat among Warriors* (Garden City, N.Y.: Doubleday, 1964), p. 255; Summersby, *Eisenhower,* p. 231.

11. DDE to Harry Hopkins, April 14, 1945, DDE MSS, Pre-Presidential, Box 146; Ann Whitman MS Diary, March 21, 1955; Eisenhower, *Crusade in Europe,* pp. 409–10. See, too, John Toland, "The Day a Generation Wept," *Ladies' Home Journal,* June 1966, p. 64. On July 10, 1945, he laid a wreath on FDR's tomb at Hyde Park (*The Papers of Dwight David Eisenhower: Occupation, 1945,* ed. Alfred D. Chandler, Jr., and Louis Galambos [Baltimore: Johns Hopkins Press, 1978], 6:163).

12. Archibald B. Roosevelt to Douglas MacArthur, November 30, 1947, MacArthur MSS, RG-10: Personal Correspondence, VIP file.

13. Earl Blaik to Douglas MacArthur, July 12, 1952, MacArthur MSS, VIP File, Box 1.

14. DDE MS Diary (Butcher), December 6, 1943, DDE MSS, Pre-Presidential, Box 144; Clifton Brock, *Americans for Democratic Action: Its Role in National Politics* (Washington, D.C.: Public Affairs Press, 1962), p. 91; Irwin Ross, *The Loneliest Campaign: The Truman Victory of 1948* (New York: New American Library, 1968), pp. 73–74, 112–13; Claude Pepper MS Diary, July 6–8, 1948. Americans for Democratic Action seized on a quite unrevealing letter from Eisenhower to James Roosevelt as the "most convincing" proof that the general could be drafted (DDE to James Roosevelt, March 29, 1948, "Memorandum Re the Availability of General Eisenhower," n.d., ADA MSS, Admin. File, Box 34). In 1952 Eleanor, FDR, Jr., and the others remained loyal to their father's party, but Ike's huge majority in the Dallas area was attributed to effective campaigning by John Roosevelt, FDR's lone Republican son (Herbert S. Parmet, *Eisenhower and the American Crusades* [New York: Macmillan, 1972], p. 145).

15. Harold Isaacs, quoted in John M. Fenton, *In Your Opinion . . . : The Managing Editor of the Gallup Poll Looks at Polls, Politics, and the People from 1945 to 1960* (Boston: Little, Brown, 1960), p. 103.

16. Milton S. Eisenhower, *The President Is Calling* (Garden City, N.Y.: Doubleday, 1974), pp. 69, 75; FDR to Milton S. Eisenhower, September 25, 1943, FDRL PPF 8516; John Gunther, *Eisenhower: The Man and the Symbol* (New York: Harper, 1952), p. 72. Years later, Milton Eisenhower said, "FDR was a master of communicating with the people; because he made the causes of problems clear to citizens, they were prepared to follow him when he outlined solutions compatible with causes" (Milton S. Eisenhower to Louis Galambos, October 23, 1980, The Papers of Dwight David Eisenhower, Johns Hopkins University). In commenting on this letter, Dr. Eisenhower said, "It does leave something of a wrong impression of my total view. I admired him for many

things and we were good friends, even though he knew I disagreed with many of his economic policies. . . . Believe me, I liked the man and admired much about him. I have lived long enough to see the unfortunate results of some of the things he set in motion, mainly a preposterous uncontrolled fiscal policy" (Milton S. Eisenhower to the author, October 21, 1982).

17. William S. White, *The Taft Story* (New York: Harper, 1954), pp. 173, 189–91.

18. Richard H. Rovere, *Affairs of State: The Eisenhower Years* (New York: Farrar, Straus & Cudahy, 1956), p. 115; Tyler Abell, ed., *Drew Pearson Diaries, 1949–1959* (New York: Holt, Rinehart & Winston, 1974), p. 209 (see, too, p. 154). When in 1957 Eisenhower made two broadcasts asking the public to back his program, his talks were likened to fireside chats (Elmo Richardson, *The Presidency of Dwight D. Eisenhower* [Lawrence: Regents Press of Kansas, 1979], p. 50).

19. Sherman Adams, *Firsthand Report* (New York: Harper & Row, 1961), pp. 166–67; Bertrand Snell to Clarence E. Kilburn, February 22, 1957, Snell MSS, C 2.3, Box 2. Three years later, Barry Goldwater dismissed Eisenhower's proposed budget as a "dime-store New Deal" (Barry M. Goldwater, *With No Apologies* [New York: Morrow, 1979], p. 11).

20. Richard Rovere to Arthur Schlesinger, Jr., September 22, 1952, Rovere MSS, Box 3; Samuel Shaffer, *On and Off the Floor* (New York: Newsweek, 1980), pp. 63–78; White, *Taft Story*, pp. 242–47; Adams, *Firsthand Report*, p. 108; Allan H. Ryskind, *Hubert: An Unauthorized Biography of the Vice President* (New Rochelle, N.Y.: Arlington House, 1968), p. 198; Emmet John Hughes, *The Ordeal of Power: A Political Memoir of the Eisenhower Years* (New York: Atheneum, 1963), pp. 86–87; William Bragg Ewald, *Eisenhower the President: Crucial Days, 1951–1960* (Englewood Cliffs, N.J.: Prentice-Hall, 1981), pp. 26, 27; Ann Whitman MS Diary, March 21, 1955. "Nothing could have stopped Yalta," Eisenhower said at one point (James C. Hagerty MS Diary, January 25, 1954). For an extensive account of the issue, see Athan G. Theoharis, *The Yalta Myths* (Columbia, Mo.: University of Missouri Press, 1970). See, too, Edward R. Stettinius, Jr., to Isaiah Bowman, February 16, 1949, Bowman MSS. The editor of the Eisenhower papers has suggested to me that Eisenhower would have been reluctant to attack Roosevelt because he disliked to personalize issues. Furthermore, his experience under MacArthur reinforced his instinct to stay out of trouble, and he knew that the reputation of FDR still weighed heavily (interview with Louis Galambos, October 4, 1982).

21. Richardson, *Presidency of Dwight D. Eisenhower*, p. 156; Milton Eisenhower, *The President Is Calling*, p. 71.

22. Edgar Kemler, "New Deals and Old: Outlook in Congress," *Nation*, January 21, 1956, p. 45; Fred I. Greenstein, "Eisenhower as an Activist President: A Look at New Evidence," *Political Science Quarterly* 94 (Winter 1979–80):594. Shortly after Eisenhower left office a prominent historian wrote: "In the 1950s, the New Deal ceased to be an active political issue and became an accepted part of the American past. No other figure could have achieved that transformation"

(Oscar Handlin, "Eisenhower Administration: A Self-Portrait," *Atlantic Monthly,* November 1963, p. 68). This point is made also in Vincent P. De Santis, "Eisenhower Revisionism," *Review of Politics* 38 (April 1976):190. See, too, penciled note, April 22, 1958, Robert E. Merriam Papers; "Statement by the President," White House press release, August 1, 1956, Bryce N. Harlow MSS, Box 21; Carl T. Curtis to I. Jack Martin, December 28, 1953, Martin MSS, Box 3; Oveta Culp Hobby to Carl Albert, January 24, 1955, Hobby MSS, Box 26; *Washington Star,* August 14, 1960, clipping, Frank Carlson MSS, Box 168; Norris Cotton, "A Congressman Reports," June 10, 1954, Cotton MSS; Dean Albertson, "Introduction," *Eisenhower as President,* ed. Albertson (New York: Hill & Wang, 1963), pp. xv–xvi.

23. Hughes, *Ordeal of Power,* p. 128; Arthur Larson, *Eisenhower: The President Nobody Knew* (New York: Scribner's, 1968), p. 8.

24. Ewald, *Eisenhower,* p. 27; telephone interviews by the author with Meade Alcorn.

25. Joseph P. Lash, *Eleanor: The Years Alone* (New York: Norton, 1972), p. 211; Eleanor Roosevelt to Doris Fleeson, January 12, 1954, Fleeson MSS, Box 9.

26. Mary Lord COHC, pp. 27–29; Roger Baldwin COHC, pp. 97–98; Lash, *Eleanor,* pp. 212, 214. For evidence, though, of the pleasure a member of the Eisenhower circle could take in a sign of her approval, see Lewis W. Douglas COHC, p. 38.

27. Bela Kornitzer, *The Great American Heritage: The Story of the Five Eisenhower Brothers* (New York: Farrar, Straus & Cudahy, 1955), pp. 82, 168, 256, 276–79; Sherwood, *Roosevelt and Hopkins,* pp. 913, 915; A. Merriman Smith, *Meet Mr. Eisenhower* (New York: Harper, 1954), p. 283. "President said that he remembered saying to Hopkins that had he voted he would probably have voted against Roosevelt in the first three terms, but he did not see how anyone could have failed to vote for Roosevelt in the fall of '44 (because of conduct of war)" (interview with Merriman Smith, November 23, 1954, DDE MS Diary [Ann Whitman File], Box 8).

28. *The Papers of Dwight David Eisenhower: The War Years,* ed. Alfred D. Chandler, Jr. (Baltimore: Johns Hopkins, 1970), 4:2321.

29. Harsch, "Eisenhower's First Hundred Days," *Reporter,* May 12, 1953, p. 12.

30. Sherwood, *Roosevelt and Hopkins,* p. 648; Gunther, *Eisenhower,* p. 72; Sixsmith, *Eisenhower as Military Commander,* pp. 137–38; White, *In Search of History,* pp. 349, 406–7.

31. Richard E. Neustadt, *Presidential Power* (New York: Wiley, 1960), p. 165.

32. Hughes, *Ordeal of Power,* pp. 346–47.

33. Ibid., p. 131; Earl Mazo and Stephen Hess, *Nixon: A Political Portrait* (New York: Harper & Row, 1968), p. 207; DDE to Thomas E. Dewey, October 8, 1954, DDE Diary, Box 8.

34. James C. Hagerty MS Diary, January 24, 1954.

35. "Or," he added, "the partisan yipping of a Truman" (Hughes, *Ordeal of Power,* p. 194).

36. Ann Whitman MS Diary, March 21, 1955. See, too, William Lee Miller, *Yankee from Georgia: The Emergence of Jimmy Carter* (New York: Times Books, 1978), p. 217.

37. Gary W. Reichard, *The Reaffirmation of Republicanism: Eisenhower and the Eighty-third Congress* (Knoxville: University of Tennessee Press, 1975), p. 10; Richard M. Dalfiume, "Introduction," in *American Politics Since 1945*, ed. Dalfiume (Chicago: Quadrangle, 1969), p. 14; Hughes, *Ordeal of Power*, pp. 333–34. See, too, Edwin L. Dale, Jr., *Conservatives in Power* (Garden City, N.Y.: Doubleday, 1960), p. 12; Bernard Sternsher, *Themes of the Fifties: Truman, Eisenhower, and the Fonz*, University Professor Lecture Series (Bowling Green, O.: Bowling Green State University, 1980), p. 9; Gary W. Reichard, "Eisenhower as President: The Changing View," *South Atlantic Quarterly* 77 (Summer 1978):279. Even revisionist historians who insist that Eisenhower was an activist president acknowledge that he was activist for conservative ends (Greenstein, "Eisenhower," p. 580).

38. *Seattle Times*, June 12, 1949, clipping, in Frank E. Holman to DDE, July 2, 1949, DDE MSS, Pre-Presidential, Box 57; *The Eisenhower Diaries*, ed. Robert H. Ferrell (New York: Norton, 1981), p. 374.

39. Larson, *Eisenhower*, p. 69; *Eisenhower Diaries*, ed. Ferrell, p. 231.

40. *Eisenhower Diaries*, ed. Ferrell, p. 374.

41. James L. Sundquist, *Politics and Policy: The Eisenhower, Kennedy, and Johnson Years* (Washington, D.C.: Brookings Institution, 1968), p. 24.

42. Jack L. Bell HSTL OH, p. 35; Gordon R. Clapp to David E. Lilienthal, June 18, 1953, Clapp MSS, Box 2; Hughes, *Ordeal of Power*, p. 152; Richardson, *Presidency of Dwight D. Eisenhower*, p. 50. See, too, Statement of Mr. Joseph M. Dodge before the Antitrust and Monopoly Subcommittee, Committee on the Judiciary, August 2, 1955, Dodge MSS, Box 8; press release, April 27, 1959, Henry Roemer McPhee, Jr., MSS, Box 8; press release draft, August 6, 1959, James C. Hagerty MSS, Box 8. For a contrary view, see Arnold Roosevelt Jones, DDE OH, 2:11.

43. Claude Wheeler DDE OH, p. 106; Ezra Taft Benson, *Cross Fire: The Eight Years with Eisenhower* (Garden City, N.Y.: Doubleday, 1962), pp. 9–11, 55, 108–9, 259; Edward L. Schapsmeier and Frederick H. Schapsmeier, *Ezra Taft Benson and the Politics of Agriculture: The Eisenhower Years, 1953–1964* (Danville, Ill.: Interstate, 1975), p. 219; Dean Albertson, *Roosevelt's Farmer: Claude R. Wickard in the New Deal* (New York: Columbia University Press, 1961), p. 400; clipping, Rice Millers' Association MSS, Box 6; Ewald, *Eisenhower the President*, p. 290; Adams, *Firsthand Report*, pp. 2, 90; Burns to Eisenhower, August 11, 1953, Burns MSS, Box 20.

44. *Eisenhower Diaries*, ed. Ferrell, p. 233; James C. Hagerty MS Diary, March 3, July 14, and February 18, 1954. Even someone as well disposed toward FDR as Milton Eisenhower observed that "President Roosevelt was not a good administrator" and that his brother had to deal with "this vast inefficiency" (Milton Eisenhower DDE OH, pp. 5–6). See, too, Milton S. Eisenhower, *The Wine Is Bitter* (Garden City, N.Y.: Doubleday, 1963), p. 9. Attacks on Roosevelt

were a staple of right-wing Republican speeches in the Eisenhower era ("Senatorial Race 1954, Undated Speeches," Joseph T. Meek MSS, Box 3; *Congressional Record*, 83d Cong., 2d sess., pp. 1868, 15397). In February 1955 Congressman B. Carroll Reece of Tennessee stated, "Someday, somehow, Yalta must be undone. God's mankind will not continue forever in the toils and chains there spun by barbaric communism about the broken body and shattered mind of a President recently elected for a fourth term by the most gigantic and egregious public fraud in the history of the world" (*Congressional Record*, 84th Cong., 1st sess., pp. 1524–25).

45. Louis L. Gerson, *John Foster Dulles* (New York: Cooper Square, 1967), pp. 18–19; Townsend Hoopes, *The Devil and John Foster Dulles* (Boston: Little, Brown, 1973), p. 47; Richard Goold-Adams, *John Foster Dulles: A Reappraisal* (New York: Appleton-Century-Crofts, 1962), p. 35; John Robinson Beal, *John Foster Dulles: A Biography* (New York: Harper, 1957), pp. 90, 96, 101–2; Deane Heller and David Heller, *John Foster Dulles: Soldier for Peace* (New York: Holt, Rinehart & Winston, 1960), pp. 103–5.

46. *Public Papers of the Presidents of the United States: Dwight D. Eisenhower, 1954* (Washington, D.C.: U.S. Government Printing Office, 1960), pp. 210–11, 903; James C. Hagerty MS Diary, February 1, 1954. When Eisenhower signed the 1956 social security legislation, he did so only with the greatest reluctance (Gerald D. Morgan to Elmer Hess, August 23, 1956, Morgan MSS, Box 23).

47. Bert Cochran, *Harry Truman and the Crisis Presidency* (New York: Funk & Wagnalls, 1973), p. 150; John Franklin Carter to "Donald," July 13, 1953, Carter MSS, Box 1.

48. Samuel Lubell, *Revolt of the Moderates* (New York: Harper, 1956), p. 4; Eugene Burdick, *The Ninth Wave* (Boston: Houghton Mifflin, 1956), p. 286.

49. Harold K. O'Brien to Paul H. Douglas, August 26, 1957, Douglas MSS, Box 564; "The Late President Franklin Delano Roosevelt," clipping, April 12, 1955, Barratt O'Hara MSS, Folder 1257; *Calais* (Me.) *Advertiser*, August 16, 1962, clipping, Clifford G. McIntire MSS, Box 905; Eric F. Goldman, "The American Liberal: After the Fair Deal, What?" *Reporter*, June 23, 1953, p. 25. A civic leader who sought financing for the bridge from Maine to Canada wrote his congressman, "It seems to me that the Democrats would give us some support because of the late Franklin Roosevelt connection" (M. B. Pike to Clifford McIntire, February 1, 1957, McIntire MSS, Box 905).

50. *Congressional Record*, 84th Cong., 1st sess., pp. 4308–19.

51. Ibid., pp. 1081, 4317.

52. Henry Cabot Lodge, *As It Was: An Inside View of Politics and Power in the '50s and '60s* (New York: Norton, 1976), pp. 49, 56. At the end of 1953, however, when the question of what kind of campaign to mount against recalcitrant Republicans arose, Lodge told Sherman Adams: "The President should not appear in it at all. I recall President Roosevelt's failure to purge Millard Tydings (D., Md.) and 'Cotton Ed' Smith (D., S.C.)" (ibid., p. 130).

53. *Congressional Record*, 84th Cong., 2d sess., p. 15631.

54. *New York Times*, January 3, 1954; clippings from the Washington Bureau

of the *New York Times,* Box 15. See, too, A. Merriman Smith, *Meet Mr. Eisenhower* (New York: Harper, 1954), pp. 3, 277. For contrasts between the two more favorable to Eisenhower, see Gunther, *Eisenhower,* p. 20; Parmet, *Eisenhower,* p. 59.

55. Norris Cotton, "Your Congressman Reports," May 7, 1953, Cotton MSS.

56. Harsch, "Eisenhower's First Hundred Days," p. 9.

57. Dalfiume, "Introduction," *American Politics since 1945,* p. 15; Fenton, *In Your Opinion,* pp. 48–49; E. Frederic Morrow, *Black Man in the White House: A Diary of the Eisenhower Years by the Administrative Officer for Special Projects, The White House, 1955–1961* (New York: Coward McCann, 1963), p. 95.

58. Thomas A. Bailey, *Presidential Greatness: The Image and the Man from George Washington to the Present* (New York: Appleton-Century-Crofts, 1966), p. 22; Fenton, *In Your Opinion,* p. 219; Peter Karsten, *Patriot-Heroes in England and America: Political Symbolism and Changing Values over Three Centuries* (Madison: University of Wisconsin Press, 1978), pp. 104–5.

59. Michael Medved, *The Shadow Presidents* (New York: Time Books, 1979), p. 258. See, too, R. Gordon Hoxie, *Command Decision and the Presidency* (New York: Reader's Digest, Crowell, 1977), pp. 249–50.

60. Arthur M. Schlesinger, "Our Presidents: A Rating by 75 Historians," *New York Times Magazine,* July 29, 1962, pp. 12, 40–41.

61. Dwight D. Eisenhower, *Waging Peace,* p. 654.

62. George E. Reedy, *Twilight of the Presidency* (New York: World, 1970), p. 62.

3. John F. Kennedy

1. Kennedy to FDR, March 14, 1933, FDRL PPF 207.

2. "Visit to Europe—1938," Henry Stimson MS diary.

3. James MacGregor Burns, *John Kennedy: A Political Profile* (New York: Harcourt Brace, 1960), p. 25.

4. At Choate "young Jack Kennedy was about as remote as possible from the New Deal idealism of most Americans" (Herbert S. Parmet, *Jack: The Struggles of John F. Kennedy* [New York: Dial, 1980], p. 30).

5. Arthur M. Schlesinger, Jr., *Robert Kennedy and His Times* (Boston: Houghton Mifflin, 1978), p. 15.

6. One of his biographers has concluded, "The New Deal simply did not touch him," and Kennedy himself recalled, "I never had any particular interest in political subjects in those days" (Richard Whalen, *The Founding Father: The Story of Joseph P. Kennedy* [New York: New American Library, 1964], pp. 227, 170). See, too, Burns, *John Kennedy,* pp. 25–31.

7. Burns, *John Kennedy,* p. 32.

8. Kennedy, Spalding said, admired such romantic figures as Churchill and Byron, but not the president, perhaps "because of Mr. Roosevelt's handicaps—

I mean the polio—that sort of removed him from a younger man" (Spalding JFKL OH, pp. 11–12).

9. For a wry account of the Prague mission, see George F. Kennan, *Memoirs, 1925–1950* (Boston: Little, Brown, 1967), pp. 91–92.

10. Harold J. Laski to Joseph P. Kennedy, August 20, 1940, FDRL PPF 207.

11. John F. Kennedy, *Why England Slept* (New York: Wilfred Funk, 1940), pp. xv–xxi.

12. Jack Kennedy had only a marginal relationship to FDR. In August 1962 he remarked, "My earliest recollection, really, of President Roosevelt was a picture I saw after his nomination in 1932 when he came with his sons and sailed along the coast of Maine, and a very magic picture of him sitting at the wheel of a sailboat" (*Public Papers of the Presidents of the United States: John F. Kennedy, 1962* [Washington: Government Printing Office, 1962], p. 609). In 1938 he visited Hyde Park to leave with the superintendent of the estate a submarine gun he thought the president might use on a fishing cruise, and two years later he sent Roosevelt a copy of *Why England Slept,* and got an acknowledgment ("John F. Kennedy Presents Franklin D. Roosevelt with a Submarine Gun"; in John F. Kennedy to FDR, August 12, 1940, and FDR to Kennedy, August 27, 1940, FDRL PPF 5787).

13. Whalen, *Founding Father,* p. 49.

14. Francis Russell, *The President Makers* (Boston: Little, Brown, 1976), p. 347.

15. Parmet, *Jack,* p. 12.

16. Hank Searls, *The Lost Prince* (New York: World, 1969), p. 70; Donald C. Lord, *John F. Kennedy: The Politics of Confrontation and Conciliation* (Woodbury, N.Y.: Barron's, 1977), p. 10; David E. Koskoff, *Joseph P. Kennedy: A Life and Times* (Englewood Cliffs, N.J.: Prentice-Hall, 1974), pp. 44–47. For substantial contributions to the campaign not only by Kennedy but by Frank Walker, William Woodin, and Edward Flynn, see "Pre-Convention Campaign Committee for the nomination of Governor Franklin D. Roosevelt for President of the United States: Records of the Democratic National Committee," Franklin D. Roosevelt Library, Hyde Park, N.Y. On the final day of the campaign, Felix Frankfurter walked into Roosevelt's suite with a "very attractive" man who "was unmistakably Irish, with his copper colored hair, and a beaming smile that exposed his shining teeth." He said, "I've put some money into Mr. Roosevelt's campaign, and I'd like to go along with you all and take part in the fun" (Kay Halle JFKL OH, pp. 1–2).

17. Howard to Baker, July 12, 1932, Baker MSS, Box 122. Years later, John F. Kennedy passed an excerpt from this letter that had come to him on to his father. For the excerpt, see C. H. Cramer to John F. Kennedy, April 17, 1959, JFKL POF, Box 136.

18. Whalen, *Founding Father,* p. 131; Gloria Swanson, *Swanson on Swanson* (New York: Random House, 1980), p. 426; Raymond Moley with the assistance of Elliot A. Rosen, *The First New Deal* (New York: Harcourt Brace & World, 1966), p. 381; Russell, *President Makers,* pp. 319–20.

19. Technically, the commissioners were free to choose the chairman, but Roosevelt made clear that they were to elect Kennedy.

20. Victor Lasky, *J.F.K.: The Man and the Myth* (New York: Macmillan, 1963), p. 48; John Henry Cutler, *"Honey Fitz"* (Indianapolis: Bobbs-Merrill, 1962), p. 267; Harold Brayman, ed., *The President Speaks Off-The-Record: From Grover Cleveland to Gerald Ford . . . Historic Evenings with America's Leaders, the Press, and Other Men of Power, at Washington's Exclusive Gridiron Club* (Princeton: Dow Jones, 1976), p. 788.

21. Raymond Moley, *After Seven Years* (New York: Harper, 1939), p. 288; Ralph F. De Bedts, *The New Deal's SEC: The Formative Years* (New York: Columbia University Press, 1964), p. 111. See, too, Chester Lane COHC, pp. 282–83.

22. Arthur Krock JFKL OH, p. 2; Nancy Gager Clinch, *The Kennedy Neurosis* (New York: Grosset & Dunlap, 1973), p. 33; Edward Gallagher JFKL OH, p. 20; Whalen, *Founding Father*, pp. 156–57.

23. Eddie Dowling COHC, pp. 249–50; James P. Warburg COHC, p. 1259; interview with Arthur M. Schlesinger, Jr., December 29, 1979. The 1938 purge got under way after a call Claude Pepper paid to Jimmy Roosevelt at Joe Kennedy's Palm Beach home (Claude Pepper MS diary, February 2, 1938).

24. Kenneth P. O'Donnell and David F. Powers with Joe McCarthy, *"Johnny, We Hardly Knew Ye"* (Boston: Little, Brown, 1970), p. 58; Burns, *John Kennedy*, p. 46. In his last years, Fitzgerald, who had known every president since Grant, when asked who was the best of the lot, answered unhesitatingly, "Franklin Delano Roosevelt," the man who "was for the underdog" (Cutler, *"Honey Fitz,"* pp. 285, 318–19).

25. Or at least he put his name on the author's page; much of the volume was actually drafted by Arthur Krock. Joseph P. Kennedy to FDR, September 6, 1935; *Boston Post*, August 16, 1936, clipping, FDRL PPF 207; Joseph P. Kennedy, *I'm for Roosevelt* (New York: Reynal & Hitchcock, 1936); Arthur Krock, *Memoirs: Sixty Years on the Firing Line* (New York: Funk & Wagnalls, 1968), p. 332; Koskoff, *Joseph P. Kennedy*, pp. 82–85, 505; Ernest G. Draper, "Domestic Economic Policies of the Democratic Administration," address, October 23, 1936, Draper MSS, Box 2.

26. Joseph P. Kennedy to Bernard Baruch, March 4, 1937, Baruch MSS; Lord, *John F. Kennedy*, p. 11; Parmet, *Jack*, p. 55.

27. Charles D. Hilles to Lord Knollys, January 15, 1938, Hilles MSS, Box 214; Claude Pepper MS diary, October 12, 1938. I have altered slightly the punctuation and spelling for greater clarity.

28. Whalen, *Founding Father*, p. 205; Koskoff, *Joseph P. Kennedy*, pp. 115–17; Parmet, *Jack*, p. 56.

29. John Morton Blum, *From the Morgenthau Diaries: Years of Crisis, 1928–1938* (Boston: Houghton Mifflin, 1959), p. 518. See, too, Cordell Hull to FDR, March 14, 1938, FDRL OF 3060.

30. Harold L. Ickes, *The Secret Diary of Harold L. Ickes*, 3 vols. (New York: Simon & Schuster, 1954–55), 2:712. In October 1939, Roosevelt told another

cabinet officer that Kennedy "always has been an appeaser and always will be an appeaser. . . . He's just a pain in the neck to me" (Robert Dallek, *Franklin D. Roosevelt and American Foreign Policy, 1932–1945* [New York: Oxford University Press, 1979], p. 207).

31. Ickes, *Secret Diary,* 3:147; Harold J. Laski to FDR, January 15, 1939, FDRL PPF 3014. Curiously, though, Kennedy announced in December 1939 that he favored Roosevelt's nomination for a third term (Bernard F. Donahoe, *Private Plans and Public Dangers* [Notre Dame, Ind.: Notre Dame University Press, 1965], p. 125). He also said he was using signature cards of the president as prizes to induce his children to improve their grades (Joseph P. Kennedy to Marguerite Le Hand, March 27, 1939, FDRL PPF 207).

32. Ickes, *Secret Diary,* 2:415, 676; Homer S. Cummings MS diary, October 15, 1938. On August 24, 1939, Adolf Berle recorded in his diary that Joe Kennedy had phoned Sumner Welles his response to FDR's message to the king of Italy: "He said it was lousy. . . . He said the only proper procedure should have been a strong message to Poland urging her to make the necessary concessions to Germany." Berle added, "I am not quite clear how you would word a strong message to Poland. It would have to begin, 'In view of the fact that your suicide is required, kindly oblige by' etc." (Adolf A. Berle, *Navigating the Rapids,* ed. Beatrice Bishop Berle and Travis Beal Jacobs [New York: Harcourt Brace Jovanovich, 1973], p. 243).

33. Parmet, *Jack,* p. 67; Searls, *Lost Prince,* p. 165; Joseph P. Kennedy to James A. Farley, July 19, 1940, Farley MSS, Box 9. See, too, Arthur Krock JFKL OH, p. 5; Charles Garabedian JFKL OH, p. 2.

34. *New York Daily News,* December 10, 1937, clipping, Republican National Committee Papers; Ickes, *Secret Diary,* 2:676; Max Lerner, *Ted and the Kennedy Legend: A Study in Character and Destiny* (New York: St. Martin's Press, 1980), pp. 19, 24. For the view that in 1940 Roosevelt raised another Irish possibility, James Forrestal, to frustrate the ambitions of Kennedy and Farley, see Eliot Janeway, *The Economics of Crisis: War, Politics, and the Dollar* (New York: Weybright & Talley, 1968), p. 207.

35. Michael R. Beschloss, *Kennedy and Roosevelt: The Uneasy Alliance* (New York: Norton, 1980), p. 16; William Stevenson, *A Man Called Intrepid: The Secret War* (New York: Harcourt Brace Jovanovich, 1976), p. 149; Breckinridge Long MS diary, October 11, 1940; Walter Trohan HSTL OH, p. 73; George Bilainkin, *Diary of a Diplomatic Correspondent* (London: Allen & Unwin, 1942), p. 252; Schlesinger, *Robert Kennedy,* p. 35; Koskoff, *Joseph P. Kennedy,* pp. 185, 270–71; Arthur Krock JFKL OH, p. 7; C. L. Sulzberger, *The Last of the Giants* (New York: Macmillan, 1970), pp. 629–30.

36. Tom Wicker, *On Press* (New York: Viking, 1978), p. 78. See, too, Grace Tully LBJL OH, I, 29.

37. Koskoff, *Joseph P. Kennedy,* pp. 296–97; James F. Byrnes, *All in One Lifetime* (New York: Harper, 1958), pp. 125–26; Russell, *President Makers,* p. 358.

38. Russell, *President Makers,* p. 358; S. K. Ratcliffe to Felix Frankfurter, November 1, 1940, Frankfurter MSS, Box 92; Raymond E. Lee, *The London*

Journal of General Raymond E. Lee, ed. James Leutze (Boston: Little, Brown, 1971), p. 115.

39. Harold Laski even referred to "Joe Kennedy's suicide" (Laski to Felix Frankfurter, November 20, 1940, Frankfurter MSS, Box 74).

40. Cutler, *"Honey Fitz,"* p. 286; Edward Gallagher JFKL OH, p. 21; Ickes, *Secret Diary,* 3:386; Beschloss, *Kennedy and Roosevelt,* p. 223. The interview was not the direct cause of his resignation, for he had already told the president of his intention to leave (James M. Landis to Joseph P. Kennedy, February 8, 1952, Landis MSS, LC, Box 51). The publication of the interview, however, removed any possibility that he might stay on and curdled relations with the Roosevelt family. It has generally been overlooked, then and since, that he also referred to Mrs. Roosevelt as a "wonderful woman" who was "marvelously helpful" (Whalen, *Founding Father,* pp. 340–44).

41. Joseph P. Kennedy to FDR, December 7, 1941, and March 4, 1942; FDR to Joseph P. Kennedy, March 7, 1941; Kennedy to FDR, March 12, 1941, FDRL PPF 207; Bill Cunningham in *Boston Herald,* August 16, 1942, clipping, Republican National Committee Papers; Joseph P. Kennedy to Frank R. Kent, March 2, 1943, Kent MSS, Box 6.

42. "You have maligned me," Honey Fitz yelled at his opponent, Joseph Casey, during the campaign. "You have told the people of Massachusetts that I'm an octogenarian, and that's false." Dumfounded, Casey asked, "Well, how old are you?" Fitzgerald retorted, "I'm seventy-nine" (Parmet, *Jack,* p. 140).

43. Schlesinger, *Robert Kennedy,* p. 48. Honey Fitz concentrated much of his campaign on criticism of the Roosevelt government, and when Casey defeated him, Joe Kennedy made a sizable contribution to Casey's Republican opponent, Henry Cabot Lodge.

44. Beschloss, *Kennedy and Roosevelt,* p. 256.

45. Merle Miller, *Plain Speaking* (New York: Berkley, 1973), p. 186. Though Truman told this story some years later, and there is no way of verifying it absolutely, it is highly plausible. That Truman and Kennedy met in Boston in 1944 is confirmed by Joseph Casey JFKL OH, p. 12, and Edward Gallagher JFKL OH, p. 25. In 1945 Harold Ickes recorded in his diary: "Kennedy continues to speak of the President in the most unfitting language. One of his choice expressions is 'that son of a bitch.' But he uses other expressions that I do not even feel like putting down in a private memorandum." He added, "I know that the President hates Kennedy" (Beschloss, *Kennedy and Roosevelt,* p. 246). For Joseph Kennedy's deep grief over the death of his son, see Kennedy to Eugene Meyer, September 11, 1944, Meyer MSS, Box 30.

46. Beschloss, *Kennedy and Roosevelt,* p. 257. For Joseph Kennedy's concern about "the growing Jewish influence in the press" in the World War II era, see Joseph P. Kennedy Memoirs, typescript, James M. Landis MSS, LC, Box 51. Kennedy's prewar reputation as a man disloyal to President Roosevelt continued to plague him after the war. In the spring of 1946, Robert Hannegan wrote the secretary of the Treasury: "I do hope it will be possible for you to give further consideration to Joe Kennedy for appointment as President of the World Bank. I do believe he would go along with you and be a team player,

regardless—and I say this fully conscious of many things that have happened in the past" (Hannegan to Fred M. Vinson, May 31, 1946, Vinson MSS, Box 139). A year later, Joe Kennedy wrote a British friend that Truman would try "to carry out the policies of a man who is dead who, even if he were alive, couldn't carry them out himself" (Koskoff, *Joseph P. Kennedy,* p. 366). For Joe Kennedy's closeness to Herbert Hoover, see James A. Fayne JFKL OH, p. 8. "Of my knowledge I can say there never was the intimacy with Roosevelt that there was with Mr. Hoover—never," Fayne stated.

47. *New Orleans Times-Picayune,* April 13, 1945, clipping, Mrs. Sidney N. Pelayo Papers; Schlesinger, *Robert Kennedy,* p. 59; William Manchester, *Portrait of a President: John F. Kennedy in Profile* (Boston: Little, Brown, 1967), p. 21.

48. Ralph G. Martin and Ed Plaut, *Front Runner, Dark Horse* (Garden City, N.Y.: Doubleday, 1960), p. 148; Lord, *John F. Kennedy,* pp. 41–42; *Congressional Record,* 81st Cong., 1st sess., p. A993.

49. Schlesinger, *Robert Kennedy,* pp. 82–83; Robert F. Kennedy to the editor, January 26, 1954, in *New York Times,* February 3, 1954.

50. Victor Lasky, *Robert F. Kennedy: The Myth and the Man* (New York: Trident, 1968), pp. 55, 74–75. See, too, Phil Fine JFKL OH, pp. 2–6; Jackson J. Holtz JFKL OH, p. 3; "From Kennedy for Senator Headquarters," press release, n.d., mimeographed, JFK MSS, Pre-Presidential Papers, Box 105.

51. Americans for Democratic Action approved of his votes on eleven of thirteen issues in 1947–48, on twenty of twenty-eight in the next Congress (John Osborne, "The Economics of the Candidates," *Fortune,* October 1960, p. 138). As a graduate student at Johns Hopkins in 1954, Stephen Hess wrote an article highlighting a shift in Kennedy's voting record; "namely that after six years of straight 'Fair Deal' voting on domestic expenditures in the House of Representatives, he had reversed himself and opposed almost all increased domestic appropriations legislation in his first two years in the Senate" (Stephen H. Hess, "Memorandum for Mr. Bob Merriam," August 8, 1960, Hess MSS, Box 2). (*The Reporter* rejected the article; there was not enough interest in Kennedy, it said.) Another, later analysis stated that the Eisenhower administration "never received any support from Senator Kennedy when the chips were down, if at all" (George H. Becker, Jr., to Oliver Gale, August 16, 1960, Hess MSS, Box 2). A study of his Senate performance from 1957 to 1960 concluded that he was "a strong supporter of liberal labor, housing, and welfare programs, a moderately strong backer of public power programs, an advocate of high agricultural price supports, an active though recent convert to civil rights legislation" (Charles H. Gray, "A Scale Analysis of the Voting Records of Senators Kennedy, Johnson and Goldwater, 1957–1960," *American Political Science Review* 59 [September 1965]:621). In general, see Americans for Democratic Action, "Voting Record of Senator John F. Kennedy," Eleanor Roosevelt MSS, Box 4415.

52. John F. Kennedy, "What's Wrong with Social Security," *American Magazine,* October 1953, p. 19; Parmet, *Jack,* pp. 269–70.

53. William F. Swindler, *Court and Constitution in the Twentieth Century: The New Legality, 1932–1968* (Indianapolis: Bobbs-Merrill, 1970), p. 154.

54. The phrase is Ferdinand Lundberg's in *Cracks in the Constitution* (Secaucus, N.J.: Lyle Stuart, 1980), p. 246. See, too, Clinton Rossiter, *The American Presidency* (New York: Harvest, 1960), p. 233; Senator Capper on S. J. Res. 10, September 27, 1945, Arthur Capper MSS, Box 58. Harold Ickes thought the movement for an amendment derived not from principle but out of "the spitefulness of those who, for personal or partisan reasons, hated President Roosevelt and what he stood for." He added, "Of course, a James A. Farley, as a part of his campaign of malice and envy, is for a limitation of Presidential tenure on 'principle,' but who ever sought Mr. Farley's counsel on any historical, legal or constitutional issue?" Without his ghost writers, Farley "would be as inarticulate as a wooden Indian" (press release, February 7, 1949, Records of the National Committee against Limiting the Presidency, Box 1).

55. Theodore Sorensen, *Kennedy* (New York: Harper & Row, 1965), pp. 17–18.

56. Burns, *John Kennedy,* p. 155; Osborne, "Economics of the Candidates," p. 138.

57. Whalen, *Founding Father,* pp. 402–3.

58. Ibid., p. 402; Jeanne M. Luboja, "John F. Kennedy and the McCarthy Issue: A Study in the Politics of Liberalism (1925–1960)," M.A. thesis, Columbia University, 1974, p. 27.

59. Burton Hersh, *The Education of Edward Kennedy* (New York: Morrow, 1972), p. 89. See, too, David Halberstam, *The Best and the Brightest* (Greenwich, Conn.: Fawcett, 1973), p. 19.

60. Luboja, "John F. Kennedy and the McCarthy Issue," is thorough and perceptive. Kennedy was also damaged by an article that reported that he had caused "anguish" among "New Deal Democrats" by expressing McCarthyite views at a 1950 Harvard seminar (John P. Mallan, "Massachusetts: Liberal and Corrupt," *New Republic,* October 13, 1952, pp. 10–12). Theodore Sorensen subsequently complained that these charges were "still being circulated a decade after they had been thoroughly discredited" (*Kennedy,* p. 4).

61. Tyler Abell, ed., *Drew Pearson Diaries, 1949–1959* (New York: Holt, Rinehart & Winston, 1974), p. 248.

62. Philip A. Grant, Jr., "Catholic Congressmen, Cardinal Spellman, Eleanor Roosevelt, and the 1949–1950 Federal Aid to Education Controversy," *Records of the American Catholic Historical Society of Philadelphia* 90 (March–December 1979), 3–13; Joseph P. Lash, *Eleanor: The Years Alone* (New York: Norton, 1972), p. 158; James Wine JFKL OH, pp. 4–6; Burns, *John Kennedy,* p. 88; Parmet, *Jack,* p. 206.

63. Lawrence Fuchs JFKL OH, pp. 40–41. See, too, Charles W. Cole JFKL OH, p. 37; Jack L. Bell JFKL OH, pp. 14–15; Robert Benjamin JKFL OH, pp. 9–10; James M. Landis COHC, pp. 606–8.

64. Parmet, *Jack,* pp. 368–69. For Eleanor Roosevelt's prestige at the 1956 convention, see Cass Canfield COHC, p. 308. To compound difficulties with FDR's family, James Roosevelt also opposed Kennedy's candidacy (Thomas Rees JFKL OH, pp. 2–3; Dore Schary JFKL OH, pp. 5–6).

65. Eleanor Roosevelt, "On My Own, Conclusion: Of Stevenson, Truman and Kennedy," *Saturday Evening Post,* March 8, 1958, pp. 32–33, 72–74; James Tracy Crown, *The Kennedy Literature: A Bibliographical Essay on John F. Kennedy* (New York: New York University Press, 1968), p. 127.

66. "College News Conference," December 7, 1958, ABC Television, Theodore Sorensen MSS, Box 25.

67. JFK to Mrs. Franklin D. Roosevelt, December 11, 1958; Eleanor Roosevelt to JFK, December 18, 1958; JFK to Mrs. Franklin D. Roosevelt, December 29, 1958; JFK to Philip L. Graham, December 29, 1958, Theodore Sorensen MSS, Box 25.

68. Eleanor Roosevelt to JFK, January 6, 1959; JFK to Mrs. Franklin D. Roosevelt, January 10, 1959; Eleanor Roosevelt to JFK, January 20, 1959; JFK to Mrs. Franklin D. Roosevelt, January 22, 1959; JFK to Philip L. Graham, January 22, 1959; Graham to JFK, January 21, 1959, Theodore Sorensen MSS, Box 25; Eleanor Roosevelt to JFK, January 29, 1959, JFKL POF 32. Graham's letter was written before he had received this latest piece of evidence.

69. Lawrence H. Fuchs, "The Senator and the Lady," *American Heritage* 25 (October 1974):59–60. "In effect, he was saying to me, 'Look, Fuchs, you're a liberal, intellectual, New York Jew. Why aren't there more guys like you for me?'" (Fuchs JFKL OH, p. 6). See, too, Fuchs to Sheldon M. Stern, August 30, 1977, Fuchs JFKL OH.

70. Gore Vidal, "The Holy Family," *Esquire,* April 1967, p. 202.

71. Gore Vidal, review of Joseph P. Lash, *Eleanor and Franklin,* in *New York Review of Books,* November 18, 1971, p. 8. Doubt has been raised about the accuracy of the story. See Koskoff, *Joseph P. Kennedy,* p. 571. If in fact Kennedy was not at Hyde Park at this time, Mrs. Roosevelt may well have been spinning a yarn about something that happened earlier and tying it to her recollection of Kennedy's interview. If so, the tale adds to the sense of how deeply Joe Kennedy's words wounded her.

72. Lash, *Eleanor: The Years Alone,* p. 287. See, too, Robert Nathan JFKL OH, p. 4. A prominent Democrat has observed: "Mrs. Roosevelt, interestingly enough, I think quite late in life developed a very strong obstinate streak that you could not deal with. First of all, I think she had a relationship with President Kennedy's father which left its mark. And no matter what was said it could not be dislodged from her mind. . . . And she just didn't have any use for his son, and she couldn't believe that there could be any disassociation from generation to generation, which was very narrow minded of her, but was rather typical" (Katie Louchheim JFKL OH, p. 37). Mrs. Roosevelt was not the only prominent Democrat to be worried about the influence of Jack Kennedy's father on his son. Harry Truman told an interviewer, "It's not the Pope I'm afraid of, it's the Pop" (Miller, *Plain Speaking,* p. 187).

73. Schary, *Heyday: An Autobiography* (Boston: Little, Brown, 1979), p. 366; Schary JFKL OH, p. 7. In 1960 Schary wrote Arthur Schlesinger, Jr.: "I got a telephone call from someone who said that I have just finished adding a sequence to *Sunrise at Campobello* in which Roosevelt talks about the right of a

Catholic to be elected President. When I explained that this scene was in the play when it opened in January of 1958, my accuser said that was a lie" (quoted in Schlesinger to JFK, August 8, 1960, JFK MSS, Pre-Presidential, Box 747).

74. Theodore H. White, *The Making of the President, 1968* (New York: Atheneum, 1969), p. 187.

75. Emmet John Hughes, *The Ordeal of Power* (New York: Atheneum, 1963), p. 312.

76. O'Donnell and Powers with McCarthy, *"Johnny,"* p. 155.

77. The drafts of Kennedy's speeches are in JFKL Presidential, Boxes 900, 915.

78. "Excerpts from Speeches by Senator John F. Kennedy," Americans for Democratic Action, Southeastern Pennsylvania Chapter MSS, Box 24.

79. Cyrus Rice JFKL OH, pp. 3–4; Ira Kapenstein JFKL OH, p. 2; Ralph de Toledano, *R.F.K.: The Man Who Would Be President* (New York: Putnam's, 1967), p. 137.

80. Hugh Sidey, *A Very Personal Presidency: Lyndon Johnson in the White House* (New York: Atheneum, 1968), p. 105.

81. Albert Eisele, *Almost to the Presidency: A Biography of Two American Politicians* (Blue Earth, Minn.: Piper, 1972), p. 25.

82. Ibid., pp. 50, 57; Hubert H. Humphrey, *The Political Philosophy of the New Deal* (Baton Rouge: Louisiana State University Press, 1970); Charles W. Bailey II, "Never Stop Running: Hubert H. Humphrey," in *Candidates 1960*, ed. Eric Sevareid (New York: Basic Books, 1959), p. 159.

83. Richard J. Walton, *Henry Wallace, Harry Truman, and the Cold War* (New York: Viking, 1976), p. 32; Allan H. Ryskind, *Hubert: An Unauthorized Biography of the Vice President* (New Rochelle, N.Y.: Arlington House, 1968), p. 59.

84. Winthrop Griffith, *Humphrey: A Candid Biography* (New York: Morrow, 1965), p. 245; Ryskind, *Hubert*, p. 230. See, too, Michael Amrine, *This Is Humphrey: The Story of the Senator* (Garden City, N.Y.: Doubleday, 1960), pp. 19, 248; "The Democratic Presidential Possibilities," *New Mexican* (Santa Fe, 1960), Hunt Unger Papers, Folder 37.

85. William Richardson JFKL OH, p. 15; Charles Love JFKL OH, p. 12; William Chilton III JFKL OH, p. 6; Andrew Houvouras JFKL OH, p. 5; John E. Amos JFKL OH, pp. 20–21; Peter Lisagor JFKL OH, p. 19. See, too, M. L. Wilson COHC, p. 1341; Lawrence E. Tierney, Jr. JFKL OH, p. 3; Lawrence F. O'Brien, *No Final Victories: A Life in Politics—From John F. Kennedy to Watergate* (Garden City, N.Y.: Doubleday, 1974), p. 72.

86. Sidney Christie JFKL OH, p. 3.

87. Lasky, *J.F.K.*, p. 339; Frank Fischer JFKL OH, p. 3. At a summit meeting of sixteen campaign workers Robert Kennedy asked, "In summary, what is your opinion regarding the religious problem in the area that you know?" He was told, "Must . . . show that there is something more important to those people than anything to do with religion. Got to have something like the feeling they had for FDR." Meeting Re West Virginia Primary, April 8, 1960, Robert F. Kennedy MSS, Pre-Administration, Political Files, Box 39. In

adopting such a strategy, Kennedy could capitalize on the fact that at least some West Virginians had already begun to think of him in connection with Roosevelt. Louis Harris and Associates, "A Study of Issues and Images in West Virginia," June 1958, JFKL Pre-Presidential, Box 818; William Bruce Hoff JFKL OH, p. 36.

88. Hubert H. Humphrey, *The Education of a Public Man: My Life and Politics,* ed. Norman Sherman (Garden City, N.Y.: Doubleday, 1976), p. 475. Humphrey added bitterly, "Beneath the image, however, there are no beneficent comparisons."

89. Lasky, *Robert F. Kennedy;* O'Donnell and Powers with McCarthy, *"Johnny,"* p. 165.

90. Victor Lasky, *It Didn't Start with Watergate* (New York: Dial, 1977), pp. 23–24; William Lawrence JFKL OH, p. 6; Edward Morgan JFKL OH, p. 6. For resentment at the charges of FDR, Jr., see Robert Nathan JFKL OH, p. 13; John Blatnik JFKL OH, pp. 17–18; Orville L. Freeman JFKL OH, p. 7; Frank Thompson JFKL OH, p. 21. Hyman Bookbinder JFKL OH, pp. 26–27, quotes an indignant letter from Humphrey. See, too, Ludwig Teller COHC, p. 328.

91. Lasky, *J.F.K.,* p. 345; Sorensen, *Kennedy,* p. 167; Lawrence H. Fuchs, *John F. Kennedy and American Catholicism* (New York: Meredith Press, 1967), p. 174; Andrew Houvouras JFKL OH, p. 21. I have slightly altered the Humphrey quotation for greater accuracy in transcription.

92. Robert Sherrill and Harry W. Ernst, *The Drugstore Liberal* (New York: Grossman, 1968), p. 154; Claude Ellis JFKL OH, pp. 5–6; Michael G. Gretchen JFKL OH, p. 4; Andrew Houvouras JFKL OH, p. 21; Marshall G. West JFKL OH, p. 7. See, too, Arch Riley JFKL OH, p. 35; Jennings Randolph JFKL OH; Esther Peters JFKL OH, p. 9; Dick Wright JFKL OH, p. 1; Miles Stanley JFKL OH, p. 8; Bill Lawrence, *Six Presidents, Too Many Wars* (New York: Saturday Review Press, 1972), pp. 232–33.

93. Charles Peters JFKL OH, pp. 11–12. See, too, Edward Morgan JFKL OH, p. 7; William Lawrence JFKL OH, p. 5; Carl Vickers JFKL OH, p. 17. For skepticism, see William Chilton III JFKL OH, p. 6; Walter Hart JFKL OH, p. 20; Sidney Christie JFKL OH, p. 11. Instead of being a liability, Kennedy's patrician Yankee mannerisms turned out to be an asset, "because they were used to the late President Roosevelt speaking, and their accents are similar," a native explained. "They were used to that accent in West Virginia, because President Roosevelt was the saviour of West Virginia" (Anne Hearst JFKL OH, p. 13).

94. Burns, *John Kennedy,* p. 243. For her unwillingness to commit herself, see Eleanor Roosevelt to Ellen S. Woodward, April 14, 1958, Woodward MSS, Box 9. The economist Paul Samuelson has recalled, "Mrs. Roosevelt was very upset, particularly about Arthur, of whom she was very fond" (Council of Economic Advisers JFKL OH, p. 76). Robert Kennedy's intervention in New York politics had also irritated the reform group of which she was a leader (Ralph de Toledano, "In Washington," in Stephen H. Hess MSS, Box 2). For the division among liberals, see Chester Bowles JFKL OH, pp. 4, 98.

95. Lash, *Eleanor,* pp. 284–85. For the claim that she was not hostile to

Kennedy, but merely believed he was not yet experienced enough for the presidency, see Lawrence Fuchs JFKL OH, pp. 14–16, 27–28; Dore Schary JFKL OH, p. 10. Fuchs surmised that she thought Stevenson "a bigger man in some respects than her husband." But he added, "It's just a feeling, just a feeling, and she never said anything in words" (Fuchs JFKL OH, p. 29).

96. Lasky, *J.F.K.*, p. 350; James Roosevelt with Bill Libby, *My Parents: A Differing View* (Chicago: Playboy Press, 1976), p. 332.

97. Lasky, *J.F.K.*, p. 395; Lash, *Eleanor*, pp. 289–91; Norman Mailer, *The Presidential Papers* (New York: Putnam's, 1963), p. 36. See, too, Margaret Dixon JFKL OH, p. 5; Arthur Chapin JFKL OH, p. 6; Mike Monroney, Jr. COHC, p. 50; Barry Bingham COHC, p. 96.

98. He added, "They saw Lyndon Johnson, who had some of F.D.R.'s political skill and acumen but not his audacity; they saw Adlai Stevenson, who had the sense of history but not his decisiveness; and they saw Stuart Symington, who had Roosevelt's ambition but not his exciting talent for capturing the public attention" (*Newsweek,* July 18, 1960, p. 28).

99. James A. Farley LBJL OH, p. 21; Arthur M. Schlesinger, Jr., *A Thousand Days* (Boston: Houghton Mifflin, 1965), p. 57; Helen Fuller, *Year of Trial* (New York: Harcourt Brace & World, 1962), p. 12; *Christian Science Monitor,* July 14, 1960. When liberals objected to the choice of Johnson as Kennedy's running mate, Galbraith circulated among the liberal delegates saying, with his characteristic irony, "This is the kind of political expedient Franklin Roosevelt would never have used—except in the case of John Nance Garner." Others, too, pointed out that in 1932 Roosevelt had chosen to round out the ticket with a conservative Texan, Speaker Garner (John Kenneth Galbraith, *A Life in Our Times: Memoirs* [Boston: Houghton Mifflin, 1981], pp. 381, 384).

100. Sulzberger, *Last of the Giants,* p. 681; David E. Lilienthal, *The Journals of David E. Lilienthal,* 6 vols. (New York: Harper & Row, 1964–76), 5:103.

101. *New York Times,* July 16, 1960. A British historian, though, has called Kennedy's acceptance address "almost a paraphrase of a speech delivered over the wireless by President Roosevelt on 24th August 1935" (David K. Adams, "Roosevelt and Kennedy," *Bulletin of the British Association for American Studies* 7 [December 1963]:30).

102. Robert Keith Gray, *Eighteen Acres under Glass* (Garden City, N.Y.: Doubleday, 1962), p. 318; "Excerpts from Speeches by Senator John F. Kennedy," Americans for Democratic Action, Southeastern Pennsylvania Chapter MSS, Box 24; Whalen, *Founding Father,* pp. 459–60. See, too, Byron G. Lander, "Group Theory and Individuals: The Origin of Poverty as a Political Issue in 1964," *Western Political Quarterly* 24 (September 1971):516–17; Sorensen, *Kennedy,* p. 225; O'Donnell and Powers with McCarthy, *"Johnny,"* p. 217; Fuchs, *John F. Kennedy and American Catholicism,* p. 217; J. K. Galbraith to JFK, October 20, 1960, Galbraith MSS, Box 74; Henry Fairlie, *The Kennedy Promise: The Politics of Expectation* (Garden City, N.Y.: Doubleday, 1973), p. 9.

103. *Senate Report 994,* 87th Cong., 1st sess., 3 vols. (Washington, D.C.: Government Printing Office, 1961), 3:115, 120–22.

104. Ibid., pp. 75, 92.

105. Richard L. Strout, *TRB* (New York: Macmillan, 1979), p. 197; O'Donnell and Powers with McCarthy, *"Johnny,"* p. 210; *Senate Report 994*, 3:42; Schlesinger, *Kennedy or Nixon*, p. 24. See, too, "If There's Another 'New Deal'—What's It to Be Like," *U.S. News & World Report*, August 8, 1960, pp. 71–73. Admiral John Harllee, who served as an aide to Kennedy on Capitol Hill, later said: "During the period that I was in his office I was tremendously impressed with him and believed that he was so similar to Franklin Roosevelt in personal magnetism and political pragmatism that I became absolutely certain that he would someday be President of the United States and that he would be a great President. I thought it was interesting to note that he also had many superficial resemblances to F.D.R., such as his connection with the Navy, health problems, wealth, prep school and Harvard background, and the Democratic party faith" (John Harllee JFKL OH, p. 7). "Much in the same way that polio mellowed Franklin Roosevelt, Kennedy's physical pain deepened his compassion," observed Claude Pepper, who served in Congress during the administrations of both men (Lewis J. Paper, *The Promise and the Performance: The Leadership of John F. Kennedy* [New York: Crown, 1975], p. 57).

106. T.R.B., "From Washington," *New Republic*, January 9, 1961, p. 2; Burns, *John Kennedy*, p. 103. See, too, Murray B. Levin, *Kennedy Campaigning: The System and the Style as Practiced by Senator Edward Kennedy* (Boston: Beacon Press, 1966), pp. 23, 83.

107. Charles Love JFKL OH, p. 12. For an account placing Mrs. Roosevelt's behavior in a more favorable light, see Lash, *Eleanor*, p. 291.

108. John A. Stover to John K. Galbraith, July 19, 1960, Galbraith MSS, Box 74. For the exclusion of Mrs. Roosevelt from the New York delegation, see Bert E. Swanson, "The Presidential Convention as a Stage in the Struggle for Political Leadership: The New York Democratic Delegation," *Inside Politics: The National Conventions, 1960*, ed. Paul Tillett (Dobbs Ferry, N.Y.: Oceana, published for the Eagleton Institute of Politics at Rutgers, 1962), pp. 197–98.

109. Fuchs, "Senator and the Lady," pp. 81–82.

110. Lash, *Eleanor*, p. 293; Hyman Bookbinder JFKL OH, pp. 58–59; Arthur Schlesinger, Jr., to JFK, August 8, 1960, JFKL Pre-Presidential, Box 747; Halberstam, *Best and the Brightest*, p. 32; Eleanor Roosevelt to Mary Lasker, August 15, 1960; Eleanor Roosevelt to JFK, August 16, 1960, JFKL POF, Box 32.

111. JFK to Eleanor Roosevelt, September 3, 1960, JFKL POF, Box 32; Lawrence Fuchs JFKL OH, p. 27; John Jay Hooker JFKL OH, p. 55; Kay Halle JFKL OH, p. 13. See, too, Carl Vickers JFKL OH, p. 17; Harris Wofford, *Of Kennedys and Kings: Making Sense of the Sixties* (New York: Farrar, Straus & Giroux, 1980), pp. 63–64.

112. Eleanor Roosevelt to JFK, October 24, 1960, JFKL POF, Box 32.

113. Memo, "To: Bobby, From: Senator Kennedy," dictated by phone, September 3, 1960, Robert F. Kennedy MSS, Pre-Administration, Political Files, Box 39; Schlesinger, *Robert Kennedy*, p. 91.

114. Whalen, *Founding Father,* pp. 458–59.
115. James L. Sundquist, *Politics and Policy: The Eisenhower, Kennedy, and Johnson Years* (Washington, D.C.: Brookings Institution, 1968), pp. 469–70. Sundquist draws upon Herbert McClosky, Paul J. Hoffmann, and Rosemary O'Hara, "Issue Conflict and Consensus among Party Leaders and Followers," *American Political Science Review* 54 (June 1960):406–27. See, too, Michael V. Di Salle JFKL OH, p. 20; Robert F. McDonough JFKL OH, p. 22; James Hilty, *John F. Kennedy: An Idealist without Illusions* (St. Louis: Forum Press, 1976), p. 7. There was, of course, one notable difference between 1960 and the Roosevelt elections. The early returns on Election Night 1960 led commentators to say that Kennedy was headed for "a landslide of Rooseveltian proportions," but when all the returns were in it was clear that Kennedy, unlike Roosevelt, had won only narrowly. Raymond Price, *With Nixon* (New York: Viking, 1977), p. 37. For one explanation of the decline in the Democratic share of the vote in such areas as California's Central Valley, see Kevin P. Phillips, *The Emerging Republican Majority* (New Rochelle, N.Y.: Arlington House, 1969), pp. 456–58.
116. T.R.B., "From Washington," *New Republic,* January 9, 1961, p. 2.
117. Arthur M. Schlesinger, Jr., to JFK, November 14, 1960, JFKL POF, Box 165.
118. Burns, "John F. Kennedy, Candidate on the Eve: Liberalism Without Tears," *New Republic,* October 31, 1960, pp. 14–16. See, too, "A Size-Up of Kennedy: An Interview with His Biographer James MacGregor Burns," *U.S. News & World Report,* November 28, 1960, p. 76.
119. Burns, *Kennedy,* pp. 280–81.
120. *Public Papers of the United States: John F. Kennedy, 1961* (Washington, D.C.: Government Printing Office, 1962), p. 28; Strout, *TRB,* pp. 217–18.
121. Schlesinger, *Thousand Days,* p. 676.
122. Robert F. Kennedy, *We Must Meet Our Duty and Convince the World That We Are Just Friends and Brave Enemies* (New York: Harper & Row, 1962), p. 54.
123. Richard E. Neustadt, "Memorandum on Staffing the President-Elect," October 30, 1960, Theodore Sorensen MSS, Box 18; Schlesinger, *Thousand Days,* pp. 123–24. In addition, Brookings put together a study on the transition which included an account of how Franklin Roosevelt used his cabinet (Bradley Patterson JFKL OH, p. 4). See, too, Arthur M. Schlesinger, Jr., *The Imperial Presidency* (Boston: Houghton Mifflin, 1973), pp. 464–65.
124. Richard E. Neustadt, "Approaches to Staffing the Presidency: Notes on FDR and JFK," *American Political Science Review* 57 (December 1963):861; William J. Hopkins JFKL OH, pp. 27–28; Hugh Sidey, *John F. Kennedy, President: A Reporter's Inside Story* (New York: Atheneum, 1963), p. 8; Theodore H. White, *In Search of History* (New York: Warner, 1979), p. 497. See, too, George F. Gilder and Bruce K. Chapman, *The Party That Lost Its Head* (New York: Knopf, 1966), p. 29; Charles Lam Markham and Mark Sherwin, *John F. Kennedy: A sense of purpose* (New York: St. Martin's, 1961), pp. 4–5; M. J.

Rossant, "The Economic Education of John F. Kennedy," *Reporter,* February 14, 1963, p. 23. James M. Landis served as a link between the New Deal and the New Frontier. Roosevelt's choice to succeed Joe Kennedy as chairman of the SEC, he had become legal adviser and political consultant for the Kennedy clan after the war. One of the first things John Kennedy did after the 1960 election was to ask Landis to prepare a report on the regulatory commissions, and within a month Landis completed the task (Landis, "The President's Reorganization Program for the Regulatory Agencies," address, November 9, 1961, Landis MSS, LC, Box 148; see, too, Landis MSS, JFKL, especially Box 19; Donald A. Ritchie, "Reforming the Regulatory Process: Why James Landis Changed His Mind," *Business History Review* 54 [1980]:283–302).

125. Schlesinger also supervised the list of invitees to the opening. He noted that the president wanted people associated with Roosevelt to be asked, but emphasized, "I see no point, however, in inviting people who hate FDR's guts (Clare Hoffman or John Taber, for example)," and he asked a White House legislative aide to "have someone look at the list and strike off the names of all unregenerate Roosevelt haters" (Arthur Schlesinger, Jr., "Memorandum for Mike N. Manatos," June 12, 1962, Schlesinger MSS, Box 19). See, too, typescript manuscript draft, "F.D.R.'s 'Old Navy': An Informal Introduction by John F. Kennedy"; Schlesinger, Memorandum for the President, August 21, 1961, June 27, 1962; Schlesinger to Eleanor Roosevelt, May 24, 1962, idem. Kennedy presided over cabinet meetings at a table designed by Jesse Jones for Roosevelt (Hale Boggs JFKL OH, p. 12).

126. Schlesinger to Seymour Harris, September 22, 1961, Schlesinger MSS, Box 11; Schlesinger to the President, December 8, 1962, JFKL POF, Box 65a; August Heckscher JFKL OH, p. 42; Lord, *John F. Kennedy,* p. 125.

127. Felix Frankfurter JFKL OH, p. 41. For greater clarity, I have slightly altered the wording.

128. Fred Dutton, Memorandum for the President, January 27, 1961; January 31, 1961, JFKL POF 63.

129. *Public Papers of the Presidents: 1962,* pp. 414, 389–90.

130. Richard Bolling to Robert L. Melan, April 26, 1961, Bolling MSS, Box 11; John Blatnik JFKL OH, p. 24; Tom Wicker, *JFK and LBJ: The Influence of Personality upon Politics* (New York: Morrow, 1968), pp. 45, 67–68; Henry Z. Scheele, *Charlie Halleck: A Political Biography* (New York: Exposition Press, 1966), p. 205; Edmund S. Ions, *The Politics of John F. Kennedy* (New York: Barnes & Noble, 1967), p. 162.

131. *Public Papers of the Presidents of the United States: John F. Kennedy, 1963* (Washington, D.C.: Government Printing Office, 1964), p. 193.

132. David T. Stanley, *Changing Administration: The 1961 and 1964 Transitions in Six Departments* (Washington, D.C.: Brookings Institution, 1965), p. 94; Don F. Hadwiger and Ross B. Talbot, *Pressures and Protests: The Kennedy Farm Program and Wheat Referendum of 1963* (San Francisco: Chandler, 1965), pp. 4–5; Stewart L. Udall, *The Quiet Crisis* (New York: Holt, Rinehart & Winston, 1963), p. xiii; "The REA Electrification Program," in Council of

State Chambers of Commerce, *Federal Spending Facts,* Bulletin no. 203, May 13, 1963, Horace R. Kornegay MSS, Box 24.

133. *Business Week,* March 30, 1963, p. 79; Leonard Mayo JFKL OH, p. 3. See, too, Alvin Shuster, "Back to the Woods: The New Youth Conservation Corps follows a 30-year-old trail blazed by the C.C.C.," *New York Times Magazine,* August 18, 1963, pp. 32, 34, 36. On the other hand, Republican members of the Education and Labor Committee opposed the administration's Youth Conservation Corps bill for failing to heed "the one basic lesson of the old CCC . . . that education and conservation work are cumbersome partners" (Charles E. Goodell to "Dear Colleague," March 11, 1963, Clifford G. McIntire MSS, Box 95).

134. Benjamin C. Bradlee, *Conversations with Kennedy* (New York: Norton, 1975), p. 227. See, too, Robert F. Kennedy JFKL OH, p. 5; Stan Opotowsky, *The Kennedy Government* (New York: Popular Library, 1961), pp. 9–11; Henry L. Trewhitt, *McNamara: His Ordeal in the Pentagon* (New York: Harper & Row, 1971), p. 11; Sidey, *John F. Kennedy,* p. 44; William V. Shannon, *The Heir Apparent: Robert Kennedy and the Struggle for Power* (New York: Macmillan, 1967), p. 187; Roosevelt with Libby, *My Parents,* p. 315; Jack Newfield, *Robert Kennedy: A Memoir* (New York: Dutton, 1969), pp. 156–57; Dorothy Goldberg, *A Private View of a Public Life* (New York: Charterhouse, 1975), p. 126; Traphes Bryant with Frances Spatz Leighton, *Dog Days at the White House: The Outrageous Memoirs of the Presidential Kennel Keeper* (New York: Macmillan, 1975), p. 42; and the oral history memoirs of Roswell L. Gilpatric, Albert Zack, Luther Hodges, Claiborne Pell, and William Batt, JFKL. On January 18, 1961, Adolf Berle entered in his diary, "Dean Rusk telephoned to ask whether it would be thinkable to appoint Franklin D. Roosevelt, Jr. as Assistant Secretary of State for Latin American Affairs. I told him it would be fatal" (Berle, *Navigating the Rapids,* p. 728).

135. Lash, *Eleanor: The Years Alone,* pp. 313–15; Eleanor Roosevelt to JFK, July 22, 26, 1961; JFK to Eleanor Roosevelt, July 28, 1961, JFKL POF, Box 32.

136. Eleanor Roosevelt to JFK, July 22, 1961, JFKL POF, Box 32; Eleanor Roosevelt to JFK, September 25, 1961, Eleanor Roosevelt MSS, Box 4469.

137. Eleanor Roosevelt to JFK, July 26, 1961, JFKL POF, Box 32; William Manchester, *The Death of a President: November 20–November 25* (New York: Harper & Row, 1967), p. 351.

138. Laura Bergquist, "What Women Really Meant to JFK," *Redbook,* November 1973, p. 54. FDR's first term had turned Jacqueline Kennedy's father from a man of Democratic inclinations to a confirmed anti–New Deal Republican (John H. Davis, *The Bouviers* [New York: Avon, 1969], p. 205).

139. August Heckscher, JFKL OH, p. 51; Jacqueline Kennedy to Eleanor Roosevelt, May 31, 1962, Eleanor Roosevelt MSS, Box 1962.

140. Eleanor Roosevelt to JFK, February 1, 1962; March 2, 1961; April 7, 1961; Transcript of an Introductory Interview with Mrs. Eleanor Roosevelt and the President to Be Included in the *Prospects of Mankind* Series for National Educational Television, April 22, 1962, JFKL POF, Box 32; John F. Macy JFKL OH, p. 57; Prescott Bush COHC, pp. 417–18.

141. Fuchs, "Senator and Lady," pp. 73, 83; Fuchs JFKL OH, pp. 35–38.

142. Hyman Bookbinder JFKL OH, pp. 60–61; John F. Macy JFKL OH, p. 59; Berle, *Navigating the Rapids,* pp. 776–77.

143. Bradlee, *Conversations with Kennedy,* p. 42; Burns, *John Kennedy,* p. 273. In his relations with Great Britain he managed to overcome the handicap of suspicion engendered by memories of his father (Arthur Krock JFKL OH, p. 8; Dean Rusk JFKL OH, p. 3).

144. Markham and Sherwin, *John F. Kennedy,* p. 56; *As Others See Us: American History in the Foreign Press,* ed. Ralph E. Weber (New York: Holt, Rinehart & Winston, 1972), pp. 286–87.

145. Sorensen, *Kennedy,* p. 258; Sulzberger, *Last of the Giants,* pp. 800–801. In the summer of 1963, a Connecticut congressman charged that "President Kennedy, refusing to heed the lessons of history, is evidently preparing to follow exactly the same course with Khrushchev that Franklin Roosevelt took with Stalin." He feared "the outcome of any treaty negotiated now with Khrushchev by Averell Harriman who, you remember, also played an important part in Roosevelt's negotiations with Stalin" (*Congressional Record,* 88th Cong., 1st sess., p. 12786).

146. Burns, *Kennedy,* p. 271. During the fourth debate with Nixon in 1960, Kennedy said, "If the United States had stronger prestige and influence in Latin America it could persuade, as Franklin Roosevelt did in 1940, the countries of Latin America to join in an economic quarantine of Castro" (*Senate Report 994,* 3:266).

147. Lincoln Gordon, *A New Deal for Latin America: The Alliance for Progress* (Cambridge: Harvard University Press, 1963). In framing this plan, Kennedy relied a great deal on Adolf Berle, who had been FDR's assistant secretary of state and ambassador to Brazil. As he did with regard to other aspects of Kennedy's administration, Schlesinger called to mind continuities with Roosevelt's Good Neighbor policy. See, for example, Schlesinger, Memorandum for the President, March 10, 1961, JFKL POF, Box 65. See, too, Robert F. Smith, "Decline of the Alliance for Progress," in *The Great Society Reader,* ed. Marvin E. Gettleman and David Mermelstein (New York: Random House, 1967), p. 379.

148. James Daniel and John G. Hubbell, *Strike in the West* (New York: Holt, Rinehart & Winston, 1963), p. 66; Sorensen, *Kennedy,* p. 766; Donald M. Wilson JFKL OH, p. 78. One Latin American leader thought that Kennedy's attitude toward the region was a distinct improvement on FDR's (Juan Bosch JFKL OH, pp. 2–3, 8).

149. *Public Papers of the Presidents: 1961,* pp. 805–6, 811.

150. *Public Papers of the Presidents: 1963,* pp. 271–72.

151. Manchester, *Portrait,* p. 215; White, *The Professional: Lyndon B. Johnson* (Boston: Houghton Mifflin, 1964), p. 258. See, too, Sander Vanocur, "Kennedy's Voyage of Discovery," *Harper's,* April 1964, p. 42; George E. Mowry, "The Uses of History by Recent Presidents," *Journal of American History* 53 (June 1966):11.

152. Burns, *John Kennedy,* p. 266; Schlesinger, *Thousand Days,* p. 99;

Schlesinger, *The Vital Center: The Politics of Freedom* (Boston: Houghton Mifflin, 1962), p. xiv; Fairlie, *Kennedy Promise,* p. 241. David Halberstam has written that liberals cherished Chester Bowles because "he was a comfortable throwback to the Roosevelt era," which was precisely what the Kennedy circle did not care for. "The liberals liked him because he kept saying the old enduring things that had bound them together in the thirties; the Kennedy people did not like the old slogans and ideas and wanted to get on with the more modern world" (Halberstam, *Best and the Brightest,* p. 24).

153. *Public Papers of the Presidents: 1962,* pp. 420, 424.

154. Though by 1935 Roosevelt was losing faith in the possibility of cooperation with business, he started out in 1933 by sponsoring a vast government-business collaboration in the National Industrial Recovery Act. That did not prevent him even then, though, from advocating such programs as the TVA, which invaded the domain of the private utilities, or from recommending legislation that, for the first time, resulted in federal regulation of the financial markets. On the other hand, even when he turned against Big Business in 1935, he continued to hold orthodox economic views, such as the necessity for a balanced budget. Still, when all the constraints on FDR's economic thinking are duly noted, it nonetheless must be said that his administration constituted a considerably more radical break with his predecessors than did Kennedy's.

155. Charles Spalding JFKL OH, p. 93; Fairlie, *Kennedy Promise,* p. 240. The economist Seymour Harris, who frequently advised the president, even troubled to send him Lord Keynes's 1938 letter scolding Roosevelt for being too hostile to business. Harris' reason for doing this is not clear, for he said, "I do not send this letter to you in the thought that you are needlessly harassing businessmen. You have been most fair and anxious to secure their cooperation. They will never love a Democratic President" (Seymour E. Harris to JFK, November 9, 1962, JFKL POF 90, Treasury 11/12/62; see, too, Harris JFKL OH, p. 20).

156. "A Second Look at Economic Policy in 1961," Council of Economic Advisers, March 17, 1961, in Walter H. Heller, Memorandum for the President, JFKL POF (Departments and Agencies), Council of Economic Advisers 1/61–3/61. See, too, Robert J. Lampman, "What does it do for the poor?—a new test for national policy," in *The Great Society: Lessons for the Future,* ed. Eli Ginzberg and Robert M. Solow (New York: Basic Books, 1974), p. 66. For the claim that Kennedy's views were more advanced than those of Roosevelt and Morgenthau, see Seymour E. Harris, "Kennedy's Economics," *New Republic,* September 18, 1961, p. 110. Regret is expressed that Kennedy's economic experts did not point out to him the value of FDR's precedent on gold policy in Council of Economic Advisers JFKL OH, pp. 62–63.

157. Jim F. Heath, *John F. Kennedy and the Business Community* (Chicago: University of Chicago Press, 1969), pp. 135, 155; Schlesinger, *Thousand Days,* p. 634.

158. Barbara Blumberg, *The New Deal and the Unemployed: The View from New York City* (Lewisburg, Pa.: Bucknell University Press, 1979), pp. 303–4;

Paper, *Promise and Performance,* p. 127; Sundquist, *Politics and Policy,* p. 133.

159. Neustadt, "Approaches to Staffing," p. 861.

160. Edward Folliard JFKL OH, p. 18; William Lawrence JFKL OH, p. 21. For a contrary view, see Marshall Fishwick, *The Hero, American Style* (New York: David McKay, 1969), p. 235. Fishwick writes of the Kennedy press conferences: "Here was the old Roosevelt 'Fireside Chat,' made visible, with prince charming doing the chatting."

161. Richard Tanner Johnson, *Managing the White House* (New York: Harper & Row, 1974), p. 129. See, too, Schlesinger, *Thousand Days,* p. 686; Frederick Dutton JFKL OH, p. 60. This is the consensus. For dissents, see Roger Hilsman, *To Move a Nation* (Garden City, N.Y.: Doubleday, 1967), p. 535; George McGovern JFKL OH, p. 45.

162. Heath, *John F. Kennedy,* p. 6; Sidey, *John F. Kennedy,* p. 17; T.R.B., "From Washington," *New Republic,* January 9, 1961, p. 2.

163. Nathan Pusey JFKL OH, p. 26.

164. Joseph Rauh JFKL OH, pp. 100–101. He added, though, "But I want you to keep this up. It's very helpful now for you to keep pushing me this way." See, too, Mort Myerson, "New Dealer Views the New Frontier," *Christian Century* 79 (April 4, 1962):424.

165. Only a few days after the election, a congressman wrote him, "I think there should be two legislative items developed from the work of our committee included in your '100 days'" (Frank E. Smith to JFK, November 14, 1960, Smith MSS, Box 1).

166. William Proxmire JFKL OH, p. 14; "The 87th Congress and the Kennedy Administration," typescript essay, Richard Bolling MSS, Box 11; John C. Donovan, *The Politics of Poverty* (New York: Pegasus, 1967), p. 20; Manchester, *Portrait,* p. 23.

167. WWR, Memorandum to the President, "The Hundred Days," April 19, 1961, Theodore Sorensen MSS, Box 38; *U.S. News & World Report,* March 18, 1963, pp. 38–39. "Today some liberals see in John Fitzgerald Kennedy much of the greatness of Franklin Delano Roosevelt," wrote one analyst in 1962. "Some, while willing and eager to see signs of a second coming, think present political conditions so different from those of the 1930's that even Roosevelt would be of little help to their cause in the 1960's" (Clifton Brock, *Americans for Democratic Action: Its Role in National Politics* [Washington, D.C.: Public Affairs Press, 1962], p. 2).

168. Felix Frankfurter JFKL OH, pp. 67–68.

169. Lasky, *Robert F. Kennedy,* p. 305; telephone conversation with Lasky, July 19, 1982. Such, at least, is the story as reported by the UPI's White House correspondent, Merriman Smith. It appears to be substantiated by Felix Frankfurter's recollection of a visit to the White House on June 17, 1963, at which the president, after asking who the "Mr. Buttinsky of this administration" was, gestured at Schlesinger, an episode that Frankfurter took to mean that Schlesinger was intruding with unwanted advice (Felix Frankfurter JFKL OH, pp. 41–42; Felix Frankfurter MSS, Box 71). Furthermore, a national news

magazine noted Kennedy's irritation at "one of the best-known liberal intellectuals on his staff" (*Newsweek,* April 16, 1962, p. 31). Though these remarks have a bite to them, Kennedy's affection for Schlesinger cannot be doubted, and the comments are in keeping with the putdown humor of the New Frontier. Schlesinger has noted that after finishing Theodore White's account of the 1960 campaign, Kennedy told him, "When I read your Roosevelt books, I thought what towering figures those men around Roosevelt were—Moley and Tugwell and Berle and the others. Then I read Teddy's book and realized that they were just Sorensen and Goodwin and you" (Schlesinger, *Thousand Days,* p. 481). The main significance of the episode is that it indicates how resistant Kennedy was to suggestions that he emulate FDR.

170. Press Panel, JFKL OH, p. 68.

171. Schlesinger, Memorandum for the President: "The Administration and Public Information," March 16, 1961, JFKL POF Schlesinger, 3/61–4/61.

172. Pierre Salinger, *With Kennedy* (New York: Avon, 1967), p. 83; Schlesinger, *Thousand Days,* pp. 722–23; Sorensen, *Kennedy,* p. 365; Fowler Hamilton JFKL OH, p. 46; Schlesinger, Memorandum for the President: "FDR's 'Fireside Chats,'" November 21, 1961, JFKL POF Schlesinger, 10/61–12/61. See, too, *Television Digest,* March 13, 1961, p. 4; J. Edward Day, *My Appointed Round: 929 Days as Postmaster General* (New York: Holt, Rinehart & Winston, 1965), p. 136; Alan Shank, *Presidential Policy Leadership: Kennedy and Social Welfare* (Lanham, Md.: University Press of America, 1980), p. 258.

173. Beer to Schlesinger, February 5, 1963, quoted in Schlesinger, Memorandum for the President, February 9, 1963, JFKL POF 65a.

174. Lincoln Gordon JFKL OH, p. 72. Gordon points a finger at Schlesinger in particular, but Schlesinger was in fact more understanding of Kennedy's problems than Gordon acknowledges.

175. Carl M. Brauer, "Origins of the War on Poverty," delivered to American Historical Association convention, New York, December 29, 1979; Strout, *TRB,* pp. 225, 227; *Newsweek,* July 16, 1962, p. 18; Leslie Lipson, "The Character of American Politics Today," *Political Quarterly* 33 (April 1962):159. See, too, Kent M. Beck, "The Kennedy Image: Politics, Camelot, and Vietnam," *Wisconsin Magazine of History* 58 (Autumn 1974):47. Not every comparison was unfavorable. Raymond Moley commented, "In my four years of association with FDR I never knew him to read a serious book, indeed any book. . . . I have no direct knowledge of the Kennedy reading habits but the evidence shows that he is well read" ("FDR-JFK: A Brain Truster . . . Compares Two Presidents, Two Programs," *Newsweek,* April 17, 1961, p. 33).

176. *Public Papers of the Presidents: 1962,* p. 894; August Heckscher JFKL OH, p. 42.

177. When Kennedy flew to Dallas in November, he was seeking to heal a division among Texas Democrats that was a legacy of the Roosevelt era. One of the conspiracy theories about Kennedy's assassination centered on the presence at the murder scene of an "umbrella man." But the Texan who carried the open umbrella that day did so, he has said, not to signal a second assassin but as a way

of taunting Kennedy about his father's past, in particular Joe Kennedy's association with Neville Chamberlain, whose umbrella had come to symbolize the appeasement of Hitler at Munich (*Raleigh News and Observer,* September 26, 1978).

178. Schlesinger, *Thousand Days,* p. 98; Manchester, *Death of a President,* p. 160; Janet Travell, *Office Hours: Day and Night* (New York: New American Library, 1968), pp. 361–62.

179. Charles Earl JFKL OH, p. 9; Charles Roberts JFKL OH, p. 21. One official recalled, "I happen to be one who was never given much to demonstrative adulation of leaders. I did go down to Constitution Avenue for the funeral procession of Franklin D. Roosevelt and was always glad I did. So, in the same way I went out twice to watch the passing of the catafalque during that weekend in November 1963" (Arthur T. Thompson JFKL OH, p. 26).

180. Wilbur Schramm, "Communication in Crisis," in *The Kennedy Assassination and the American Public: Social Communication in Crisis,* ed. Bradley S. Greenberg and Edwin B. Parker (Stanford: Stanford University Press, 1965), pp. 2, 19; Paul B. Sheatsley and Jacob J. Feldman, "A National Survey on Public Reactions and Behavior," in ibid., p. 169. See, too, David Kirschner, "The Death of a President: Reaction of Psychoanalytic Patients," *Behavioral Science* 10 (January 1965):1–6.

181. Schramm, "Communication in Crisis," p. 3.

182. Vance Bourjaily, *The Man Who Knew Kennedy* (New York: Bantam, 1967), pp. 76–77. The contrast was even more striking in the first draft of the novel, in which a critical sentence read: "Roosevelt's death had been ten minutes of sadness, for an old, sick hero, gone to rest" (Vance Bourjaily MSS.)

183. Lilienthal, *Journals,* 5:523.

184. Paul Douglas JFKL OH, p. 26; William L. Benton JFKL OH, p. 28. A reporter for the *Washington Post* remarked, "I heard Roosevelt's first Inaugural speech with its 'The only thing we have to fear is fear itself,' which wasn't terribly original. And I'd say Kennedy's Inaugural was far better than any of Roosevelt's" (Edward Folliard JFKL OH, p. 26).

185. David Riesman, "Kennedy and After," *New York Review of Books,* December 26, 1963; also in "The Meaning of the Life and Death of John F. Kennedy," ed. Sidney Hertzberg, *Current,* January 1964, pp. 36–37; George Meany JFKL OH, p. 24. See, too, W. Walter Neeley JFKL OH, p. 6. Kennedy, wrote Joseph Alsop, was loved not as Roosevelt was, merely by the masses, but by the men who knew him best; "Roosevelt did not command the love of his closest collaborators" ("The Legacy of John F. Kennedy," *Saturday Evening Post,* November 21, 1964, p. 18).

186. Leopold Senghor JFKL OH, p. 5. (I have corrected a minor error in transcription.) For more than a decade after his death Kennedy outranked Roosevelt in opinion surveys. In a 1973 Harris poll, FDR was placed highest by Americans over fifty; Kennedy prevailed among those under thirty (*Yonkers* (N.Y.) *Herald Statesman,* January 22, 1973; Hedley Donovan, "Fluctuations on the Presidential Exchange," *Time,* November 9, 1981, p. 122). For other com-

parisons, especially in regard to the capacity to inspire confidence, see Cesar Chavez JFKL OH, p. 16; Robert C. Goodwin JFKL OH, p. 30; John F. Henning JFKL OH, p. 16; Ray Fitzgerald JFKL OH, p. 12; Seymour Harris JFKL OH, p. 79; William R. Hearst, Jr. JFKL OH, p. 7.

187. *Time,* November 29, 1963, p. 29; Schlesinger, *Thousand Days,* p. 1030; David Bazelon, "Reflections on the Fate of the Union: Kennedy and After," *New York Review of Books,* December 26, 1963, p. 9; John F. Kennedy, "Foreword," in Theodore Sorensen, *Decision-Making in the White House: The Olive Branch or the Arrows* (New York: Columbia University Press, 1963), p. xii. See, too, Arthur Link in Sidney Hertzberg COHC, p. 14; Lincoln Gordon JFKL OH, p. 3.

188. Burns JFKL OH, pp. 14–15, 53. If, in the eyes of historians, Kennedy's reputation soon began to fade, the reason lay in part in disaffection with the ideology of the Roosevelt era. As one historian summed up the attitude of critics, "Roosevelt-style liberalism seemed conservative and ill prepared to cope with new perplexities, and they recalled that Kennedy had been rather reluctant to join even the liberal vanguard" (Jim F. Heath, *Decade of Disillusionment: The Kennedy-Johnson Years* [Bloomington: Indiana University Press, 1975], p. 159). David Dempsey has made a different point: "The issue of Union, from which Lincoln took his mandate, will never be separated from its most eloquent spokesman, nor will the Great Depression and World War II be remembered without F.D.R. By comparison, Kennedy lacked a clear-cut and dramatic confrontation with a turning point in history" (*New York Times Book Review,* June 7, 1964, p. 2). It is arguable, though, that the civil rights struggle offered such an opportunity, particularly if Kennedy had seized it early enough and forcefully enough.

189. White, *In Search of History,* pp. 517–18.

190. *Saturday Review,* December 12, 1964, p. 44; Eric F. Goldman, *The Tragedy of Lyndon Johnson* (New York: Knopf, 1969), p. 13; *Newsweek,* November 30, 1964, p. 26; James Reston, "What Was Killed Was Not Only the President but the Promise," *New York Times Magazine,* November 15, 1964, pp. 24, 127. See, too, Karl E. Meyer, "John F. Kennedy," *New York Journal-American,* November 22, 1964.

191. Gerald W. Johnson, "'Once Touched by Romance,'" *New Republic,* December 7, 1963, p. 15; William G. Carleton, "Kennedy in History: An Early Appraisal," in *John F. Kennedy and the New Frontier,* ed. Aida Di Pace Donald (New York: Hill & Wang, 1966), p. 210. One writer has suggested that Lord Raglan's paradigm (in *The Hero: A Study in Tradition, Myth and Drama*) can be applied profitably to John F. Kennedy. "His father was called to a royal court (as Ambassador to the Court of Saint James['s] and the son was educated by (presumably) wise men (at Harvard). Then he went off to fight an evil dragon (the Japanese navy) and after a bloody fracas (PT 109) triumphed and returned to marry the beautiful princess (Jackie). Having inherited his father's kingdom (politics) he fought and defeated a second contender (Nixon) before taking over as ruler (President). For a time he suddenly lost favor (the Bay of Pigs

crisis), tried to rally his people, and died a sudden and mysterious death (did Oswald really shoot Kennedy?). Amidst great mourning (the first worldwide television funeral) he was buried on a sacred hillside (Arlington). Now he has many shrines (a cultural center, airport, library, highway, and a space launching site)" (Fishwick, *Hero, American Style,* pp. 11–12).

4. Lyndon B. Johnson

1. *New York Times,* April 13, 1945; interview by the author with William S. White; Rowland Evans and Robert Novak, *Lyndon B. Johnson: The Exercise of Power* (New York: Signet, 1968), p. 31; Richard Harwood and Haynes Johnson, *Lyndon* (New York: Praeger, 1973), p. 165.

2. *New York Times,* April 13, 1945.

3. Dorothy Palmie Alford in Max Starcke with Mrs. Max Starcke and Dorothy Palmie Alford LBJL OH, p. 11; Sam Houston Johnson, *My Brother Lyndon* (New York: Cowles, 1970), pp. 72–73. On the day of FDR's funeral, Johnson asked his House colleague Helen Gahagan Douglas to his office. "We were both very depressed," she remembered. "We sat very quietly during the time of the funeral reminiscing about our President. In this way we became friends. Mutual admiration of President Roosevelt" (Helen Gahagan Douglas LBJL OH, p. 11). Lady Bird Johnson has said, "The day Roosevelt was buried the whole town was just immobile, frozen, stunned, almost disbelieving, almost angry that it could have happened to them. Lyndon actually went to bed" (Merle Miller, *Lyndon: An Oral Biography* [New York: G. P. Putnam's Sons, 1980], p. 105). The most recent contention that Johnson was a conservative or a man of no principles appears in Robert A. Caro, *The Years of Lyndon Johnson: The Path to Power* (New York: Knopf, 1982), especially pp. 271–75, 768. Caro has unearthed a remarkable amount of new material, but the weight of evidence, including much of Caro's own evidence, leads to a contrary conclusion.

4. Turner Catledge oral history interview, University of Southern Mississippi, copy at Mississippi State; John Kenneth Galbraith, *A Life In Our Times: Memoirs* (Boston: Houghton Mifflin, 1981), p. 446. Galbraith added: "Nothing so endured in his memory as his appointment by F.D.R. in 1935, when he was twenty-seven, to head the National Youth Administration in Texas and his service from 1937 on as Roosevelt's favorite young congressman. There were many later occasions when Lyndon Johnson, deferring to Texas wealth, folk rites, oil or cupidity, thought it wise to subdue his liberal convictions. But he never abandoned them, and he was particularly concerned to prove to himself and to others that he had not."

5. *New York Times,* April 13, 1945.

6. *New York Herald Tribune,* February 16, 1937; *New York Times,* February 25, 1937; Senator Tom Connally as told to Alfred Steinberg, *My Name Is Tom Connally* (New York: Crowell, 1954), p. 188; George Sutherland to Tom Connally, June 5, 1937, Sutherland MSS, Box 6; Stephen Early, Confidential

Memorandum for the President, February 8, 1937, FDRL PSF Supreme Court; Harold L. Ickes, *The Secret Diary of Harold L. Ickes* (New York: Simon & Schuster, 1954), 2:75–81; *Austin American,* February 20, 1937, scrapbook clipping, Ickes MSS, Box 477; Lionel V. Patenaude, "Garner, Sumners, and Connally: The Defeat of the Roosevelt Court Bill in 1937," *Southwestern Historical Quarterly* 74 (July 1970):44. See, too, George Van Slyke, "Politics on Parade," *New York Sun,* March 6, 1937, scrapbook clipping, James A. Farley MSS, Box 16; John Henry Kirby to R. B. Dresser, February 12, 1937, Grenville Clark MSS, Series VII, Box 1; *New York American,* February 10, 1937, clipping, *New York Journal-American* files; L. L. James to Louis D. Brandeis, April 2, 1937, Brandeis MSS, G 14, Folder 1.

7. Henry Hirshberg LBJL OH, pp. 11–12; Daniel Quill LBJL OH, p. 15; Claude C. Wild, Sr., LBJL OH, p. 7; Caro, *Years of Lyndon Johnson,* p. 263; Marvin Jones LBJL OH, pp. 5–6; Mary Rather LBJL OH, II, pp. 13–14; Doris Kearns, *Lyndon Johnson and the American Dream* (New York: Harper & Row, 1976), p. 84; Harwood and Johnson, *Lyndon,* p. 30.

8. Clarke Newlon, *L.B.J.: The Man from Johnson City* (New York: Dodd, Mead, 1970), pp. 57–68; John H. Binns to Lyndon B. Johnson, February 3, 1964, LBJ MSS, Gen FG 2/FDR, Box 48; Keith Wheeler and William Lambert, "The Man Who Is the President," *Life,* August 14, 1964, p. 18; Ronnie Dugger, *The Politician: The Life and Times of Lyndon Johnson: The Drive for Power, from the Frontier to Master of the Senate* (New York: Norton, 1982), p. 189; Gene Latimer LBJL OH, p. 16.

9. Alfred Steinberg, *Sam Johnson's Boy: A Close-Up of the President from Texas* (New York: Macmillan, 1968), p. 110; Caro, *Years of Lyndon Johnson,* p. 417. See, too, Oscar L. Chapman LBJL OH, I, pp. 37–38; Sam V. Stone LBJL OH, p. 6; Welly Kenon Hopkins LBJL OH, p. 20; Arthur E. Goldschmidt and Elizabeth Wickenden LBJL OH, p. 8; Emmette S. Redford LBJL OH, pp. 10–11; Malcolm Bardwell LBJL OH, p. 15; "Someone the Tenth District Needs," radio address, former state senator Fleetwood Richards of Lockhart, KNOW, Austin, 7:15–30, April 1, 1937, LBJ MSS. For conflicting accounts of how Johnson came to run, see Sim Gideon LBJL OH, p. 7; Mary Rather, Interview II, LBJL OH, pp. 11–12; Henry A. Zeiger, *Lyndon B. Johnson: Man and President* (New York: Popular Library, 1963), p. 22; Steinberg, *Sam Johnson's Boy,* p. 105; Max Starcke with Mrs. Max Starcke and Dorothy Palmie Alford LBJL OH, p. 6; Daniel Quill LBJL OH, pp. 11–14; Daniel J. Quill LBJL OH, pp. 11–12; Willard Deason LBJL OH, p. 24; Kearns, *Lyndon Johnson,* pp. 85–86; Ray E. Lee LBJL OH, pp. 3–6. The notion that Johnson was the lone advocate of Roosevelt's Court plan has been perpetuated by any number of writers. See, among others, Robert Sherrill, *The Accidental President* (New York: Grossman, 1967), p. 107; David Halberstam, *The Best and the Brightest* (Greenwich, Conn.: Fawcett, 1973), p. 547; Clarke Newlon, *L.B.J.,* p. 66.

10. Booth Mooney, *The Lyndon Johnson Story* (New York: Farrar, Straus & Cudahy, 1956), p. 36; leaflet in Mrs. W. S. Birdwell Scrapbook, LBJ MSS, House of Representatives, Box 193. See, too, Percy Bones to Constitutional

Democracy Association, n.d. [March 1937], and B. H. Broiles to Richmond P. Hobson, n.d. [March 1937], Hobson MSS, Box 107.

11. Elliott Roosevelt to James A. Farley, April 5, 1937, Farley MSS, Box 5; Steinberg, *Sam Johnson's Boy,* p. 11. According to one source, Roosevelt sent Johnson money for the campaign (Daniel Quill LBJL OH, p. 13). So closely was FDR identified with Johnson's first campaign that more than one source subsequently reported erroneously that Roosevelt had publicly endorsed Johnson or had asked him to run. See, for example, William S. White, *The Professional: Lyndon B. Johnson* (Boston: Houghton Mifflin, 1964), p. 138; Tom C. Clark LBJL OH, pp. 8–9; Helen Gahagan Douglas LBJL OH, p. 9.

12. *New York Times,* April 11, 1937; *San Marcos Record,* April 16, 1937; clipping from Wichita Falls newspaper, April 11, 1937, LBJ MSS, House of Representatives, Scrapbook 1. See, too, Claude C. Wild, Sr., LBJL OH, p. 10; Caro, *Years of Lyndon Johnson,* p. 445; LBJ to C. N. Avery, n.d., and LBJ to Polk Shelton, n.d., LBJ MSS, House of Representatives, Box 1; Reese B. Lockett to FDR, April 11, 1937, LBJ MSS, White House Famous Names, Box 7. For skepticism that Johnson's victory showed all of Texas was for the plan, see Joe Burns, "World Comment," *Gatesville News,* April 16, 1937, scrapbook clipping, Tom Connally MSS, Box 602; Leonard Baker, *Back to Back: The Duel Between FDR and the Supreme Court* (New York: Macmillan, 1967), p. 189. Johnson received little more than one-quarter of the vote in the Tenth District.

13. John Callan O'Laughlin to Herbert Hoover, April 17, 1937, O'Laughlin MSS: Caro, *Years of Lyndon Johnson,* pp. 446–48; clipping, LBJ MSS, House of Representatives, Scrapbook 1; Ray E. Lee LBJL OH, p. 26; Claude C. Wild, Sr., LBJL OH, p. 14. It is sometimes said that Johnson was invited only because of the governor's intervention, but in fact that is not so. See Memorandum for the Trip File, April 20, 1937, LBJ MSS, White House Famous Names, Box 7.

14. Bascom Timmons LBJL OH, pp. 6–7; Steinberg, *Sam Johnson's Boy,* pp. 118–20.

15. Newlon, *L.B.J.,* pp. 72–73; Arthur E. Goldschmidt and Elizabeth Wickenden LBJL OH, p. 11; Grace Tully LBJL OH, I, 2; Oscar L. Chapman LBJL OH, II, 12, I, 37; Caro, *Years of Lyndon Johnson,* p. 449; Harwood and Johnson, *Lyndon,* p. 36. See, too, Jim Bishop, *FDR's Last Year* (New York: Morrow, 1974), p. xii; *The Road to the White House: The Story of the 1964 Election by the Staff of the New York Times,* ed. Harold Faber (New York: New York Times, 1965), p. 128; A. S. Mike Monroney LBJL OH, pp. 8–9; John W. McCormack LBJL OH, p. 3; Allen J. Ellender LBJL OH, p. 2; H. Jerry Voorhis LBJL OH, p. 3; Tom [Corcoran] to M. A. Le Hand, July 8, 1938, FDRL PPF 6149; Eliot Janeway, *The Economics of Crisis: War, Politics, and the Dollar* (New York: Weybright & Talley, 1968), pp. 208–9.

16. FDR to LBJ, August 2, 1939, LBJ MSS, White House Famous Names, Box 7. See, too, Harold Ickes MS Diary, July 24, 1939, Miscellaneous Pages, Ickes MSS, Box 25.

17. Harwood and Johnson, *Lyndon,* p. 105; Zeiger, *Lyndon B. Johnson,* pp.

23–25; Theodore H. White, *The Making of the President 1964* (New York: Atheneum, 1965), pp. 39n–40n.

18. Caro, *Years of Lyndon Johnson,* pp. 572–93, 654; Ickes, *Secret Diary,* 2:693–99; Zeiger, *Lyndon B. Johnson,* pp. 26–27; LBJ memorandum, LBJ to FDR, November 14, 1940, LBJ MSS, White House Famous Names, Box 7. See, too, A. Willis Robertson LBJL OH, p. 7. A document boosting Lyndon Johnson as a presidential candidate in 1960 stated, "In 1940, when Democratic control of the House of Representatives was threatened, FDR personally asked Johnson to take charge of the national campaign to elect Democrats to the House. Johnson, then only 32, surprised the experts by actually increasing the House Democratic majority" ("Some Legislative Accomplishments of Senator Lyndon B. Johnson," Americans for Democratic Action, Southeastern Pennsylvania Chapter MSS, Box 24).

19. Caro, *Years of Lyndon Johnson,* p. 677; press conference transcript, LBJ MSS, White House Famous Names, Box 7. Johnson subsequently embroidered the tale. In 1964 he said, "You know, down in Texas in 1941 President Roosevelt was very popular and he asked me to run for the Senate, because he said he needed me to help him" (*Public Papers of the Presidents of the United States: Lyndon B. Johnson, 1963–64,* 2 vols. [Washington, D.C.: Government Printing Office, 1965], 2:1488).

20. Elster M. Haile to Stephen Early, June 25, 1941, FDRL OF 300, Box 33; Caro, *Years of Lyndon Johnson,* p. 678. See, too, Robert N. Hall, "Lyndon B. Johnson's Speaking in the 1941 Senate Campaign," *Southern Speech Journal* 30 (Fall 1964):15–23; Roland Young, "Lone Star Razzle Dazzle," *Nation,* June 21, 1941, p. 722.

21. Telephone message from Tom Corcoran, May 24, 1941; FDR to LBJ, May 26, 1941; LBJ to FDR, May 31, 1941; James Rowe, Jr., Memorandum for the President: Lyndon Johnson, June 3, 1941; FDR to LBJ, June 4, 1941, LBJ MSS, White House Famous Names, Box 7.

22. FDR to LBJ, June 5, 1941; FDR to D. C. McCord, June 21, 1941, LBJ MSS, White House Famous Names, Box 7.

23. Charles R. Ashman, *Connally: The Adventures of Big Bad John* (New York: Morrow, 1974), p. 60; Evans and Novak, *Lyndon B. Johnson,* p. 23; FDR to Maury Maverick, Jr., June 4, 1941, FDRL PPF 3446.

24. Robert E. Kintner, Memorandum for the President, August 12, 1966, LBJ MSS, White House Famous Names, Box 7; Evans and Novak, *Lyndon B. Johnson,* pp. 14–15; Dugger, *Politician,* pp. 254–55. Johnson appears to have needed some persuasion to accept FDR's foreign policy. In the spring of 1940 his chief adviser wrote him that Lindbergh was "preaching your doctrine: just don't bother Hitler and Hitler won't bother you. . . . I will admit you are a whiz on domestic problems but I still think that on international problems you should listen to the elder statesmen" (A. J. Wirtz to LBJ, May 20, 1940, Wirtz MSS, Box 6). Johnson was capable of carrying his emulation of Roosevelt to an absurd point. One of his secretaries has remembered a day when she was called into his office to take dictation: "I almost came literally unglued. . . . I

looked up and saw Lyndon with pince-nez glasses with a ribbon-FDR type. I wanted just to scream, you know, with laughter but I was afraid that his sense of humor would not exactly go along with mine" (Dorothy Palmie Alford in Max Starcke with Mrs. Max Starcke and Dorothy Palmie Alford LBJL OH, p. 12).

25. Caro, *Years of Lyndon Johnson,* pp. 764–67; Jim F. Heath, *Decade of Disillusionment: The Kennedy-Johnson Years* (Bloomington: Indiana University Press, 1975), pp. 34–35; Halberstam, *Best and the Brightest,* pp. 547–49; Harry McPherson, *A Political Education* (Boston: Little, Brown, 1972), pp. 6–7; Lyndon B. Johnson to Mrs. Thos. P. Caughlin, April 28, 1950, Edwin E. Willis MSS, Box 62; James C. Hagerty MS Diary, February 15, 1954.

26. Sherrill, *Accidental President,* pp. 108–9, 99.

27. Samuel I. Rosenman to Harry S. Truman, June 19, 1956, Rosenman MSS, Box 11; Richard H. Rovere, "A Man for This Age, Too," *New York Times Magazine,* April 11, 1965, pp. 119–20; Rovere MSS, Box 10; Elizabeth Wickenden Goldschmidt LBJL OH, Tape 1, p. 24.

28. Grace Tully LBJL OH, p. 14; LBJ to Mrs. Franklin D. Roosevelt, August 12, 1957, LBJ MSS, White House Famous Names, Box 7.

29. Anthony Lewis, review of Merle Miller, *Lyndon: An Oral Biography, New York Times Book Review,* August 10, 1980, p. 1; Tyler Abell, ed., *Drew Pearson Diaries, 1949–1959* (New York: Holt, Rinehart & Winston, 1974), p. 502; Sherrill, *Accidental President,* p. 167. See, too, *New York Post,* March 22, 1959, clipping, Robert Bendiner MSS, Box 22.

30. *Senate Report 994,* 87th Cong., 1st sess. (Washington, D.C.: Government Printing Office, 1961), 3:396, 96, 182, 168. See, too, "Summary of the Voting Record of Senator Lyndon B. Johnson," Allen J. Ellender MSS, Misc., Box 66.

31. Arthur M. Schlesinger, Jr., *A Thousand Days: John F. Kennedy in the White House* (Boston: Houghton Mifflin, 1965), p. 20; Robert L. Riggs, "The South *Could* Rise Again: Lyndon Johnson and Others," in *Candidates 1960: Behind the Headlines in the Presidential Race,* ed. Eric Sevareid (New York: Basic Books, 1959), p. 317.

32. Victor Lasky, *J.F.K.: The Man and the Myth* (New York: Macmillan, 1963), p. 395; Helen Fuller, *Year of Trial: Kennedy's Crucial Decisions* (New York: Harcourt, Brace & World, 1962), pp. 15, 17; Evans and Novak, *Lyndon B. Johnson,* p. 328; Schlesinger, *Thousand Days,* p. 704; George E. Reedy LBJL OH Tape 3, p. 5.

33. *Public Papers of the Presidents of the United States: Lyndon B. Johnson, 1963–64,* 2 vols. (Washington, D.C.: Government Printing Office, 1965), 1:250; Toinette Bachelder LBJL OH, p. 5. I have corrected an error in transcription. See, too, Memorandum for Juanita Roberts: Roosevelt Portrait for the Cabinet Room, January 24, 1964, LBJ MSS, White House Famous Names, Box 7; Walter Heller, "Notes on Meeting with President Johnson," November 23, 1963, Heller MSS, Box 7.

34. *Public Papers of the Presidents, 1963–64,* 1:592; Henry Graff, "How Johnson

Makes Foreign Policy," *New York Times Magazine,* July 4, 1965, p. 20; Eric F. Goldman, *The Tragedy of Lyndon Johnson* (New York: Dell, 1969), p. 67; Theodore H. White, *The Making of the President 1968* (New York: Atheneum, 1969), pp. 100–101; Jack Valenti, *A Very Human President* (New York: Norton, 1975), p. 308; Sherwin Goldman in "Lyndon Johnson and Vietnam: Perceptions of War and Peace," study group conducted by Doris Kearns, January 20, 1974, Lehrman Institute, New York City. See, too, Fred R. Harris, *Potomac Fever* (New York: Norton, 1977), p. 101. As late as 1966, a White House aide wrote him, "I had some research material gotten up in regard to the relationship of the President to President Roosevelt, in case it could be useful in identification with President Roosevelt" (Robert E. Kintner, Memorandum to the President, August 12, 1966, LBJ MSS, White House Famous Names, Box 7).

35. *Public Papers of the Presidents, 1963–64,* 2:1559; Jack Bell, *The Johnson Treatment: How Lyndon B. Johnson Took Over the Presidency and Made It His Own* (New York: Harper & Row, 1965), p. 283; Frank Cormier, *LBJ: The Way He Was* (Garden City, N.Y.: Doubleday, 1977), p. 14; Lady Bird Johnson, *A White House Diary* (New York: Holt, Rinehart & Winston, 1970), p. 485; Graff, "How Johnson Makes Foreign Policy," p. 20; Hugh Sidey, *A Very Personal Presidency: Lyndon Johnson in the White House* (New York: Atheneum, 1968), pp. 244–45. See, too, George Christian, *The President Steps Down: A Personal Memoir of the Transfer of Power* (New York: Macmillan, 1970), p. 40.

36. *Public Papers of the Presidents of the United States: Lyndon B. Johnson, 1965,* 2 vols. (Washington, D.C.: Government Printing Office, 1966), 2:919, 604, 897; *Public Papers of the Presidents, 1963–64,* 2:640. For the contributions of FDR, Jr., to Johnson's program for Appalachia, see William Batt JFKL OH, pp. 181, 188–89.

37. *Public Papers of the Presidents, 1965,* 2:681.

38. *Public Papers of the Presidents, 1965,* 2:807, 1:458; *Public Papers of the Presidents, 1963–64,* 1:335–36.

39. Cormier, *LBJ,* p. 46; *The Road to the White House,* ed. Harold Faber, pp. 7–8; Elizabeth Wickenden Goldschmidt LBJL OH, Tape 1, p. 3; Goldman, *Tragedy of Lyndon Johnson,* p. 606. Remarking on a clipping from the *Boston Globe,* Johnson's personal secretary wrote, "In that particular pose, the likeness to his beloved President Roosevelt is indeed amazing" (Juanita D. Roberts to Ethel E. Murphy, July 27, 1964, LBJL, Gen FG 2/FDR, Box 48). See, too, A. W. Moursund to LBJ, December 2, 1963, LBJL Ex FG 2, Box 42; Elinor Graham, "Poverty and the Legislative Process," in *Poverty as a Public Issue,* ed. Ben B. Seligman (New York: Free Press, 1965), p. 254.

40. Graff, "How Johnson Makes Foreign Policy," p. 18; interview by the author with Bill Moyers, November 18, 1965.

41. William S. White, *Professional,* pp. 151–52; *Public Papers of the Presidents, 1965,* 1:343. As an example of Johnson's going out of his way to quote FDR, see LBJ to William L. Dawson, November 3, 1965, Dawson MSS, Box 1.

42. Valenti, *Very Human President,* p. 105.

43. McPherson, *Political Education,* p. 88.

44. Carl M. Brauer, "Origins of the War on Poverty," typescript of paper, American Historical Association, New York, N.Y., December 29, 1979.

45. Fred I. Greenstein, "College Students' Reactions to the Assassination," in *The Kennedy Assassination and the American Public: Social Communication in Crisis,* ed. Bradley S. Greenberg and Edwin B. Parker (Stanford: Stanford University Press, 1965), p. 236; "Notes on Meeting of the President with Senator Robert Kennedy, April 3, 1968," Charles S. Murphy MSS, HSTL, Box 66. See, too, Tom Wicker, "Lyndon Johnson vs. The Ghost of Jack Kennedy," *Esquire,* November 1965, pp. 87–93, 145–72; Garry Wills, *Nixon Agonistes: The Crisis of the Self-Made Man* (New York: New American Library, 1979), p. 114.

46. White, *Making of the President 1964,* pp. 389–90; interview by the author with Richard Goodwin, Middletown, Conn., December 13, 1965; notes, "The Politics of Upheaval," in speech file, Richard Goodwin MSS.

47. Richard L. Strout, *TRB* (New York: Macmillan, 1979), p. 276, reprinting his column of March 20, 1965; Richard Rovere, "A Man for This Age, Too," *New York Times Magazine,* April 11, 1965, p. 118; Joseph A. Califano, Jr., *A Presidential Nation* (New York: Norton, 1975), p. 8; Joseph S. Clark, "Pennsylvania and the Great Society," remarks at Roosevelt Day Dinner, Pittsburgh, press release, February 19, 1966, Clark MSS, Box 7 (B); Hubert H. Humphrey, *The Education of a Public Man: My Life and Politics,* ed. Norman Sherman (Garden City, N.Y.: Doubleday, 1976), p. 266; William L. Batt, Jr., JFKL OH, pp. 78–79. A contemporary libertarian critic saw Johnson's program as derivative of the state-sanctioned cartelization fostered by the National Recovery Administration. "The formal corporatism of the NRA is long gone, but the Great Society retains much of its essence," wrote Murray Rothbard. "The usual tripartite *rapprochement* of big business, big unions, and big government symbolizes the organization of society by blocs, syndics, and corporations, regulated and privileged by the federal, state, and local governments" (Murray N. Rothbard, "The Great Society: A Libertarian Critique," in *The Great Society Reader,* ed. Marvin E. Gettleman and David Mermelstein [New York: Random House, 1967], p. 507). Johnson developed the Great Society program not in the orthodox way, through government channels, but by independent task forces, a procedure based on his own experience as a member of the committee Roosevelt appointed to survey economic conditions in the South (Lyndon Baines Johnson, *The Vantage Point: Perspectives of the Presidency, 1963–69* [New York: Holt, Rinehart & Winston, 1971], pp. 326–27). On the task forces, see William E. Leuchtenburg, "The Genesis of the Great Society," *Reporter* 34 (April 21, 1966):36–39.

48. "Remarks on the 82d Anniversary of the Birth of Franklin D. Roosevelt," *Public Papers of the Presidents, 1963–64,* 1:251; Elizabeth Wickenden Goldschmidt LBJL OH, Tape 1, p. 3; Britt Brown to Frank Carlson, May 18, 1964, Carlson MSS, Box 352; Thomas E. Cronin, "Small Programs, Big Troubles: Policy Making for a Small Great Society Program," in *American Politics and Public Policy,* ed. Walter Dean Burnham and Martha Wagner Weinberg (Cambridge: MIT Press, 1978), p. 80; Joseph A. Kershaw, with the assistance of

Paul N. Courant, *Government against Poverty* (Washington, D.C.: Brookings Institution, 1970), p. 26; Johnson, *Vantage Point,* pp. 80–81; James L. Sundquist, *Politics and Policy: The Eisenhower, Kennedy, and Johnson Years* (Washington, D.C.: Brookings Institution, 1968), p. 73; Sargent Shriver, *Point of the Lance* (New York: Harper & Row, 1964), p. 18; *Public Papers of the Presidents, 1963–64,* 2:535, 1206. The martial imagery of a *war* on poverty recalled the pervasive use of that metaphor in the 1930s. See William E. Leuchtenburg, "The New Deal and the Analogue of War," in *Change and Continuity in Twentieth Century America,* ed. John Braeman, Robert H. Bremner, and Everett Walters (Columbus: Ohio State University Press, 1964).

49. *Public Papers of the Presidents, 1963–64,* 1:652–53.

50. Goldman, *Tragedy of Lyndon Johnson,* pp. 241, 256.

51. *Public Papers of the Presidents, 1963–64,* 2:1296.

52. Ibid., p. 1495.

53. Barry M. Goldwater, *With No Apologies: The Personal and Political Memoirs of the United States Senator Barry M. Goldwater* (New York: Morrow, 1979), pp. 44–45. See, too, Frank Annunziata, "The Revolt Against the Welfare State: Goldwater Conservatism and the Election of 1964," *Presidential Studies Quarterly* 10 (Spring 1980):254–63.

54. *New York Times,* October 23, 1964.

55. James R. Wason, "Labor-Management under the Johnson Administration," *Current History* 48 (August 1965):66; *Public Papers of the Presidents, 1965,* 2:1080, 1013; *New York Times,* September 8, 1966. See, too, *To Heal and to Build: The Programs of Lyndon B. Johnson,* ed. James MacGregor Burns (New York: McGraw-Hill, 1968), p. 253. One political analyst wrote: "The political events of 1964 make possible, and all but ensure, the early completion of the New Deal" (David T. Bazelon, *Power in America: The Politics of the New Class* [New York: New American Library, 1967], p. 91).

56. *Public Papers of the Presidents, 1965,* 2:813. Johnson's proposal for a National Foundation on the Arts and Humanities owed an obvious debt to the Federal Arts Project of the New Deal, and in the field of conservation and public power he carried on the Roosevelt program (Dorothy Rockwell Clark, "The Legacy of the Federal Theatre Project," *George Washington Magazine* 2 [Summer 1965]:22; *Public Papers of the Presidents, 1963–64,* 2:1033; Abner P. Wood to Edwin E. Willis, October 13, 1964, Willis MSS, Box 141).

57. *Public Papers of the Presidents, 1965,* 1:414–15.

58. Goldman, *Tragedy of Lyndon Johnson,* p. 21; Harwood and Johnson, *Lyndon,* p. 177. See, too, Valenti, *Very Human President,* p. x.

59. Sidey, *Very Personal Presidency,* pp. 71, 87; Kearns, *Lyndon Johnson,* pp. 282–83, 286, 374. See, too, George D. Aiken LBJL OH, p. 20; Arthur E. Goldschmidt and Elizabeth Wickenden LBJL OH, p. 77.

60. LBJ to FDR, July 21, 1941, LBJ MSS, White House Famous Names, Box 7; George Tindall, *The Emergence of the New South, 1913–1945* (Baton Rouge: Louisiana State University Press, 1967), p. 728; Harwood and Johnson, *Lyndon,* p. 36. (I have corrected a spelling error in Johnson's letter to Roosevelt.) A

member of the White House bureaucracy overheard some of Kennedy's aides talking of replacing Johnson as vice-president on the 1964 ticket. He has written: "The Kennedy 'brains' cited FDR as their precedent for dumping LBJ. Roosevelt had changed Vice Presidents in midstream, they said, so the country wouldn't hold it against Kennedy if he followed that example and turned from LBJ to someone else" (Traphes Bryant with Frances Spatz Leighton, *Dog Days at the White House: The Outrageous Memoirs of the Presidential Kennel Keeper* [New York: Macmillan, 1975], p. 66).

61. Joseph P. Lash, *Eleanor: The Years Alone* (New York: Signet, 1973), pp. 275, 280; telephone conversation from Mrs. Franklin Roosevelt to Senator Johnson, May 28, 1959, LBJ MSS, White House Famous Names, Box 7; Grace Tully LBJL OH, p. 32.

62. Harris, *Potomac Fever,* p. 102; David E. Lilienthal, *The Journals of David Lilienthal* (New York: Harper & Row, 1976), 6:485. Years later, Mrs. Johnson, asked whether she consciously modeled her role on any predecessor, said no. The questioner persisted: "Did you particularly admire any previous First Lady? Eleanor Roosevelt, for instance?" She replied: "I had an awful lot of respect for her hard work, and her caring, and her knowledge. But then I had a very sympatico feeling for Dolley Madison" (Barbara Klaw, "Lady Bird Johnson Remembers," *American Heritage* 32 [December 1980]:6–8).

63. Valenti, *Very Human President,* p. 308. There is some evidence that the relationship was reciprocal. FDR often spoke of himself as "Papa," and it was said that "President Roosevelt loved Lyndon Johnson as one loves his own son" (Richard Tanner Johnson, *Managing the White House: An Intimate Study of the Presidency* [New York: Harper & Row, 1974], p. 18; Memorandum for George Christian, October 11, 1967, LBJ MSS Ex FG 2, Container 42).

64. Kearns, *Lyndon Johnson,* p. 371. There is much on the theme of surrogate fathers elsewhere in Kearns as well as, in different ways, in Steinberg, Caro, and other writers. See, too, Elizabeth Wickenden Goldschmidt LBJL OH, Tape 1, p. 14; George E. Reedy LBJL OH, Tape 1, p. 24. For a cautionary note, see Ross K. Baker, *Friend and Foe in the U.S. Senate* (New York: Free Press, 1980), pp. 21–22. Johnson, it has been suggested to me by James Olney, cannibalized Roosevelt, and in two ways. He fed off him in developing his policies, and, in seeking to swallow up FDR's achievements, he devoured him. Moreover, Johnson's unusual public references to Roosevelt's paralysis might be related to his own anxiety that he might be stricken by the same affliction that had crippled one of his grandparents. One can only speculate about what Johnson thought when in June 1936, at a gathering of NYA state directors at Hyde Park, Roosevelt dispensed with his braces and wheelchair, and Johnson saw the president carried in by two men (Kearns, *Lyndon Johnson,* pp. 30–33, 342–43; John H. Binns to Lyndon B. Johnson, February 3, 1964, LBJ MSS, Gen FG 2/FDR, Box 48). Some of the writing about Johnson's psyche seems to me to outrun the evidence, and I have been reluctant to add to that genre, but no one can write seriously about Johnson without contemplating the "daddy" phenomenon. For a warning about the cannibalizing rubric, see Erik H.

Erikson, *Life History and the Historical Moment* (New York: Norton, 1975), pp. 92–93.

65. Goldman, *Tragedy of Lyndon Johnson,* p. 301. See, too, Bell, *Johnson Treatment,* p. 283.

66. W. Averell Harriman, Memorandum for the President, November 9, 1964, NSF, Memos to the President, LBJL, Box 7; *New York Times,* November 8, 1964; Rovere, "Letter from Washington," *New Yorker* (January 16, 1965), p. 126. See, too, *Arkansas Gazette,* November 12, 1964.

67. Evans and Novak, *Lyndon B. Johnson,* p. 517; *Public Papers of the Presidents, 1965,* 1:369. Lady Bird Johnson has insisted that President Johnson, unlike FDR, was scared of the White House, and both she and her daughter Lynda Bird have said that Johnson's assertions of superiority to Roosevelt should be dismissed as braggadocio (interview of the author with Lady Bird Johnson and Lynda Bird Robb).

68. Goldman, *Tragedy of Lyndon Johnson,* p. 395; interview by the author with Lyndon B. Johnson, White House, September 22, 1965. See, too, Cormier, *LBJ,* p. 46; Samuel Shaffer, *On and Off the Floor* (New York: Newsweek, 1980), p. 221; *Public Papers of the Presidents, 1963–64,* 1:250, 779; Sidey, *Very Personal Presidency,* pp. 61–63; Adolf A. Berle, *Navigating the Rapids,* ed. Beatrice Bishop Berle and Travis Beal Jacobs (New York: Harcourt Brace Jovanovich, 1973), p. 825. For an examination of the idea that "the War on Poverty is not just the New Deal in different dress," see S. M. Miller and Martin Rein, "The War on Poverty: Perspectives and Prospects," in *Poverty as a Public Issue,* ed. Ben B. Seligman (New York: Free Press, 1965), p. 278; Daniel Patrick Moynihan, "The Professionalization of Reform," in *The Great Society Reader,* ed. Gettleman and Mermelstein, pp. 463–65. Johnson was proud that he had found sources of expertise independent of the New Dealers. "How did we know what to do?" he asked. "We got the best thinkers in fields that had been neglected—transportation, fiscal policy, science, medical care. We got men from Johns Hopkins, elsewhere. The program wasn't drafted by Corcoran and Cohen. It came from the best thinkers. Quality went into it" (interview by the author with Lyndon B. Johnson, White House, September 22, 1965).

69. Interview by the author with Henry Wilson, White House, September 22, 1965; Lawrence F. O'Brien, *No Final Victories: A Life in Politics—from John F. Kennedy to Watergate* (Garden City, N.Y.: Doubleday, 1974), p. 195.

70. Johnson, *Vantage Point,* pp. 323–24; Charles Halleck JFKL OH, p. 28; interview by the author with Senator Mike Mansfield, U.S. Senate, September 22, 1965. In a book published while Johnson was still in office, one scholar even scored Johnson's legislative achievements *before* 1965 above FDR's. John C. Donovan wrote: "The Johnson legislative performance in 1964, coming before his impressive landslide victory over Senator Goldwater, ranks with Woodrow Wilson's monumental record as 'parliamentary' leader during his first term and in respects outshines FDR's famous one hundred days in the sense that Johnson had neither the congressional voting strength nor the atmosphere of crisis which so aided Roosevelt in 1933" (*The Politics of Poverty* [New York: Pegasus,

1967], pp. 21–22). See, too, Robert J. Lampman, "What Does It Do for the Poor?—A New Test for National Policy," in *The Great Society: Lessons for the Future*, ed. Eli Ginzberg and Robert M. Solow (New York: Basic Books, 1974), pp. 66–67; Clinton P. Anderson with Milton Viorst, *Outsider in the Senate: Senator Clinton Anderson's Memoirs* (New York: World, 1970), p. 318; James H. Duffy, *Domestic Affairs: American Programs and Priorities* (New York: Simon & Schuster, 1978), p. 190.

71. Kearns, *Lyndon Johnson*, p. 96; interview by the author with Lyndon B. Johnson, White House, September 22, 1965. See, too, Sidey, *Very Personal Presidency*, p. 72. Twice in one telephone conversation in 1963, Johnson, while vice-president, cited the Roosevelt administration as a bad example (telephone conversation, LBJ–Theodore Sorensen, June 3, 1963, George Reedy Office Files, Box 1).

72. Interview by the author with Bill Moyers, White House, November 18, 1965. See, too, *New York Herald Tribune*, February 2, 1965; Bell, *Johnson Treatment*, pp. 43, 83; Sherrill, *Accidental President*, pp. 10–11, 89; "Norris Cotton Reports to You from the United States Senate," January 28, 1965, August 5, 1965, Cotton MSS; "Kennedy, Johnson, and the Intellectuals," in John P. Roche, *Sentenced to Life* (New York: Collier Macmillan, 1974), p. 40; Patrick Anderson, *The President's Men: White House Assistants of Franklin D. Roosevelt, Harry S Truman, Dwight D. Eisenhower, John F. Kennedy, and Lyndon B. Johnson* (Garden City, N.Y.: Doubleday, 1968), p. 300; Evans and Novak, *Lyndon B. Johnson*, p. 10; Johnson, *Managing the White House*, p. 175.

73. Johnson, *Vantage Point*, pp. 447–48.

74. *Public Papers of the Presidents, 1963–64*, 1:684.

75. Interview by the author with Douglass Cater, White House, September 22, 1965; interview by the author with Lyndon B. Johnson, White House, September 22, 1965; interview by the author with Bill Moyers, White House, November 18, 1965. Similarly, Larry O'Brien stated, "Johnson often mentions the 1937 experience of FDR as an example to be avoided" (interview by the author with Lawrence F. O'Brien, White House, September 22, 1965). See, too, Marcus Cunliffe, *American Presidents and the Presidency* (London: Fontana, 1972), p. 271; Bell, *Johnson Treatment*, p. 284. The memory of what had befallen Franklin Roosevelt in 1937 haunted the president. "Johnson was warned that Home Rule for the District of Columbia could be his Supreme Court fight," said another member of the White House staff (interview by the author with Hayes Redmon, September 22, 1965). See, too, *New Republic*, November 21, 1964, p. 1; Norris Cotton Newsletter, July 25, 1968, Cotton MSS.

76. Goldman, *Tragedy of Lyndon Johnson*, pp. 307–8; *New York Times*, December 16, 1964; Philip Geyelin, *Lyndon B. Johnson and the World* (New York: Praeger, 1966), p. 146; Douglas Ross, *Robert F. Kennedy: Apostle of Change* (New York: Pocket Books, 1968), p. 30.

77. Evans and Novak, *Lyndon B. Johnson*, pp. 514–15; Halberstam, *Best and the Brightest*, p. 547. See, too, Johnson, *Vantage Point*, p. 323; W. W. Rostow, *The Diffusion of Power* (New York: Macmillan, 1972), pp. 333–34. Johnson's

allusion to FDR's paralysis is curious; presidents do not go door to door soliciting votes on Capitol Hill. Theodore White noted after talking to McGeorge Bundy: "Mac's final thought: the fantastic impression on LBJ of the election. . . . LBJ was mesmerized not by the war, but [by] making real the dream of FDR. He kept saying to the White House 'I got only three months to get this work through.' All his attention, all his energy, all his leverage were pressed on getting his domestic programs through." "Conversation with Mac Bundy," December 15, 1967, Theodore White MSS, Box 32.

78. Tom Wicker, *JFK and LBJ: The Influence of Personality upon Politics* (New York: Morrow, 1968), pp. 235, 276.

79. Goldman, *Tragedy of Lyndon Johnson,* pp. 449–51.

80. Graff, "How Johnson Makes Foreign Policy," pp. 18–20. Similarly, Doris Kearns has recorded that Johnson said to her, "You see, I deeply believe we *are* quarantining aggressors over there just like smallpox. Just like FDR and Hitler, just like Wilson and the Kaiser. . . . I was taught in Congress and in committees on defense preparedness and by FDR that we in Congress were constantly telegraphing the wrong messages to Hitler and the Japanese—that the Wheelers, the Lindberghs, the La Follettes, and the America Firsters were letting Hitler know he could move without worrying about Uncle Sam" (Kearns, *Lyndon Johnson,* p. 329).

81. Christian, *President Steps Down,* pp. 102–3.

82. Henry F. Graff, *The Tuesday Cabinet: Deliberation and Decision on Peace and War under Lyndon B. Johnson* (Englewood Cliffs, N.J.: Prentice-Hall, 1970), p. 105; Frances FitzGerald, *Fire in the Lake: The Vietnamese and the Americans in Vietnam* (Boston: Little, Brown, 1972), p. 234; Kearns, *Lyndon Johnson,* p. 267.

83. *Public Papers of the Presidents of the United States: Lyndon B. Johnson, 1966,* 2 vols. (Washington, D.C.: Government Printing Office, 1967), 1:288.

84. *Department of State Bulletin* 55 (September 12, 1966):371–72.

85. Roscoe Drummond, "The New Isolationists," *Washington Post,* April 12, 1967.

86. *Public Papers of the Presidents, 1967,* 2:1051.

87. Alexander Kendrick, *The Wound Within: America in the Vietnam Years, 1945–1974* (Boston: Little, Brown, 1974), p. 20. See, too, Anthony Austin, *The President's War: The Story of the Tonkin Gulf Resolution and How the Nation Was Trapped in Vietnam* (Philadelphia: Lippincott, 1971), p. 325.

88. Janeway, *The Economics of Crisis,* p. 290; Sherrill, *Accidental President,* pp. 229–30, 232. See, too, Larry L. King, *Of Outlaws, Con Men, Whores, Politicians, and Other Artists* (New York: Viking, 1980), p. 257; Charles L. Mee, Jr., *Meeting at Potsdam* (New York: M. Evans, 1975), p. 311; Tom Hayden, "Welfare Liberalism and Social Change," in *Great Society Reader,* ed. Gettleman and Mermelstein, pp. 483–84. For a prophetic view, see David Riesman, "Kennedy and After," *New York Review of Books,* December 26, 1963, p. 3.

89. Kearns, *Lyndon Johnson,* p. 285.

90. Herbert Y. Schandler, *The Unmaking of a President* (Princeton: Princeton University Press, 1977), p. 269. See, too, Address by Senator Edward M.

Kennedy Before the Massachusetts Chapter of Americans for Democratic Action, Boston, March 4, 1967, Donald Richard Larrabee MSS, Box 543. Johnson did drop a hint of what he would do by telling a story about the 1940 campaign when Franklin Roosevelt, in refusing to compete with John Nance Garner for Texas' votes, said, "Maybe I won't run at all" (Theodore C. Sorensen JFKL OH [RFK], p. 35).

91. White, *Making of the President 1968*, pp. 114–16; interview by the author with James H. Rowe, Jr.

92. Kearns, *Lyndon Johnson*, p. 322; *Congressional Record*, 88th Cong., 2d. sess., pp. 1953–54. See, too, Eric F. Goldman, Memorandum for the President, December 4, 1964, Ex CO 305, LBJL, Box 75.

93. Rovere, "Letter from Washington," *New Yorker*, January 16, 1965, p. 122.

94. Lilienthal, *Journals*, 6:325; William O. Douglas, *The Court Years, 1939–1975* (New York: Vintage, 1981), pp. 336, 312, 333.

95. Hubert H. Humphrey, *The Cause Is Mankind: A Liberal Program for Modern America* (New York: Praeger, 1964), p. 24; Larry L. King, *Of Outlaws*, pp. 271, 273.

96. Interview by Hugh Sidey of *Time* with the President, May 16, 1967, DB, LBJL, Box 65; *Public Papers of the Presidents, 1967*, 2:1164; *Public Papers of the Presidents, 1966*, 2:1360, 1452. See, too, "Notes of the Meeting of the President with Hugh Sidey," August 9, 1967, DB, LBJL, Box 73.

97. *Public Papers of the Presidents, 1967*, 2:1080–81.

98. Albert Eisele, *Almost to the Presidency* (Blue Earth, Minn.: Piper, 1972), p. 248.

99. Philip Reed Rulon, *The Compassionate Samaritan: The Life of Lyndon Baines Johnson* (Chicago: Nelson-Hall, 1981), p. 290. Gus Tyler has written of "the Roosevelt Era that ran from 1932–68," while Herbert Parmet has commented, "It does not take much exaggeration to consider the night of March 31, 1968, as a landmark for the post–New Deal Democratic Party, as the moment when the old coalition finally yielded to the new fragmentation, when the old politics gave way to the new. . . . Finally, after a quarter of a century, the Democratic Party was left to confront the reality that had been building ever since Roosevelt's death, the failure of the realignment to survive in any permanent, meaningful sense" (Dugger, *Politician*, p. 14; Parmet, *The Democrats: The Years after FDR* [New York: Oxford, 1976], p. 248).

100. Goldman, *Tragedy of Lyndon Johnson*, pp. 623–25.

101. White, *Making of the President 1968*, p. 68.

102. Sidey, *Very Personal Presidency*, pp. 105–6.

103. Harwood and Johnson, *Lyndon*, pp. 178–82. See, too, Ross, *Robert F. Kennedy*, pp. 50–51; Jack Newfield, *Robert Kennedy: A Memoir* (New York: Dutton, 1969), p. 65; Robert A. Divine, "The Johnson Literature," in *Exploring the Johnson Years*, ed. Divine (Austin: University of Texas Press, 1981), p. 21.

104. Goldman, *Tragedy of Lyndon Johnson*, pp. 623–25; Kendrick, *The Wound Within*, pp. 37, 44; George Herring, *America's Longest War: The United States and Vietnam, 1950–1975* (New York: Wiley, 1979), pp. 5–6; Daniel Yergin, *Shat-*

tered Peace: The Origins of the Cold War and the National Security State (Boston: Houghton Mifflin, 1978), p. 88; Chester L. Cooper, *The Lost Crusade: America in Vietnam* (New York: Dodd, Mead, 1970), pp. 28–35. Hubert Humphrey wrote, "Our support of French colonialism in Indochina was a mistake begun by the Truman administration (against the views of his predecessor, FDR)" (Hubert H. Humphrey, *The Education of a Public Man: My Life and Politics,* ed. Norman Sherman [Garden City, N.Y.: Doubleday, 1976], p. 66). For a more critical view of FDR's policies, see Walter LaFeber, "Roosevelt, Churchill, and Indochina: 1942–45," *American Historical Review* 80 (December 1975):1277–95; Gary R. Hess, "Franklin Roosevelt and Indochina," *Journal of American History* 59 (September 1972):353–68.

105. George Reedy, *Lyndon B. Johnson: A Memoir* (New York: Andrews & McMeel, 1982), p. 43.

106. C. H. Sulzberger, *an Age of Mediocrity: Memoirs and Diaries, 1963–1972* (New York: Macmillan, 1973), p. 6; Kearns, *Lyndon Johnson,* p. 301; Valenti, *Very Human President,* pp. 380–81; Samuel Shaffer, *On and Off the Floor* (New York: Newsweek, 1980), pp. 220–21.

107. Harris poll MS data for December 1972 and February 1976. See, too, *Yonkers Herald Statesman,* January 22, 1973.

5. Second Republican Interlude: Richard Nixon and Gerald Ford

1. Dan Rather and Gary Paul Gates, *The Palace Guard* (New York: Harper & Row, 1974), p. 302. William Buckley referred to "Franklin D. Roosevelt, McGovern's patron saint" (William F. Buckley, Jr., *Inveighing We Will Go* [New York: Putnam's, 1972], p. 38.)

2. Garry Wills, *Nixon Agonistes: The Crisis of the Self-Made Man* (New York: New American Library, 1979), p. 83.

3. Richard Harris, California State Fullerton Richard Nixon OH, p. 18; Richard Nixon, *RN: The Memoirs of Richard Nixon* (New York: Grosset & Dunlap, 1978), p. 7; George Johnson, *Richard Nixon: An Intimate and Revealing Portrait of One of America's Key Political Figures* (Derby, Conn.: Monarch, 1961), p. 37; Bela Kornitzer, *The Real Nixon: An Intimate Biography* (Chicago: Rand McNally, 1960), p. 78. In 1934 Frank Nixon, after driving east from California to drop his son off at Duke Law School, said that his next stop would be Washington. "I'm going to see the President," he announced. "I want to tell him about the Townsend Plan. I don't think he understands it" (Fawn M. Brodie, *Richard Nixon: The Shaping of His Character* [New York: Norton, 1981], p. 50).

4. Transcript of David Brinkley interview with Richard Nixon, ABC News Closeup, c. November 1981.

5. Lyle Otterman, California State Fullerton Richard Nixon OH, p. 14; Milton Viorst, "Nixon of the O.P.A.," *New York Times Magazine,* October 3, 1971, pp. 70–77; Nixon to H. C. Horack, April 23, 1942, Nixon MSS, Duke University Archives.

6. Raymond Price, *With Nixon* (New York: Viking, 1977), pp. 51, 64.

7. Theodore H. White, *Breach of Faith: The Fall of Richard Nixon* (New York: Atheneum, 1975), p. 252, and *The Making of the President, 1972* (New York: Bantam, 1973), p. 18.

8. Brinkley interview. On April 12, 1945, Nixon was dining with his wife, Pat, at Bookbinders in Philadelphia when a waiter told him that he had just heard on the radio of Roosevelt's death. "Like everyone else, we were shocked and saddened by the news," Nixon has written (*RN,* p. 33).

9. Brodie, *Richard Nixon,* pp. 108, 154; Nixon, *RN,* p. 25; Viorst, "Nixon of the O.P.A.," pp. 70–77.

10. *Life,* November 6, 1970, p. 66; Gerald Kepple California State Fullerton Richard Nixon OH, p. 6.

11. Earl Mazo, *Richard Nixon: A Political and Personal Portrait* (New York: Harper & Row, 1959), pp. 286–87; Nixon to Charles H. Percy, March 21, 1959, Percy MSS, Box 9.

12. Nixon, *RN,* p. 99.

13. Lester David, *The Lonely Lady of San Clemente: The Story of Pat Nixon* (New York: Crowell, 1978), pp. 80–81.

14. Price, *With Nixon,* pp. 45–46.

15. *Public Papers of the Presidents of the United States: Richard Nixon, 1969* (Washington, D.C.: Government Printing Office, 1971), pp. 1–2.

16. William Safire, *Before the Fall: An Inside View of the Pre-Watergate White House* (Garden City, N.Y.: Doubleday, 1975), p. 54, and *Safire's Washington* (New York: Times Books, 1980), p. 244; *Public Papers of the Presidents of the United States: Richard Nixon, 1970* (Washington, D.C.: Government Printing Office, 1971), p. 257. Nixon's economic initiatives were often compared to FDR's. When in the summer of 1971 Nixon announced "the most comprehensive New Economic Policy to be undertaken by this nation in four decades," *Time* wrote that he was initiating "the most sweeping changes since the Hundred Days of the New Deal in 1933, when Franklin Roosevelt took the U.S. off the gold standard" (*Time,* August 30, 1971, p. 4). In commenting on Nixon's decision for devaluation, Jerry Voorhis, whom Nixon had ousted from Congress, wrote, "So it was that Richard Nixon followed in the footsteps of Franklin D. Roosevelt, whose action in raising the dollar price of gold as an anti-depression measure had been so roundly attacked through the years by that same Richard Nixon" (Jerry Voorhis, *The Strange Case of Richard Milhous Nixon* [New York: Eriksson, 1972], p. 235). See, too, William M. Leiter, "The Presidency and Non-Federal Government: The Benefactor-Aversion Hypothesis: The Case of Public Assistance Policies in the New Deal and Nixon Administrations," *Presidential Studies Quarterly* 10 (Fall 1980):636–44. For calls during Nixon's first term for a revival of the New Deal, see Cabell Phillips, "It Wasn't All Leaf Raking: Why Not Another WPA?," *New Republic,* February 6, 1971, pp. 19–20; *New York Times,* November 8, 1972. A shrewd observer who later served in Ford's cabinet has recalled being impressed by the extent to which Nixon in the White House modeled himself on Roosevelt (interview by the author with Edward Levi, April 24, 1980).

17. *Public Papers of the Presidents of the United States: Richard Nixon, 1971* (Washington, D.C.: Government Printing Office, 1972), pp. 1212–13.

18. Nixon, *RN,* pp. 610, 1034.

19. *Public Papers of the Presidents: 1971,* pp. 448–49.

20. Buckley, *Inveighing We Will Go,* pp. 265–66, 293.

21. Milton S. Eisenhower, *The President Is Calling* (Garden City, N.Y.: Doubleday, 1974), p. 321; Richard L. Strout, *TRB* (New York: Macmillan, 1979), pp. 356–57.

22. Strout, *TRB,* p. 346; Wills, *Nixon Agonistes,* pp. 72–73; White, *Breach of Faith,* p. 252.

23. Price, *With Nixon,* pp. 121–23. See, too, Safire, *Before the Fall,* p. 50.

24. Safire, *Before the Fall,* p. 549. In 1972 James Roosevelt endorsed Nixon (Charles R. Ashman, *Connally: The Adventures of Big Bad John* [New York: Morrow, 1974], p. 269).

25. White, *Making of the President, 1972,* pp. 13, 403. Nixon and Roosevelt received almost identical shares of the total vote, but, as Nixon foresaw, FDR got a somewhat larger proportion of the two-party vote.

26. Rather and Gates, *Palace Guard,* p. 301; Barry M. Goldwater, *With No Apologies* (New York: Morrow, 1979), p. 247; Price, *With Nixon,* pp. 127–28; Clayton Fritchey quoted in Walter F. Mondale, *The Accountability of Power: Toward a Responsible Presidency* (New York: David McKay, 1975), p. 179.

27. White, *Making of the President, 1972,* p. 18.

28. Nixon, *RN,* p. 761. See, too, Leonard Lurie, *The Running of Richard Nixon* (New York: Coward, McCann & Geoghegan, 1972), p. 21.

29. Memo by Raymond Price cited in Price, *With Nixon,* pp. 77–78.

30. Safire, *Safire's Washington,* pp. 134, 137. This statement badly distorts the historical evidence.

31. J. Anthony Lukas, *Nightmare: The Underside of the Nixon Years* (New York: Viking, 1976), pp. 285–86. The outcry over Nixon's firing of Archibald Cox was likened to the reaction to FDR's Court-packing message (Elizabeth Drew, *Washington Journal: The Events of 1973–1974* [New York: Vintage, 1976], pp. 148–49). For parallels drawn by other writers between Roosevelt and Nixon with regard to the Supreme Court, see Safire, *Before the Fall,* pp. 493–94; Gerald Gunther, "The Nixon-Burger Court: Where Is It Going?," prepared for Stanford Club and Law Society joint meetings, Long Beach and Santa Ana, Calif., June 8, 1972, mimeo, Alexander M. Bickel MSS, Box 3. I have corrected a minor typographical error in the Gunther paper.

32. Victor Lasky, *It Didn't Start with Watergate* (New York: Dial, 1977), pp. 143–61; Price, *With Nixon,* pp. 285–86.

33. Fawn Brodie, *Richard Nixon,* p. 19; Price, *With Nixon,* pp. 229, 235. See, too, Maurice H. Stans, *The Terrors of Justice: The Untold Side of Watergate* (New York: Everest, 1978), pp. 455–56. A Democrat, Maurice Stans voted for FDR in 1936, then was alienated by the Court-packing plan and drifted to the Republicans because they believed "in restraints on national government spending to produce balanced budgets (a promise Roosevelt had made and broken)" (p. 114).

34. For criticism of Nixon's claim that the covert operations of the FBI had been authorized by previous presidents, see Frank Mankiewicz, *Perfectly Clear: Nixon from Whittier to Watergate* (New York: Quadrangle, 1973), p. 3. One writer has stated that Nixon's huge, structured staff invited intrigue, as FDR's small, more intimate staff did not (John Herbers, *No Thank You, Mr. President* [New York: Norton, 1976], pp. 169–70). There are revelations about the Roosevelt presidency that are disturbing, though, and I think some historians and political scientists have been too quick to dismiss them. I expressed thoughts about the comparison between Watergate and FDR's administration in "The Roots of Watergate Cannot Be Found in the Age of Franklin Roosevelt," *Los Angeles Times,* September 18, 1973, sec. 2, p. 7, and, with less assurance, in "Appraising the Legacy of Richard Nixon," *Newsday,* June 14, 1982, sec. 2, pp. 2–5, a panel discussion in which I participated with James David Barber, Eric Goldman, J. Anthony Lukas, and members of the *Newsday* staff, particularly Murray Kempton.

35. Safire, *Before the Fall,* pp. 688–89.

36. Brinkley interview.

37. In the summer of 1974 William Safire wrote in praise of Gerald Ford: "Mr. Nixon wound up with a lifetime batting average of .500 in picking Vice Presidents, better than F.D.R.'s .333" (*Safire's Washington,* p. 29)..

38. "But," he added, "many of my former close friends from high school days were directly affected by WPA—by other New Deal programs. . . . There was hardly a family in Grand Rapids that in one way or another didn't have a direct relationship to the problems of the economy—jobs, WPA, etc." (transcript of David McCullough interview with Gerald Ford, December 2, 1981).

39. Only when he was reminded when Roosevelt died did Ford say, "I had very, very emotional reactions to his death because he had taken the United States through some very difficult economic problems and some very challenging experiences internationally" (McCullough interview). McCullough has emphasized to me the utter absence of spirit in Ford's replies, in marked contrast to the gusto of another man he interviewed about Roosevelt, Ronald Reagan. I have also drawn upon David McCullough, "The Legacy: The President They Can't Forget," *Parade,* January 31, 1982, pp. 4–6. At a conference at the LBJ Library on March 4, 1983, the fiftieth anniversary of the New Deal, Ford revealed how vague his recollections of the age of Roosevelt were. He even thought that FDR had been at Potsdam.

40. Jerald F. terHorst, *Gerald Ford and the Future of the Presidency* (New York: Okpaku, 1974), pp. 7–9; Philip W. Buchen Gerald R. Ford OH, p. 8; interview by the author with Gerald R. Ford.

41. Speech by Representative Gerald R. Ford, Jr., at annual Lincoln Day dinner, 15th Congressional District, Detroit, February 14, 1950, Gerald Ford MSS, Congressional Papers, Speeches and Press Release Files.

42. Ron Nessen, *It Sure Looks Different from the Inside* (New York: Playboy Press, 1978), pp. 77–78; Gerald R. Ford, *A Time to Heal: The Autobiography of Gerald R. Ford* (New York: Harper & Row, 1979), p. 232.

43. *Congressional Record,* 94th Cong., 2d sess., p. 23419. See, too, Tip

O'Neill's comparison of Ford to Hoover in the *Washington Post,* February 20, 1976, clipping, William H. Harsha MSS.

44. Interview by the author with Donald Rumsfeld, April 23, 1982; *Public Papers of the Presidents of the United States: Gerald Ford, 1974* (Washington, D.C.: Government Printing Office, 1975), pp. 228–29; Richard Reeves, *A Ford, Not a Lincoln* (New York: Harcourt Brace Jovanovich, 1975), p. 160; Frank Freidel, "Responses to Economic Crisis: Hoover and Ford," paper read at conference, "The Relevance of the New Deal to the Present Situation," June 23–25, 1975, City University of New York.

45. Dom Bonafede, "White House Report/Ford's First 100 Days Find Skepticism Replacing Euphoria," *National Journal* 6 (November 16, 1974):1711–14; Myra MacPherson, *The Power Lovers: An Intimate Look at Politics and Marriage* (New York: Putnam's, 1975), p. 35; John Osborne, *White House Watch: The Ford Years* (Washington, D.C.: New Republic Books, 1977), p. 171; John J. Casserly, *The Ford White House: The Diary of a Speechwriter* (Boulder: Colorado Associated University Press, 1977), p. 65. One Ford watcher, noting that the president, in accordance with the principle of "competitive redundancy," assigned two or more people to the same task, speculated, "Perhaps he retained a youthful memory of Franklin D. Roosevelt's artful playing of Cabinet officers and would-be Vice Presidents against one another" (Robert T. Hartmann, *Palace Politics: An Inside Account of the Ford Years* [New York: McGraw-Hill, 1980], p. 382).

46. Transcript of David Brinkley interview with Gerald Ford, ABC News Closeup, November 17, 1981.

47. McCullough interview.

6. Jimmy Carter

1. Martin Schram, *Running for President, 1976: The Carter Campaign* (New York: Stein & Day, 1977), pp. 272–74; Kandy Stroud, *How Jimmy Won: The Victory Campaign from Plains to the White House* (New York: Morrow, 1977), p. 344; Jules Witcover, *Marathon* (New York: Signet, 1977), pp. 581–82; Victor Lasky, *Jimmy Carter: The Man and the Myth* (New York: Richard Marek, 1979), pp. 277–78; William Lee Miller, *Yankee from Georgia: The Emergence of Jimmy Carter* (New York: Times Books, 1978), p. 84.

2. Jimmy Carter, *A Government as Good as Its People* (New York: Pocket Books, 1977), pp. 162–63.

3. *Atlanta Constitution,* September 7, 1976.

4. Witcover, *Marathon,* pp. 581–82; Lasky, *Jimmy Carter,* p. 277; Elizabeth Drew, *American Journal: The Events of 1976* (New York: Random House, 1978), p. 412.

5. Will Alexander COHC, p. 581.

6. Schram, *Running for President,* pp. 314–15.

7. Transcript of telephone interview of Jimmy Carter by David McCullough, November 23, 1981.

8. Carter, *Government as Good,* p. 126; James Wooten, *Dasher: The Roots and the Rising of Jimmy Carter* (New York: Summit, 1978), p. 17.

9. Jimmy Carter, *Why Not the Best?* (Nashville: Broadman Press, 1975), p. 77; Carter, *Government as Good,* p. 230.

10. Carter, *Government as Good,* p. 84; Drew, *American Journal,* p. 421; Carter, *Why Not the Best?,* p. 15.

11. Carter, *Government as Good,* pp. 169–70.

12. George F. Will, "Odd Man In?" *Newsweek,* July 26, 1972, p. 32; Schram, *Running for President,* p. 319; *U.S. News & World Report,* September 13, 1976, p. 20; Ron Nessen, *It Sure Looks Different from the Inside* (New York: Playboy Press, 1978), p. 251n.

13. Betty Glad, *Jimmy Carter: In Search of the Great White House* (New York: Norton, 1980), pp. 359, 353, 356.

14. Stroud, *How Jimmy Won,* p. 127.

15. *Washington Post,* October 25, 1976; *New York Post,* July 19, 1976; Richard L. Strout, *TRB* (New York: Macmillan, 1979), p. 451. It was even suggested facetiously, because each had a toothy smile, that Carter was "Eleanor Roosevelt's illegitimate son" (Wooten, *Dasher,* p. 23).

16. *Washington Post,* October 25, 1976; Robert S. McElvaine, "Franklin and Jack . . . and Jimmy?" *America* 135 (October 23, 1976):247; Stroud, *How Jimmy Won,* p. 191. In a well-publicized interview in *Playboy* in 1976, Robert Scheer remarked, "Not everybody's sure whether you're a conservative in liberal clothing or vice versa. F.D.R., for instance, turned out to be something of a surprise to people who'd voted for him, because he hadn't seemed as progressive before he was elected as he turned out to be. Could you be a surprise that way?" Carter rejected the parallel, for the 1976 Democratic platform was "very progressive, very liberal, very socially motivated," and he intended to carry it out as he had fulfilled his pledges in the past ("Jimmy Carter: a candid conversation with the Democratic Candidate for the presidency," *Playboy,* November 1976, p. 64).

17. *Newsweek,* November 15, 1976, p. 29; "The Fortune 500 Presidential Poll," *Fortune,* October 1976, p. 125; *New York Times,* November 12, 1976. See, too, Robert Shogan, *Promises to Keep: Carter's First Hundred Days* (New York: Crowell, 1977), pp. 55–56; Haynes Johnson, *In the Absence of Power* (New York: Viking, 1980), p. 22.

18. Gerald W. Johnson, "Carter on Trial: Following in FDR's Footsteps?" *New Republic,* December 4, 1976, p. 10.

19. Johnson, it should be said, acknowledged that. He wrote, "This is not to assert, even by implication, that James Earl Carter is another Franklin D. Roosevelt. He isn't" (ibid.).

20. Robert Coles, "Jimmy Carter: Agrarian Rebel?: The Southern Paradox," *New Republic,* June 26, 1976, pp. 15, 19; Wooten, *Dasher,* pp. 119, 133–34; *Washington Post,* October 24, 1976 (William Greider); Bruce Mazlish and Edwin Diamond, *Jimmy Carter: A Character Portrait* (New York: Simon & Schuster, 1979), p. 30; Glad, *Jimmy Carter,* p. 86; *Los Angeles Times,* January 24, 1980. A historian who has written on Carter has remarked: "I have a feeling that

Earl Sr.'s views were pretty much those of the Carter household. Therefore, I would guess that Jimmy Carter grew up with a favorable attitude toward many of the New Deal programs, especially REA, but with a vaguely negative attitude toward Roosevelt" (Numan V. Bartley to the author, April 25, 1979).

21. Julia L. Coleman to Eleanor Roosevelt, January 11, 1934, Eleanor Roosevelt MSS, Box 92.

22. *Addresses of Jimmy Carter: Governor of Georgia, 1971–1975,* ed. Frank Daniel (Atlanta: Ben W. Fortson, Jr., distributed by Georgia Department of Archives and History, 1975), p. 55.

23. It has been suggested to me that Carter was too young, and the youthful Georgians around him too young, for FDR to mean much (interview by the author with Hedley Donovan). Clearly, neither Carter nor his aides had the intimate association with Roosevelt that a Johnson did. Yet Carter was twenty in Roosevelt's last year, surely old enough to have been influenced, and youth had no effect on the capacity of a Bill Moyers to relate to the Roosevelt era.

24. Witcover, *Marathon,* pp. 265, 284; Drew, *American Journal,* pp. 127, 134.

25. Hugh Sidey, "New Lineup, New Ball Game," *Time,* July 26, 1976, p. 28; Mark I. Gelfand, "Historical Perspectives on Carter's Urban Policy: The View from the New Deal Era," paper delivered at the convention of the Organization of American Historians, San Francisco, April 1980, typescript.

26. *New York Times,* June 3, 1977. When, shortly after he received the 1976 nomination, Carter listed "the finer aspects of previous Administrations" he intended to emulate, he made no mention of Roosevelt's (Glad, *Jimmy Carter,* p. 353).

27. Schram, *Running for President,* p. 184; Drew, *American Journal,* p. 41; *New York Times,* October 20, 1976.

28. Stroud, *How Jimmy Won,* pp. 350, 370, 388–89; Schram, *Running for President,* p. 297; Drew, *American Journal,* p. 519. See, too, Morris Janowitz, *The Last Half-Century: Societal Change and Politics in America* (Chicago: University of Chicago Press, 1978), p. 532; Arthur M. Schlesinger, Jr., "The Shambles of '76," *Wall Street Journal,* November 1, 1976, p. 14; Miller, *Yankee from Georgia,* p. 84.

29. Richard H. Rovere, "Letter from Washington," *New Yorker,* November 15, 1976, p. 199; *U.S. News & World Report,* July 19, 1976, p. 29; Walter Dean Burnham, "The 1976 Election: Has the Crisis Been Adjourned?" in *American Politics and Public Policy,* ed. Burnham and Martha Wagner Weinberg (Cambridge: MIT Press, 1978), pp. 8, 9, 13, 14.

30. Johnson, "Carter on Trial," p. 11. See, too, Aaron Wildavsky and Jack Knott, "Jimmy Carter's Theory of Governing," in *American Politics and Public Policy,* ed. Burnham and Weinberg, p. 71.

31. *New York Times,* February 3 and March 20, 1977. For subsequent fireside chats by Carter, see ibid., February 2, 1978; Johnson, *In the Absence of Power,* p. 285.

32. *Public Papers of the Presidents of the United States: Jimmy Carter, 1980–81* (Washington, D.C.: Government Printing Office, 1981), 1:397; Mazlish and

Diamond, *Jimmy Carter,* p. 175; *Public Papers of the Presidents of the United States: Jimmy Carter, 1979* (Washington, D.C.: Government Printing Office, 1980), p. 2025. When in Indianapolis in 1979 Carter encouraged his listeners not to fear the future, his admonition was likened to FDR's "The only thing we have to fear is fear itself" (Richard Reeves, "The Real Estate Panic," *Esquire,* July 3–19, 1979, p. 9). One Washington correspondent compared Carter's relationship to Bert Lance to that between Franklin Roosevelt and Harry Hopkins (Johnson, *In the Absence of Power,* p. 200).

33. Stroud, *How Jimmy Won,* p. 114; Gail Sheehy, "Ladies and Gentlemen, "The Second President—Sister Rosalynn," *New York,* November 22, 1976, p. 52; Hugh Carter as told to Frances Spatz Leighton, *Cousin Beedie and Cousin Hot: My Life with the Carter Family of Plains, Georgia* (Englewood Cliffs, N.J.: Prentice-Hall, 1978), pp. 185, 188.

34. *Miami Herald,* March 18, 1977; *Hartford Courant,* May 29, 1977; *New York Times,* November 2, 1977, August 22, 1979, August 14, 1980. See, too, Richard P. Nathan et al., "Monitoring the Public Service Employment Program: The Second Round," in National Commission for Manpower Policy, Special Report no. 32, March 1979, mimeo; Dewey Grantham, *The Regional Imagination: The South and Recent American History* (Nashville: Vanderbilt University Press, 1979), p. 22.

35. *New York Times,* May 29, 1979.

36. *Washington Post,* October 24, 1976 (William Greider); *New York Times,* July 8, 1979; *Public Papers, 1979,* p. 1235. See, too, *New Orleans Times Picayune,* September 2, 1979.

37. Gladys B. Santo, "Listening to Carter, but Hearing F.D.R.," *New York Times,* August 1, 1979.

38. Miller, *Yankee from Georgia,* p. 84; Hugh Sidey, "Washington: Rites of Passage," *Time,* March 14, 1977, p. 18. My account of that evening is based largely on personal observation.

39. TRB, "Temps Perdu," *New Republic,* March 19, 1977, p. 2; *Washington Post,* March 6, 1977; *Miami Herald,* March 19, 1977.

40. *Congressional Record,* 95th Cong., 1st sess., March 15, 1977, p. 7575; David Broder, "It Was a Shame Carter Couldn't Come," *Washington Post,* March 9, 1977.

41. *New York Times,* July 18, 1978, and March 19, 1979; Lawrence Halprin to the author, December 5, 1977. I served as a consultant to Mr. Halprin on this project.

42. Lasky, *Jimmy Carter,* p. 14; Stuart E. Eizenstat, Remarks, Women's National Democratic Club, Washington, D.C., January 4, 1979.

43. *New York Times,* January 29, 1977; Shogan, *Promises to Keep,* pp. 225–26.

44. TRB, "Temps Perdu," p. 38. In his memoir published after Carter left office, Attorney General Griffin B. Bell wrote: "There are those, such as Thomas E. Cronin, a scholar on the presidency, who contend that the Twenty-second Amendment is a mistake because it would not permit a man like Franklin D. Roosevelt to continue serving in a unique period like the early 1940s. I reject

that view. It is unthinkable that anyone could be a good President beyond eight years. The job is so incredibly difficult that a President burns out. I voted against Roosevelt for that reason" (Griffin B. Bell with Ronald J. Ostrow, *Taking Care of the Law* [New York: Morrow, 1982], p. 227).

45. *Washington Star,* April 30, 1979.

46. *Durham Morning Herald,* January 2, 1979; *New York Times,* November 19, 1978, and August 8, 1980; "Statement of Senator William D. Hathaway on the Regional Development Act of 1978," typescript, Hathaway MSS, Box 1031; transcript of interview of Jimmy Carter by David Brinkley, ABC News, December 18, 1981. See, too, Paul Light, "Passing Nonincremental Policy: Presidential Influence on Congress, Kennedy to Carter," *Congress & the Presidency* 9 (Winter 1981–82):80; Robert Scheer, "Playboy Interview: Dennis Kucinich," *Playboy,* June 1979, p. 108. Kucinich, Cleveland's "boy mayor," rejected Great Society programs as elitist, but said, "The last time we had any domestic programs in this country that had a favorable impact was during Roosevelt's WPA."

47. *New York Times,* June 5, 1977; B. Drummond Ayres, Jr., "The Importance of Being Rosalynn," *New York Times Magazine,* June 3, 1979, pp. 39, 44. It was noted that she was the first president's wife since Eleanor Roosevelt to testify publicly before a congressional committee. Senator Jennings Randolph, the last survivor of the Hundred Days Congress, told her, "I vividly remember Eleanor Roosevelt when she came up here. She had a shrill voice and you have a soft voice. But you both have the same quality" (Ayres, "Importance of Being Rosalynn," p. 56). See, too, Tom Wicker in *New York Times,* July 24, 1979.

48. Gail Sheehy, "Ladies and Gentlemen," p. 52.

49. Elizabeth Drew, "Constituencies," *New Yorker,* January 15, 1979, pp. 52–53.

50. Transcripts of Brinkley and McCullough interviews.

51. *U.S. News & World Report,* September 13, 1976, p. 19; interview with Hedley Donovan; *Public Papers of the President of the United States: Jimmy Carter, 1978* (Washington, D.C.: Government Printing Office, 1979), p. 90; transcript of Brinkley interview.

52. Interview by the author with Jody Powell; Stroud, *How Jimmy Won,* p. 108; Daniel Yergin, "Harry Truman revived and revised," *New York Times Magazine,* October 24, 1976, p. 40; interview by the author with Hedley Donovan; interview by the author with Madeleine Albright.

53. Transcripts of Brinkley and McCullough interviews; David McCullough, "A Presidential Appraisal of FDR," typescript of manuscript to be published in *Parade.*

54. Jerome Angel, "If You Had Three Wishes . . . ," *New York Times Magazine,* May 15, 1977, p. 84; John Osborne, "No Laurel Wreaths Yet," *New Republic,* January 22, 1977, p. 5; comment by Edwin Diamond in Mazlish and Diamond, *Jimmy Carter,* p. 266; "The White House News Summary," July 21, 1979, mimeo.

55. Larry L. King, *Of Outlaws, Con Men, Whores, Politicians and Other Artists*

(New York: Viking, 1980), p. 205; *New York Times,* April 29, 1977, August 23, 1979, October 16, 1979. Similarly, Carter's labor secretary, Ray Marshall, described the president's labor record as the best since the New Deal (*Durham* (N.C.) *Morning Herald,* February 8, 1979). Not since the Great Depression, it was said, had a president been called upon to face problems of such magnitude (*Binghamton Evening Press,* July 17, 1979, quoted in "White House News Summary," July 21, 1979).

56. *New York Times,* August 23, 1979; Johnson, *In the Absence of Power,* p. 296; Edward F. Prichard, Jr., in Neal Peirce column, August 13, 1978, Washington Post Writers Group, mimeo. See, too, Louis W. Koenig, "Historical Perspective: The Swings and Roundabouts of Presidential Power," in *The Tethered Presidency: Congressional Restraints on Executive Power,* ed. Thomas M. Franck (New York: New York University Press, 1981), p. 50. When Senator William Proxmire criticized the choice of Griffin Bell as attorney general, he said that Carter should have followed the model set by Franklin Roosevelt in naming Homer Cummings (Clark R. Mollenhoff, *The President Who Failed: Carter Out of Control* [New York: Macmillan, 1980], p. 40). To metropolitan journalists Carter was a much more elusive figure than Roosevelt. As a feature writer for the *Washington Post* observed: "Jimmy Carter is harder to understand because he is truly an unfamiliar type in presidential politics—a Southerner, an engineer, a businessman, a pious Baptist. FDR was a Victorian aristocrat, much easier to know than a small-town peanut warehouseman who did not even go to law school" (William Greider in *Washington Post,* October 24, 1976).

57. *New York Times,* June 25, 1979; Emmet John Hughes, "The Presidency vs. Jimmy Carter," *Fortune,* December 4, 1978, p. 63. Two of Carter's junior cabinet officials observed, "Jimmy Carter had enormous difficulties in his term—difficulties for a man who was hardly Rooseveltian in his ability to communicate with the nation or to operate tactically" (Ben W. Heineman, Jr., and Curtis A. Hessler, *Memorandum for the President: A Strategic Approach to Domestic Affairs in the 1980s* [New York: Random House, 1980], p. 50). See, too, Russell Baker, "Music Man in the White House," *New York Times Magazine,* June 22, 1980, p. 14. After dismissing Carter's Economic Revitalization Program as a "humdrum little New Deal," one writer declared, "If in name, hoopla and some content the ERP is a very modest New Deal, no one will ever confuse Carter with FDR" (Sidney Weintraub, "Carter's Economic Doodling: A Little New Deal," *New Leader,* September 22, 1980, pp. 5–6). Carter's energy "war," complained George Will, was like the bore war of 1940, in sorry contrast to Roosevelt's record. "When F.D.R. wanted to galvanize the nation, he went on a hundred-day dash, doing things like closing the banks. Bang! Three days after he took office his impact was visible on Main Street" (column of July 22, 1979, reprinted in *The Pursuit of Virtue and Other Tory Notions* [New York: Simon & Schuster, 1982], p. 185).

58. *New York Times,* January 24 and 25, 1979.

59. Ibid., July 14, 1979; memorandum to the writer from James L. Baugh-

man, April 5, 1977; Edwin Diamond, "President Carter On the Airwaves—Echoes of F.D.R.," *New York Times,* March 20, 1977; Johnson, *In the Absence of Power,* p. 285. Some critics thought that Carter's fireside chat was overproduced. Sander Vanocur wrote that the performance brought to mind Oscar Levant's comment on Hollywood: "You have to sweep away the surface tinsel to get to the real tinsel underneath" (Shogan, *Promises to Keep,* p. 130).

60. Arthur Schlesinger, Jr., "If FDR Were President: His Vitality, Activism Missing Today," *Washington Post,* March 12, 1978; John Rosenberg, "'If FDR Were Alive Today . . .'" *Nation,* April 15, 1978, p. 420; Arthur Schlesinger, Jr., "The Great Carter Mystery," *New Republic,* April 12, 1980, p. 21. Asked "Do Carter's first days in the White House remind you at all of FDR's?" Tommy Corcoran replied mischievously, "Franklin Roosevelt was just as ambivalent as Mr. Carter is now" ("New Dealer 'Tommy the Cork' Recalls F.D.R. and Justice Holmes—And Has a Warning for Jimmy Carter," *People,* April 18, 1977, p. 66).

61. Johnson, *In the Absence of Power,* p. 295; Baughman memorandum; *Cleveland Plain Dealer,* April 12, 1980; Emmet John Hughes, "The Presidency vs. Jimmy Carter," *Fortune,* December 4, 1978, pp. 53–54; James Fallows, "The Passionless Presidency: The Trouble with Jimmy Carter's Administration," *Atlantic,* May 1979, p. 44.

62. Interviews by the author with Hedley Donovan.

63. See, for example, Seymour Melman, "Jimmy Hoover?" *New York Times,* February 7, 1979; Sidney Weintraub, "Carter's Hoover Syndrome," *New Leader,* March 24, 1980, p. 5. One letter to an editor observed: "During the Depression, Herbert Hoover kept assuring us that prosperity was just around the corner. This week, Jimmy Carter told us that we finally turned the corner—to find unemployment high, production low and inflation astronomical. Either it was the wrong corner or Mr. Hoover was spoofing us" (Eugene Shapiro to the editor, May 1, 1980, in *New York Times,* May 8, 1980).

64. Hughes, "The Presidency vs. Jimmy Carter," pp. 52–53.

65. *Washington Post,* December 24, 1978.

66. Drew, "Constituencies," p. 70; Garry Wills, "How Carter Hangs On," *New York Review of Books,* February 8, 1979, p. 17; Bob Carolla, "From Memphis, a Liberal Message to Carter," *Washington Post,* December 20, 1978; *Newsweek,* January 29, 1979, p. 25. See, too, Robert S. McElvaine, "Jimmy Carter: Populist or Politician?" *Intellect* 106 (April 1978):371.

67. Murray B. Levin and T. Repak, *Edward Kennedy: The Myth of Leadership* (Boston: Houghton Mifflin, 1980), p. 157; *New York Times,* July 29 and December 18, 1979, March 20, 1980; Timothy B. Clark, "Kennedy's Socioeconomic Record," *Journal of the Institute for Socio-Economic Studies* 5 (Spring 1980):2.

68. *New York Times,* May 21, 1980; December 9, 1979; November 9, 1979; November 8, 1979; September 14, 1979.

69. Ibid., April 9 and 11, 1980; *Durham* (N.C.) *Morning Herald,* May 18, 1980.

70. Elizabeth Drew, "A Reporter at Large; 1980: The Final Round," *New Yorker,* June 23, 1980, p. 68.

71. Drew, "Constituencies," p. 74; Wills, "How Carter Hangs On," p. 20; Drew, "Reporter at Large," pp. 73–74; Elizabeth Drew, *Portrait of an Election:*

The 1980 Presidential Campaign (New York: Simon & Schuster, 1981), p. 182; Levin and Repak, *Edward Kennedy*, p. 181. See, too, William R. Shaffer, "A Discriminant Function Analysis of Position-Taking: Carter vs. Kennedy," *Presidential Studies Quarterly* 10 (Summer 1980):451–68.

72. Eizenstat, Remarks, Women's National Democratic Club, January 4, 1979.

73. *Wall Street Journal*, June 6, 1979.

74. *New York Times*, August 13, 15, 16, 1980; TRB, "Do We Need This?" *New Republic*, August 23, 1980, p. 3; *Washington Post*, August 13, 1980, including a column by Richard Cohen, "Ted Kennedy and the Art of Oratory"; Rowland Evans and Robert Novak, "Carter's Dilemma Persists," *Durham* (N.C.) *Morning Herald*, August 19, 1980. When a young Massachusetts delegate told Kennedy that the delegation opposed a move to make Carter's nomination unanimous, the senator ordered him to fall into line. The young man, who promptly complied, was FDR's grandson, James Roosevelt, Jr. (*Newsweek*, August 25, 1980, p. 30).

75. *New York Times*, August 15, 1980; *Raleigh News and Observer*, August 15, 1980.

76. Neil Goldschmidt, quoted by David S. Broder in *Raleigh News and Observer*, January 26, 1981; *New York Times*, August 10 and October 16, 1980. In the same fashion, David Broder wrote, "If Harold Ickes were alive, Jimmy Carter would have a better chance of being re-elected president." Noting that FDR's secretary of the interior had once leveled Wendell Willkie's pretensions by calling him "the barefoot boy from Wall Street," Broder observed, "If Ickes were around today, watching ex-Democrat Ronald Reagan campaigning in the steel mills of Youngstown and other industrial cities, he would know what to say: 'Ah, Ronnie Reagan . . . the Hollywood hard-hat. The populist from Pacific Palisades!'" Alas, he concluded, "Carter is incapable of the light touch—and instead uses blunderbuss tactics that always end up backfiring on him. And that is one reason Reagan is still out front in this election" (*Durham* (N.C.) *Morning Herald*, October 13, 1980).

77. William E. Leuchtenburg, "Landslide of Jumping to Conclusions," *Washington Star*, November 16, 1980; *New York Times*, November 9, 1980; Ferrel Guillory, "Did 50.7 percent give Reagan a mandate?" *Raleigh News and Observer*, May 8, 1981. See, too, Warren E. Miller and J. Merrill Shanks, "Policy Directions and Presidential Leadership: Alternative Interpretations of the 1980 Presidential Election," *British Journal of Political Science*, 12 (July 1982), 299–356.

78. *Time*, November 17, 1980, p. 44.

79. Frank Annunziata, "Jimmy Carter and the Death of the Welfare State," *USA Today*, November 1980, p. 607.

7. Ronald Reagan

1. *New York Times*, July 20, 1980. As he observed the crowd sitting in silence while Reagan quoted FDR, David Broder wrote, "They're saying, come on,

Ronnie, don't give us any of that New Deal guff" (Lou Cannon, *Reagan* [New York: Putnam's, 1982], p. 270).

2. *Time,* July 28, 1980, pp. 29, 31.

3. Frank Van Der Linden, *The Real Reagan: What he believes; What he has accomplished; What we can expect from him* (New York: William Morrow, 1981), p. 164.

4. *New York Times,* July 20, 1980.

5. Ibid., July 18, 1980.

6. David McCullough, "The Legacy: The President They Can't Forget," *Parade,* January 31, 1982, pp. 4–6.

7. Joseph Lewis, *What Makes Reagan Run?: A Political Profile* (New York: McGraw-Hill, 1968), p. 93; transcript of "Ben Wattenberg at Large," no. 113, Reagan interview, December 1981; I. David Wheat, "Energy: Security with Confidence," in *The Future Under President Reagan,* ed. Wayne Valis (Westport, Conn.: Arlington House, 1981), p. 84.

8. Transcript of interview of Ronald Reagan by David Brinkley, ABC, December 22, 1981.

9. *New York Times,* October 29, 1980; transcript of Brinkley interview.

10. Transcript of interview of Ronald Reagan by David McCullough, December 1, 1981.

11. Jules Witcover, *Marathon: The Pursuit of the Presidency, 1972–1976* (New York: Viking, 1977), p. 99; Cannon, *Reagan,* p. 18; Robert Lindsey, "Creating the Role," in Hedrick Smith et al., *Reagan the Man, the President* (New York: Macmillan, 1980), p. 26; transcript of McCullough interview.

12. George H. Smith, *Who is Ronald Reagan?* (New York: Pyramid, 1968), p. 52; Edmund G. (Pat) Brown and Bill Brown, *Reagan: The Political Chameleon* (New York: Praeger, 1976), p. 137; transcript of McCullough interview.

13. Transcript of McCullough interview.

14. Transcript of McCullough and Brinkley interviews.

15. Ronald Reagan with Richard G. Hubler, *Where's the Rest of Me?* (New York: Duell, Sloan & Pearce, 1965), p. 139; *Newsweek,* July 21, 1980, p. 35; Witcover, *Marathon,* p. 99.

16. Materials in Americans for Democratic Action MSS, Chapter Files, Box 1, Admin. Files, Box 53; James Loeb, Jr., to Charles A. Wellman, October 25, 1947, ibid., Chapter Files, Box 4; Loeb to Reagan, October 25, 1947, ibid., Box 1. However, a prominent Hollywood writer in California ADA wrote, "Who pulled that neat trick of placing Ronald Reagan in as national board member of California? I like Reagan but he's not national board material" (Emmet Lavery to Joseph Rauh, February 25, 1948, ibid.).

17. *Washington Post,* October 24, 1947; *New York Times,* October 24, 1947; Philip Dunne, *Take Two: A Life in Movies and Politics* (New York: McGraw-Hill, 1980), p. 206; Cannon, *Reagan,* pp. 18, 70.

18. Lee Edwards, *Reagan: A Political Biography* (San Diego: Viewpoints, 1967), p. 51; Cannon, *Reagan,* pp. 79, 88; James M. Perry in *National Observer,* June 19, 1976. In the summer of 1948 Reagan wrote, "I'm convinced ADA offers

the only voice for real liberals and I look forward to the time when I can be of more help" (Reagan to Leon Henderson, July 15, 1948, Americans for Democratic Action MSS, microfilm, University of North Carolina at Chapel Hill).

19. Cannon, *Reagan*, p. 74; Theodore H. White, *America in Search of Itself: The Making of the President, 1956–1980* (New York: Harper & Row, 1982), p. 309; Allen Rivkin to "Ed," December 20, 1949, press release, March 21, 1950, Helen Gahagan Douglas MSS, Boxes 177, 194; Helen Gahagan Douglas, *A Full Life* (New York: Doubleday, 1982), p. 323; Colleen M. O'Connor to the author, August 25, 1982; *Time*, October 7, 1966, p. 32.

20. Cannon, *Reagan*, p. 88; *Time*, October 7, 1966, p. 32.

21. White, *America in Search of Itself*, p. 242; Bill Boyarsky, *The Rise of Ronald Reagan* (New York: Random House, 1968), p. 25; Brown and Brown, *Reagan*, p. 161; Wayne Valis, "Ronald Reagan: The Man, the President," in *The Future under President Reagan*, ed. Valis, p. 33; Cannon, *Reagan*, p. 18.

22. *U.S. News & World Report*, February 1, 1982, p. 55.

23. Witcover, *Marathon*, p. 407; transcript of Wattenberg interview.

24. *The Public Papers and Addresses of Franklin D. Roosevelt*, ed. Samuel I. Rosenman (New York: Random House, 1938), 4:20–21; William E. Leuchtenburg, *Franklin D. Roosevelt and the New Deal* (New York: Harper & Row, 1963), pp. 124–33; Thomas H. Eliot to the editor, February 4, 1982, in *New York Times*, February 14, 1982.

25. Transcript of Wattenberg interview; *U.S. News & World Report*, February 1, 1982, p. 55; *New York Times*, December 23, 1981; *Congressional Record*, 78th Cong., 2d sess., p. 6.

26. The closest Reagan ever approached to a direct criticism of Roosevelt came in an interview with David Brinkley when he said that "Roosevelt himself believed that he could persuade Stalin, and that Stalin wasn't"—he laughed— "a bad fellow" (transcript of Brinkley interview).

27. Transcript of McCullough interview; White, *America in Search of Itself*, p. 308; *U.S. News & World Report*, February 1, 1982, p. 55; transcript of Wattenberg interview.

28. *Time*, May 17, 1976, p. 19.

29. *New York Times*, August 13, 1980; Morton Kondracke, "Politics: The Dream Is Dead," *New Republic*, August 23, 1980, p. 7. See, too, Dale Larson, "Reagan Rewrites the Record," *American Federationist* 87 (October 1980):12.

30. *New York Times*, August 15, 1980.

31. Ibid., August 17, 1980. See, too, Melvyn B. Krauss, "Reagan's Comments on Fascism and the New Deal," *Wall Street Journal*, September 9, 1980.

32. Hugh Johnson, *The Blue Eagle from Egg to Earth* (Garden City, N.Y.: Doubleday, Doran, 1935), pp. 123–33; John P. Diggins, *Mussolini and Fascism: The View from America* (Princeton: Princeton University Press, 1972), p. 280; John A. Garraty, "The New Deal, National Socialism, and the Great Depression," *American Historical Review* 78 (October 1973):908, 914; Bernard Sternsher, *Rexford Tugwell and the New Deal* (New Brunswick, N.J.: Rutgers University Press, 1964), pp. 15, 325; Ellis W. Hawley, *The New Deal and the*

Problem of Monopoly (Princeton: Princeton University Press, 1966), p. 43; Richard Collier, *Duce!: A Biography of Benito Mussolini* (New York: Viking, 1971), pp. 65, 93; William L. Shirer, *20th Century Journey: A Memoir of a Life and the Times* (New York: Simon & Schuster, 1976), p. 398; Benito Mussolini, "Roosevelt e il Sistema," *Bolletino del R. Ministero degli Affari Esteri* 40 (Luglie 1933):715–17, in FDRL PPF 432.

33. Transcript of McCullough interview; George H. Smith, *Who is Ronald Reagan?*, p. 52; Robert Lindsey, "Creating the Role," in Hedrick Smith et al., *Reagan the Man, the President*, p. 31; Reagan with Hubler, *Where's the Rest of Me?*, p. 139.

34. Reagan with Hubler, *Where's the Rest of Me?*, pp. 167–69.

35. It has also been said that his views were shaped by his second wife, Nancy, who shared the outlook of her archconservative adoptive father, the Chicago surgeon Dr. Loyal Davis. See, for example, James M. Perry in *National Observer,* June 19, 1976; Lindsey, "Creating the Role," p. 33. This allegation, however, has been denied by his most painstaking biographer (Cannon, *Reagan,* p. 78). Oddly, in 1932 a Chicago tabloid ran on its first page a photograph from the 1932 Democratic convention that nominated FDR, showing a little girl seated on the lap of her mother. The child would one day be Nancy Reagan (*Washington Post,* April 26, 1981).

36. Cannon, *Reagan,* p. 82. See, too, Michael Miles, "Reagan and the Respectable Right," *New Republic,* April 20, 1968, p. 26.

37. Boyarsky, *Rise of Ronald Reagan,* p. 101; Smith, *Who Is Ronald Reagan?,* p. 74.

38. Lewis, *What Makes Reagan Run?,* p. 50; Gerald R. Ford, *A Time to Heal: The Autobiography of Gerald R. Ford* (New York: Harper & Row, 1979), p. 387.

39. Boyarsky, *Rise of Ronald Reagan,* p. 263.

40. Witcover, *Marathon,* p. 97; transcript of Brinkley interview.

41. Elizabeth Drew, *Portrait of an Election: The 1980 Preisdential Campaign* (New York: Simon & Schuster, 1981), p. 292; Van der Linden, *Real Reagan,* p. 194; Leonard Silk, "On the Supply Side," in Smith et al., *Reagan the Man, the President,* p. 53; Smith, "Mr. Reagan Goes to Washington," in Smith et al., *Reagan the Man, the President,* p. 149; telephone interview, Myron Waldman, February 16, 1983.

42. Cannon, *Reagan,* p. 88.

43. Van der Linden, *Real Reagan,* pp. 149, 198–99. See, too, White, *America in Search of Itself,* p. 381; David S. Broder, *Changing of the Guard: Power and Leadership in America* (New York: Simon & Schuster, 1980), p. 461.

44. Jack Kemp, *An American Renaissance: A Strategy for the 1980s* (New York: Harper & Row, 1979), pp. 13–14; Kemp, "Economics, Inflation, Productivity— and Politics," in *Future under President Reagan,* ed. Valis, pp. 62–63.

45. *Washington Post,* November 6, 1980; *Christian Science Monitor,* November 6, 1980; *Durham Morning Herald,* November 20, 1980. See, too, C. David Sutton, "Appalachia and the 1980 Election," *Appalachian Journal* 8 (Winter 1981):153.

46. *New York Post,* November 5, 1980; *Washington Post,* December 27, 1980; Ronald Steel, "Franklin D. Reagan," in *New York Times,* January 18, 1981.

47. *New York Times,* January 11, 1981.

48. Ibid., December 11 and 19, 1980; Chalmers M. Roberts, "A Second '100 Days'?" *Washington Post,* December 27, 1980. Roberts added: "One can see a parallel between FDR's budget director, Lewis W. Douglas—who wanted to slash government spending 25 percent and who stood up to, and temporarily defeated, the most powerful lobby of the day, the World War I veterans—and Reagan's budget chief, Stockman. Both resigned House seats to take the job—Douglas was 38, Stockman 34—and both had a passion for economy."

49. Edward W. Chester, "Shadow or Substance?: Critiquing Reagan's Inaugural Address," *Presidential Studies Quarterly* 11 (Spring 1981):172.

50. Dom Bonafede, "From a 'Revolution' to a 'Stumble'—The Press Assesses the First 100 Days," *National Journal* 13 (May 16, 1981):882; Steven R. Weisman, "Reagan's First 100 Days: A Test of the Man and the Presidency," *New York Times Magazine,* April 26, 1981, p. 51. One careful study concluded that though the "Reagan Counterrevolution" aimed to roll back history to the era before FDR, the administration's attitude toward welfare programs expressed "a New Deal concept of 'the deserving poor'" in turning away from the broader emphases of the Great Society (John L. Palmer and Isabel V. Sawhill, "Perspectives on the Reagan Experiment," in *The Reagan Experiment: An Examination of Economic and Social Policies under the Reagan Administration,* ed. Palmer and Sawhill [Washington, D.C.: Urban Institute Press, 1982], pp. 24–26).

51. *New York Daily News,* February 6, 1981; *Newsweek,* March 2, 1981, p. 22; Cannon, *Reagan,* p. 417. See, too, *Los Angeles Times,* June 25, 1981; Mary McGrory in *Raleigh News and Observer,* August 3, 1981; Hugh Sidey, "The Presidency: Scripture for a New Religion," *Time,* March 2, 1981, p. 15.

52. *Charlotte Observer,* March 5, 1982.

53. George F. Will, "1981: The Last Word," *Newsweek,* January 4, 1982, p. 68; Cannon, *Reagan,* pp. 422–23.

54. *Raleigh News and Observer,* March 24, 1982.

55. Robert Lekachman, *Greed Is Not Enough: Reagonomics* (New York: Pantheon, 1982), p. 3; *Newsweek,* March 2, 1981, p. 33; Robert S. McElvaine, "Reagan's Mellon Slices," *New York Times,* May 21, 1981; Frank Freidel, "Roosevelt in Reagan's eyes, and in history's," *Boston Globe,* January 24, 1982. See, too, *San Jose Mercury,* May 24, 1981; *New Orleans Times-Picayune,* September 1, 1980; Robert J. Donovan, "Conservative coalition rooted in FDR years," *Kansas City Times,* July 9, 1981. For Reagan's misconstruing of FDR's record, see Francis L. Loewenheim, "Reaganscribing History," *New York Times,* March 23, 1981.

56. TRB, "Reagan's Gamble," *New Republic,* May 9, 1981, p. 3; *Durham Morning Herald,* May 11, 1981. See, too, Joseph Kraft, "Reagan's Sixty Days," *Washington Post,* March 19, 1981; *Christian Science Monitor,* February 19 and May 1, 1981; Elizabeth Wehr in *Durham Morning Herald,* February 4, 1981; Jack W. Germond and Jules Witcover, "A Little Story Reagan Told About The Poor," *Washington Star,* March 13, 1981.

57. *New York Times,* January 21, 1981; Mary McGrory in *Raleigh News and Observer,* August 10, 1981. One newspaper account carried the subhead: "Roosevelt's Rural Electrification Administration helped form scores of small power companies. Reagan thinks they can now go it alone" (*New York Times,* March 29, 1981). See, too, *Christian Science Monitor,* March 30, 1981.

58. Cannon, *Reagan,* p. 425; Robert L. Heilbroner, "In Hoover's Wake, Helmsman Reagan," *New York Times,* October 19, 1981; "The New Old Deal," *New York Times,* January 28, 1982. See, too, Saul Bernstein to the editor, May 31, 1981, ibid., June 7, 1981; George F. Will, "1981: The Last Word," *Newsweek,* January 4, 1982, p. 68. Some conservatives and libertarians, however, expressed skepticism that Reagan was carrying out a "180 degree turn in the course of government" (George F. Will, "So This Is a Revolution?" *Manchester Guardian Weekly,* October 4, 1981, p. 17; Murray N. Rothbard, "The Reagan Fraud," *Reason* 13 [June 1981]:84).

59. Barbara Mikulski, ADA Speech. I am indebted to Congresswoman Mikulski for sending me the typescript of her address, which was delivered to a convention of Americans for Democratic Action. Reagan's insistence that in 1980 the United States was in a "severe depression" opened him to the charge that he had no awareness of what the Great Depression was like. See, for example, Mike Royko's column, *Madison* (Wis.) *Capital Times,* September 5, 1980.

60. The account of the luncheon derives from personal observation as a guest at the affair, which was attended not only by luminaries of the Roosevelt era but by four historians and the television news commentators Walter Cronkite and Eric Sevareid. That FDR's centennial came in the administration of a president who appeared intent on dismantling the New Deal was widely noted. See, for example, *Baltimore Sun,* August 30, 1981.

61. *Wall Street Journal,* November 18, 1981; Michael J. Copps, "Defending FDR's Legacy," *Washington Post,* January 29, 1982; *National Review,* September 4, 1981, p. 999.

62. This account is based mainly on my own observations at the White House on that day, but also on the *New York Times* and the *Washington Post,* January 29, 1982. When Reagan returned to his office after speaking at the luncheon, he told his aides, "I am still for the New Deal; it is the Great Society I object to" (confidential White House source). FDR, Jr., though, refused to come to the White House luncheon, saying, "The Reagan Administration is undoing steps that my father's administration took 40 to 50 years ago" (*New York Times,* January 29, 1982).

8. Waiting for Franklin D.

1. Lloyd Lewis, *Myths after Lincoln* (New York: Harcourt, Brace, 1929), p. 394; George B. Forgie, *Patricide in the House Divided: A Psychological Interpretation of Lincoln and His Age* (New York: Norton, 1979), p. 6; Rexford G. Tug-

well, *Off Course: From Truman to Nixon* (New York: Praeger, 1971), p. 7. "Nostalgia for a lost presence" has been said to characterize Heidegger's work. See Jacques Derrida, *Of Grammatology* (Baltimore: Johns Hopkins University Press, 1976), p. xvi. Mrs. Roosevelt noted the parallel between FDR and Lincoln in a column written shortly after her husband's death. Alfred Haworth Jones, *Roosevelt's Image Brokers: Poets, Playwrights, and the Use of the Lincoln Symbol* (Port Washington, N.Y.: Kennikat Press, 1974), p. 113. On April 13, 1945, the Associated Press circulated a story on the theme "Lives of Roosevelt and Lincoln Strange Parallel." It stated, "They led their people through war to the promised land of peace. They were not permitted to enter. They died on the edge of it. . . . The two great wartime presidents died 80 years apart, almost to the day" (*Asheville Citizen-Times*, April 13, 1945, clipping Zebulon Weaver MSS, Box 80-8.4, Folder 75). In 1984, a Philadelphian, still a faithful New Dealer, remembered how as a boy he had gone on April 13, 1945, to a synagogue where, in tribute to FDR, a rabbi read "Captain, My Captain" (telephone interview, Isador Kranzel).

2. Tugwell, *Off Course*, pp. 3, 10 See, too, Marshall W. Fishwick, *American Heroes: Myth and Reality* (Washington, D. C.: Public Affairs Press, 1954), p. 17.

3. W. Jackson Bate, *The Burden of the Past and the English Poet* (Cambridge: Belknap Press, Harvard University Press, 1970), pp. 3, 32. See, too, Forgie, *Patricide in the House Divided*, p. 7.

4. Bate, *The Burden of the Past and the English Poet*, pp. 39n, 122; Robert Louis Stevenson, *Memories and Portraits* (New York: Scribner's, 1894), p. 59. See, too, Alan Weinblatt, "T. S. Eliot and the Historical Sense," *South Atlantic Quarterly*, 77 (Summer 1978), 282–95.

5. Paul Henry Lang, *George Frederic Handel* (New York: Norton, 1966), p. 703; Donal Henahan, "The Mystery of the Dropout Composer," *New York Times*, March 14, 1982, 2:3; George R. Marek, *Beethoven: Biography of a Genius* (New York: Funk & Wagnalls, 1969), p. 638. In her excellent catalogue essay, Barbara Haskell has explained the development of a new aesthetic in the late 1950s as a reaction against the awesome shadow cast by the Abstract Expressionists. She noted, in particular, Tom Wesselmann's *cri de coeur*: "De Kooning had already painted all my paintings" (Barbara Haskell, *Blam!: The Explosion of Pop, Minimalism, and Performance, 1958–1964* [New York: Whitney Museum of American Art, 1984], p. 13).

6. Harold Bloom, *The Anxiety of Influence: A Theory of Poetry* (New York: Oxford University Press, 1973); Ulrich Wilcken, *Alexander the Great* (New York: Norton, 1967), pp. 270–71; Robert K. Massie, *Peter the Great: His Life and World* (New York: Knopf, 1980), pp. 853–54; Pieter Geyl, *Napoleon For and Against* (New Haven: Yale University Press, 1949), pp. 71–72; Geyl, "Latter-Day Napoleon Worship," in *Debates with Historians* (New York: Meridian, 1958). For other examples, see Wilbur Cortez Abbott, "The Fame of Cromwell," in *Conflicts with Oblivion* (New Haven: Yale University Press, 1924), p. 192; Erik H. Erikson, *Life History and the Historical Moment* (New York: Norton, 1975), p. 126.

7. Merrill D. Peterson, *The Jefferson Image in the American Mind* (New York:

Oxford University Press, 1960), pp. 25, 34; David Donald, *Lincoln Reconsidered: Essays on the Civil War Era* (New York: Knopf, 1956), p. 6.

8. *The Best Known Works of Nathaniel Hawthorne* (Garden City, N.Y.: Blue Ribbon, 1941), p. 228.

9. William Alfred Bryan, *George Washington in American Literature* (New York: Columbia University Press, 1952), pp. 41–42; Brant, *Fourth President*, p. 442; Glyndon G. Van Deusen, *The Jacksonian Era, 1828–1848* (New York: Harper, 1959), p. 115. Jefferson showered so much advice on President Monroe that on one occasion the president replied apologetically, "I have to acknowledge three letters from you of the 8th, 13th, and 16th of this month" (W. P. Cresson, *James Monroe* [Chapel Hill: University of North Carolina Press, 1946], p. 192). For Jackson's influence on President Polk, see Charles Sellers, *James K. Polk: Continentalist, 1843–1846* (Princeton: Princeton University Press, 1966), pp. 164, 184.

10. Bryan, *George Washington,* p. 48; Marcus Cunliffe, *George Washington: Man and Monument* (Boston: Little, Brown, 1958), p. 15.

11. Theodore Roosevelt to Maria Storer, December 8, 1902, in *The Letters of Theodore Roosevelt*, ed. Elting E. Morison et al., 8 vols. (Cambridge: Harvard University Press, 1951–54), 3:391; Anne O'Hare McCormick, "Where in the Next Four Years?," *New York Times Magazine*, November 8, 1936, p. 26.

12. James Oliver Robertson, *American Myth*, *American Reality* (New York: Hill & Wang, 1980), p. 320; Geoffrey Blodgett, "The Political Leadership of Grover Cleveland," *South Atlantic Quarterly*, 82 (Summer 1983), 288. To achieve consistency, I have changed the punctuation in the long quotation.

13. Bryce Nelson, "The Best Memorial for FDR," *Washington Post*, June 14, 1981; Finlay Lewis, *Mondale: Portrait of an American Politician* (New York: Harper & Row, 1980), pp. 24, 36. In the Polish crisis of December 1980, a Republican congressman from Georgia read FDR's quarantine address into the record as a hornbook for dealing with the Soviet Union (*Congressional Record*, 96th Cong., 2nd sess., p. E5493). The congresswoman from Hawaii, Patsy Mink, recalled that the most important influence on the formation of her political views was the series of captivating fireside chats she heard as a girl in Maui (Patsy Mink OH, Former Members of Congress, pp. 2–3, Mink MSS, Box 1).

14. Bate, *Burden of the Past*, p. 3.

15. Paul Roazen, *Freud and His Followers* (New York: Knopf, 1975), pp. 36–37.

16. Lawrence J. Friedman, *Inventors of the Promised Land* (New York: Knopf, 1975), p. 77. See, too, Howard N. Rabinowitz, "The Washington Legend, 1865–1900: The Heroic Image in Flux," *American Studies*, 17 (Spring 1976), 5–24.

17. Richard Tanner Johnson, *Managing the White House* (New York: Harper & Row, 1974), p. 150. See, too, Harry M. Caudill, *The Watches of the Night* (Boston: Little, Brown, 1976); John Rosenberg, "If FDR Were Alive Today . . . ," *Nation*, April 15, 1978, p. 421. For a skeptical attitude toward the applicability of the New Deal to the problem of modern unemployment, see John A. Garraty, "Against Federal Creation of Jobs," *New York Times*, January 3, 1978.

18. For the latter contention, see Harry Truman, "A Message from the Presi-

dent of the United States," January 13, 1951, in Americans for Democratic Action, *1951 Roosevelt Day*, Dorothy Kenyon MSS, Box 13.

19. John Morton Blum in *Journal of American History*, 71 (June 1984), 177; *Los Angeles Times*, September 8, 1972; *New York Times*, October 4, 1972; interview with Franklin D. Roosevelt, Jr., October 13, 1984.

20. Herbert Stein, *Presidential Economics: The Making of Economic Policy from Roosevelt to Reagan and Beyond* (New York: Simon & Schuster, 1984), p. 312. For the similarities and dissimilarities of Reagan and FDR, see Fred I. Greenstein, "Reagan and the Lore of the Modern Presidency: What Have We Learned?" in *The Reagan Presidency: An Early Assessment*, ed. Greenstein (Baltimore: Johns Hopkins University Press, 1983), pp. 168–69; Irving Louis Horowitz, "From the New Deal to the New Federalism: Presidential Ideology in the U.S. from 1932 to 1982," *American Journal of Economics and Sociology*, 42 (April 1983), 129–48; Samuel H. Beer, "Ronald Reagan: New Deal Conservative?," *Society*, 20 (January–February 1983), 40–44.

21. Stephen B. Baxter, "The Myth of the Grand Alliance in the Eighteenth Century," in Paul R. Sellin and Baxter, *Anglo-Dutch Cross Currents in the Seventeenth and Eighteenth Centuries* (Los Angeles: William Andrews Clark Memorial Library, UCLA, 1976), p. 43. For the attempt to maintain a political fiction, see Harold L. Kahn, *Monarchy in the Emperor's Eyes: Images and Reality in the Ch'ien-lung Reign* (Cambridge: Harvard University Press, 1971), p. 5.

22. Donald R. McCoy, "Trends in Viewing Herbert Hoover, Franklin D. Roosevelt, Harry S. Truman, and Dwight D. Eisenhower," *Midwest Quarterly*, 20 (1979), 125; Mel Elfin to the writer, July 10, 1980; Lewis, *Mondale*, p. 51; *Wall Street Journal*, November 20, 1980; Bryce Nelson, "Best Memorial for FDR"; Peter Kovler, "Franklin Who?," *Kansas City Times*, July 6, 1981.

23. Morton Keller, "Reflections on Politics and Generations in America," *Daedalus*, 107 (Fall 1978), 123–35; José Ortega y Gasset, *The Modern Theme* (New York: Harper & Row, 1961), p, 15. See, too, Paul R. Abramson, *Generational Change in American Politics* (Lexington, Mass.: D. C. Heath, 1975); Samuel P. Huntington, "Paradigms of American Politics: Beyond the One, the Two, and the Many," *Political Science Quarterly*, 89 (March 1974), 22–26; Alan B. Spitzer, "The Historical Problem of Generations," *American Historical Review*, 75 (December 1973), 1362; Rene Wellek and Austin Warren, *Theory of Literature* (New York: Harcourt, Brace, 1949), pp. 278–79.

24. *New York Times*, April 1, 1979. For questioning of the usefulness of the New Deal legacy, see *New York Times*, January 23, 1981; *U.S. News & World Report*, September 14, 1981, p. 88.

25. *New Republic*, January 27, 1982, p. 9; Randall Rothenberg, *The Neo-Liberals: Creating the New American Politics* (New York: Simon & Schuster, 1984), p. 28.

26. Paul Tsongas, address to Americans for Democratic Action, reprint of *Congressional Record*, 126 (June 16, 1980), courtesy of Senator Tsongas; Tsongas, *The Road from Here: Liberalism and Realities in the 1980s* (New York: Vintage, 1982), p. 38; *New York Times*, October 20. 1981.

27. Rothenberg, *The Neo-Liberals*, p. 129; Sidney Blumenthal, "Hart's Big

Chill," *New Republic*, January 23, 1984, p. 19; *Raleigh News and Observer*, March 7, 1984; *Wall Street Journal*, April 6, 1984; Ben Keppel in *Sacramento Bee*, April 29, 1984.

28. *New York Times*, July 22, 1984; Blumenthal, "Hart's Big Chill," p. 22. The choice of Geraldine Ferraro for the vice-presidential slot was also perceived, in part, to be an "attempt to win back for the Democratic party its old New Deal working class ethnic base" (*Asheville Citizen*, July 13, 1984).

29. *Washington Post*, July 20, 1984, and August 23, 1984.

30. Walter F. Mondale, "The Legacy of the New Deal: The Role of Government in American Life," *Minnesota Law Review*, 68 (December 1983), 265–71; *International Herald Tribune*, August 25–26, 1984; *New York Times*, October 11, 1984; *Raleigh News and Observer*, September 26, 1984.

31. Gerald M. Pomper, *Elections in America: Control and Influence in Democratic Politics* (New York: Dodd, Mead, 1970), p. 162; Walter Dean Burnham, "Death of the New Deal," *Commonweal*, December 9, 1966, pp. 285–86; David S. Broder, *Changing of the Guard: Power and Leadership in America* (New York: Simon & Schuster, 1980), pp. 228, 233; Ross Baker on the MacNeill/Lehrer Report, November 17, 1980.

32. Joseph Kraft in *New York Post*, November 15, 1984.

33. *U.S. News & World Report*, November 19, 1984, p. 38; *Time*, November 19, 1984, p. 72; *Raleigh News and Observer*, December 23 and December 8, 1984.

34. William R. Schulz to Walter Mondale, November 25, 1983. I am indebted to Mr. Schulz for sending me a copy of this letter and his statement.

35. *Spectator Magazine* (Raleigh, N.C.), August 2, 1984, p. 3.

36. Wilson Carey McWilliams, "Under Cover: Memories and Heroes," *Worldview*, 27 (January 1984), 2. He added, though, "However, our political memory is failing, . . . the old allegiances thinning out." For the complaint that there are no longer the giants of bygone days, see C. H. Sulzberger, *An Age of Mediocrity: Memoirs and Diaries, 1963–1972* (New York: Macmillan, 1973), p. 8. That perception is challenged in Lewis J. Edinger, "Where Are the Political Superstars?," *Political Science Quarterly*, 89 (June 1974), 249–50.

37. Joe Mysak in *Credit Markets*, January 3, 1984.

38. Paul Simon, *The Once and Future Democrats: Strategies for Change* (New York: Continuum, 1982), pp. 14, 37–38; "Address by Bill Clinton, Governor of the State of Arkansas, Democratic National Convention—1980," mimeo. I am indebted to Governor Clinton for providing me with the text of his remarks.

39. *Washington Post*, November 26, 1984.

40. Quoted in Peterson, *Jefferson Image*, p. 332.

41. Quoted in Nina Tumarkin's outstanding study, *Lenin Lives!: The Lenin Cult in Soviet Russia* (Cambridge: Harvard University Press, 1983), p. 248.

42. McCormick, "Where in the Next Four Years?," p. 26.

43. Donald, *Lincoln Reconsidered*, p. 14; George E. Mowry, "The Uses of History by Recent Presidents," *Journal of American History*, 53 (June 1966), 10–11; Torbjorn Sirevag, "Franklin D. Roosevelt and the Use of History," *Americana Norwegica*, 2 (1968), 299–342; Jones, *Roosevelt's Image Brokers*, p. 64. For the no-

tion that FDR sought to "out-Roosevelt Theodore Roosevelt," see Turner Catledge OH, pp. 38–39.

44. Jones, *Roosevelt's Image Brokers,* pp. 42, 65–73, 109–10.

45. Rexford G. Tugwell, *The Brains Trust* (New York: Viking Press, 1968), p. 442; John Morton Blum, *V Was for Victory: Politics and American Culture during World War II* (New York: Harcourt Brace Jovanovich, 1976), p. 8; Ernest R. May, *"Lessons of the Past": The Use and Misuse of History in American Foreign Policy* (New York: Oxford University Press, 1973), p. 11; Robert E. Sherwood, *Roosevelt and Hopkins: An Intimate History* (New York: Harper, 1948), p. 697; H. R. Baukhage MS Diary, September 6, 1946

46. *The Public Papers and Addresses of Franklin D. Roosevelt* (New York: Random House, 1938), 1:627–39, 745–46.

47. Statement of the Jeffersonian Democrats of Virginia, Thomas Lomax Hunter MSS; Peterson, *Jefferson Image*, pp. 332–33, 355; Frank Freidel, "Roosevelt in Reagan's Eyes, and in History's," *Boston Globe*, January 24, 1982; Charles M. Wiltse, *The Jeffersonian Tradition in American Democracy* (New York: Hill & Wang, 1960), p. 266. One of FDR's speech writers recorded in his diary the president's campaign plan for 1936: "July 6th, open the Skyline Drive near Washington—non-political and therefore the best politics; July 7—Charlottesville, Va.—Monticello—Jefferson. He will speak on theme that Jefferson's opposition to privilege—which led him to stand for states rights in his day [—] would lead him to stand for just the opposite today" (Stanley High MS Diary, May 18, 1936).

48. William B. Rhoads, "The Artistic Patronage of Franklin D. Roosevelt: Art as Historical Record," *Prologue*, 15 (Spring 1983), 8–12. The memorial was completed under FDR's sponsorship "in requital," it was said, for his destruction of his predecessor's philosophy of government.

49. FDR to E. M. House, March 10, 1934, House MSS; Peterson, *Jefferson Image*, pp. 360–63, 448.

Index

Library of Congress Cataloging in Publication Data

Leuchtenburg, William Edward, 1922–
    In the shadow of FDR.

    Includes bibliographical references and index.
    1. United States—Politics and government—1945–   . 2. Roosevelt, Franklin D.
(Franklin Delano), 1882–1945—Influence. I. Title. II. Title: In the shadow of F.D.R.
E743.L49 1983   973.92   83-45147
ISBN (cloth) 0-8014-1387-7
ISBN (paper) 0-8014-9303-X

Women, violence and male power

Feminist activism, research and practice

edited by
Marianne Hester, Liz Kelly and Jill Radford

Open University Press
Buckingham · Philadelphia

Open University Press
Celtic Court
22 Ballmoor
Buckingham
MK18 1XW

and
1900 Frost Road, Suite 101
Bristol, PA 19007, USA

First Published 1996

A catalogue record of this book is available from the British Library

ISBN 0 335 19506 7 (pb) 0 335 1507 5 (hb)

Library of Congress Cataloging-in-Publication Data
Hester, Marianne, 1955-
    Women, violence, and male power : feminist activism, research, and practice / Marianne Hester, Liz Kelly, and Jill Radford.
        p. cm.
    Includes bibliographical references (p.   ) and index.
    ISBN 0–335–19507–5 (hb). — ISBN 0–335–19506–7 (pb)
    1. Women—Crimes against—Great Britain.   2. Sexual abuse victims—Great Britain.   3. Sex crimes—Great Britain.   4. Patriarchy—Great Britain.   5. Feminist theory—Great Britain.   I. Kelly, Liz. II. Radford, Jill, 1947-   .   III. Title.
HV6250.4.W65H47   1995
362.82′92′0941—dc20   95–15786
                                                                              CIP

Typeset by Graphicraft Typesetters Ltd, Hong Kong
Printed in Great Britain by St Edmundsbury Press Ltd,
Bury St Edmunds, Suffolk

Contents

Acknowledgements

We want to thank Sage Publications Ltd for permission to reprint Chapter 5, Jill Radford's and Elizabeth Stanko's 'Violence against Women and Children: the Contradictions of Crime Control under Patriarchy' originally published in K. Stenson and D. Cowell (eds) (1991), *The Politics of Crime Control*; and the editors of *Critical Social Policy* for permission to reprint Liz Kelly and Jill Radford's (1990) '"Nothing Really Happened": the Invalidation of Women's Experiences of Sexual Violence' originally published in *Critical Social Policy*, Volume 30. We also want to thank Jacinta Evans at the Open University Press for her support, all the women involved in the British Sociological Association Women's Caucus Violence Against Women Study Group, and Bernie, Kate and Rosemary whose help made this book possible.

Notes on contributors

Marian Foley has been actively involved in Rape Crisis work for many years. She is currently employed by the Merseyside Sexual Assault Centre Development project, which is trying to establish services for women who have experienced sexual violence.

Terry Gillespie is a senior lecturer and course leader of BA Criminology at the Nottingham Trent University. She is researching support services for survivors of rape and sexual assault and has worked with survivors at a rape crisis centre. Her publications include *Working with Violence* (with Carol Lupton).

Marianne Hester has a longstanding interest in the links between women's experiences, feminist theory and political action. She has been involved in feminist activity since the early 1970s and in campaigns against violence against women since the early 1980s, including support work in Rape Crisis in the North and South West of England. She has carried out research into various forms of male violence and power, in history and in present day Britain and Denmark. She is lecturer in the School for Policy Studies at the University of Bristol.

Liz Kelly has been a feminist activist for over 20 years and a feminist researcher for 14. She has worked in a refuge with children and women, in Rape Crisis and many local and national campaigns. The British Sociological Association (Women's Caucus) Violence Against Women Study Group was born at the time she needed it most – finishing her PhD. Since 1987 she has been privileged to work at the Child and Women Abuse Studies Unit, University of North London, developing feminist research methods, training and policy. She lives in Manchester, Dalston (and on British Rail).

Sue Lees is professor of women's studies at the University of North London.

She has a longstanding interest in women and the law and has conducted several research projects into the judicial treatment of rape and sexual assault. Her book *Carnal Knowledge: Rape on Trial* is to be published by Hamish Hamilton in 1996.

Michelle McCarthy has always worked with people with learning disabilities. She trained as a social worker, and for the last five years has specialized in the area of sexuality. She has a personal and political commitment to working with women with learning disabilities, particularly on matters of sexual health and sexual abuse. She has written widely about this work and is now a lecturer in learning disability at the University of Kent.

Jo Moran-Ellis is a lecturer in sociology at the University of Surrey, working in the area of childhood and child protection. She has researched organizational responses to child abuse referrals, focusing recently on health professionals.

Maggie O'Neill is a senior lecturer in women's studies and sociology at the University of Staffordshire. She is on the management committee of POW, Prostitute Outreach Worker project. She is currently continuing ethnographic research with female prostitutes focusing on the rights and needs of women.

Jill Radford has spent the last 20 years on the interface of feminist activism and academe working at the Wandsworth policing campaign, LESPOP, and Rights of Women, as well as teaching sociology, criminology and women's studies at the South Bank University, University of Westminster, and the Open University. She was one of the founding members of the British Sociological Association (Women's Caucus) Violence Against Women Study Group and has published widely in the field. Her daughter is a New Age traveller and her son has a degree in Business.

Lorraine Radford is senior lecturer in social policy and women's studies at the Roehampton Institute in London. She is an experienced researcher of the law, social policy and violence against women and has published a number of articles in this area. She has been an active member of a woman's refuge support group for the past 15 years.

Elizabeth A. Stanko, reader in criminology, Brunel University, Uxbridge has explored gender and justice for the past 15 years. Her work explores violence against women, men's experiences of violence, and how the criminal justice system intersects with women's and men's experiences of violence. She has published widely in the areas of violence against women, gender, safety and policing.

1
Introduction

Jill Radford, Liz Kelly and Marianne Hester

Our starting point for *Women, violence and male power: feminist activism, research and practice* is to share the many exciting ideas, discussions and developments arising from the work of the BSA Violence Against Women Study Group between the mid-1980s and the early 1990s. We see the book as an important contribution not only to debates around violence and male power, but also as a means of encouraging further feminist research and activity in this area. The book reflects a shared commitment to research that centres on the material reality of women's lives and contributes to the generation of strategies for change.

The Study Group

The Violence Against Women Study Group was set up at the time of the British Sociological Association (BSA) annual conference 'War, Violence and Social Change' in 1985. This conference saw the first major discussions of violence against women at an academic conference in the UK. Many of the papers from that conference were later published in *Women, Violence and Social Control*, edited by Jalna Hanmer and Mary Maynard (1987). The present book can be seen as continuing the project of that earlier volume. It provides insights on new issues and questions that have become important to our understanding of abuse, and reflects the new directions in which research in this area has developed subsequently.

What the earlier book did not address in any great depth were the many and varied ways in which differences between women affected their experiences of violence, and the options available to them in coping with it. More recent feminist research, policy and practice has been more nuanced, exploring these areas of complexity and contradiction.

In supporting a study group around sexual violence the BSA provided an important forum for feminists working in and outside higher education, those who had already done research and others just beginning, to meet and network with each other. This has been significant in encouraging more feminist work, especially legitimizing feminist dissertations and funded research projects in universities and colleges in the area of women and violence. The membership of the group has spanned a wide range of experiences and locations. It has included community based women's groups and organizations, local authority policy makers and women from universities and colleges. This maintenance of links and connections between academics, activists and those with a remit to develop policy in the community (not mutually exclusive categories) both reflects the central second wave Women's Liberation Movement principle of the necessary connection between theory and practice and has created a process in the group which is less fragmented and more accountable than most other academic study groups.

An illustration of these links in action is the development of feminist approaches to familial homicide. One study group meeting brought together groups concerned with both the ways the provocation defence is used to defend/excuse violent men and campaigning for women who had killed their abusive partners (McNeill 1991; Justice for Women 1993; Southall Black Sisters 1994). This dialogue prompted exploration of current legal defences and led to the proposal for a new defence of 'self-preservation' (Radford and Kelly 1991; Radford and Kelly 1995).

Like most groups, the Violence Against Women Study Group has had a changing membership over the years. While there has been a core of regular members, other women have used the group in a variety of ways depending on the stage of their research and the usual limitations on women's time. For convenience the group has often met in London but its members come from across the UK. Since its inception the study group has had a predominantly white membership whilst committed to working in ways which are anti-racist, alongside questioning and challenging other forms of dominance and privilege. The study group has been more representative in terms of class, age, sexuality and health/disability. The contributions to the book reflect the perspectives of the membership as a whole. Whilst aware that it largely constitutes a First World standpoint and one based in Britain, this volume contributes to an increasingly global feminist response to male violence.[1]

The context

It is important to identify some of the recent theoretical and practical developments and the changed political and socioeconomic contexts within which this work has been undertaken. An understanding of the 'personal as political' has been central to feminist work on violence against women. Theorizing, research, campaigning and support work has taken women's experiences of sexual violence as its starting point. As a consequence this work challenges traditional views of what counts as knowledge, raising complex discussions of epistemology including the questions of 'how we know' and 'who decides what we know'. Within a feminist framework, researchers' own experiences of sexual violence are recognized as significant to the research process, both in terms of the effect we may have on the ways and extent to which women articulate and name their experiences of sexual violence, and our knowledge and understanding of our own experiences.

Over the past couple of decades campaigns around, and increasingly also research into, sexual violence have not only placed violence on the public agenda but have shown sexual violence to be a key element in male power over and control of women. The term 'sexual violence' recognizes that violence is a gendered phenomenon within the context of patriarchal social relations (Kelly 1988). It is also a recognition that violence from men to women is likely to be sexual, as in rape or sexual assault, or sexualized, that is a power 'turn on' for men (MacKinnon 1982; Hester 1992). The terminology reflects the development of knowledge and theorizing about male violence against women during the late 1970s and 1980s. In this chapter we also use the term 'women and violence' to include violence *by* women, situating all such violence analytically within a 'sexual violence approach'.

Since women began to speak out about domestic violence and rape in the late 1960s and 1970s (see Griffin 1971; Russell and Van de Ven 1976; Dobash and Dobash 1979) we have, with increasing confidence, spoken out and named the many ways women of different ages, races, sexualities, classes and dis/abilities experience sexual violence and abuse (see also rhodes and McNeill 1985). We have identified many forms of sexual violence, the commonalities and differences between women's experiences of such violence. Liz Kelly developed the concept of 'continuum' within the Violence Against Women Study Group to express these connections (1988). Women's experiences of sexual violence as brought to light through, for instance, consciousness-raising groups, the work of rape crisis centres, refuges and advice projects, have made it possible to document otherwise hidden events and social relations. This has enabled feminist researchers and activists to piece together an increasingly realistic and dynamic picture of the nature of sexual violence and abuse. It is now incontestable that sexual violence is extensive and that most, if not all, women in Britain (let alone elsewhere) have at some time experienced violence, harassment and abuse from men (Radford 1987; Kelly *et al.* 1991).

Feminist theorizing of sexual violence has also engaged with existing analyses of the family and the state, and in particular analyses of gender and sexuality. More complex analyses have been developed which take into account the myriad, often hidden, power relations and changing, gendered, meanings which sexual violence entails – whether in the context of the family or the legal and social institutions of the state or elsewhere (Kelly and Radford, Chapter 2, this volume). In-depth feminist critiques of existing policy and practice within state agencies have also emerged.

As the prevalence of various forms of sexual violence were acknowledged outside feminism, a response, and an increasingly popular one, has been to de-emphasize the gendered distribution of both victimization and abusing. This undermining of feminist knowledge takes a number of forms including: focusing on the less common sexual assault experienced by men and boys; emphasizing female perpetration of violence; collapsing of all forms of abuse and assault into the ungendered overarching category of 'violence'; or separating forms of violence against women from one another so their cumulative meaning is lost. Work undertaken by women in the study group is based on a feminist analysis which insists that sexual violence is not a question of '*people raping/battering/abusing people*'. The way violence is used and acted out in relationships, encounters and institutions is specifically gendered and constructed by, as well as a reflection of, the power relations which constitute hetero-patriarchy (Hester 1992). We maintain that it is possible to locate all forms of interpersonal violence within this framework, although currently undertheorized for example are interpersonal violence between men, men and boys and women's use of violence. The chapters by Gillespie (Chapter 10) and Kelly (Chapter 3) in this volume address these issues.

There is no doubt that feminist critiques, coupled with campaigns for change, have had some impact on the formulation of policy and practice. An obvious case in point are the changes in police policy and procedures regarding domestic violence, rape and sexual abuse of children. The setting up of 'rape examination suites' and responding to situations of violence from husbands/male partners as crimes are just some examples. In the mid-1980s television exposure of police practice provided graphic and public witness to the criticisms feminists had been making for some time, creating a necessity for change (Radford 1987).

However, these developments are also problematic, in that while appropriating feminist concerns, the state, whether as social services practitioners or the police, tend to redefine the issues within non-feminist discourses. It is also important to locate these changes in a broader context; it is not simply coincidence that improved police responses came in the wake of a need on the part of the police to re-establish legitimacy following uprisings in British inner cities during 1981 and 1985, and the miner's strike of 1984–5. Domestic violence units and rape examination suites, initially established in London and West Yorkshire, are now commonplace.[2] While these changes have improved initial police responses for many women, feminists have remained critical, since police practice remains variable, both within and between police divisions. Women in refuges, women who call rape crisis centres, and those participating in research still report that some police are hostile and do not take their complaints seriously. Moreover, changes in policing have yet to be reflected in other sections of the criminal justice system, particularly the courts and the Crown Prosecution Service. As yet, there are very few international examples of integrated and consistent reforms in justice systems.

Recording women's experiences of violence, naming and giving voice to them, is only a first step in challenging existing ideas, policies and practices. The link between theory and practice is a central one. This process can be conceptualized as a spiral in which each turn of the circle moves us across another dimension, beyond the point where we previously were, changing both how we understand and act on our experiences. Catharine MacKinnon (1987) has reminded us that what defines 'feminist method' is the practice of 'consciousness raising'. This is one of the names given by feminists to the sharing of women's individual and personal experiences, not in itself sufficient for the building of theory but as the basis from which to develop theoretical understanding and analysis *in order* to take action. The placing of women's experiences at the centre of feminist research practice can, however, become a form of exclusion, if the question 'which women' is not addressed.

This potential exclusion became more apparent in the 1980s. As women insisted that their different experiences of oppression were recognized within feminism, responses to these challenges were reflected in theory and practice. How sexual violence was understood and responded to was no exception to this wider process of attention to inclusion. The complexity of sexual violence, its many different forms, and its potentially variable meanings and impacts in terms of race, ethnicity, culture, class, sexuality, dis/ability and age, emerged (Mama 1989; Southall Black Sisters 1990).

The question of *which* women's experiences are included and which are excluded has been recognized as crucial; research on violence against women has begun to explore differences in women's experiences and how these connect to different ways of coping with men's violence. For example, a cursory glance at advice offered to women about personal safety reveals a reliance on strategies which depend upon privileged access to wealth and/or resources. Access to private transport can provide some limited protection to women who can afford it at the same time as lack of access adds to other women's sense of isolation and vulnerability. While domestic violence and sexual abuse makes the home one of the most dangerous places for women, homeless women are amongst the most vulnerable (Hendessi 1991). Globally, women escaping violence are similarly vulnerable in refugee and relocation camps. Sexual violence has been used as a weapon by men on all sides in war and social dislocation (McCollom *et al.* 1994).

Differences in women's positions in relation to the power structures of race, class and sexuality inform the responses to violence against women by the state, professionals and the voluntary sector. For example, class shapes the experiences of women making complaints of sexual violence. While women from all backgrounds are open to abuse, class influences the amount of respect a woman is accorded when dealing with professionals like solicitors, social workers and psychologists. Middle-class women are likely to receive more respect and be taken more seriously. At the same time being middle-class can also be a negative factor in dealings with police and other authorities in that it can produce scepticism stemming from prejudiced and stereotyped beliefs; that middle-class men (for liberals, 'new' men with 'reconstructed masculinities') do not do this sort of thing. Poorer, working-class and minority ethnic women often encounter other obstacles in seeking support and similarly encounter stereotyped responses which in this instance draw on notions of the commonness and even acceptance of abuse in certain social groups.

Acknowledging the complexity of ways in which race and racism structure women's experiences of violence have raised important and difficult issues for both black and white feminist activists and researchers. Some white feminists have learnt from black women the inseparability of racism and sexism when black women are attacked by white men, and that for black women making complaints to the police or pursuing a case through the courts requires them to engage with institutions that are both sexist and racist. The general racism in public representations of crime and criminality can inform white women's perceptions of safety and danger, encouraging an attribution of more danger to black men. The complex interrelationship of sexism and racism in contemporary society, informed by the legacies of colonialism and imperialism, also create huge problems for black women in researching and speaking out against violence from men in their own communities (Mama 1989; Wilson 1993; Southall Black Sisters 1994). Loyalty to communities in the face of racist ideas and practices creates deep concerns that reporting violence may result in racist and punitive reactions against an already overpoliced section of the community (Mama 1989; Southall Black Sisters 1990; Dobash and Dobash 1992).

As awareness of racism has seeped into white consciousness, some institutions and professional training programmes have adopted 'equal opportunities' and even 'anti-discriminatory' policies. The impacts of these policies on practice can be confusing and unpredictable. For example, versions of 'cultural awareness' and 'multiculturism' have become justifications for a non-interventionist stance (Southall Black Sisters 1994). One (probably unintended) outcome of this is that black and ethnic minority women and children who are victimized are afforded less protection than their white counterparts. At the same time, it is essential that the variation in cultural and familial constraints experienced by different groups of black and ethnic minority women are recognized and understood, for instance by women of Asian and Afro-Caribbean descent and Arab, Irish and Jewish women.

Lesbian feminists have been active participants in developing and conducting research on sexual violence. Research *on* lesbians and violence initially focused on anti-lesbian violence and harassment of lesbians in public places, identifying an increased vulnerability in a political climate shaped by legitimized homophobia; such as Section 2A of the Local Government Act of 1988 (Lespop 1989). Recently more complex issues have emerged. Women have begun to speak out about experiences of abuse within lesbian relationships, forcing an uncomfortable recognition in relation to women's use of violence (Taylor and Chandler 1995 and Kelly, Chapter 3, this volume).

Feminist research has also focused on age in terms of child abuse, both sexual and physical. This was a question women had previously placed on the public agenda in first wave feminism (Jeffreys 1985; Gordon 1988). More recently, and beginning from the testimony of adult survivors, feminists have been instrumental in putting child sexual abuse back on the public agenda.

In this context feminists have awakened the professional conscience as those working in social work and psychology have begun to address the problem, although, as suggested earlier, not necessarily within a feminist analysis. Professional approaches have tended to be wary of gendered analyses, preferring to locate the problem of sexual abuse in terms of family and individual pathology. The feminist challenge to family systems and family dysfunction explanatory models has been particularly influential in shifting how mothers are perceived – in the case of incest, from a 'collusive participant' to 'non-abusing parent' (MacLeod and Saraga 1988; Hooper 1991). The most recent variant of the ungendered professional approach is the popularized 'cycle of abuse'. Feminist analysis has pointed to the gendered distribution of offending and victimization which this model makes both invisible and inexplicable (Kelly 1991). 'Cycle of abuse' models also change the grounds on which support is provided to children who have been victimized from a matter of need and rights to a presumed model of future offending.

Whilst there has been some work, especially in the US, on the rape of elderly women (Koss and Harvey 1991), as yet feminist analysis of what has become known as 'elder abuse' is undeveloped (but see Mastrocola-Morris 1989). This is an area where work is needed, given that women constitute the majority of the elderly, and that they are predominantly cared for by other women, be they relatives or nursing/care workers. Exploratory discussions have prompted awareness that elderly women are most likely to be abused by a male living in the household. Some of these men are sons who have returned to live with parents after their female partners have excluded them because of domestic violence.

Exploring disabled women's experiences of sexual violence is also a recent phenomenon, and more developmental and research work has been conducted in other western countries than in Britain. Margaret Kennedy has been a key figure in Britain in developing awareness of the abuse of children with disabilities (Kennedy and Kelly 1992) and in arguing for support services for adults who have been abused. Some refuges and rape crisis lines have devoted time and resources to making their services more accessible, and feminists working in service provision, especially in relation to learning difficulties, have opened up the issue of women's experiences of violence (Jacobsen 1992). Michelle McCarthy's Chapter 8 in this volume is part of this emergent literature.

The many developments of what may be termed 'identity politics', which we have mentioned only briefly, have forced recognition of differences within women's experiences of sexual violence, highlighting limitations in earlier analyses. They also indicate the importance of identity politics to the project of feminism; in bell hooks's words:

> Identity politics emerges out of the struggles of . . . exploited groups to have a standpoint on which to critique dominant structures, a position that gives purpose . . . to struggle.
>
> (1991: 180)

The study group is committed to developing our understanding of the ways in which violence is implicated in multiple structures of power relations, and the effects this has on access to sources of support and protection. Understanding these complexities is essential for feminist theory and practice.

The 'backlash'[3] and the fightback for feminism

Dale Spender (1983) reflecting on the years following the 1914–18 war in Europe, has suggested that every wave of feminism is followed by a period of anti-feminist reaction, in which concerted attempts are made to marginalize, distort and discredit feminist perspectives. Susan Faludi (1992) and Marilyn French (1992) have detailed what they define as a current anti-feminist backlash in malestream US politics and culture. By the end of the 1980s and early 1990s, feminist activists in the UK were also noting this process as the Lesbian Custody Project's (1989) briefing paper *Backlash Against Lesbian Parenting* illustrates.

While it is not difficult to identify specific illustrations of anti-feminism, for example populist media notions of post-feminism, the ridiculing of political correctness, and the representation of campaigns against sexual violence as a form of victimization, it has been harder to locate it theoretically. For one thing, while attacks on feminism and feminists are central to these events, reaction is broader, directed at anti-racism, lesbian and gay rights politics, radical community work and progressive politics generally. What is particularly interesting is that this reaction, where work on violence against women is concerned, appears to have its origins in two very different quarters: one arising from a particular strand within feminism; the other from more traditionally reactionary forces in the form of a challenge by male academics to both the substance and content of feminist research (Kelly *et al.* 1994).

The challenge from within feminism has primarily taken the form of theoretical analysis, especially poststructuralist perspectives drawing on psychoanalysis and 'postmodernism'. The most public expression of this challenge can, ironically many would think, be found within much of women's studies, where throughout the 1980s a series of separations occurred: of women's studies from feminism; of theoretical writing from women's lived experience; of knowledge creation from activism. The dominant theoretical perspectives in women's studies are no longer developed within feminism, but draw on male gurus ('dead white men'): Freud, Lacan and Foucault. Psychoanalytic and postmodern feminism have become the order of the day, and those holding to 'modernist' notions like the existence of material reality are often summarily dismissed as 'essentialist'.[4]

This challenge appears in its most public and explicit form in the debates on pornography (Kelly 1985, 1990; Chester and Dickey 1988; Rogerson and Semple 1992), but has taken a more insidious and unhelpful form in general, and repeated phrases, which are read as critique. These include the suggestion that work on sexual violence is 'essentialist' and that it constructs and positions women as inevitable 'victims'. The potency of these assertions can be seen in the frequency with which they are repeated in both published work (especially introductory women's studies texts) and student essays. This charge is made with little serious attention being given to the actual substance of feminist research and support work.

It is both the power and frequency of such assertions which makes it necessary for us to unpack (or 'deconstruct') them here. At a straightforward level the criticism is directed at the entire project of documenting women's experiences of systematic victimization through sexual violence. At a more complex level the critique is a challenge to the theories of male power and social change generated by feminist work on sexual violence. In our view, these criticisms fail to engage with the actual, material realities of women's and children's lives, as outlined for instance in this and the previous BSA volume (Hanmer and Maynard 1987). What is noticeably absent is reference to and awareness of feminist practice in providing support to women and children who have been abused, which has been based on the concepts of survival/survivor. This absence is particularly worrying given that the feminist perspective on survival and survivors has been enormously influential in changing both research, policy and practice agendas globally.

A central tenet of poststructuralism is that material power does not reside primarily in structures of contemporary western society, such as the patriarchal relations of oppression and subordination, class relations of capitalism or the racism of post-colonial societies. Instead power is represented as diffuse, infusing all social and personal relationships. Being everywhere, but nowhere in particular, it dissolves in complex and confusing ways within the subjectivity of unique individuals. Consequently, within postmodern theory, it is now a matter of debate whether it is even possible to talk about 'women'. This effectively precludes any feminist project, as Tania Modleski's (1991) revealing book title *Feminism Without Women* illustrates (see also Hester 1992). In poststructuralism the emphasis shifts to an individualized idealist world of representations and texts (which are what women's accounts of their experiences of oppression are taken to be), to be 'deconstructed' through notions of subjectivity, identity and discourse.

Central to the claims of poststructuralists is the recognition that it is no longer possible to speak of women as a social category. Generally, however, postmodernist work on difference remains underdeveloped and rarely explored empirically or politically. Difference becomes a variety or mixture, as applicable to a box of chocolates as to groups of human beings.

Recognizing differences between women does not preclude the possibility of feminist analysis. This book asserts that central to feminism is the task of understanding how within patriarchal societies women's oppression is experienced by women who may be simultaneously privileged and/or oppressed by the power structures of race, class, sexuality, age and/or dis/ability while being oppressed by gender. Our concern is to understand the ways in which sexual violence as a major expression of male power in women's lives is a source of both commonality and difference between women (McKiernan and McWilliams 1994).

As feminists our concern goes beyond attempting to understand this particular expression of male power to finding ways of challenging it and securing progressive changes in the lives of *all* women. For such change to benefit all women we must begin by mapping out the differences between women, and what their consequences are in legislation, policy and practice. The dynamic of working with both commonality and difference is the only strong foundation on which networks, alliances and coalitions can be sustained. Without some commonality the connections are tenuous and/or situational; without acknowledgement of difference whole groups of women are marginalized or even forgotten.

Critical male reaction to feminist work on sexual violence has been muted until recently. In the early 1990s, however, direct challenges emerged to the extensive knowledge built over the last two decades. Central to this challenge is how violence and abuse are defined. The prevalence findings in research conducted by feminists on both rape and sexual abuse have been disputed by Gilbert (1991) and Howitt (1992). At issue are the ways feminist researchers have chosen to ask about experiences of victimization. For feminists the decision to ask more open-ended questions was informed by recognition of how frequently experiences are minimized, reflecting meanings in dominant discourses such as the law (Kelly and Radford, Chapter 2 and Stanko, Chapter 4, this volume). Yet it is precisely this opening up of definitions that these male academics are resisting. They seek to return us to previous certainties, where men – as scientists, judges and the/rapists – set the boundaries of what was and was not violating, what was and was not 'serious'. These concerns are not solely academic. Some men have been revealingly open about the unease such questioning of male behaviour creates. Journalists, including editorial writers, have not been slow to join the chorus of masculine defensiveness, most clearly articulated in the media-constructed furore over 'date rape' in 1993.

Government research funded by the Home Office has attempted to redefine the problem of men's violence as one of women's excessive and irrational fear of crime. In the British Crime Survey, for instance, Home Office criminologists asked women how safe they felt walking alone in their neighbourhoods after dark and compared the findings to the lower numbers of women who disclosed incidents of crime. They concluded that women's fear of crime was excessive, and therefore, irrational. This reinterpretation of the problem led to crime prevention policies aimed at reducing women's fear of crime, rather than attempting to reduce men's perpetration of it. Policy initiatives drew on victimization surveys which claimed to have learnt from feminist research, but actually paid little attention to it. The outcome has been a redefinition of the issues within a non-feminist discourse, producing 'woman-blaming' policies of individual responsibility for personal safety (Stanko 1993).

Alongside the 'crime control' professionals have emerged the 'damage control' experts. Here again the starting point was feminist research and practice, transformed and appropriated into what Louise Armstrong (1991), in the case of sexual abuse in childhood, has called the 'incest industry'. What was in the 1970s a feminist struggle for recognition of the prevalence and social meaning of sexual violence has in the 1990s become an arena of increasingly individualized frameworks and practices. Sexual violence has become the vehicle for the production of a multitude of syndromes and disorders, all of which require 'treatment'. They also serve to dis-locate such violence from its social, powered, context. As the list of diagnoses expands, and the variety of therapies to help us 'recover' or 'heal' mushroom, some feminists are asking 'how did we get here?' (Armstrong 1994). Rather than enabling women and children different ways to understand their experiences, allowing them to see themselves as one of many, and encouraging them to become part of a collective resistance to sexual oppression, what is increasingly on offer are personal (and even lifelong) 'journeys from victim to survivor' (Kelly *et al.* 1994).

Contents

The contributions in this book have come out of ideas, working papers or discussions in the study group in the late 1980s and early 1990s. While each chapter is written by and reflects the approach of its individual author(s), all have benefited from discussion and feedback from members of the group.[5] The group provided a supportive forum for early discussions and the sharing of ideas in a feminist context.

The book comprises three parts. The first focuses on theoretical and methodological issues; the second addresses the law, protection and criminal justice; and the third centres on researching experience and supporting women, reflecting current debates about provision of feminist support services in a period of popularist anti-feminism and economic recession. Throughout the book, the need to maintain and re-establish connections across boundaries is emphasized.

Part I, Making Sense: Theory and Conceptualization, opens with '"Nothing Really Happened": The Invalidation of Women's Experiences of Sexual Violence', in which Liz Kelly and Jill Radford explore the implicit meanings of a remark women frequently make about experiences of physical and sexual abuse. They discuss how this minimizing and discounting of events that did indeed happen is both reflected in, and constructed by, the criminal justice system. The implications of inclusion and exclusion in definitions of sexual violence are explored, especially in relation to campaigns for legal reform.

In the next chapter Liz Kelly addresses what has become an area of intense debate: women's use of violence. In 'When Does the Speaking Profit Us?: Developing a Feminist Analysis of Violent and Abusive Women' she explores the data on women's abusive behaviour and outlines both useful and unhelpful ways in which this can be accommodated in feminist theory and practice.

Elizabeth Stanko draws on her own experience of systematic sexual harassment, emphasizing that feminist researchers are neither inoculated against abuse, nor immune to the impacts it has at the time and over time. The fact of being an 'academic' working in the field does not preclude the struggle to 'make sense', to be able to speak. Her account also illustrates the catch-22 for women; we are left with irresolvable questions and conflicts whether we choose to resist or not, whether we make official reports or not.

Part II, Law, Protection and Criminal Justice, extends feminist analysis of legal and legislative processes and their consequences. It opens with Jill Radford and Elizabeth Stanko's discussion of 'Violence Against Women and Children: The Contradictions of Crime Control under Patriarchy'. This chapter analyses some of the tensions arising from feminist commitment to eradicating male violence and securing women's safety in the long term and the short term necessity of easing women's everyday lives by developing practical prevention and support strategies. At a theoretical level, the chapter examines the conceptual problems, compromises and contradictions arising from competing definitions and understandings of sexual violence.

Marianne Hester and Lorraine Radford take issue with the representation of the Children Act as a landmark in British legal history. The title, 'Contradictions and Compromises: The Impact of the Children Act on Women and Children's Safety', highlights the inconsistent, and even paradoxical, consequences of the legislation in letter and practice. They illustrate how elements of the Children Act work against previous legislation designed to provide women with protection from domestic violence; compromising both women's and children's safety and well-being. They discuss the problems arising for a feminist professional practice where private and public law intersect.

In the last chapter in this section, Sue Lees revisits earlier feminist debates about the treatment by the criminal justice system of women who have been raped. The chapter is based on court observations. She finds that rape trials are as difficult, if not more so, than in the earlier period of feminist campaigning in this area.

Part III, Researching Experience and Supporting Women, combines chapters about ongoing feminist action research and examinations of the dilemmas currently facing the provision of feminist support services established by and for women. The section opens with Michelle McCarthy's documentation of the sexual violence experienced by women with learning difficulties. She provides an account of the methodological challenges that she faced as both a researcher and practitioner and the barriers women with learning difficulties face in having their abuse recognized and responded to.

Maggie O'Neill's chapter focuses on women working as prostitutes, and it shares a number of concerns with the previous one: methodological and ethical dilemmas; a marginalized and stigmatized group of women who are particularly targeted for abuse; and an action/change orientated framework. 'Researching Prostitution and Violence: Towards a Feminist Praxis' includes detailed accounts of the violence women experienced, a discussion of routes into prostitution which goes beyond previous models, and an account of the local interagency work which takes female empowerment as its starting point.

In the next chapter Terry Gillespie examines what she defines as two faces of backlash currently facing rape crisis centres. She defines rape crisis centres as feminist voluntary groups offering a confidential needs-based support service 'for women, by women'. Drawing on her ongoing research into rape crisis centres and their relationship to other agencies offering support to 'victims' of sexual assault, she explores current pressures to compromise and/ or fundamentally change principles and practice. The two issues addressed here are providing services to men who have been raped or sexually abused and pressure to disclose confidential information to the police and lawyers.

Marian Foley also focuses on rape crisis centres, but here she draws on her research comparing feminist-run services with a police-funded sexual assault centre based in a hospital, heralded as a model of 'good practice'. She draws out the implications of the medicalization of rape, whilst also noting that the initial fears which feminists had concerning sexual assault, have not, as yet, materialized. The pressures on rape crisis centres to 'professionalize' are located within a discussion of both competition for funding, and dilemmas concerning structures and what constitutes feminist support work.

Jo Moran-Ellis's chapter 'Close to Home: The Experience of Researching Child Sexual Abuse' concludes the book and examines the impact of researching sexual violence on feminist researchers. It has been an important principle of feminist research to locate ourselves within the topics we study. In honestly documenting her rage, grief and personal dilemmas, she highlights that being a feminist and doing feminist research can be painful and disturbing whilst at the same time illuminating and powerful.

Taken as a whole the book demonstrates an increasing sophistication in feminist theory and practice, and exciting developments in feminist methodology, which draw on radical traditions within action and participatory research.

Notes

1 For instance, men's use of rape against women in war situations has again been made public through the war in the former Yugoslavia and recent conflicts in Somalia, Rwanda and Haiti (see McCollum, Radford and Kelly 1994).

2 Distribution of rape examination suites is patchy, and notably absent in the six counties called Northern Ireland (McKiernan and McWilliams 1993).

3 We have put the term 'backlash' in inverted commas because in our view the concept oversimplifies and in some sense misrepresents the processes at work. Feminist historians have documented periods of time, which vary across cultures and contexts, where the struggles and gains of earlier women's movements have been resisted; periods in which men have had to reconstruct their power over women in order not to lose it (Hester 1992). The term, as it has been used, tends to be understood as a one-off event, and fails to make connections with previous struggles.

4 It ought to be a matter of some concern to committed postmodern feminists that their rejection of basic feminist precepts has been welcomed, even embraced, by many longtime anti-feminists, both individuals and institutions. They revel in the new language of dismissal and mystification, which has arisen from post-modernism and has added new life to their misogyny.
5 Two of the chapters have been previously published, one in a journal and one in a criminology book. The rest have been written specifically for this volume.

References

Armstrong, L. (1991) Surviving the incest industry, *Trouble and Strife* 21: 29–32.

Armstrong, L. (1994) *Rocking the Cradle of Sexual Politics: What Happened when Women said Incest.* New York: Addison-Wesley Publishing Company.

Chester, G. and Dickey, J. (eds) (1988) *Feminism and Censorship: The Current Debate.* London: Prism Press.

Dobash, R. and Dobash, R. (1979) *Violence Against Wives: A Case Against the Patriarchy.* New York: Free Press.

Dobash, R. and Dobash, R. (1992) *Women, Violence and Social Change.* London: Routledge.

Faludi, S. (1992) *Backlash: The Undeclared War Against Women.* London: Chatto and Windus.

Feminist Review (1980) Issue 36.

French, M. (1992) *The War Against Women.* London: Hamish Hamilton.

Gilbert, N. (1991) The phantom epidemic of sexual assault, *Public Opinion*, 103: 54–65.

Gordon, L. (1988) *Heroes in Their Own Lives: The Politics and History of Family Violence, Boston 1880–1960.* London: Virago.

Griffin, S. (1971) Rape: the all-American crime, *Ramparts*, 10(3): 26–35.

Hanmer, J. and Maynard, M. (eds) (1987) *Women, Violence and Social Control.* London: Macmillan.

Hendessi, M. (1991) *4 in 10: The Links Between Sexual Abuse and Young Women's Homelessness.* London: CHAR.

Hester, M. (1992) *Lewd Women and Wicked Witches: A Study of the Dynamics of Male Dominance.* London: Routledge.

hooks, b. (1991) *Yearning: Race, Gender, and Cultural Politics.* London: Turnaround.

Hooper, C. A. (1991) *Mothers Surviving Child Sexual Abuse.* London: Routledge.

Howitt, D. (1992) *Child Abuse Errors: When Good Intentions Go Wrong.* London: Harvester.

Jacobsen, Y. (1992) Women first: a national speakout for women with learning difficulties, *Trouble and Strife*, 24: 35–40.

Jeffreys, S. (1985) *The Spinster and her Enemies: Feminism and Sexuality 1880–1930.* London: Pandora.

Justice for Women Collective (1993) *Justice for Women: Information Pack.* London: Justice for Women.

Kelly, L. (1985) 'Feminist v. feminist', *Trouble and Strife*, 7: 4–10.

Kelly, L. (1988) *Surviving Sexual Violence.* Cambridge: Polity Press.

Kelly, L. (1990) Abuse in the making, *Trouble and Strife*, 19: 32–7.

Kelly, L. (1991) Outrageous injustice, *Community Care Supplement*, 25 June, ii–iii.

Kelly, L., Burton, S. and Regan, L. (1994) 'Beyond victim or survivor: Sexual violence, feminist theory and identity,' paper at British Sociological Association Conference, Preston, May.

Kelly, L., Regan, L. and Burton, S. (1991) *An exploratory study of the prevalence of sexual abuse in a sample of 1244 16–21 year olds*, Final Report to the ESRC. London: Child Abuse Studies Unit, University of North London.

Kennedy, M. and Kelly, L. (guest eds) (1992) *Child Abuse Review*, 1(2) (entire issue).

Koss, M. and Harvey, M. (1991) *The Rape Victim: Clinical and Community Responses*. Beverley Hills, CA: Sage.

Lesbian Custody Project (1989) *Backlash Against Lesbian Parenting*, briefing paper. London: Lesbian Custody Project.

Lespop (1989) *Annual Report*. London.

McCollom, H., Radford, J. and Kelly, L. (1994) Wars against women, *Trouble and Strife*, 28: 12–19.

McKiernan, J. and McWilliams, M. (1994) Domestic violence in a violent society: the implications for abused women and children, *Rights of Women Bulletin*, spring: 13–19.

MacKinnon, C. (1982) Feminism, marxism, method and the state: an agenda for theory, *Signs*, 7: 515.

MacKinnon, C. (1987) *Feminism Unmodified: Discourses on Life and Law*, Cambridge, MA: Harvard University Press.

MacLeod, M. and Saraga, E. (eds) (1988) Family secrets: child sexual abuse, *Feminist Review*, 28 (entire issue).

McNeill, S. (1991) Change the law (1), *Trouble and Strife*, 22: 7–11.

Mama, A. (1989) *The Hidden Struggle: Statutory and Voluntary Sector Responses to Violence Against Black Women in the Home*. London: London Race and Housing Research Unit.

Mastrocola-Morris, E. (1989) *Woman Abuse: The Relationship Between Wife Assault and Elder Abuse*, Toronto: Canadian National Clearinghouse on Family Violence.

Modleski, T. (1991) *Feminism Without Women: Culture and Criticism in a 'Postfeminist' Age*. New York: Routledge.

Radford, J. (1987) Policing male violence, policing women. In J. Hanmer and M. Maynard (eds) *Women, Violence and Social Control*. London: Macmillan.

Radford, J. (1993) The lesbian custody project, backlash against lesbian parenting: First it was Clause 28 and then . . . In P. Noerager Sterne (ed.) *Lesbian Health: What Are the Issues?* Washington DC: Taylor and Francis.

Radford, J. and Kelly, L. (1991) Change the law (2), *Trouble and Strife*, 22: 12–14.

Radford, J. and Kelly, L. (1995) Self-preservation: feminist activism and feminist jurisprudence. In M. Maynard and J. Purvis (eds) *Self Preservation: Feminist Activism and Feminist Jurisprudence*. London: Taylor and Francis.

Radford, J. and Russell, D. (eds) (1992) *Femicide: The Politics of Woman Killing*. Milton Keynes: Open University Press.

rhodes, d. and McNeill, S. (eds) (1985) *Women Against Violence Against Women*. London: OnlyWomen Press.

Rogerson, G. and Semple, L. (1992) Who watches the watchwomen?: Feminists against censorship, in F. Bonner *et al.* (eds) *Imagining Women: Cultural Representations and Gender*. Cambridge: Polity Press.

Russell, D. and Van de Ven, N. (eds) (1976) *The Proceedings of the International Tribunal of Crimes Against Women*. Millbrae, CA: Les Femmes.

Southall Black Sisters (1990) *Against the Grain: A Celebration of Survival and Struggle 1979–1989*, London: Southall Black Sisters.

Southall Black Sisters (1994) *Domestic Violence and Asian Women: A Collection of Reports and Briefings*. London: Southall Black Sisters.

Spender, D. (1983) *Women of Ideas (And What Men Have Done to Them)*. London: Ark.

Stanko (1993) Ordinary fear: women, violence and personal safety, in P. Bart and E. Moran *Women and Violence*. London: Sage.

Taylor, J. and Chandler, T. (1995) *Lesbians Talk: Violent Relationships*. London: Scarlet Press.

Wilson, M. (1993) *Crossing the Boundary: Black Women and Sexual Abuse*. London: Virago.

Part I
Making sense: theory and conceptualization

2

'Nothing really happened': the invalidation of women's experiences of sexual violence[1]

Liz Kelly and Jill Radford

Introduction

In this chapter we explore the social processes through which women's experiences of sexual violence are invalidated, and the impact this has on our own understandings of our experiences of men's violence and the implications for social policy. Understanding these processes not only makes sense of these experiences, and how we, as women, cope with and respond to them, but also sheds light on the low rate of reporting such events to the police, and the police and courts' responses to violence against women, which has been addressed elsewhere (Radford 1986; Kelly 1988a; Hanmer et al. 1989). It is also essential for an understanding of current concern with 'fear of crime' and of significance for research methodology. Further, we are concerned with the ways in which man-made law has been explicitly constructed to exclude from 'crimes against the person' all but 'extreme' forms of sexual violence. Through comparing and connecting the formal construction of the law and women's understandings of the violence they experience from men we argue that the law not only reflects but also constructs a very limited definition of sexual violence, and thereby plays a significant role in denying or trivializing women's experience of male sexual violence. Recent criminological research is also implicated in this process of exclusion.

A central theme in our argument is that as women we tend, and indeed are systematically encouraged, to minimize the violence that we experience from men. That women (and children) have been unable to speak about their experiences of sexual abuse, coercion, exploitation and assault has been an important theme in recent feminist writing. What has been referred to as 'silencing' is, however, a complex process. In order to be able to speak about something, one must first be able to name and define it. It is these two separate, but interlinked processes which underlie our argument.

One of the most significant aspects of feminist theory and practice has been to find/create/redefine words which reflect and record women's experiences. Concepts which are now commonplace simply did not exist before the present wave of feminist activism, for example, domestic violence, sexual harassment, child sexual abuse. Whilst these behaviours undoubtedly existed – they were revealingly referred to by first wave feminists as 'unspeakable outrages' (Radford 1989) – what women lacked were social definitions. Names provide social definitions, make visible what is invisible, define as unacceptable what was accepted; make sayable what was unspeakable (Kelly 1988a). Naming also involves an implicit analysis which challenged the view that men's behaviour was 'natural'; what has come to be known as 'social construction theory' had some of its origins in first wave questioning of essentialist notions of masculinity and femininity. The fundamental issue for feminists then, as now, was to locate men's abusive behaviour within a framework of women's oppression by, and resistance to, male power.

A second strand of feminist reconstruction of language has been to transform the meaning of words that did exist, here rape and pornography are the most obvious examples. Pornography is no longer discussed only in terms of 'obscenity' and 'public decency', and the stereotype of rape as a brutal attack by a stranger has long been a subject of feminist critique. A slightly different illustration is the way feminists have substituted the word 'survivor' for 'victim', in order to both challenge victim-blame and make visible women and children's resistance and coping strategies.

In the currently popular language of 'radical' sociologists and criminologists, feminists have been engaged in the dual project of deconstructing patriarchal 'discourses' and a feminist reconstruction.

There are numerous ways in which women's experiential knowledge is denied, invalidated and forced underground, ways which change and adapt to cultural and political circumstances. Men, who as the perpetrators of sexual violence have a vested interest in women's silence, have, in a range of ways and in a range of contexts, constructed 'knowledge' about sexual violence, crime and women's sexuality: through institutions such as the law, medicine, psychiatry as much as the 'common sense' that is promoted by the media, including pornography. In each of these sites the mythology of rape is recreated, albeit in slightly different form and using different language. What malestream knowledge has attempted to do is limit what counts as abuse – it operates by the strategy of inclusion and exclusion, including what men define as violating/abusive and excluding much of what women experience as violating/abusive.

As Catharine MacKinnon has often pointed out (MacKinnon 1988) one of the major problems in proving rape in court is that much so called consensual heterosex is coercive, if not forced. 'Real' rape (see Estrich 1987) according to the law, enforced by the police and reinforced by the mass media, is an attack at night, in a public place, by a stranger who uses force (preferably a weapon). If there is any suggestion of a prior relationship of any kind between the woman and her rapist, then consent becomes an issue. Even the British Home Office has had to admit recently what feminists and women more generally have known for years: that the majority of rapes are committed by men women know (Smith 1989).

Yet the law requires a clear distinction between rape and not-rape; a 'no win' situation for women reporting and feminists trying to envisage legal reform. One of the reasons why feminists have campaigned to have rape in marriage criminalized is that it highlights this legal paradox, whilst at the same time recognizing that few cases would ever be prosecuted since the rape/not-rape line would only be marginally revised. However, rather than broaden the definition of rape, the preferred strategy of our most senior judges has been to move in the opposite direction. In 1986 (four years after the Rape in Marriage Campaign) Lord Lane introduced new guidelines for sentencing convicted rapists (it is significant to note that most judicial reviews focus on sentencing, the concluding stage of a legal process which at every stage filters out incidents which don't accord with narrow malestream definitions of rape and which women find distressing throughout). The basic premise of Lord Lane's guidelines was a notion of two degrees of rape which turn on a definition of seriousness which reflects the 'real' rape model: use of 'excessive' violence; use of a weapon; repeated rape; rape of elderly women or young children. In the process, the majority of rapes are once again defined as 'less serious' and therefore even less likely to come to court (Radford 1986). Here, rape, as is often the case, provides a paradigm case for feminist analysis.

We now move on to examine how malestream strategies of inclusion and exclusion function to deny women's reality and influence the perceptions of women themselves.

The law plays the central role in constructing 'what counts' as crime, and in the case of sexual violence (unlike, for example, public order offences) it focuses almost entirely on extremes, thereby discounting many women's experiences. Thus only a proportion of women's complaints are seen as legitimate, according to the law – legitimacy here defined in terms of the actions, behaviour and relationships of the male assailant and the female he victimizes. Thus the law suggests that clear distinctions can be made between violence and not violence, and thereby between abusive and 'normal' men. It is this assumed clarity which constrains and constructs the framework through which women have to make sense of events. As we will illustrate, many women find themselves caught between dominant malestream definitions and their own experiential knowledge. Women's struggle to negotiate these tensions and conflicts has a range of possible outcomes. Some involve adoption of aspects of the dominant meaning (not naming behaviour as abusive, forgetting it or minimizing it), whilst others constitute an explicit challenge to them. Most include a complicated mix of both.

When women say 'nothing really happened' – a frequent remark which prefaces accounts of things which did indeed happen – they are minimizing or denying experiences. Very real things happen when we are followed or chased on the street, when male partners insist on sex or engage in systematic emotional abuse – we do not feel safe, our trust is betrayed.

In the sections which follow we want to illustrate the ways in which competing interpretations and meanings inform the ways in which women talk about and respond to so called 'minor' offences. The data we will use is drawn from two research projects: a community survey of 314 women in Wandsworth, contacted by random street selection (Radford 1987); a sample of 60 women who chose to take part in a study on sexual violence and who were interviewed twice (Kelly 1988a). Women's own words demonstrate both the complexity of their responses and the ways in which malestream 'discourses' influenced their accounts and perceptions.

While we are aware that male sexual violence may occur in any social space women and men share, and that the most frequent abuse occurs in a woman's own home from a man she knows, we have organized our discussion to begin in the public arena of the streets, moving from there to consider sexual harassment in the work place and then into the private sphere of women's homes. In this way we are again emphasizing the connections which exist between the various forms of sexual violence occurring in the public world, the public–private world of work and the private space of a woman's home.

Public space

Whilst the 'real' rape model focuses on public space, it at the same time discounts events there which do not involve actual or attempted sexual assault. The events women describe below include kerb-crawling, being followed and other intimidatory encounters with men. Each woman either explicitly or implicitly connects the event to the possibility of rape; indeed it is often precisely the fact that they were not raped which permits them to say 'nothing really happened'. This linkage is precisely what is denied in legal and criminological thinking, as evidenced in the recent suggestions that women's 'fear of crime' is exaggerated and unfounded (see Hanmer and Saunders 1984; Stanko 1990 for a critique). This point is made and taken further in Sandra McNeill's (1987) study of flashing in Leeds. Having been exposed to the threat posed by Peter Sutcliff, the 'Yorkshire Ripper', the fear women felt on being flashed at was linked not only to the possibility of rape but also death. 'Time and time again women mentioned "what he was going to do next" as the reason for their fear. And at the back or the front of their minds was death' (McNeill 1987 7: 102).

The following quotations are drawn from Jill Radford's community study of violence against women in Wandsworth. They illustrate the contradictions facing women in negotiating experiences of sexual violence. Whilst recounting these experiences to interviewers asking about their experience of this violence, they at the same time and repeatedly say 'nothing really happened'.

> I was kerb-crawled too, earlier this week. I hate this sort of thing. It happened again later in the day, when I was walking home. I was in tears by the time I got home, nothing happened, just comments, but I was intimidated.

> I've been frequently harassed by kerb-crawlers. It happened even when I was pregnant. There were several incidents about a fortnight ago, though nothing actually happened. The assumptions men make – their arrogance. It makes me sick and angry. I don't go out much alone now. I resent that enormously.

Nothing actually happened – that is if you discount intimidation, feeling sick and angry, being in tears, being unable to safely inhabit public space.

These kinds of intimate intrusions can take a number of forms, and the example which follows is one of the most frequent women experience – other variants are 'give us a smile' and 'cheer up luv, it might never happen' – statements which in themselves have made 'it' happen.

> A stranger, a man passing in the street pulled a contorted face and hissed something at me. Nothing happened, but I was unsettled for a while. It was pure menace, out of the blue. You wander along thinking your own thoughts and suddenly this invades your space, your life with menace. I have the right to daydream in the street sometimes. One can't live in a constant state of alertness, awaiting the violence of men.

The next woman, like the one before her, understands the intention behind these intrusions into women's personal space.

> Yes, I often get angered by men's comments and at nights. Nothing happens, but it's a form of terror. You can tell they know it's terror by the way they laugh and that. Cowards, they only do it in groups.

Nothing happens because:

> All these things are everyday harassment, the background against which our lives are lived. Not much ever happens but it's threatening and calculated to intimidate women – to terrorize us.

Nothing much ever happens – apart from a form of terrorism, in response to which women have to manage the daily threat, the calculated everyday harassment. Women's capacity to cope with and manage this everyday reality is affected by our physical and mental abilities.

> I came out of a shop and a man was looking at me. I crossed the road to the butchers and waited in a queue. As I left the shop, the man was there and opened the door for me. I'm disabled and he offered to help me with the shopping. He asked if I lived far. I refused to let him carry my shopping. In spite of my refusals, he pushed my chair all the way home and followed me into my flat and insisted on coming in. I didn't want him to, but didn't quite know how to say 'no', after all he had walked me home and I didn't want to seem ungrateful. I made him a cup of tea and he chatted. He asked to sit near me. I refused and decided I had to get rid of him. Nothing had happened, but I was uncomfortable. I said the doctor was coming and got rid of him without more difficulty. He's come up the street since, and once tried to kiss me. He still comes to my flat and asks me to take my clothes off. I think it's dreadful. Because they force their 'help' on you, they expect sex or something, it makes me sick.

Nothing happened – apart from a potential sexual assault, orchestrated through taking advantage of this woman's particular vulnerability. For black women sexual and racial abuse from white men often combine in forms of compounding humiliation and threat.

> Last week I was shopping with the kids in the Arndale Centre, when four white boys started making racist comments and made as if to grab the pram. They may have been just messing about, but I was scared. It happened last Wednesday, about 11.30 in the morning. I was scared, though nothing actually happened. Afterwards I was angry, but what can you do?

> I was in the tube the other day and a man was making racist and insulting sexual remarks. He was white and said I was a snobbish black tart and he knew what was good for me, all that sort of talk you know, but he didn't do anything. It makes me really sick.

They didn't do anything – apart from assert white male supremacy over black women and children.

On one level all of these women were clear that something had happened – they told their stories for that reason, including what the impacts of these encounters were. They are saying 'nothing' happened because they know that their perceptions of 'something' are unlikely to be validated, except by researchers concerned about sexual violence, and possibly other women.

> I was followed down the street. I heard footsteps and looked to see who it was. He was definitely following me because whenever I walked faster, or slowed down, he did. He spoke to me, asked me why I had changed my bag from one hand to the other. I was afraid of him, I was angry, I will fight back if any man attacks me, I won't give in easily.

I didn't tell the police, they would have gone over and over it, asking me all sorts of questions about what I was doing making out it was all my fault, and then in the end tell me nothing happened and I'm silly to make a fuss over nothing.

It is the effect of these perceptions women have of the responses of others which lead to assaults being defined as 'nothing': not worthy of concern.

I was molested by a man who grabbed hold of me and pushed himself against me in the tube when it was crowded. I screamed as loudly as I could. He slapped my face, but then got off as we got to a station. I suppose I was lucky that nothing actually happened.

Two evenings ago, I was terrified. I was coming in from the car park and this man sprang up out of the bushes and ran very fast towards me. Nothing happened, but I was terrified, shaking, my legs turned to jelly and I thought what might have happened. Men don't realize how terrifying they are, though perhaps they do.

Public-private space

The next series of experiences are also drawn from the Wandsworth study and focus on women's experience of sexual harassment at work. As a result of feminist work within and outside of the trade unions, sexual harassment at work is now recognized as a form of abuse experienced by women which can occur in any context of paid work in which women work with or for men. The men might be women's employers, managers, supervisors, work colleagues, clients or customers. The Wandsworth study showed that while there are some work situations in which dealing with this form of abuse is almost a routine part of the job (see also Kelly 1988a), sexual harassment is widespread in work contexts in which women have dealings with men for example, bar work, canteen work, childcare, cleaning, civil service, community work, hospital work, library work, shop work, social work, teaching and transport work.

The incidents reported again demonstrate how women both understand that something has happened to cause them anxiety, fear and undermine their confidence in their work, yet by saying 'nothing happened' they recognize that in malestream ideology nothing untoward would be deemed to have occurred. This minimizing or even negating of their experience may well also serve as a coping strategy which, for the time being at least, allows them to remain at work. Other women in the survey reported that experiences of sexual harassment caused them to give up their jobs.

I work as a live in nanny and I'm 17 years old. It's just that I feel nervous at the way he looks at me when his wife is out. It happens regularly, she goes out at least once a week. He's not done anything yet, but the way he looks at me makes me nervous.

I'm a nurse and work mostly with women, but sometimes with men, and I'm quite often harassed by them – it's happened three times in the last couple of weeks. They get bored I suppose, you get the 'come here darling' or they make passes at you when you make their beds. It's regular and I suppose you have to put up with it as best you can. I do get seriously worried when I'm on the ward alone on the night shift – that's happening more and more with the cuts. I don't know how much longer I'll be able to stand it, even assuming nothing worse happens.

Yes I've experienced harassment at work in a lot of subtle, that is not physically violent, ways. Nothing violent has ever happened – touch wood, but verbal harassment is regular and a constant reminder.

The men in the office are forever having a go – sort of half joke/half propositioning me. They know I don't like it, but they never give up. It's nothing really. I can handle it, or I have so far, but it pisses me off. I'm exhausted by the end of the day.

These accounts all show that 'nothing' happens on a very regular basis. Precisely because these experiences can in fact be defined, in malestream thinking as 'nothing', women find them so difficult to deal with. Malestream thinking is full of clichés about women making a 'fuss about nothing', so it's not surprising that sometimes as women we silence our experiential knowledge. (Each of the accounts suggests that it is the regularity of the harassment which adds to the threat it poses, a threat which each of the women clearly links to a potential for more 'serious' violence.) As the following account shows, the threat can be very explicit, but because in this instance she was able to contain it, still – 'nothing happened'.

Before the baby was born, I had a job. This man, a colleague, wanted to take me out. I was pregnant. I refused. He threatened to hit me if I didn't. I was frightened but talked to him to calm him down, so in the end nothing happened.'

Like stranger violence in a public place, sexual harassment at work is compounded by racism in the experience of black women. Here again the power of white malestream ideology is such that these incidents, involving the assertion of white male supremacy, can be described as nothing.

I've been attacked in the library – young white boys fooling around in a threatening and racist way. Nothing's actually happened to me, but I've had to call the police to have them removed. It's always distressing. It's a good job I've got and I can't afford to lose it, but the violence of men, together with their racism, is a real problem for me.

I clean at a university, the classic role for black women. We're all women and a lot of us are black. My boss, a man, has no respect for us at all. We have to play our role as women. Because I object and refuse to take their comments – it's abuse really, though nothing's happened yet – I'm often in trouble, but I don't like the way they carry on and I'll say so.

The last account in this section points to the additional issues sexual harassment at work holds for lesbians, resulting in fear, isolation, and humiliation while those responsible for the abuse can still be said to have 'not actually done anything'. Again the response of others, ranging from collusion to refusal to see, compound the difficulties of naming, understanding and dealing with the experience.

I'm a part-time teacher and teach 17 year olds. There's about 10 of them in one particular group who harass me as a lesbian. I've felt very frightened, very humiliated, though they've not actually done anything, well they have, they've done plenty, but you know what I mean. I refused to work with them. I've also been harassed by male colleagues on the staff and had no support from other women, that's upset me. It's very difficult when my head of department harasses me, verbally and touches my shoulders, nothing I can complain about. I need the work, so it's hard to protest effectively and I've had no support from the other women on the staff.

Intimate relationships

We now want to illustrate how similar processes occur within intimate relationships: that ideologies, stereotypes and limited definitions combine with women's own coping strategies to prevent them naming and defining men's behaviour as violent and abusive. The experiences we refer to here come from interviews done for *Surviving Sexual Violence* (Kelly 1988a). There, and elsewhere (see Kelly 1988b), how definitions of forms of sexual violence operate through inclusion and exclusion is discussed.

Whilst the phrase 'nothing really happened' does not appear as frequently or as explicitly in women's accounts of 'private' sexual violence, forms of denial and minimizing which parallel those we have already described can be discerned. The occurrence of sexual violence within ongoing heterosexual relationships makes naming even more complex, since many women have an investment, at least in the short term, in not defining men's behaviour as abusive. They may also be influenced by romanticized public representations of intimate relationships which encourage them to view abuse as an, albeit distorted, form of caring.

Specific groups of women have further practical and material reasons for minimizing the abuse they are experiencing. For women with disabilities leaving a violent partner involves the loss of her 'carer' and for some the prospect of a future in institutional care. For black women the reality of racism can create a tension between their experience of abuse, and a felt need to protect the community from intervention by white institutions, especially the police. Migrant women, the majority of whom are black, fear having their immigration status, their 'right to stay' investigated – and women may have 'no recourse to public funds' stamped on their passports. Lesbians may fear risk losing custody of their children if they leave abusive men. Moreover, these forms of oppression are not mutually exclusive. Each can function as a powerful reinforcer of the cultural injunction not to name men's violence and abuse.

Just as the stereotype of 'real rape' highlights the issues we are raising here, so too does the way in which 'domestic violence' is represented and understood. Despite feminist campaigns and services, to most women the word 'battered' implies frequent, systematic physical violence – if this is not their experience then they are not 'battered women'. The wider definitions used by women's aid groups – including physical, sexual and mental abuse – have not yet reached most women. Consequently many women dismiss their own experiences as not being 'real' or 'serious' violence, despite how real and serious the events, and the impacts of them, might be.

> I remember my first responses were dismissing it and disbelief. I nearly did it again today, because I'm still at the point where I think 'well it's not really violence'. Then I think 'come on be straight with yourself'. It did start out in minor ways with pushing and it wasn't till near the end of the marriage that he got into things that you think of as being attacked. That went a long way before I thought *this* is violence – a hell of a long way.

> I kept quiet about it partly because of this business of not accepting it as violence – and there was a *very* strong sense that because you were married you didn't say anything. I was depressed for a long time, I accepted that label, that it was my personality and nothing to do with the marriage, the violence.

> I didn't think of it as – it wasn't until really late on that I thought there was violence . . . I can't remember any major acts of violence until about four years ago, any real sort of *injuries* but the threat was there.

For each of these women until there were visible 'injuries', they did not define the acts as an attack or their partner's behaviour as violent. The complexity of recognizing and naming men's actions as abuse is one important, but neglected, reason why many women do not seek outside support and stay with abusive men. It is not that women accept or expect abuse, but that it takes them 'a long time' to name what is happening to them as violence.

Women also minimize violent incidents where there were injuries; it was 'serious', but not frequent. A range of reasons may be given for this: not wanting to acknowledge what was happening; not seeing any alternatives and so focusing on getting through each day/week; that they (as white middle-class professional women and/or as strong capable women) and/or their partner (as white middle-class and/or respected member of the community) did not fit the stereotypes of abused women and abusive men. This was illustrated most clearly by a woman who was working to set up a refuge in her home town. At the time she was being abused by her husband, but she saw no connection between her 'few' experiences and those of the women she was seeking to support.

The focus on 'serious' violence is reflected in legal and police practice; it is the presence and extent of visible injuries which determine whether acts of violence are classified as common assault, actual bodily harm or grievous bodily harm. Harm is defined in relation to whether the surface of the body has been 'violated'. Violation of the person, of their will, of their ability to act through the use of intimidation and threat are not criminal (apart from the threat to kill) and therefore not 'serious'.

> Quite a lot of the time he wasn't physically violent, but there was just this *threat* all the time you see . . . It was a mental cruelty as there was always the threat of physical violence. You don't see it as serious at the time, it's only when you get out that you realize how much it affected you.

Women's accounts reveal again and again that the more subtle violations of the person have long-term repercussions. Violence and the threat of violence are used by men to control women – either to enforce their will or punish women for perceived transgressions. Control over and limitation of women's daily lives is a central feature of 'domestic violence'. Actual and threatened violence is usually accompanied by forms of degrading and belittling talk. Living in this reality can sap women's strength, autonomy and sense of self. Yet many women do more than simply get through each day – they hold down jobs, care for their children and (if not prevented) maintain relationships with relatives and friends. Stereotypes of women who are being abused which suggest that they are weak and passive miss the range and complexity of women's responses to 'domestic violence'. Policy and practice which simply reproduces these stereotypes will fail to offer meaningful support to many women.

Many women recall confusing and distressing events in childhood which they were unable to make sense of at the time. Some may now name these experiences as incest or sexual abuse, but there are a range of experiences and aspects of relationships that women do not find easy to name.

> I remember uncles coming over at family gatherings and me just feeling uncomfortable about them. Now I know they were rubbing themselves up against me and things like that.

Or with fathers

> As I got older how he kissed me changed – on the lips and for longer . . . He used to have this 'joke' – he'd come into my room in the morning to wake me with a cup of tea and say 'It's raping time'!

> When I think about it now there was something very creepy about him . . . a kind of sexual innuendo. I think I've blocked a lot out that

I could do well to get in touch with again, it comes out in dreams, it really sort of shouts at me in dreams.

What women are struggling with here is whether the 'something' they remember is 'anything' or 'nothing'. As children and young women they lacked the knowledge and experience to make sense of such behaviour, as adults they are ambivalent about what sense to make of it. If they name it as abuse, that also means naming their male relative an abusive man, an 'abuser'.

Several women during the course of their interviews redefined such experiences as abuse, and one woman who now defines herself as an incest survivor described how that process of redefinition had taken her over 10 years, partly because the abuse her father practised (he was a lawyer) never involved breaking the law. It was what Linda Herman has defined as 'seductive'. What women's accounts of childhood sexual abuse demonstrate is that we know when we are being abused – it makes us feel uncomfortable, dirty, used, confused, upset – but because definitions of abuse tend to refer to specific acts, not our feelings, we find it difficult to name many of these experiences as abusive – we weren't 'really' or 'seriously' abused.

The question of what counts as rape is also one women have to frequently negotiate in heterosexual relationships. We have already noted the stereotype of 'real' rape and how it disguises the fact that most women are raped by someone they know. When women talk about their experiences of non-consensual heterosexual sex they refer to this stereotype and in so doing minimize their own experiences as adolescents and adult women. Whilst the women we quoted earlier say 'nothing really happened' because they were not coerced or forced to have sex, women who were forced or coerced say 'it wasn't really rape'. The closer women's relationship is to the man, the less likely she is to name forced sex as rape. Thus the most common form of rape according to Diana Russell (1982) – marital rape – is neither recognized in English and Welsh law, nor easily named by women[2]. In order to name it women have to struggle with the dissonance between their own feelings and reactions and public discourse.

> I just laid on the bed and let him try, and of course he couldn't keep his erection and he was getting really mad about that . . . so I wasn't actually raped as such, he didn't – but I was as far as I was concerned. You blindly go on accepting so called legal definitions so that if there is no intercourse it's not rape, it's 'indecent assault'. But *it is rape* to the woman it happens to. Rape is – it's a violation of your . . . self. It's trying to kill the self, what better way to do it than to say you've got no power, no autonomy, if I want to do this to you I can just do it.

Inclusion and complexity

The examples we have quoted here are just a few from the many documented in our research which illustrate the range of abusive behaviour women encounter from men which is minimized, not named directly. In attempting to reflect this complexity one of us has used the concept of a continuum of sexual violence (Kelly 1988a). It is one way of including rather than excluding the 'normal' actions of men which women experience as abusive, as well as those which are currently criminalized. However, the analysis underlying this concept – that categories are not mutually exclusive, that seriousness cannot be assessed through a hierarchy of acts – is the opposite of that which informs the construction and implementation of law. When women say 'nothing really happened' they are making a statement about how much worse it could have been. When the law says 'nothing really happened' it implies that a woman has not been violated/abused. A revealing example of this process at work is the fact that Metropolitan Police do not refer women who withdraw their complaint of rape to counselling services; if there is no investigation/prosecution then 'nothing really happened'.

Recent feminist campaigns have focused on achieving public recognition of the extent of sexual violence and more inclusive definitions. However, despite appearances to the contrary, the opposite trend can also be discerned. One new strategy for maintaining limits on the intervention of the law is the increasing use in the USA, Canada and Australia of 'diversion' programmes for men charged with incest or 'domestic violence' offences. Abusive men are 'diverted' into treatment programmes, all criminal charges against them are dropped if they complete the treatment. Thus the law recognizes that a crime of assault against the person has been committed, whilst abrogating to itself the right to define and treat it differently from similar offences which take place outside the family or offences against property. There is powerful support for 'diversion' in Britain. Diversion suggests that 'nothing really happened' or that the 'something which happened' is less deserving of legal sanction than other offences. We are not arguing here against 'treatment' (although we have yet to see convincing evidence that it works), but against the privileging of men who abuse women and children in their families.

What these policies suggest is that where positive reform or increased recognition appears at the front door, new strategies to maintain the status quo are brought in through the back, deflecting attention from the extent of abuse which occurs within heterosexual relationships and families. It is not only the rehabilitation of abusers that is at stake here, but also the rehabilitation of heterosexuality and the nuclear family.

One implication of our analysis is the limitation of the law, and legal reform in the struggle to control sexual violence. It is simply impossible to legislate against all forms of male behaviour which women experience as abusive – that would involve criminalizing much of the interaction between men and women. The law cannot eliminate patriarchal attitudes and behaviours – that requires the mass resistance of women. Despite this, however, we do not think that feminists should abandon legal reform, rather that this strand of activism must begin from a recognition that gains will be extremely limited if our campaigns are not informed by an understanding of how the law functions to limit what 'counts' as violence against women and children.

Campaigns for legal reform must, therefore, be directed at creating more inclusive definitions, and attempts at exclusion or decriminalization must be resisted. The Rape in Marriage Campaign, which we were both involved in, is an example of working for a less exclusionary definition of rape. The two central planks of the campaign were achieving legal recognition that women's consent cannot be presumed and that sexual violence should be defined in relation to the form of the assault, not the relationship between the man and the woman. It would also validate many women's experiences which are currently denied by the law in England and Wales. The history of resistance to this reform (some change was first mooted by the Criminal Law Revision Commission in 1980) is itself evidence of the desire of many to keep legal definitions of rape as limited as possible: protecting the mythology of hetero-sexuality and the nuclear family, cornerstones of the patriarchal status quo. In this context the decision in January 1990 by the Home Office to refer the matter to Law Commission, with the stated intention of accepting some form of criminalization of rape in marriage is a surprising move. Until the Law Commission has completed its deliberations, which we understand will be later in 1991, it is impossible to judge how inclusive any new proposal will be (for more details see Radford 1990).

The proposed reform must be placed in context of events which occurred within weeks of the Home Office's decision. On 10 April, Judge Raymond Dean stated in his summing up in a rape trial in which the man and woman knew each other: 'When women say no they don't always mean no' (*Daily Mail* 11 April 1990). Whilst this statement produced outrage and disbelief from feminist groups, there were more alarming responses. For example, Valerie Grove argued in a feature article in the *Sunday Times* (15 April 1990) that rape laws should be limited to offering protection to women in relation to stranger rape in public places, that there was no role for the criminal law in policing sexual encounters between friends.

> What I ponder is this. All rape is deplorable; but surely a distinction should be drawn between the rapist who knows his victim and the random rapist who attacks any woman, and therefore threatens all women. One kind of rape is a private dispute between acquaintances, former lovers etc. Why should such a matter of personal distress be examined in open court?

We suspect her views are widely held, and mirror those of MPs and judges who view men who kill their wives as 'no threat to the community'. If legal reform is not accompanied by public debate about definitions of 'violence' we will yet again witness the one step forward two steps back phenomenon.

Notes

1 This chapter was previously published in *Critical Social Policy* (1990–1) Volume 30, winter issue, pp. 39–53.

2 Since this chapter was first published, case law (RvR [1991] 2 WLR 1065) has established that it is possible to bring a case of rape against a husband in England and Wales. This was already possible in Scotland, but the situation is yet to be clarified by reform of statute law.

References

Estrich, S. (1987) *Real Rape*. Cambridge, MA: Harvard University Press.

Hanmer, J. and Maynard, M. (eds) (1987) *Women, Violence and Social Control*. London: Macmillan.

Hanmer, J., Radford, J. and Stanko, E. (eds) (1989) *Women, Policing and Male Violence*. London: Routledge.

Hanmer, J. and Saunders, S. (1984) *Well Founded Fear*. London: Hutchinson.

Kelly, L. (1988a) *Surviving Sexual Violence*. Cambridge: Polity Press.

Kelly, L. (1988b) What's in a name?: defining child sexual abuse, *Feminist Review*, 28: 65–73.

MacKinnon, C. (1988) *Feminism Unmodified: Discourses on Feminism and the Law*. Cambridge, MA: Harvard University Press.

McNeill, S. (1987) Flashing: its effects on women. In J. Hanmer and M. Maynard (eds) *Women, Violence and Social Control*. London: Macmillan.

Radford, J. (1986) 'Thanks for nothing, Lord Lane', unpublished paper from the Critical Legal Studies Conference, London: June.

Radford, J. (1987) Policing male violence: policing women. In J. Hanmer and M. Maynard (eds) *Women, Violence and Social Control*. London: Macmillan.

Radford, J. (1989) Women and policing: contradictions old and new. In J. Hanmer, J. Radford and E. Stanko (eds) *Women, Policing and Male Violence*. London: Routledge.

Radford, J. (1990) Rape in marriage: make it a crime, *Rights of Women Bulletin*, spring: 12–14.

Russell, D. H. (1982) *Rape in Marriage*. London: Macmillan.

Smith, L. (1989) *Concerns About Rape*, Home Office Research Study No. 109. London: HMSO.

Stanko, E. A. (1990) *Everyday Violence: How Women and Men Experience Sexual and Physical Danger*. London: Pandora.

3

When does the speaking profit us?: reflections on the challenges of developing feminist perspectives on abuse and violence by women

Liz Kelly

The title of this chapter draws on an Audre Lorde poem (Lorde 1984). A prominent theme in her life and work was to challenge the silence that has surrounded much of women's experiences. She was deeply committed to finding ways to speak and communicate which did justice to the range, depth and complexity of women's lives and circumstances. It is now over four years since I decided to talk about women's use of violence at a meeting of Sappho, a London lesbian discussion group. I took that decision, despite many misgivings and apprehensions, because I believed that refusing to discuss difficult issues has never profited feminism. Silence has been a major weapon in men's arsenal which has prevented women and children from talking about their experiences of sexual violence, let alone finding ways to get support and join in campaigns and movements for justice.

Since that talk was revised and published (see Kelly 1991), it has been the basis for a number of discussions and workshops, and a television programme used parts of it to set the context for a documentary on abuse by women.[1] Two national conferences have also been organized on the issue and a book of papers published.[2] The issue struck a chord (or number of chords) within and outside the women's movement, and in important senses some of the reticence which existed previously has shifted.

However, many of my original concerns remain. This chapter develops the original paper, and discusses the conditions which are necessary if public debate and discourse on abuse by women is to profit both those who have experienced it and the Women's Liberation Movement.

The current context

The reluctance of most lesbians and/or feminists to discuss women's use of violence reflected a justified anxiety; that the issue would be used to undermine the grudging acceptance of the extent and range of men's use of violence towards women and children and/or to reinforce negative stereotypes of lesbians. Feminists have never totally denied that women could be abusive. Our use of statistics, for example, that 95 per cent of child sexual abuse is committed by men (the figure common to many studies and commentaries) contains an implicit acknowledgement that 5 per cent is committed by women. It is possible, therefore, to argue that reluctance to focus on the 5 per cent was a strategic political decision; that only by drawing attention to the scale of men's actions were we ever likely to shift public perception. At the same time, though, there was some avoidance of the difficult and challenging questions which abuse by women raises. Both these factors informed, and continue to inform, feminists' responses to this issue.

During the early 1990s we have witnessed some individuals in the professions and the media seizing upon emerging evidence about women's use of violence to make outspoken attacks on feminist analysis. Research findings, however spurious, which suggest that women are as, or even more, violent than men or that men are as, or even more, likely to be victimized are paraded before us, as if they invalidate dozens of previous studies. Each new case involving women as perpetrators of violence provides an opportunity for media features and speculations. For example, in two cases, Aileen Wounros and Beverley Allitt[3], the reporting turned in part on authors vying for the dubious privilege of designating the women 'the first' female serial killer. This climate is not conducive to thoughtful exploration and reflection; it frequently confirms our worst fears. Refusing to participate in the media circus can appear to be the best option in an impossible situation, where either including or excluding women's use of violence places it at the centre of discussions.

If we fail to develop a feminist analysis of abuse by women we are handing over this issue to the professionals and the media. Silence also means that we will continue to fail women and children who have suffered at the hands of women, and risk losing the clarity we need in order to hold on to what we have learnt and built in the last two decades. For example, as evidence of abuse by women emerges, and evidence grows of boys and men's experiences of sexual victimization (predominantly at the hands of other men), women's organizations are being asked to justify in new ways why they continue to provide support *for* women *by* women (see Gillespie, Chapter 10, this volume). In attempts to demonstrate their 'awareness', policy makers, local councillors and officials, and many professionals have begun suggesting that victimization ought to be discussed and responded to in gender neutral ways. We need a strong, secure position from which to defend our frameworks and services; rather than seeing acknowledging abuse by women and victimization of men and boys as a challenge to our hard-won knowledge base, we need to approach them as extensions of what we already know.

To build this security we must move on from the defensive posture many of us (including me) have previously adopted. Whilst not disputing that there has been a strong reluctance amongst many feminist/lesbian groups and communities to take on this issue, it has been constructed as an ongoing 'collective feminist refusal' by professionals and journalists outside the movement. I accepted this charge until recently; on reflection I want to acknowledge that there were informal communities and feminist organizations which attempted in the past, and which are continuing to address violence in lesbian relationships. There were, and are, rape crisis lines and refuges which support/ed women who had been abused by women, and/or work with women who were being violent to children. But this work is either not publicly documented, or only available in the form of annual reports and statistics in applications for funding. The fact that activists were often too busy to write their own history, has provided fertile ground for outsiders to invent a past which supports their current arguments.

The complexity of relationships between women, including issues of violence and abuse, is a strong theme in the writings of many African and Asian women.[4] Whilst this may not have been the norm, we do our movement a great disservice when we participate in the rewriting of its history. As Kum-Kum Bhavhnani notes, what we are trying to create are feminist ways 'of writing [and speaking] history [in which] conflicting interests between women are made *visible*' (1993: 96, original emphasis). It is not as though everyone else was tackling the issue, and we were alone, steadfastly refusing to notice! The crucial question today is not whether feminists will face up to the issue of abuse by women, but *how* we use feminist politics to make sense of, and respond to it.

What was missing in the past, and in my view is not that well developed now, is thoughtful, collective reflection on what abuse by women means for us: how we locate it in our theoretical framework; how we approach naming, defining and studying it; what kinds of support are needed for those who have been abused by women, and more contentiously, for women who have used violence. The remainder of this chapter explores my concerns about these issues.

The theory issue

The insecurity that many feminists and/or lesbians experience when beginning to address women's use of violence reflects a profound concern that it will undermine feminist analysis of both sexual violence and heterosexuality. But feminist theory is not that fragile. It has developed over time, become broader, more inclusive and (sometimes unnecessarily) more complex. Including women's use of violence is only a threat to a version of feminism which views men and women, masculinity and femininity as fixed, unchanging, biologically based, which defines violence as an inherent potentiality in men. A feminism which begins from understanding gender as a social construct, which recognizes the variability with which gendered selves and individual biography combine, can locate women's use of violence within its existing framework.

The linkage of power, violence and sexuality has been one of the foundations of feminist analyses of male domination; we have argued that, as in other political systems, men's gender power is ultimately backed by force, that force is used when power is in jeopardy. Hence sexual violence is the outcome of men's power as men and women's resistance to it (Kelly 1988). An extension and development of this analysis involved mapping how patriarchal relations were constructed through (hetero) sexuality and sexuality constructed through gender (Coveney *et al.* 1984; MacKinnon 1989). This theoretical work involved adapting and applying perspectives on public politics and violence to the interpersonal and private. Whilst women's use of violence was not a focus in early theoretical development, complex discussions developed, which are still the subject of debate. Explorations of our relationship to notions of 'femininity' included both a rejection of traditional constructions of it, alongside a reclamation and redefinition of what were termed 'women's virtues' (West 1991); feminists were interested in creating the possibility for women to be strong and tender, caring and angry, connected to others and autonomous. Revisiting these discussions in order to explore the reality of women's relationship to anger, aggression and violence would benefit us at this point.

The use of violence as a means of maintaining systems of oppression is not confined to gender relations. However, the use of interpersonal violence is more characteristic of women and children's oppression than that of other groups, and sexualized violence is differentially targeted at women and girls. What has not been done within or outside feminism is systematic comparison of the structures, forms and justificatory ideologies of all forms of political violence.[5] Mapping the variations of state, institutional, organized and individual violence and noting particularly the cross-cutting examples where multiple power hierarchies are in operation – for example, war, rape and strip-searching of women political prisoners – might provide us with a wider framework for understanding both men's and women's uses of violence (see McCollom *et al.* 1994 for a beginning). For example, in other systems of domination we easily recognize that violence can be a reaction to/product of powerlessness. Disenfranchised groups may view violence as the only/a legitimate way to resist domination, although this too tends to be gendered, with the majority of those taking up arms being men and the forms of insurgency frequently becoming a reflection of the actions of the dominating group (Morgan 1989).

Toni Morrison's novel *Beloved* (1987) is an impassioned account of how a black woman who has escaped slavery decides that killing her children is preferable to them being re-enslaved; an illustration of how context can create choices which are no choices, where the only power she feels she has, the only protection she can offer her children, is death. Her use of the power she has as an adult and mother is overdetermined by an oppressive context which is itself violent and violating. To use violence from a position of powerlessness cannot have the same foundation or the same meanings as that from a position of powerfulness, even though the consequences for those it is directed towards may be the same.

If we begin from the current structures of social power then the least likely targets of violence for women are men, and it is usually only in extreme circumstances that women use violence interpersonally towards men: circumstances in which the woman (or her child, and in some cases sibling) has been abused/violated by the man in question (Justice for Women 1993). Women's violence to men is overwhelmingly responsive to prior abuse: acts of self-preservation, self-defence or responses to injustice. The most likely target for women's violence is children, over whom women have power by virtue of being adults. Mothers are also expected to 'control' their own children. The use of physical violence by women towards children has not been problematic for feminist frameworks, although it has not received the attention it should have (Wise 1984).

What has been problematic is evidence of sexual abuse of children by women, since the sexual is not constructed as a form of 'power over' for women. It is only problematic if we take the connections between masculinity, femininity and sexuality as 'naturalistic' essential qualities, which are inherent to people by virtue of their sex, rather than being the outcome of complex personal biographies in historical, social and cultural contexts. The stereotyped expectations of men and women, the creation of gendered selves affects all men and women, but its influences and outcomes are not uniform. Feminist theorists have created powerful criticisms of 'dualistic' thinking, whereby opposing characteristics are attributed to men and women, as if they apply universally and without variation (Hare-Mustin and Marecek 1990). At the level of massive generality they may be descriptive of gender stereotypes but lived experience is more complex. It is entirely possible for women to identify with, even want, the kind of 'power over' that the sexual frequently provides for men. Having access to it is more complex than for men, and we have not yet explored the conditions and circumstances which would facilitate this 'power over' for women; but logically we are most likely to find instances of it involving children.

Accounting for violence between girls and adult women is not necessarily problematic for feminism; factors involved here include the use of violence to create/impose hierarchies in groups, especially where other resources are not available, the ways in which divisions between women are encouraged and sometimes even created by men – one of the most common causes of fights between girls and women are heterosexual relationships. Again, we may have paid limited attention to these issues, but they are not in principle, outside our framework.

What has proved far more taxing is violence between lesbians, especially within lesbian relationships. It represented a profound threat to the feminist promotion of lesbianism as offering the possibility of non-hierarchical relationships. Acknowledging that some lesbians use violence does not undermine the fact that the power they hold within a relationship is not, and cannot, be the same as that held by men in heterosexual relationships. It is an interpersonal use of 'power over', not backed up by social systems outside the relationship.

Understanding lesbians' use of violence also requires taking account of the context in which lesbian relationships exist. It is one of marginalization at best, and secrecy, deceit and fear at worst. Lesbians frequently have to manage contradictory public and private identities and meanings, and struggle to develop positive identities and meanings for themselves and their relationships in a context of invisibility, being defined as 'abnormal' and frequent subjection to hostility and abuse. This raises the complex issue of how to make sense of the use of 'power over' in contexts of relative powerlessness, how violence can be used as an interpersonal resource when not backed up by social power. We also need to explore how 'internalized oppression' affects the ways individuals see themselves and others, the ways we conduct relationships. One recurrent theme in accounts of abuse in lesbian relationships is the fear the abusive woman has of losing her partner; her controlling behaviour is directed towards ensuring she stays. This is not necessarily the same as a heterosexual man's sense of 'rightful ownership'; it could be connected to profound dread of isolation in a hostile world.

To make feminist sense of women's various uses of violence and abuse we need to begin from understanding that dominant constructions of masculinity and femininity are ideologies/discourses which influence rather than determine self-concept, beliefs and behaviour. It is possible that the most powerful men have so much control that they can afford to behave 'nicely', the most disadvantaged women have always had to act in 'unfeminine' ways simply to survive. The fact that an individual man is gentle and nurturant does not mean he no longer has social power as a man, the fact that an individual woman is strong and challenging, not to mention violent, does not alter the structures which maintain and reproduce male dominance and female subordination.

Some implications of thinking seriously

Women's use of violence and strategies of power and control are issues which resonate in women's groups where the difficulty in naming and resolving conflict and power relationships remains little theorized; there are very few published accounts, and hardly any written collectively. We need accounts which address the potential difficulties and contradictions between the goal of increasing women's individual power and control in their lives and the creation of collective/communal ethics and contexts.

Some of the very early second wave feminist writings about structure addressed these issues. Joleen's 'The tyranny of structurelessness' (1973) was a reflection on how simplistic conceptions of non-hierarchy create situations in which power is routine – but operating in covert and implicit ways which makes it far harder to name and challenge. Our continued and repeated failure either self-reflexively, and/or group-reflexively to tackle controlling and manipulative actions has created ongoing difficulties in women's organizing. Whilst attention has been paid to how institutionalized forms of 'power over' such as race, class, sexuality and disability, affect the perspective of and actions within women's groups, not all 'power plays' in groups are reducible to these structures. Developing a more complex model of interpersonal power, the use of manipulation to control, would be a valuable resource which would have applications within group, friendship and partnership contexts.

We must also find ways of exploring the question of why some women use violence and abuse. In a number of recent discussions women have expressed strongly felt resistance to my suggestion that we need to ask why, arguing that this constitutes a search for ways to excuse women's behaviour. I find this both alarming and disconcerting, since for me 'why' has always been a fundamental feminist question; unless we understand why and how women's oppression is so tenacious, we cannot hope to know how to end it. This unwillingness to explore various explanations has, at times, been so strong that differences between men and women's experiences (such as the fact that a high proportion of women who sexually abuse children have been coerced to it by a man who is abusing her) have been seen as tantamount to denying the women's actions. This simplified either/or position is not helpful; being victimized does not remove all responsibility, but it places actions and choices in a particular, constrained context. Men who coerce women into abusing children do so in the full knowledge that this will damage the relationship between mother and child, aware that the fact of their coercion will make little or no difference to the child's feelings about their mother at the time. Rejecting an analysis which sees differences between the position of the coerced woman and the coercive man means we remain within his construction of meaning, and as such are unable to locate him as the architect of the situation.

When discussing coercion of women to abuse, we must make connections to the experience of children and young people abused in organized networks, in which the recruitment and/or abuse of other children is a deliberate strategy used by the adults to entrap them. We have developed a clearer perspective in these cases; we can neither respond by saying that they had no choice, nor can we do the injustice of holding them as accountable as the adults who entrapped them in the first place and orchestrated and enforced subsequent behaviour. It matters whether women who have abused in coercive contexts experience the sex/power/pleasure connection which men do, or whether they experience it as another form of assault on them. We can only discover the answer to this question if we are willing to ask why.

The anger which has surfaced in discussions of this issue led me to reflect on the extent and depth of woman hating in western cultures. This woman hating is never far below the surface, and has been internalized in a variety of ways by all women. Internalized woman hatred was something consciousness raising enabled us to explore and struggle with. Women's use of violence seems to be a powerful activator of submerged woman hatred.

The ambivalent relationship many feminists have to women's use of violence is also illustrated by an almost opposite response; a 'heroizing' of women who 'fight back'. Women who kill abusive husbands seldom view their actions at the time, or later, as self-conscious political resistances to patriarchal domination, and many continue to be troubled by what they did. Aileen Wournros (a poor white American woman, tried in the early 1990s for the murders of a number of men) is not an 'amazon warrior' revenging her wrongs and the wrongs experienced by all prostituted women, but a woman who experienced serial abuse throughout her life, who lived on the margins of survival. To not recognize the damage male violence, in all too many forms, has done to her is to create a feminist mythology as a counter-point to the 'woman/lesbian serial killer' mythology the mainstream media invented. Neither construction does justice to the reality of this woman's life.

The definition and prevalence issue

Naming violence and abuse by men has been a central principle and arena of creative development in this wave of feminism; unlike our foresisters last century we were determined that our experiences of violation should not be 'unspeakable'.[6] It is, therefore, fitting that the first volume of accounts by lesbians about their experiences of abuse in relationships should be entitled *Naming the Violence* (Lobel 1986). Without a name, behaviour remains an individual concern, it lacks social reality, social meaning or social recognition. Within this central principle though are complex issues which require us to do our thinking and research with clarity and thoughtfulness.

When I first wrote about this issue I drew attention to the ways in which non-feminist researchers and commentators were defining sexual abuse more broadly when women were the actual, or hypothesized, per-petrators. I questioned the ways in which women's routine caring for the bodily needs of babies and children was being constructed as offering un-paralleled opportunities for abuse. Since that time I have been witness to, and been told other accounts, of women, some of whom would identify themselves as feminists, using different definitions of abuse when women are identified as abusers. For example, one woman recently attended an incest survivors group in which everyone but her said they had been abused by their father and their mother. Her initial shock at this rapidly transformed into dismay when it became apparent that none had been sexually abused by their mothers, and all were defining their mother's 'failure to protect' as equivalent to repeated assaults by their fathers.[7] I have had several discussions with women researching abuse in lesbian relationships, in each case their definition of abuse is far broader than that used in relation to violence in heterosexual relationships, including manipulative behaviour, dishonesty and disrespectful treatment.

Clearly the behaviours of these mothers and lovers were experienced as hurtful, forms of betrayal even, and in that sense they are problematic. But I am deeply concerned by the implications of using such wide definitions that all mother/daughter, and/or lesbian relationships come within the remit of abuse. I have never supported exclusionary definitions, but we are in danger of the very concepts we have striven to imbue with powerful meaning becoming devoid of it. We need to devote serious feminist attention to what the words violence, assault, abuse, conflict and disrespect mean and where the boundaries (however fuzzy) are between them. When I proposed using the concept of a continuum to cover both the range of, and connections between, the violations women and girls experience at the hands of men (Kelly 1988) I never intended that be understood as suggesting that all events were the same. In that work, and subsequent research with other women in the Child Abuse Studies Unit, we have challenged the presumption that impacts of violence can be 'read off' from the form of assault. Nonetheless, there are differences in physical and emotional damage. We must find ways at the same time to notice connections, similarities and differences between forms of violence and abuse.

Within this discussion we must explore the consequences of transferring the concepts we have created or redefined in the last two decades from abuse by men to abuse by women. Erin Solaro, writing in the US feminist newspaper *Off Our Backs* (1993), uses word 'rape' to name sexual assaults by women without comment. In the context of the US a number of reforms of the law on rape defined it in gender neutral terms. In Britain this issue was debated in the early 1980s within a coalition of women's groups who were preparing a submission to the Criminal Law Revision Commission (Ginsberg and Lerner 1989). Although there was no absolute consensus, that group agreed that the definition of rape (penetration of a vagina by a penis) remain, since it was (and remains) the only gender specific crime against women on the statute book. The group suggested changing the relative importance – in terms of sentencing tariffs – of other offences, but rejected removing the word rape from statute or changing its definition (see Gillespie, Chapter 10, this volume for a discussion of this issue in relation to 'male rape'). What are the implications of changing the law in the interests of 'equality' so that women can be charged with rape? Do women who have been sexually assaulted by women think that it is only if the word 'rape' can be used that their experiences will be taken seriously?

Whilst recognizing that the evidence we currently have about women's use of violence is limited, we do have some, and it is crucial that it is used appropriately. I am going to focus here on the two most problematic areas: women's sexual abuse of children, and violence in lesbian relationships.

At a recent conference (see note 2) Michelle Elliot claimed that the reason we do not have data recording a greater prevalence of sexual abuse by women is that researchers have not asked the 'gender question'. This is simply not true. All of the broad sample prevalence studies in the US and Britain (see, for example, Finkelhor 1979; Russell 1984; Kelly *et al.* 1991) have included questions which allow the gender of abusers to be analysed, and in each case the percentages for adult female abusers are between 5 and 7 per cent. Whilst some local figures for reported cases have been cited recently as indicating a much higher incidence, the NSPCC, in a section of their 1990 *Annual Report* (which interestingly was not picked up by the media) stated categorically that their figures did not support the popular 'tip of the iceberg' view of women as abusers. That any child is abused by a woman is sufficient for it to be taken seriously. One has to ask, however, why so many people want the prevalence to be greater than research findings, why they insist that there has to be far more than we are currently aware of, and why the iceberg of hidden cases is always gender specific.

The information we have currently about violence in lesbian relationships is even more limited. There has been an increase in personal accounts published in the women's and lesbian press and cases are being reported to formal agencies, such as police domestic violence units. Cases are also becoming more public knowledge; for example, in 1991 a very large criminal injuries compensation award was made to Susan Craker for an assault by her ex-lover (*Guardian* 11 December 1991) and an article in the US women's newspaper *Sojourner* details the case of Debra Reid, a black woman convicted of murdering her abusive lover.

The most detailed study to date is by Claire Renzetti (1992), in which 100 lesbians responded to advertisements (which specified that the study was about abuse in relationships) in the lesbian and gay press in the US (see Scott 1994 for a detailed critical review). All completed a questionnaire and 40 were interviewed. She discusses other US research, some of which involves large samples of over 1,000 participants. Many of these studies have used a problematic research instrument – the Conflicts Tactics Scale – which has been the subject of much debate in studies of violence in heterosexual relationships. The main criticisms centre on the use of composite figures covering a range of behaviour (from pushing through to 'beating up'), the lack of any assessment of the effects of behaviour – whether it created fear and/or resulted in injury – and no assessment of whether the actions of individuals were offensive or defensive (see Dobash and Dobash 1992 for a detailed critique). Relatively high proportions of lesbians, in these studies, were deemed to have abused a partner (30 per cent) and a higher percentage defined as having been abused (52 per cent). In none of the discussions of these findings have either the problems with this research instrument, or the possibility noted that lesbians may be more sensitive to, and therefore more likely to report, power imbalances in relationships, been discussed.

Renzetti recognizes that none of the studies conducted so far have been 'true prevalence studies'; that is based on a random sample of the lesbian population, and she notes how complex it would be to do such a study.[8] Yet she concludes her book by stating that violence is as prevalent in lesbian as in heterosexual relationships. There is currently no empirical base from which to make this claim. The challenge for researchers is to create methodologies which are sensitive to both similarities and differences between violence and abuse in heterosexual and lesbian relationships, and which take seriously the possibility that there may be different definitions of abuse operating which will influence naming and reporting.

The impacts issue

In many discussions of abuse by women the assertion is frequently made that it is 'worse' than abuse by men. One factor which has exacerbated this claim is the lack of public recognition offered to survivors, which in turn created a context where women who have been abused by women have felt obliged to stress the negative impacts in order to be taken seriously. It has, however, been an important feminist principle not to create hierarchies of oppression/ abuse; to insist that experiences which the law and institutions define as 'minor' may have major consequences for women and children; and to recognize that many women and children are able to marshal internal courage and strength and find external support in surviving brutal attacks without permanent or inevitable damage.

The frequency of this statement demands that we explore why and ask what sits underneath the attribution of 'worse'. Whilst not disputing that some women can be extremely vicious and cruel, the claim seldom rests on demonstrating that the forms abuse takes are 'worse'. What is at issue is what being abused by a woman means; the issues and questions it raises are deep and profound, they resonate with, and affect, our sense of ourselves as women (and in some cases as men). It is never the same at the level of meaning to be abused by a woman. This is not because it is less common, less validated, although that is part of the context in which meaning is created, but simply that it *means something different* to be abused by a man or a woman, and that meaning will have additional dimensions if the abuser is the same or different sex to the child or woman they abuse. Whilst no two experiences are the same, the meanings of abuse relate to gender, and impacts are also to some extent gendered.

As many have noted, for a man or boy to be victimized fits uneasily with stereotypes of masculinity; the most usual comment which follows this observation is that, therefore, it must be 'worse' for boys to be abused, especially by a woman. Apart from the revealing other side of this statement – the relative acceptability of the victimization of girls, and normalization of men's abusive behaviour – this is not necessarily how boys and men respond. A substantial number of young men reporting abuse in a recent prevalence study (Kelly *et al.* 1991) were able through constructions of masculinity to 'rewrite the script', defining experiences as seduction, or something they actively wanted, or initiated, or enjoyed, and this was more likely if the abuser was female. This interpretation protected these young men from the impacts which accompany defining experiences as victimization. This is not to recommend this coping strategy – it probably contributes to a belief that childhood sexual experiences are not damaging – but to highlight how central gender is to the ways events are experienced and understood. Such rewritings are not as easily available to girls or women, although there are women who report minimal impacts of coerced sexual experiences. What is important here is paying attention to the details of how and why the gender of abusers matters, how and why that influences the consequences of abuse, and building from that an awareness of differences which do not have to be hierarchically graded or compared.

Where abuse occurs within a lesbian relationship there are likely to be layers of meaning that form the context for the impacts on women. One's abuser is someone who shares not only a gender but also a sexual identity, someone from within a small and frequently beleaguered community. If the women also profess a feminist politics the presence of abuse represents a betrayal of strongly felt beliefs and principles. If the abusive woman holds other forms of advantage, such as financial, racial or educational, these may enhance her ability to control her partner. If on the other hand it is the victimized woman who occupies a position of advantage, the violence may be excused as the expression of powerlessness. The pain which many lesbians experience when abused by a lover is evident in the virtually ubiquitous statement that writing or speaking about it was one of the most difficult things the woman has ever done. It is so difficult because of the additional meanings involved, what the experience calls into question, rather than the forms of violence or abuse being 'worse'.

The practical support issue

Some principles of feminist support work with women and children who have been victimized by men apply in supporting those abused by women: belief, validation and respect. As feminist services have developed a sense of history and security in their practice, more complex formulations have emerged, whereby it is possible to acknowledge that for a variety of reasons (fear, shame, distrust) women may not always tell the truth. So belief has become a more nuanced and complex matter. Validation has been a central principle in contrast to the denial and minimizing which predominated in the mainstream. It connects to the principle of naming violation and placing responsibility on the abuser. Feminist services have, however, never worked with a principle of validating everything a woman might say; we have, for example, always attempted to question (in a supportive rather than interogatory way) ways women blame themselves for abuse. As public discourses on violence and abuse become stronger, and non-feminist explanations abound, there are many things women might say which we would seek to offer alternatives to, such as 'cycle of abuse' models through which women come to think that they will inevitably hurt a child, despite never having felt an impulse to do so.

Providing feminist support for survivors of any form of violence or abuse always involves more than belief and validation. It ought to be a mark of our respect for the woman we work with that we articulate our political understandings, and engage with her in a process through which we attempt to arrive at a 'joint interpretation of meaning'.

Feminist practice has always begun from, although not limited itself to, what women who have been abused say they want and need. Until recently belief and validation for women abused by women has not been automatically forthcoming; that is undoubtedly changing. There is a lot to be learnt from looking in detail at how women seek support. In Renzetti's (1992) study 75 per cent of the lesbians had sought help, a minority using formal sources of support such as the police and lawyers, the majority looking to counsellors and friends. What the women in her study said that they wanted most was for friends to listen to and support them, to name abuse and to encourage and help them leave the relationship. This is the challenge to the lesbian community; lesbians who are being abused, understandably and reasonably, want support from their community, from those who already know and care for them. As with abuse in heterosexual relationships, the target for change in discussions of abuse in lesbian relationships has tended to be on formal institutions, rather than informal networks (Kelly 1993). Like many other issues in this chapter this is not an either/or option, rather a both/and necessity.

We also have to face the contentious issue of who should work with women who have abused. Can we afford to take the view we have with men, that we will not work with abusers? If we think men should work with abusive men, isn't the logical corollary that women should work with abusive women? Here again the relevance of gender, and the similarities and differences between men and women's behaviour, motivations and understandings are critical. I have not yet discovered any accounts of feminist work with lesbians who have abused their partners, but the one detailed account of work with women who have sexually abused children highlights the importance of working with women as women.

Ruth Mathews and her two co-workers report on a programme they developed which has involved 16 women convicted of sexual offences against children in the US (Mathews *et al.* 1991). Almost two-thirds abused with men, most of this group being coerced to abuse. All 16 had an extensive history of victimization by men in both childhood and adulthood. They note that this is a different profile from male offenders, further illustrated by the fact that when they began the programme all but one of the women admitted what they had done and did not seek to project blame onto children. Most discussions of work with male sexual abusers report that much early work is devoted to breaking down denial and projection.

Some of the women had already failed in male orientated programmes for sex offenders. The groups used a model of women's self-development in their work, which began from a recognition that these women had no basis for a positive or autonomous sense of self. To use the frameworks underpinning work with male abusers would have stripped these women of the few resources they had which could be the basis for change.

Whilst I have been critical of the 'cycle of abuse' explanation for all sexual abuse (Kelly 1992), we do have to take seriously the persistent finding amongst women convicted of sexual offences (albeit very small samples), that they have histories of repeated victimizations by men. Why, for a minority of women this translates into becoming the victimizer and for the majority does not, is an important issue for future research. In refusing to accept simplistic cycle of abuse models, we need to leave open the possibility that in particular instances and circumstances there may be complex connections between victimization and victimizing.

Reclaiming a politics

Working on this issue has constantly involved a return to what I understand as the principles of feminism, the origins of our perspective. This revisiting has led me to ponder on the implications of the shift in feminist goals and directions, which I see as a move away from the struggle for women's liberation, and which required nothing less than transforming the societies of which we are part. We have moved towards a quest for women's equality; equal access to what in the public realm affords men power and advantage is no longer focused solely on economic areas such as pay and career opportunities, but has, for some, extended to pornography and institutions such as marriage. The 'right' of lesbians and gay men to marry is a very different goal to that of abolishing the institution altogether. How does this reduction of feminist ambition affect our expectations of, and behaviour towards, each other?

In terms of theory and explanation feminists have rightly focused on the differences between men and women in relation to power, violence and sexuality. In recent years many feminist academics have defined this work as 'essentialist' and pointed to neglected similarities between women and men. If we are to make sense of women's use of violence, whilst holding on to our hard won knowledge and clarity about male sexual violence, we must refuse this either/or option, and be courageous enough to look at both.

Notes

1 An Open Space production for BBC2, *Unspeakable Acts*, broadcast on 26 April 1993.
2 Both conferences were held in London and organized by Kidscape, in 1991 and 1993. The most recent was jointly organized with the National Children's Bureau and Childline. For the book, see Elliot 1993.

3 Aileen Wounros was convicted of the murder of a number of men in the US. She killed them in the context of prostitution. She claims that in each case she was acting in self-defence. Beverley Allitt was working as a nurse in an intensive care unit, in Britain, where a number of children died. She was found guilty of their murder, expert testimony argued that she was suffering from Munchausen's Syndrome by Proxy.

4 Relevant here is work on female circumcision and the complex relationships of kin in extended families, especially the roles of mothers-in-law in cultures where wives move into their husband's family home, and between wives in polygamous marriages.

5 I use the term 'political violence' here deliberately, drawing on the work of Joan McKiernan and Monica MacWilliams (1993) who question, in the context of Northern Ireland, the reserving of the term to the actions of the state and armed groupings from Republican and Loyalist communities.

6 For women and children with certain disabilities, abuse is literally unspeakable, since their forms of communication are not speech as conventionally defined (see also Michelle McCarthy, Chapter 8, this volume).

7 The way in which 'failure to protect' has developed into a new form of woman/ mother-blaming, following the effectiveness of feminist challenges to mothers being defined and treated as 'collusive', is an issue which needs further exploration.

8 In CASU (from summer 1994 CAWSU – Child and Woman Abuse Studies Unit) we have discussed the possibility of conducting a prevalence study of abuse in lesbian relationships. The major problem we struggle with is how to create a random, or even representative sample of a minority community which is invisible, and in which many of its members have good reasons for keeping their sexual orientation secret. To find 500 or 1,000 lesbians through the usual methods of randomized house to house calls, or random telephone dialling would be both enormously time consuming and costly, and unlikely ultimately to produce the desired representativeness.

References

Bhavhnani, K.-K. (1993) Tracing the contours: feminist research and feminist objectivity, *Women's Studies International Forum*, 16(2): 95–104.

Coveney, L. *et al.* (eds) (1984) *The Sexuality Papers*. London: Hutchinson.

Dobash, R. and Dobash, R. (1992) *Women, Violence and Social Change*. London: Routledge.

Elliot, M. (ed.) (1993) *Female Sexual Abuse of Children: The Ultimate Taboo*. Harlow: Longman.

Finkelhor, D. (1979) *Sexually Victimized Children*. New York: Free Press.

Ginsberg, E. and Lerner, S. (1989) *Sexual Violence Against Women: A Guide to the Criminal Law*, London: Rights of Women.

Hare-Mustin, R. and Marecek, J. (1990) *Making a Difference: Psychology and the Construction of Gender*. London: Yale University Press.

Joleen (Freeman, J.) (1973) The tyranny of structurelessness. In Anne Koedt, Ellen Levine and Anita Rapone (eds) *Radical Feminism*, pp. 285–9. New York: Quadrangle.

Justice for Women Collective (1993) *Information Pack*. London: Justice for Women.

Kelly, L. (1988) *Surviving Sexual Violence*. Cambridge: Polity Press.

Kelly, L. (1991) Unspeakable acts: women who abuse, *Trouble and Strife*, 21: 13–20.

Kelly, L. (1992) Outrageous injustice, *Community Care Supplement*, 25 June: ii–iii.

Kelly, L. (1993) Towards an integrated community approach to domestic violence. in Child Abuse Studies Unit (ed.) *Violence Against Women and Children – A Feminist Perspective*, London: University of North London Press.

Kelly, L., Regan, L. and Burton, S. (1991) *An Exploratory Study of the Prevalence of Sexual Abuse in a Sample of 1200 16–21 Year Olds*. Final Report submitted to ESRC, University of North London, London.

Lobel, K. (ed.) (1986) *Naming the Violence: Speaking Out About Lesbian Battering*. Boston, MA: Seal Press.

Lorde, A. (1984) The transformation of silence into language and action. In Lorde, A. *Sister Outsider: Essays and Speeches*. Truemansburg, NY: Crossing Press.

McCollom, H., Kelly, L. and Radford, J. (1994) Wars against women, *Trouble and Strife*, 28: 12–19.

MacKiernan, J. and MacWilliams, M. (1993) 'Studying domestic violence in a violent society', paper at the Fifth International Interdisciplinary Congress on Women, San José, Costa Rica (edited version in *Rights of Women Bulletin*, winter 1994).

MacKinnon, C. (1989) *Towards a Feminist Theory of the State*. Cambridge, MA: Harvard University Press.

Mathews, R., Mathews J. K. and Speltz, K. (1991) *Female Sexual Offenders: An Exploratory Study*. Orwell, VT: Safer Society Press.

Morgan, R. (1989) *The Demon Lover: On the Sexuality of Terrorism*. London: Methuen.

Morrison, T. (1987) *Beloved*. London: Chatto and Windus.

NSPCC (1990) *Annual Report*. London: NSPCC.

Renzetti, C. (1992) *Violent Betrayal: Abuse in Lesbian Relationships*. London: Sage.

Russell, D. (1984) *The Secret Trauma: Incest in the Lives of Girls and Women*. New York: Basic Books.

Scott, S. (1994) Lies, lesbians and statistics, *Trouble and Strife*, 28, 36–40.

Solaro, E. (1993) What part of no did she not understand?, *Off Our Backs*, June: 16–17.

West, R. (1991) Jurisprudence and gender. In K. Bartlett and R. Kennedy (eds) *Feminist Legal Theory: Readings in Law and Gender*. San Francisco, CA: Westview Press.

Wise, S. (1984) *Becoming a Feminist Social Worker*, Studies in Sexual Politics 6, Manchester: University of Manchester.

4

Reading danger: sexual harassment, anticipation and self-protection

Elizabeth A. Stanko

The purpose of this chapter is to explore how men's sexually harassing behaviour is *perceived* and *found to have meaning* by women in order to negotiate and affirm our relationship to personal safety. Sexual harassment is often characterized as inconsequential and harmless to women. This characterization can only be made if our experiences of daily sexual harassment (Wise and Stanley 1987), common histories of adolescent sexual pestering (Lees 1986), and legacies of sexual threat and abuse (Kelly *et al.* 1991) are ignored.

Controversy continues to rage about sexual harassment. Survey after survey documents *reported* sexual harassment. Yet commentators vehemently resist women's descriptions of men's behaviour as threatening, malicious, unwelcome and intrusive. In this age of alleged openness about sexuality, accusations of sexual harassment are met with justificatory statements such as 'it was only a joke'; 'I didn't know you didn't feel the same way'; 'you misinterpreted my intentions'; or simply, 'you're lying'. Since the publication of Lin Farley's (1978) *Sexual Shakedown*, the first book-length exposé about sexual harassment, many still belittle the existence of sexual harassment and many women are surprised and disappointed by the impact of sexual harassment on their everyday lives. Lawsuits, complaints procedures, workers' guidelines, professional statements of ethics aside, men's sexual use of women in public and private continues.

We hear the term 'sexual harassment' used more today, though, than we did 15 years ago. Predominant in the literature is the presentation of sexual harassment as something to be unproblematically understood and unproblematically resisted. It is illustrated through a documentation of women's complex reactions to a range of men's behaviour which women define as annoying and/or threatening. In response to this greater awareness, advice literature seeks to arm us with assertiveness to equip us to confront harassment.

Indeed, there is an ever-growing industry of advice material for women about sexual danger. While some of this is addressed solely to sexual assault, behaviour at work or in public, most of this advice advocates that we ready ourselves for harassment. I do not wish here to undermine the need, or even desire, of women for self-protection. What I wish to do is to raise questions about the power of acknowledging the *need* for self-defence, while, at the same time, retaining a widespread denial of the collective impact of sexual harassment on all women's lives.

My questions are informed by my own studies of women's experiences of men's violence and are connected with my own experience(s) of and my struggle against sexual harassment. I am an academic criminologist, who thinks, campaigns, and debates issues related to women and men's violence. And for the first time, after 15 years, I am locating that debate and discussion explicitly through my personal experiences. My current thinking is devoted to examining the imponderable: what is safety? This professional and personal exploration prompts me to ask: does arming oneself for protection against sexual harassment (or other forms of sexual violence) have any impact on how we see ourselves as women?

Surrounded by advice prompting us to take care in public and private, do we see ourselves as passive victims, an accusation hurled recently by Naomi Wolf (1993) or Katie Roiphe (1993)? How do different women make different sense of men's sexualized actions and behaviour? In other words, has the advice literature helped us sort out the safe from the unsafe men? Ultimately, I am exploring how we as women, now more than ever, are expected to manage men's sexualized behaviour toward us. The message of the advice literature, in effect, is every woman for herself. Collective confrontations with men's abuses, spearheaded by feminist campaigns, are pushed once again to the margins.

Personal memories

Fifteen years ago, as a young academic on the east coast of the United States, I, along with many other women, became the target of unwanted and unwelcome sexual attention by my head (or chair) of department. As I look back on it now, I am unable to describe the numerous details of my harasser's behaviour. It is my own reluctance to recall what I recalled for too long, the details of the harassment, which took place over a period of six months, and my resistance to it which ranged over a period of four years.

Briefly, the situation arose as follows. For six months or so, I was kissed in the office, my clothing and appearance were noted, commented upon, and subjected to sexual innuendo. I witnessed other colleagues experiencing similar discomfort and outrage. I complained to higher officials. I know that I experienced the harassment as threatening. I also know that I felt uncomfortable, embarrassed, angry, disempowered, imposed upon, and humiliated. His behaviour was not new, nor unique. Another faculty member had propositioned me just after I accepted my job. In that case I felt perfectly able to say 'no', and felt there were no repercussions for doing so.

But this was different. We had already worked together for two years as colleagues. As far as I could tell, he supported me enthusiastically in my first reappointment, and respected my development as a scholar and teacher. Yet, as I found out during the course of the dispute, many other women had received unwelcome 'attention', even during the time he was friendly and supportive to me. Three of eight members of a small department faculty ('the women' – two academics and the department secretary) began to share accounts of his offensive conduct.

Initially, I was surprised that the man I had respected could do such 'things'. The stories, though, became distressing. I was forced to re-evaluate my relationship with him and, ultimately, my assessment of him as an abuser of women. I had to overturn my previously uncontested opinion of him: he became an abusive man. All this was in 1978–9. While the sexualized behaviour eventually stopped, other kinds of retaliation carried on for years. The struggle to have his behaviour and its implications for the behaviour of all men and all women, taken seriously continued for another three and a half years, and took place in public debates, in the media, and in the courts.

By 1981, I (along with four others) was sued by the harasser for $23 million for defamation of character. (Personally, I was only liable for about $7.5 million!) The university's legal and management team failed to protect us when the university settled its internal grievance process with the aggressor. The harasser lodged what was one of the first counter-suits in the US against women alleging sexual harassment. The other female faculty member, then reeling from the failure of the university to renew her contract, and I countersued the university in 1981. The case was settled out of court in 1982, in our favour, accompanied by an apology from the harasser. Frightened of retaliation, I still resist using his name today.

During those four years, I was subjected to a daily barrage of comment, threatening phone calls, hostility from colleagues, attention from the media (radio, TV talk shows, and even an editorial in the local newspaper!), and professional debates and campaigns. I continued working full time in the same department as my aggressor, and was expected to carry on a professional life unscathed by the storm in my workplace. What is important to me is what, and how, I learned about sexual danger and how to cope with the process of publicly naming such behaviour as abuse. I wish to use this experience, as painful as it is, to recall, to explore some of the theoretical strands which appear within my own work about safety, and our experiences and confrontations with men's violence (see, in particular, Stanko 1985, 1990a, 1990b).

Forewarned is forearmed?: deciding to name the abuse

In a thoughtful and thought-provoking monograph, Kirsten Bumiller (1988) suggests that being a victim of discrimination is a collective phenomenon, a condition of the relationship between the powerful and the powerless. Powerlessness, she further opines, is not a *possession* of an individual, it is relational, and socially constructed. In declaring victimization, an individual must stand apart from the collective experience and announce specific effects of unequal treatment. Asserting discrimination, as an individual claimant, means separating oneself from the collective inequalities, and making a public declaration about the right not to be treated in such a way.

In demanding the right not to be sexually harassed, women are objecting to what has been and is considered to be routine: sexualized treatment at the hands of men. Many of us choose to find other ways of resisting and/or coping with the intrusion of men's sexualized comments. Liz Kelly (1988) speaks of how some women minimize the violence they have experienced. Bumiller speaks of individuals becoming engaged in 'a politics of survival – a battle designed to preserve the bare minimum of human autonomy' when one decides to cope individually without the assistance of a legal tribunal or collective or personal confrontation which might have served the purpose of validating an accusation of sexual harassment (1988: 70). In an analysis of why people who identify themselves as unequally treated fail to demand redress, Bumiller proposes that anti-discrimination laws uphold the status quo of state power rather than support the claims of those harmed. People feel ambivalent about asking the state for redress, because they feel they may be more harmed by the process of fact-finding. So too, we may question our own responses to felt discrimination, however hurtful and frightening these experiences might be. Bumiller identifies three processes which people use to justify non-confrontation with what they perceive to be unfairness: sacrifice, exclusion and distortion. Placing Bumiller's themes within knowledge about violence against women might look something like this: a woman who changes her dress, because she wishes to avoid unwanted comment, is willing to sacrifice her choice of style to some envisioned 'safe' territory. Battered women who attempt to manage the role of 'the good wife' (whatever that might actually mean in practice) are willing to give up their notions of 'good wife' and substitute those of their violent husbands. So, for instance, she wears the dress he likes, feeds him the food he wants, and keeps the children disciplined in the way he thinks is appropriate. Women then sacrifice their own sense of self, accommodating to some idealized (and almost certainly unattainable) version of good wife/satisfied husband.

Questioning power, which we do when we claim we have been harmed, means that we are often stigmatized for demanding to be treated differently, that is, not abused. Those who demand differential treatment are labelled as potential troublemakers. So, for instance, women who make allegations that comments from male employers, co-workers or clients are sexual, are questioning how men *normally* treat women in so many other public and private spaces. In effect, women who allege sexual harassment insist that they are *not* like *ordinary* women because they do not expect to be sexualized. Women who do not comply with men's overtures are often accused of 'being lesbians', that is, not 'normal', normal being defined as heterosexual in a patriarchal society.

If I demand to be treated differently from other women, as I did by naming what I experienced as harassment, then alleging harassment could be a sign that I am *refusing* to be *a woman*. I am asking for my sexuality not to be intruded. Questioning the order of things upsets many of the taken-for-granted rules for heterosexual interaction. Thus women who make allegations that the comments they receive are unwelcome, sexualized, remarks are virtually excluding themselves from the routine order of things. As Bumiller succinctly observes: 'There are no minor infractions within "normal" ranges of behaviour; there is only rebellion or submission' (1988: 74).

The final theme which Bumiller identifies is that of distortion. Victims, by the very fact that they raise questions about their treatment, challenge the 'social standards of the powerful'. Those who question the ordinary way things are are in danger of being labelled 'hysterical', 'irrational' or 'humourless'. Again, in the case of sexual harassment at work, women are to assume that the twin powers of sexuality and economic control does not exist. Sexualized comments, harassers and others allege, should be understood as if they exist *outside* the context of job evaluations and performance monitoring. Indeed, the long and protracted legal argumentation concerning the connection between sexualized treatment and economic consequences continues to be difficult to prove in sexual harassment cases. Nonetheless, the use of women's sexuality as a legal assistant has not been overlooked by the lawyers acting in such cases (see also Stanko 1982). A *Wall Street Journal* article, for instance, catalogues how civil suits in sexual harassment cases are methodically including women's sexual and medical history within the remit of legitimate questioning about the allegations of sexual harassment (*Wall Street Journal* 19 September 1994).

The very act of *claiming* unfair sexualized treatment is resistance against it. It is an act of individual defiance. But why then do critics say that feminists portray women who experience sexual violence as weak and passive recipients of men's abuse? There is, I believe, confusion here. The recurrent theme of critics, such as Naomi Wolf (1993) or Katie Roiphe (1993) fails to embrace the *process* of how, as individuals, we come to terms with our experiences. In my own situation, I found it hard to believe that I, a white, middle-class, educated, professional woman could be subjected to unwanted sexual attention. Clearly, this was naive. Of course, I received harassment as I walked on the street. Certainly, I received unwelcome attention when I travelled alone. But in my workplace, I relied upon privilege bestowed by education, whiteness, and self-assurance, to take me above womanhood. That is, I somehow believed that I could be defined primarily by my *intellect*. Instead, I was trapped within a body, a body that is female, and *as female* I could be dismissed as a professional (beyond body?) because I could be sexualized.

I had to claim I was harassed by someone I had already worked with for two years. I had little experience to assist me in anticipating how difficult it would be to explain how the meaning of his behaviour had changed, and the effect that it was having on me and other women around me. Moreover, the longer I complained and protested my treatment, the more unreasonable *I* was portrayed. I was a 'frustrated, lonely woman' who was going through a divorce. I hated men. I was hysterical. I was making it up in order to further my own career. I was just downright vindictive. Or, as surfaced in the depositions, I was an FBI agent plotting against a known leftist (after all, stated the aggressor, my research area included the police!). Anything and everything was used against me to discredit my account of the aggressor's behaviour. And I was lucky. My colleague was even more the target of vindictive retaliation. An anthropologist who occupied chairs in two universities in Santiago before the coup, she was an astute observer of culture and power. She was portrayed as someone who 'misinterpreted' American society, another 'lonely, frustrated, childless woman', and an alleged CIA agent (this was directly stated by the harasser under oath, during the time her sister was being tortured by the military regime in Chile).

She was even more a target, however. Racism fuelled the campaign against her. More insidious, she was a resident alien, without permanent immigration status. The university joined the abuse bandwagon and refused to sign her green card, casting her adrift into the immigration lottery. Structurally, she was more vulnerable than I, but she was to me a bridge to a vision of something different. She lived through the carnage that was Santiago in 1973. Her friends and family were spread over the world in an attempt to escape the mutilation of the fascist regime. She offered me an understanding of transcendence over the way I was socialized to *know* how power worked to maintain compliance. So we resisted together.[1]

The struggle against this particular harasser's behaviour was equally a confrontation with the institution within which it thrived. The issue of sexual harassment was barely surfacing within universities in the US in 1978. We refused to end our legal proceedings unless the university adopted a policy which condemned sexual harassment, and identified a process whereby all members of the university community could complain should the need arise. We knew that the failure to protect us was not really directed at us individually; we knew that no member of the university community was safeguarded against such behaviour.

Fifteen years later, when I look at the advice material which exists now to assist women to avoid sexual harassment, I cannot but notice how it glosses over the notion of *collective* impact of sexual harassment on women. It is as if we, as individual women, are expected somehow to suspend ourselves in animation, outside the extensively documented consequences of gendered stratification, and to take individual evasive action, believing it will work. So we leave jobs, change the way we dress, avoid being alone with harassers as creative avoidance strategies, in effect, we take active, individual measures to resist.

Training films, women's survival guides, and police advice converge in eschewing collective contexts of violence against women. According to these guidelines, arming oneself against sexual harassment demands a recognition of its potential, without a clear recognition of women's collective vulnerability (see also Connell 1987). Without an understanding of this wider context, however, it is very difficult to understand how we create conditions which allow individual women to name men's sexualized actions and behaviour as harassment.

I had all the advantages: white, educated, articulate, heterosexual, and I found no protection within my advantaged position. My complaints were questioned because they were *women's* complaints. As hard as I tried, I could not negotiate myself out of *being female*.

Collective and individual naming: the power of uncertainty

I have characterized some forms of sexual harassment as 'little rapes' (Stanko 1985). Briefly, men's unwanted 'attentions' range from leering, sexual teasing, comments or questions through unwanted touching, unwanted pressure for sexual favours or dates to sexual assault and implied or explicit threats for non-compliance. It is, I have suggested elsewhere, impossible to conceptualize sexual harassment outside the whole range of sexual threats, experiences and atmosphere – rape, sexual abuse of children, battering and sexual terrorism in the home, public pestering on the street – which exists for women in most of the world. Each woman defines for herself what she experiences as harassment. The research suggests a great deal of convergence of the kinds of experiences women name as harassment, and at the same time, there is divergence.

In my case, the sexual intimidation took place in my workplace, a place where I previously felt comfortable. A once safe and welcoming place became a hostile environment. What, or who, was the invader? And why would I and other women interpret the harasser's behaviour as just that, harassment, rather than friendly behaviour?

Describing scenarios of harassment often miss the depth and detail of how we experience ourselves as safe within a context of sexual unsafety. Here women's differences become paramount, though commonalities emerge. 'One woman's wine is another woman's poison' may have some resonances here. Let's say I'm offered a cup of coffee before a meeting by a colleague and he says, 'You can come to my office any time day or night for coffee'. Now this could be interpreted as a friendly, open invitation to share some caffeine. Why would any woman be wary of visiting a colleague's office? It is because I view him not only as a colleague but also as a man. Why would I be wary about one man and not another? This is a difficult task, for as an individual responsible for my own safety, and briefed about the possibility of encountering sexual harassment, I am left to sort out the so-called safe from the so-called unsafe men.

Questions about how women err and miss the signs of potential dangerous sexual encounters with men arise commonly during the questioning of women alleging rape during trials. Women are asked: why did you think that this man would *just* take you home, unmolested after meeting him at a pub? Why did you not think about men's sexual intentions when you interact with casual acquaintances? former partners? colleagues? Women are considered cultural dopes if we miss the cues which, as women, we are expected to *know* simply because we are women.

According to surveys of sexual harassment, one in two women in paid employment report such experiences. What about the other 50 per cent? Some women still interpret men's sexual attention at work and elsewhere as flattery. In May 1993, for instance, a judge in Cardiff, Wales cited a man in a court public gallery with contempt for wolf-whistling at a woman juror. The case caught the attention of the media, in part, I believe, to counteract the feminist messages about sexual harassment. Interviews with the juror revealed:

> Men sometimes whistle at me in the street and it doesn't bother me a bit. There's nothing wrong with it – it's only a way of saying they think I'm pretty. I was embarrassed [in court] at the time because it was a serious occasion, but secretly I was also very flattered.
>
> (*Sunday Telegraph* 23 May 1993)

This example illustrates the difficulty with different interpretations of sexual harassment: this woman is performing the very public role of a juror, a key member of the criminal justice system deputized for decision making. The judge (correctly, in my view) cited the man for contempt. The whistling man, in effect, sexualized her public role, invading the formal (non-sexual?) courtroom with personalized (hetero) sexuality. The woman was embarrassed, as she states, because 'it was a serious (non-sexual?) occasion'. But she had been asked later, in retrospect, *as a woman*, how she felt about being *noticed* as a woman, not as a juror.

Quite clearly some (many?) women wish to be sexually attractive to men. To me, though, it is the context which provides the clues about when and whether sexualized comments are appropriate. The power to define *which* context is appropriate is largely in men's control, however; in a largely heterosexual, male-dominated context, men's unfettered prerogative is to sexualize women any time, any place, if they so choose. Taking a stand against such treatment, and especially placing the right to define whether such comments are welcome or appropriate in the hands of those with less power, upsets the status quo. Men, many complain, no longer know when they can comment upon women's sexual appearance *when they feel like it*. Indeed, the *problem* with demanding an end to sexual harassment is that it upsets the privilege of men's propriety over women.

Sexual danger, we learn in childhood, comes from a variety of sources and people (Stanko 1990a). From childhood onwards, children are taught to 'say no, run and tell' if approached by a stranger. Strangers, we are particularly warned, will (or could) bring us harm. Too often, children are not told about those known to them. As the data shows, known men, especially family friends, authority figures and family members, pose more danger to physical and sexual health of children. For parents in Britain, the fear of abduction by strangers ranks second to traffic danger when parents worry about children's safety (Hillman 1993). We are rarely warned about our fathers, brothers, cousins, co-workers, clients or close family friends. In my situation, the sexual harasser was not a stranger; he was a man who was my boss and long standing colleague. His excuse was that he was 'creating a family atmosphere' within the department (of course, what this says about families could be the topic of many essays!).

We accumulate this knowledge about danger, and carry it into our adult life. The very complaint of Roiphe (1993) is that anxiety about the possible dangers of heterosexual encounters has become part of young women's lives (Holland *et al.* 1990). Young men continue to dominate the way young women experience heterosexuality. Indeed, the research suggests that a significant proportion of men's sexual demands are experienced by young women as coercion, and now labelled as 'date rape' or other forms of abuse. Young women still walk a fine line between sexual respectability and unrespectability. But many (some?) young women also *know* about intrusive sexuality. Young women receive unwanted sexualized attention, not only from their peers, but from older men as well, on the street, in the classroom, at work, at home and elsewhere. These experiences happen in both public and private spaces.

How does such knowledge about sexual vulnerability affect women who work? Or women who do not work? What about elderly women? young women? poor women? élite women? black women? Is it possible to be immune from the anxiety that anticipating harassment might bring?

We are expected to know and behave as if we are sexual targets. But we are not supposed to be anxious about this; we are not supposed to treat all men as if they are sexually dangerous; we are expected to sort out the safe from the unsafe men. When was the last time you, the reader, could definitively make such judgements without risking a mistake or confronting an accusation of unfairness or worse, political correctness?

So we are expected to act as if we could be victims, and indeed, many of our daily routines suggest just that. Many women already choose to interpret men's behaviours as potentially dangerous, especially in public spaces (Gardener 1980, 1988, 1990). In private, however, the negotiation is far more ambivalent. In private, women have other obligations and contradictions with which to contend (Bart and O'Brien 1985). In private, we are to treat men as if they are safe, or we are to act as if we can manage men's behaviour so that it doesn't get out of control. Everyone likes to make judgements about how others might have unnecessarily trusted someone they shouldn't have. In the abstract, I, and other women I know, have an opinion about what we would do if we encountered sexual harassment. Then it happens and we don't handle it as well as we would like. After all, we want to keep our jobs, our relationships, our respectability. So we juggle our lives as women with the way we find meaning in men's behaviour' toward us.

Present and unaccountable: managing the consequences of sexual danger

In the field of criminology, a concept of 'fear of crime' attempts to capture how women and men assess their risk of crime. It should be no surprise that women are more likely to assess their risk of personal violence, even though, according to all official statistics, far more young men report to police and crime survey researchers that they have been violently attacked. Women feel able to admit vulnerability, and this vulnerability has been variously explained as women locating themselves amongst the sexually vulnerable (see Gordon and Riger 1988). The contradiction is that the notion of fear is supposed to address how safe women feel in public (Pain 1993), while all the evidence suggests that it is women's own homes where they are the most vulnerable to physical and sexual assault. Women are thus able to express fear about public space, but, even when expressed, there is no clear explanation within criminological circles *why* such anxiety should exist. It is therefore acceptable to be afraid of the dangers brought by strangers, but not acceptable, or even understandable, why we should be afraid of those we know. Fear of crime, as a concept, is virtually useless to describe the fears harboured by, for example, battered women, incest survivors and those bullied by schoolmates.

I am now in a workplace where I feel more comfortable. The anxiety about leaving the abusive situation brought concerns about the possibility of entering yet another, unknown one. I found interviewing and accepting my next job particularly traumatic. I was unnerved, and unsettled by having to start all over again. In this job I've been lucky. I've been largely successful in avoiding harassment. But what does that mean? It means that I have not abandoned my protective shield. As much as I campaign and write to change women's collective lives, I have been forced, through my own need for personal survival, to alter my own behaviour.

The most consistent question I am asked is: knowing what you know now, would you do it (file a law suit, fight against unequal treatment) again? Probably, though I don't really know the answer. It takes courage to stand up and fight, but it doesn't mean that my choice was more noble than those who chose to do something else. Strategies for surviving abuse vary according to one's resources – emotional, financial, social and physical. Again, I was lucky. That time, I had a house I could mortgage to pay for my legal fees ('rights' are very costly in the United States); I was without children so I didn't have to worry about the effect on them; I did divorce in the middle of the dispute, but separation was in both of our best interests; my job was not secure, and it was professional failure which continually stared me in the face when I looked in the mirror each morning.

It took me years to recover from the stress brought on by such a public confrontation. Confronting men's violence leaves you feeling vulnerable in many places and spaces in your life. I felt less secure on the street; I had nightmares; I felt I was losing my mind; I aged; I harboured anger I thought few could understand; I felt that I had to hide the fact that I had sued my former employers, either because people felt sorry for you, or treated you with contempt or distrust. Those who demand to be treated differently do feel stigmatized, and some indeed are stigmatized.

The second question people ask me about the sexual harassment case is: did you win? I guess we did. There are no winners in these cases, however. The damage from the fight is real. The loss, the pain, the stress, the memories are still here. All these feelings still would be present had I not confronted the situation, I suspect. I guess I could say that it has made me stronger. But for what?

Ultimately, I left my workplace, unable to revive any commitment to teaching within an institution which took such an active part in my abuse. Of course, there are the few special people who supported me during this trying time, and I still have a strong sense of affection and loyalty toward them. But anger is quick to swell when I hear of others in similar situations.

Epilogue

It is difficult for me to separate discussions of sexual harassment from discussions about what it means to be a woman. Suddenly, in the past 15 years, and especially since the Anita Hill–Clarence Thomas hearings in 1991, sexual harassment has come to the foreground *to be managed*. Documentaries are produced, books and advice abound, professional conferences are well attended, corporations and public sector employers issue guidelines for staff. Yet the newspapers assail feminists for insisting on demanding that men stop their abuse. Such feminists are accused of so-called 'political correctness' (now a derogatory term used against those who demand a change in language as a minimum display of amending past abuses).

Sexual harassment has not stopped. Individual women's strategies, as advocated by all the advice literature, do not change men's behaviour. While, if such individual assertion works and we avoid the perpetuation of harassment, essentially we continue to manage men's unwelcome sexualized attention. I worry about this. Individual strategies which merely deflect men's behaviour do not bring an end to the collective impact of such abuse on women's lives. Too often, we are settling for a strategy of containing the effects of sexual harassment and dumping them on so-called legitimate targets – women who might not have experienced assertiveness training, women with fewer resources, women who must fend for themselves without the aid of a network of support.

As long as the term sexual harassment is divorced from the complex realities and intimacies of different women's lives, as long as it is considered a 'phenomenon', then we will fail to understand the power of sexual harassment. Each of us has a part to play in assuring that action against 'sexual harassment' is a collective one. We can each do that by supporting women who experience, in a variety of situations, men's behaviour as threatening and abusive. And we must continue to find ways of collectively confronting the systematic and intrusive abuse individual women experience. Empowering ourselves individually must also empower us collectively.

Note

1 There were indeed three other women, an undergraduate student, a postgraduate student and the former department secretary who were also sued by the harasser. Often, the five of us would seek collective support from each other. They chose to avoid the public confrontation of a countersuit, so only my colleague and I sued the university in 1981 for failing to uphold our right to complain about our conditions of work.

References

Bart, P. and O'Brien, P. (1985) *Stopping Rape: Successful Survival Strategies*. New York: Pergamon.

Bumiller, K. (1988) *The Civil Rights Society*. Baltimore, MD: Johns Hopkins University Press.

Connell, R. (1987) *Gender and Power*. Stanford, CA: Stanford University Press.

Farley, L. (1978) *Sexual Shakedown*. New York: McGraw Hill.

Gardener, C. B. (1980) Passing by: street remarks, address rights and the urban female, *Sociological Inquiry*, 50: 328–56.

Gardener, C. B. (1988) Access information: private lines and public peril, *Social Problems*, 35: 384–97.

Gardener, C. B. (1990) Safe conduct: women, crime and self in public places, *Social Problems*, 37(4): 311–28.

Gordon, M. and Riger, S. (1988) *The Female Fear*. New York: Free Press.

Hillman, M. (1993) *Children, Transport and the Quality of Life*. London: Policy Studies Institute.

Holland, J., Ramazanoglu, C. and Scott, S. (1990) Managing risk and experiencing danger: tensions between government AIDS educational policy and young women's sexuality', *Gender and Education*, July: 125–46.

Kelly, L. (1988) *Surviving Sexual Violence*. Cambridge: Polity Press.

Kelly, L., Regan, L. and Burton, S. (1991) *An Exploratory Study of the Prevalance of Sexual Abuse in a Sample of 1200 16–21 Year Olds*. Final Report to the ESRC, University of North London, London.

Lees, S. (1986) *Losing Out*. Cambridge: Polity.

Pain, R. (1993) 'Crime, social control and spatial constraint', unpublished PhD thesis, University of Edinburgh, Edinburgh.

Roiphe, K. (1993) *The Morning After: Sex, Fear and Feminism*. Boston, MA: Little Brown.

Stanko, E. A. (1982) Would you believe in this woman? In N. H. Rafter and E. A. Stanko (eds) *Judge, Lawyer, Victim, Thief: Women, Gender Roles and Criminal Justice*. Boston, MA: North Eastern University Press.

Stanko, E. A. (1985) *Intimate Intrusions: Women's Experience of Male Violence*. London: Routledge.

Stanko, E. A. (1990a) *Everyday Violence: How Women and Men Experience Physical and Sexual Danger*. London: Pandora.

Stanko, E. A. (1990b) When precaution is normal. In L. Gelsthorpe and A. Morris
    (eds) *Feminist Perspectives in Criminology*. Milton Keynes: Open University Press.
Wise, S. and Stanley, L. (1987) *Georgie Porgie*. London: Routledge.
Wolf, N. (1993) *Fire With Fire*. London: Chatto & Windus.

Part II

Law, protection and criminal justice

5

Violence against women and children: the contradictions of crime control under patriarchy

Jill Radford and Elizabeth A. Stanko

Before engaging with our title subject, we will introduce ourselves and our relationship to the issue of violence against women and children and the academic debates about crime control. Jill Radford, a British feminist, has been active in researching, theorizing and campaigning against violence against women since the late 1970s. Betsy Stanko, an American feminist now working in Britain, founded, along with other women, a shelter for battered women and children in Worcester, Massachusetts in the late 1970s. Both of us are criminologists and have struggled with issues of men's violence in our own lives. As feminists we argue that sexual violence is used by men as a way of securing and maintaining the relations of male dominance and female subordination, which are central to the patriarchal social order. We recognize that patriarchy is crossed through and is in interaction with other power structures, namely those of race, class, age and status regarding disability. These shape women's experience of sexual violence and the response of the police and others. We firmly believe that it is through challenging the patriarchal order by increasing women's autonomy that men's violence must be confronted. While this long term goal is central to our politics, we, like many feminists, are concerned with the need to address the problem in current society. It is these concerns which have drawn us into identifying, naming and working around the problem of male sexual violence. Given that our work links both the immediate problems arising from ongoing sexual violence and the practical strategies to ease women's everyday lives with the longer term goal of eradicating sexual violence, we anticipate contradictions. This chapter addresses some of the contradictions arising in recent attempts to redefine and address the problem of sexual violence in England and Wales within the paradigms of crime control operant within the policing and legal process.

Our purpose here is to articulate some of the many contradictions facing feminists who attempt to enter the crime control debates. Although our examples arise largely from the UK and USA, we feel that they illustrate the dilemmas facing feminists in other countries. We begin by examining what we refer to as 'violence against women and children'. Much of this violence is virtually ignored by criminologists and criminal justice policy makers. We then look at the more recent shift in policing sexual violence and domestic assault. The majority of violence against women and children is directed at them by men in their families. Yet dominant professional intervention tactics effectively transform feminist analysis of men's violence to a gender neutral problem of 'family violence'. We conclude by looking at the attempts to include violence against women under the rubric of crime and the resultant crime control strategies. We argue that it is this redefinition of the problem, from that of men's sexual violence to women, defined through women's experience, to that of crime, as defined by the malestream legal system, which underpins a fundamental contradiction. Throughout, we will ask how possible it is to think seriously about 'crime' to women and attempt to develop 'crime control' strategies that promote women's autonomy and safety.

Violence against women: problems of definition

Over the past 20 years, feminists have once again named and addressed the problem of men's sexual violence from the perspective of women's experience. As has been documented previously:

> through the process of naming, women have voiced their anger and expressed their commitment to struggle and survival. 'Men's violence', 'sexual violence', 'rape', 'incest', 'sexual abuse of women and children', 'woman battering', 'womanslaughter', 'woman killing', 'frawen [woman/ wife] mishandling', 'the male peril', 'sexual terrorism', 'outrage', 'unspeakable horror', 'sexual harassment' – these are some of the words women in several cultures and at different times in this century have drawn upon to describe their experiences of men's violence.
>
> (Hanmer *et al.* 1989: 1–2)

Through listening to women's experiences of behaviour they found abusive, feminist definitions expanded as women named previously unnamed forms of abuse:

> The development of feminist research and discussion over the past fifteen years can in a very real sense be seen in terms of ever-widening definitions and naming of sexual violence in general and in particular forms.
>
> (Kelly and Radford 1987: 243)

racism + sexism in separable

A significant illustration of this is Ruth Hall's (1985) use of the concept 'racist sexual violence' to highlight the fact that for black women, racism and sexism are often inseparable.

Another strand in this work is the documentation of women's experience of sexual violence. Survey after survey documents the extent to which women endure various forms of male violence as everyday features of their lives (Stanko 1988). Sexual harassment, sexual assault, physical battering, childhood sexual abuse and intimidation, obscene phone calls, and the deluge of pornographic popular literature are the backdrop for women's relationships with men.

lifetime continuum of violence

Kelly (1988) suggests that women's everyday lives exist along a continuum of sexual violence. Radford (1987) endorsed the 'circular spiral of violence', outlined earlier by Hanmer and Saunders (1984), which illustrates the ways in which dominant discourse about public violence impacts on women, often resulting in their becoming isolated within the wider community, retreating into their homes as ostensibly safe havens, where their resultant dependency on men makes them even more vulnerable to abuse.

Stanko (1985, 1990) concludes that women's understanding of physical and sexual safety is so tightly woven with their concern for sexual integrity as to render the concept of safety problematic for women. Rather than take safety for granted, women, she proposes, build strategies of precaution into their everyday lives and speak of situations as less *unsafe*.

In the first comprehensive study of black women's experience of domestic violence, Amina Mama (1989) focuses on the ways in which racism and sexism combine to exacerbate the problems black women face in this situation. In this work, she is also highly critical of previous neglect of black women's experience of violence against women. She points to the part played by racist and sexist immigration laws which define foreign-born wives of British men as dependents with no independent right of residence in the UK:

> The scandalous situation in which British men can call the immigration department to deport wives they have abused, or simply decided they have no further use for, is condemned. So is the use of the immigration service by some men to further terrorise the women with whom they live. Immigration law currently empowers individual men to torture with impunity, women with uncertain or dependent immigration status, because it enables them to have the woman deported, perhaps away from her British born children.
>
> (1989: xv)

These and many other feminist studies over the past 15 years have consistently and persistently illustrated the endemic nature of violence within women's lives (Russell 1982, 1984, 1985; Scheppele and Bart 1983). The central feminist explanation for the widespread existence of men's violence to women and children is that it is essential to a system of gender subordination (MacKinnon 1989). Much of violence against women, captured by the feminist surveys, remains outside the realm of criminological thinking about crime. This is a consequence of attempting to locate feminist definitions based on women's experiences into man-made legal categories. Basically they just don't fit. Legal definitions are drawn from dichotomies: lawful as against unlawful; crime and no crime; innocence and guilt; the good polarized against the bad (Smart 1989). Women's experiences generally, and even more so in relation to violence, are much more complex. The 1970s debates around the limited legal concept of consent/non-consent in the law of rape is one illustration.

While the most frequent and routinized forms of male sexual violence are shielded from public view, lost in the discourse of dysfunctional families and female inadequacies, what does come to the attention of the public are the crimes of the psychopathic stranger, the deranged rapist or the serial killer. The attention drawn to public danger to women is not however a commentary about the gendered nature of this danger (Cameron 1988; Caputi 1988), only that it is dangerous for women to be in public. Thus, the bulk of violence to women, that which occurs in private, rarely comes to public attention, is scorned by the police, and the women who ask for police intervention are left neglected and often abused by the very system financed by the state to protect them.

Criminological thinking about crime continues to revolve around the safety of the public and the traditional belief that the proper police role is the policing of public order. Our attention to perceived threats to community life is constantly aimed towards public order problems, to the potential threat from the deranged or evil stranger who wishes to relieve us, forcibly, of our valuables and injure us when out in public, or to the deranged killers or serial rapists striking randomly. The literature analysing risk of criminal victimization recognizes the important contribution made by the lifestyle of the 'victim' to their coming into contact with predatory crime, yet totally neglects how women are so often victimized by those they already know (Hindelang *et al.* 1978; Cohen and Felson 1979; Hough and Mayhew 1983, 1985; Gottfredson 1984; Mayhew *et al.* 1989).

What the changes in the police response to violence against women and children are about, is the pushing of some of what was classified as non-crime into the crime books. The rise in violent crime in England and Wales, for example, is largely due to the changes in the recording practices of the police concerning domestic violence and rape. In order to explore the crime control and crime prevention strategies about *crime* to women, the reader must keep in mind that, at least in the public discourse, this remains a fraction of the incidences women themselves consider to be *violent* and *threatening* situations.

Keeping feminism alive within debates about controlling violence

Our perspective is not that of dispassionate academics concerned with an anthropological or voyeuristic study of other women, that is with separating or distancing ourselves from our subject. We see the links between the provision of support and safe services, research, theorizing and campaigning as integral and necessary to confronting the oppression of patriarchy within women's everyday lives. Because we conduct our debates within the academic world as well as within the world of the everyday, we live out the contradictions in our social practice. At the same time we have a unique insight into processes through which issues feminists raised about male violence have sparked sudden interest on the part of academics, professional service providers (such as social services, psychologists, psychiatrists and counselling professionals) and also the Home Office (the central British ministry responsible for criminal justice in England and Wales), the police and the legal system.

Within academia, we have become aware of the move to make women's studies respectable, and as a part of this a growth of interest in the subject of violence against women and children. Once established on the agenda of acceptable academic issues, however, feminist concerns are often abandoned as academic success takes priority over feminist praxis. We know, for example, that feminist support services working around violence against women receive many requests from students and tutors at every level from GCSE (the first educational qualification gained by 15–16 year olds in the UK), through to postgraduate levels to supply information about violence against women, showing interest in drawing on feminist work but without any commitment to the issues or concern for the safety and well-being of all women. Within the academy the personal is divorced from the political and both are divorced from the academic in the rush for academic success and recognition. In this process, we see every day how feminist work is appropriated, but without the feminist commitment which gave it its meaning.

A similar appropriation of feminist concerns can be identified in the belated recognition on the part of some in the caring professions that violence against women and children is a serious and a legitimate area of concern/intervention. While welcoming the fact that these professional carers are recognizing issues feminists have been highlighting as of urgent concern to women, we see very real problems in the form taken by this professional, so-called 'expert', intervention. This is especially important here, because debates about crime control inevitably lead to a diversion of many cases of violence away from the criminal justice system. There is, for instance, serious discussion about the establishment of a family court in England and Wales to handle matters arising within families, including violence and sexual abuse.

We are particularly troubled by the professional redefinition of the problem. Rather than identifying male sexual violence as part of the backdrop of women's lives, conventional intervention models, using the paradigm of victimology, identify it as something that affects only a minority of women, who can then be held in some way responsible for it. This woman-blaming logic of victimology leads many social service providers to conduct support services on their own professional terms – counselling or family therapy directed at reintegrating women and children who have been abused back into active heterosexuality and family life with the abuser with minimum disruption. This is in contrast with feminist women-centred support services developed by and with survivors of male violence, whose response is unconditional support for women and children in whatever strategies they elect. Instead of forwarding women's and children's best interests, we see too many of these professionals containing women within the structures of heterosexuality and the family and building lucrative careers for themselves on the backs of male violence (Kelly 1989). These academic and professional interventions in the public discourse about violence against women mark two major ideological shifts.

A third major shift has become evident in the Home Office and police forces for England and Wales. Although feminist critiques in the UK and elsewhere through the 1970s and early 1980s constituted a continuing source of embarrassment to those responsible for law enforcement and the judicial process, the recent about-turn in UK policy, we argue, does not stem directly from the pressure of British feminists. Rather, the British police have sought advice and direction from their North American counterparts in dealing with modern management of inner-city riots as well as sexual violence and domestic assault against women. By the 1980s, the crisis in policing could no longer be hidden from public gaze. An urgent need on the part of the police to seek legitimacy from the British public was becoming apparent. After the inner-city uprisings of 1981, followed by the Scarman report, the damning PSI report on the London Metropolitan police (Smith and Gray 1983) uprisings in Broadwater Farm and Brixton in London in 1985, the police experienced a serious need to renegotiate some consensus in the inner city (Sim et al. 1987).

By shifting attention to the problem of violence against women, in their discourse crime against women, the police in adopting the mantle of protectors to women and children, attempted to renegotiate some legitimacy within the inner city. However this targeting of women in the inner city is problematic for feminists. At the most obvious level, such a move is predicated on the discredited assumption that male violence against women is more prevalent in certain areas, among certain communities, defined with reference to race and class as pathological. Further, the unresolved tensions between the police and minority ethnic communities raises a scepticism around police motivation.

The work of North American feminists confronted police practices in relation to woman battering by lobbying for legislative mandates in many US states, and through filing class action law suits in New York and Oakland, condemning the practice of entire police forces. But the individual liability case against Torrington, Connecticut (which resulted in disastrous financial consequences for the municipal government) made police forces take notice; failing to take action in domestic situations could now cost police precious tax resources. These actions opened the doors to scrutinize US policing and police practice (Ferraro 1989). Changes in the US provided examples of 'good practice' that could be adopted by British police. But the importing of these ideas about 'good' practice left out any possibility of a feminist base.

Identifying women on the one hand as a vocal source of criticism and on the other as a needy target and by drawing on internal police debates on new softer 'community policing' styles of policing (Alderson 1979), police attention has turned to the long-neglected problem of violence against women. The change of heart has been rapid indeed. For instance, in 1984 Sir Kenneth Newman attempted to shed police responsibility for what he considered 'rubbish work', or non-police matters, naming domestic violence and stray dogs as two such examples. By 1990, police forces were competing with each other to find the most creative policy to deal with domestic violence!

But the new interest in violence against women does not include a commitment to promoting women's autonomy, nor does it recognize how policing policy affects women within varying race, class, ethnic and religious contexts. The location of London's first domestic violence units in Tottenham and Brixton, as Amina Mama (1989) states, raises questions about how policing differentially affects women and their communities:

> The establishment of domestic violence response units, staffed by women police officers and resourced to do proper monitoring and follow-up work may be a good idea, but we were concerned to note that these are an initiative so far restricted to areas of black concentration which are already heavily and oppressively policed. This raises the possibility that such units have a hidden agenda, concerned with convicting more black men, underpinning the publicly proclaimed agenda which stresses supporting and following up incidents in the interests of women being subjected to violence.
>
> (Mama 1989: 304–5)

The interest of the political heart of the British ministry in violence to women is widening. The Home Office now recognizes women's 'fear of crime' as a serious problem, and has designed pamphlets to reassure women about their safety in public places. Women's fear of crime is consistently found to be much higher than that of men (Hough and Mayhew 1983, 1985; Maxfield 1984, 1988). Hough and Mayhew (1983), the two Home Office researchers responsible for the establishment of the *British Crime Surveys*, speculated that this fear was out of all proportion with their statistically estimated chances of victimization, and therefore potentially 'irrational'. In offering a feminist explanation for women's fear, Stanko (1987: 130) has suggested:

> While women's fear remains an anomaly of perception for criminologists and policy-makers, understanding women's fear of crime – which might also be read as *women's fear of men* – entails understanding the ever-present reality of women's experiences of men's threatening and/ or violent behaviour.

Women's fear of crime, however unfounded to policy makers, has become the focus of a growing number of safety campaigns. The campaigns about safety attempt to reassure women by suggesting ways to minimize the potential threat of public space through the avoidance of dangerous strangers.

Exemplified in their 'bolts and bars' approach to crime prevention, the Home Office's focus spotlights street crime, adding to the type of concern voiced by Amina Mama above. John Patten, junior minister of the Home Office and convenor of the ministerial Group on Women, would benefit from adopting a feminist explanation of sexual violence. At a conference on rape, held at the YWCA in London in the summer of 1987, he told a delegation from the Townswomen's Guilds, a group of women similar to the League of Women Voters in the US, that the problem of rape was difficult and so was prosecuting men, who frequently claimed that women 'led them on'. Patten could not suggest a practical solution to preventing rape because it was difficult to foresee, as much of it was 'on the spur of the moment' rape.

If feminism is to remain in the forefront of critiques of crime control, we must not lose sight of our politics. We must not lose sight of our starting point, the experiences of women and children; we must not separate women's experiences of violence and danger from unknown and known men; and we must not forget that men's sexual violence is part of the backdrop of all women's lives and not something experienced by a minority who can be labelled as inadequate and helpless victims. Managing sexual danger is an integral part of being female (Kelly 1988; Stanko 1990) and any understanding about crime control must place women's safety at the centre of the debate (see also MacKinnon 1989). Altering definitions of what is crime, such as changes to the law of rape and encouraging police to treat what comes to their attention as criminal violence are two approaches to confronting crime against women and children. Both strategies, we argue, may lead to some thorny contradictions in resulting approaches to crime prevention, women's safety and crime control. Let us look at the two strategies of change in more detail.

Legislative change

An illustration of legislative change is the move towards outlawing rape in marriage in England and Wales. This was the subject of a concerted feminist campaign in the early 1980s in many countries, including the US, Canada, Australia and Sweden. Feminist arguments are arguments of principle, asserting that there could be no equality for married women while in law they could be subjected to sexual violence by their husbands without redress. From a feminist perspective this present state of law represented a clear statement about the nature of marriage and a woman's place within it, and the compulsory nature of heterosexuality itself. The British government in its decision in January 1990 to refer this matter to the Law Commission, under the supervision of Professor Brenda Hoggett, QC, has indicated its welcome for a change in law. Hoggett's own views are already on the record:

> The difficulties of proving rape are indeed formidable, particularly where a woman knows her assailant well. . . . There is no reason why the difficulties of proving anti-social behaviour should make us less ready to acknowledge it as a crime.
>
> (Atkins and Hoggett 1984: 72)

What practical benefits this move will bring for women is difficult to know. We do know both that many women will welcome this legal reform and that many women are subjected to this form of abuse. The 1989 Granada Television *World in Action* survey designed by the Centre for Criminology at Middlesex Polytechnic showed that 96 per cent of the 1,000 women interviewed said there should be a law against rape in marriage. Further, 60 per cent reported there had been occasions when they had agreed with reluctance to have sex with their husbands; 15 per cent reported having been coerced by their husbands into having sex; 12 per cent reported that they had been forced into having sex, despite a clear refusal; and 5 per cent reported being beaten before being raped.

From these figures, it is clear that on the face of it there are real practical as well as ideological reasons for criminalizing rape in marriage. However, even Hoggett is concerned that in practice implementing such a law will be difficult. These difficulties were just one of the reasons why previous Law Commission reports have consistently rejected this change. The judiciary has systematically shown its reluctance to convict rapists when they are known to the abused woman. They are also reluctant to convict rapists on the testimony of women alone as shown in the corroboration warning, where judges in rape and sexual assault trials instruct juries to the effect that it is well known that women, like small children, are notorious liars. It seems again that a recommendation for change is largely symbolic. Perhaps the government is more concerned to improve the public image of marriage and heterosexuality, leaving all manner of practical difficulties in place to prevent large numbers of married men – practically one-third, taking the figures above in their most generous interpretation – being convicted of this crime. Removing the legal impediment will not automatically protect women from sexual abuse by their husbands.

Police practice

Feminist concern about the failure of police to protect them from violence is not new. The very inclusion of women within the police force, for instance, is grounded within the belief that women are best able to deal with women and their protection (Feinman 1986; Radford 1990). So when feminist criticism angrily attacked police treatment of women who reported rape or domestic violence during the 1970s in the US, the initial defensive reactions were followed by setting up special units in many forces to deal specifically with sexual assault.

Ian Blair's (1985) study of US police practices with respect to sexual assault provided the Metropolitan Police with a structure to ward off increasing public pressure about police treatment of women reporting rape. As the police began to reveal their private face to the public through Roger Graef's BBC documentary series (1982), a number of coterminous events, starkly illustrating the criminal justice insensitivity to women who had been raped, brought remarks even from (the then) Mrs Thatcher. Sir Nicholas

Fairbairn, Lord Chancellor of Scotland, resigned over a decision not to prosecute three defendants in a horrendous and violent rape case (Jeffreys and Radford 1984).

Increasingly, the police turned to their US counterparts who had already begun to alter their practice. The establishment of special examination rooms for women victimized by sexual assault, the training of women police officers in taking initial statements from women reporting rape or sexual assault and, in some jurisdictions, the referring of women to Home Office-backed victim support schemes, are examples of recent UK initiatives.

For some feminists, this last point is a site of controversy and struggle. Rape crisis centres are consciously rooted in feminist principles, women-centred, and have a unique expertise working with women whether or not they rely on police intervention into the violence they experience from men. Victim Support, a voluntary organization, contacts victims of crime through police referrals. Their government support rose in 1991 to around £4.5 million, a 200 per cent increase over four years. As the funding to Victim Support increases, rape crisis centres and Women's Aid become starved of funding. At the same time, the majority of domestic physical and sexual assaults are never reported to police, and therefore would never be referred to Victim Support. Despite the commitment of some feminist volunteers within victim support, the philosophy of the national organization, Victim Support, is actively non-feminist. For example, there has been no commitment to guarantee that the support volunteer sent to a sexually assaulted woman be female, a stance that, to feminists, is essential to the process of women coming to terms with the experience of sexual assault. With these moves, the police seem to share an unspoken assumption with policy makers that they have now radically changed their practice and all is currently satisfactory. Police recording of sexual assault complaints has risen, due, perhaps, to careful review of no-criming procedures, encouraged by the damning evidence of the excellent Scottish study of police practices in cases of sexual assault (Chambers and Millar 1983). Window-dressing reforms then have addressed the most glaring inadequacies in the police response to women reporting rape, public concern is apparently addressed and political debate is relocated elsewhere, but the question of male sexual violence and the police response to it has only been addressed on the most superficial of levels.

Attention has turned to police practice around domestic assault. Force orders in 1985 and Home Office guidelines concerning violence against women in 1986 and 1990, responded to criticisms from feminists working within the Women's Aid Federation, from feminist activists within Women Against Violence Against Women groups and by the Advisory Committee to Her Majesty's Government, the Women's National Commission report on *Violence Against Women* (Home Office 1986). Academic studies such as that by Susan Edwards (1989) in Islington, north London, showed that police response to complaints of violence within the home largely left women on their own with no legal recourse or protection against violent intimates or former intimates. In London alone, by 1991, over 40 jurisdictions have set up special units to monitor domestic violence and the Home Office guidelines of July 1990 recommend the establishment of such units in all police forces (Radford 1990).

Here also the British police looked to their American and Canadian colleagues to witness far-reaching change in policing practice. The studies of London, Ontario (Jaffe *et al.* 1982), and Minneapolis (Sherman and Berk 1984) pointed to a more aggressive policing policy to reduce violence in the home. A study by Horton and Smith (1988) of the Hampshire constabulary reinforced the need to do something about 'domestics': they reflected 10 per cent of police calls in citizen-initiated requests for assistance.

The new policing strategy is to treat the complaints they receive from women about sexual and physical violence more often as criminal violence. To this end, in London, West Yorkshire, Wolverhampton and elsewhere specialist units have been established; some, but not all, staffed by women police officers to supervise officers' handling of 'domestics' and to provide follow up support services. In addition to recommending that all police forces establish such units, the July 1990 Home Office Guidelines also inform officers that their primary concern should be the safety of the woman and any children involved and that in relation to the man, their first concern should be the possibility of arrest. These measures are new. Their impact has still to be noted, researched and evaluated. An aspect of the new guidelines which is already a subject of controversy is the recommendation that police forces set up a computerized 'at risk' register, naming women reporting domestic violence. This register, it is claimed, will assist the police in protecting the women concerned, yet keeping police files on 'victims' of crime is an entirely new departure and one which raises civil liberties implications. Many women, particularly black women and those whose residence status in this country is uncertain, may be deterred from reporting if they know this will give them a police record. Given the multi-agency approach of the guidelines, such a register, in the hands of social service professionals operating within a victimology perspective, will become a register of pathology listing inadequate women around whom professional intervention can be targeted with a view to retraining and reintegrating them within active family-structured heterosexuality. A vital and urgent task for feminists will be the monitoring of the impact of these new initiatives, particularly in terms of their class and race dynamics.

Criminal violence is private violence

The fact remains that many of women's experiences of coercive sexuality are not recognized in man-made law (Kelly 1988; Stanko 1990; Holland *et al.* 1990). Although the judicial authorities are now seeing more crime than previously, the problem of violence to women, largely located within their relationships with familiar and familial men, is still leading to some conceptual problems in relation to its redefinition in criminal discourse, and discourse concerning remedies and crime control strategies which still revolve around public, not private, violence.

When familial violence is recognized, the old stereotypes around race and class surface. Violence is assumed to be a characteristic of black and working-class families, which were then pathologized (see Ferraro 1989 on the US; Zoomer 1989 on Holland). If the violence is deemed the norm in 'pathological' families, then either no intervention is called for or alternatively black families are targeted for therapy to bring them into the white, nuclear family 'norm'. Conversely, in white middle-class families, the prevailing myth is that 'nice' professional men don't do it. The strength of this myth is such that some middle-class women find it hard to convince police and other state professionals that they need support.

What is interesting, however, is that the Home Office studies are now beginning to throw some light on the curious reality for women: that their attackers are most likely to be those near and dear rather than the shadowy stranger (Smith 1989a). The British crime survey (Mayhew *et al.* 1989) (England and Wales only) found that 56 per cent of the assaults against women were 'domestic' in origin. Smith's (1989b) study of rape found that two-thirds of those prosecuted for rape involved men known to the women. Forty-four per cent of women killed are killed by their husbands or former lovers; 8 of 10 know their killer, according to an analysis of the murders between 1984 and 1988 in England and Wales (Radford and Russell 1992).

Although there are moves within the Home Office to take this violence seriously, the policy on crime prevention has moved in the opposite direction. Crime prevention advice stems primarily from a perspective that rests prevention on situational deterrence. The 'locks and bolts' solution to crime suggests that adequate security, vigilance, and common sense reduce the likelihood of experiencing crime.

Moving the responsibility for crime prevention to the individual through adequate security and reasonable precaution means that approaches to preventing crime necessarily focus on the danger of the unpredictable stranger who awaits opportunities for criminal enterprise. (This approach leads to woman-blaming when protection fails. Not having taken self-defence classes is deemed provocation or negligence inviting attack.) Take for example the £11 million Home Office crime prevention campaign. Now in its fourth edition, *Practical Ways to Crack Crime* includes a special section advising women about safety. Although there is a paragraph about domestic violence, it appears at the end of a four-page litany addressing women's precautions at home, while on the street, and driving. (The fact that the heading for the section, 'Special Advice for Women', is subsumed under the heading 'Your Family' does deserve more than a passing mention.) Women are advised to take care, to protect themselves outside the home and inside the home from outside intrusion.

If one assumes that it is women's safety that is important, then the Home Office campaign on crime prevention misses the mark by a wide margin. So too do the efforts of the newly arrived caring professionals in the field, because, we believe, they do not offer a gendered analysis about violence against women. Physical battering, according to this thinking, is either a reflection of bad marital relations, personality disputes, or intoxicating substances, not the manifestation of unequal power and a need for control. Sexual abuse, following the same line, arises because of some men's uncontrollable lust or miscommunication with women and children, not as an exercise of patriarchal power. Women, in the tradition of victimology, are often blamed as being inadequate wives or as colluding in their own harm and that of their children. The assumption, understandable in childhood, that mothers are all-knowing, is used by professionals to find mothers of abused children guilty of either collusion or 'failure to protect'. These explanations of men's violence succeed in keeping most of the violence against women outside officially used definitions of crime, and away from the only arm of the state mandated to protect – the police and the criminal justice apparatus (Stanko 1985). Instead diversion programmes, family therapy, and men's counselling groups are the new professional growth industry. Caught up within their own paradigms, the new professionals, confident of the 'cures' they offer, are concerned with the reintegration of women and children within the family, within heterosexuality at whatever risk, and given there is little monitoring of the impact of these uncertain remedies, there must certainly be serious risks.

This then is the heart of the contradiction facing feminists. On the face of it the police and caring professions have responded – albeit for a complex range of reasons – to feminist criticisms of the 1970s, but have done so in a way which has completely negated feminist definitions, politics, research and provision of support services. Not only this, but these interventions are part of a wider attempt on the part of an authoritarian right-wing populist government to win public support for their law and order policies, and these attempts are seductive to some white middle-class women. In terms of policing the velvet glove of a caring police force goes hand-in-hand with the iron fist of riot control and militaristic policing in the 'inner city'. One feminist response has been to monitor these moves, identify and bring together these developments, with a view to understanding at the level of practice as well as ideology. In this chapter we have not attempted to solve these contradictions, but at least to identify them and their complex roots. Identifying a contradiction is a step on the road to resolving it. Certainly, within the politics of feminism, the 1990s has seen a renewed commitment to defend feminist politics and practice and identify and challenge the professional takeover.

Central to the challenge of the professional takeover must be an insistent statement of feminist politics and reinstatement of feminist practice. In relation to violence against women and children, our politics are informed by women's experiences. From feminist support and research work as cited above, we have come to understand that violence, far from being an aberrant experience in our lives or the experience of aberrant women, is in fact the backdrop against which women's lives are lived. We have come to see male sexual violence as one of the defining characteristics of patriarchal societies. While the form and nature of male sexual violence may be situationally defined and thus varied across culture and through time, the presence of male violence is, we argue, a feature of all societies characterized by male supremacy and female subordination – the social relations of patriarchy. It serves as a means of reinforcing women's role as subordinate to men, in the public world, at work and primarily, as both feminist and the Home Office's own research has documented, in the home – in the family.

The family, and the institution of heterosexuality which underpins it, is a central institution in patriarchal society, one in which the private struggles around patriarchal power relations are enacted, and hence one in which violence frequently features as a form of control of the powerless by the powerful. It is not limited to the family, however, as in the public sphere and in paid employment women who are outside heterosexuality, or give the appearance of being marginal to it, are those primarily targeted for sexual violence, abuse and harassment, as the amount of violence experienced by lesbians and other women marginal to the white middle-class, ageist and able-bodied image of heterosexual 'normality' status. This is a central point of Adrienne Rich's (1983) classic article, 'Compulsory heterosexuality and lesbian existence'.

Controlling crime against women and children, as we see it, demands policy and practice that confronts men's licence to abuse. However, the state's concern about male sexual violence in the family can be seen as an attempt at policing the family and heterosexuality in order to clean up its public face and to restore its legitimacy as a safe institution for women, by curbing that violence which it can no longer hide. So by moving towards curbing the excesses of male sexual violence within the family and hetero-sexuality, these sacred institutions of patriarchy are preserved intact and patri-archal gendered relations are reaffirmed, reproduced and represented as in the best interests of women and children. Achieving this requires a silencing of any feminist politics which asks disturbing questions about whether hetero-sexuality is the natural, normal and only possibility for women, whether it is indeed voluntary or compulsory for women living under conditions of patriarchy and whether it is in our best interests. We will continue to ask: is this new concern with violence to women on the part of the state's police and professional carers a concern with women's interests, a concern for women's autonomy, or is it a last ditch attempt at reinstating the patriarchal status quo by restoring an apparently respectable face to its central institu-tions, the family and heterosexuality?

References

Alderson, J. (1979) *Policing Freedom: a Commentary on the Dilemmas of Policing in Western Democracies*. Plymouth: McDonald and Evans.
Atkins, S. and Hoggett, B. (1984) *Women and the Law*. Oxford: Basil Blackwell.

Blair, I. (1985) *Investigating Rape*. London: Croom Helm.

Cameron, D. (1988) *Lust to Kill*. Oxford: Polity.

Caputi, J. (1988) *The Age of Sex Crime*. Ohio, NM: Bowling Green State University Press.

Chambers, G. and Millar, A. (1983) *Investigating Sexual Assault*. Edinburgh: HMSO.

Cohen, L. E. and Felson, M. (1979) Social change and crime rate trends: a routine activity approach, *American Sociological Review*, 44(4): 588–608.

Edwards, S. (1989) *Policing 'Domestic' Violence*. London: Sage.

Feinman, C. (1986) *Women and Criminal Justice*. New York: Pergamon.

Ferraro, K. (1989) The legal response to woman battering in the United States. In J. Hanmer, J. Radford and E. A. Stanko (eds) *Women, Policing and Male Violence*. London: Routledge.

Gottfredson, M. (1984) *Victims of Crime: Dimensions of Risk*. London: HMSO.

Hall, R. (1985) *Ask Any Woman*. London: Falling Wall Press.

Hanmer, J., Radford, J. and Stanko, E. A. (1989) *Women, Policing and Male Violence*. London: Routledge.

Hanmer, J. and Saunders, S. (1984) *Well Founded Fear*. London: Hutchinson.

Hindelang, M., Gottfredson, M. and Garofalo, J. (1978) *Victims of Personal Crime*. Cambridge, MA: Ballinger.

Holland, J., Ramazanoglu, C. and Scott, S. (1990) Managing risk and experiencing danger: Tensions between government AIDS educational policy and young women's sexuality, *Gender and Education*, July: 125–46.

Home Office (1986) *Violence Against Women: Treatment of Victims of Rape and Domestic Violence*, Home Office Circular 69/86. London: Home Office.

Home Office (1990) *Domestic Violence*, Home Office Circular 60/100. London: Home Office.

Horton, C. and Smith, D. (1988) *Evaluating Police Work: An Action Research Project*. London: Policy Studies Institute.

Hough, M. and Mayhew, P. (1983) *The British Crime Survey*. London: HMSO.

Hough, M. and Mayhew, P. (1985) *Taking Account of Crime*. London: HMSO.

Jaffe, P., Wolfe, P., Telford, A. and Austin, G. (1982) The impact of police charges in incidents of wife abuse, *Journal of Family Violence*, 1(1): 37–49.

Jeffreys, S. and Radford, J. (1984) Contributory negligence: being a woman. In P. Scraton and P. Gordon (eds) *Causes for Concern*. London: Penguin.

Kelly, L. (1988) *Surviving Sexual Violence*. Cambridge: Polity Press.

Kelly, L. (1989) Bitter ironies: the professionalisation of child sex abuse, *Trouble and Strife*, 16, summer: 14–21.

Kelly, L. and Radford, J. (1987) The problem of men. In P. Scraton (ed.) *Law, Order and the Authoritarian State*. Milton Keynes: Open University Press.

MacKinnon, C. A. (1989) *Toward a Feminist Theory of the State*. Cambridge, MA: Harvard University Press.

Mama, A. (1989) *The Hidden Struggle: Statutory and Voluntary Sector Responses to Violence against Black Women in the Home*. London: The London Race and Housing Research Group.

Maxfield, M. (1984) *Fear of Crime in England and Wales*. London: HMSO.

Maxfield, M. (1988) *Explaining Fear of Crime: Evidence from the 1984 British Crime Survey*. London: Research and Planning Unit Paper No. 43.

Mayhew, P., Dowds, L. and Elliot, D. (1989) *The 1988 British Crime Survey*. London: HMSO.

Radford, J. (1987) 'Policing male violence – policing women'. In J. Hanmer and M. Maynard (eds) *Women, Violence and Social Control*. London: Macmillan.

Radford, J. (1990) Sorry, sir, it's domestic. You're nicked, *Rights of Women Bulletin,* autumn: 6–8.

Radford, J. and Russell, D. E. H. (1992) *Femicide: The Politics of Woman Killing.* Milton Keynes: Open University Press.

Rich, A. (1983) *Compulsory Heterosexuality and Lesbian Existence.* London: Onlywomen Press.

Russell, D. E. H. (1982) *Rape in Marriage.* New York: Macmillan.

Russell, D. E. H. (1984) *Sexual Exploitation.* Beverly Hills, CA: Sage.

Russell, D. E. H. (1985) *Incest: The Secret Trauma.* New York: Basic Books.

Scheppele, K. and Bart, P. (1983) Through women's eyes: defining danger in the wake of sexual assault, *Journal of Social Issues,* 39(2): 63–81.

Sherman, L. and Berk, R. (1984) The specific deterrent effects of arrest for domestic assault, *American Sociological Review,* 49(2): 261–72.

Sim, J., Scraton, P. and Gordon, P. (1987) Introduction. In P. Scraton (ed.) *Law, Order and the Authoritarian State.* Milton Keynes: Open University Press.

Smart, C. (1989) *Feminism and the Power of the Law.* London: Routledge.

Smith, D. and Gray, J. (1983) *Police and People in London.* London: Policy Studies Institute.

Smith, L. J. F. (1989a) *Domestic Violence.* London: HMSO.

Smith, L. J. F. (1989b) *Concerns about Rape.* London: HMSO.

Stanko, E. A. (1985) *Intimate Intrusions.* London: Unwin Hyman.

Stanko, E. A. (1987) Typical violence, normal precaution: men, women and interpersonal violence in England, Wales, Scotland and the USA. In J. Hanmer and M. Maynard (eds) *Women, Violence and Social Control.* London: Macmillan.

Stanko, E. A. (1988) Hidden violence to women. In M. Maguire and J. Pointing (eds) *Victims of Crime: A New Deal?* Milton Keynes: Open University Press.

Stanko, E. (1990) *Everyday Violence.* London: Pandora.

Zoomer, O. (1989) Policing woman beating in the Netherlands. In J. Hanmer, J. Radford and E. A. Stanko (eds) *Women, Policing and Male Violence.* London: Routledge.

6

Contradictions and compromises: the impact of the Children Act on women and children's safety

Marianne Hester and Lorraine Radford

This chapter examines recent and contradictory developments which have taken place in Britain with regard to women, violence from known men and child contact. That is, how legislation and professional practice in relation to domestic violence – seeking to protect women against violence from male partners – is being undermined through the impact of the Children Act (1989), which focuses on contact between children and parents after parents separate or divorce. On the one hand there has been increasing recognition by the state, in terms of legislation and law enforcement, of the need for intervention where men are being violent to female partners. This has resulted in the, albeit limited, development and growth of some positive approaches to facilitating women's safety. Since the late 1980s the police in particular have claimed to be changing their attitudes and have introduced some useful initiatives. On the other hand, the new legislation on child care, which also concerns separating parents and their children, the Children Act, has tended to affect women's safety negatively. It is also, in some related ways, negatively affecting the safety of children. Specifically, professionals working in this area of family law are misinterpreting child welfare in contact cases. A child's 'right to know' a parent and to have contact with him or her is taking precedence over considerations for the mother's safety as well as the child's safety and well-being through contact with the violent father.

A central concern is the way violence from men to female partners, and the impact of such violence on any children they may have, is excluded from considerations regarding the future of the children. For example, domestic violence is no longer seen as a private domestic but a criminal matter. By contrast in child care law almost the opposite has taken place, and domestic violence is seen as an entirely separate and private matter between parents with no implications for the children.

The chapter begins by looking at the changes in state responses to domestic violence and the ideologically loaded notion of the 'protection' of women during the past couple of decades, and then goes on to discuss the problems and contradictions arising from the impact of the Children Act. It is largely based on findings from current research into domestic violence and child contact arrangements in Britain and Denmark,[1] which examines the process by which the nature of children's contact with parents is negotiated after the parents separate in circumstances with a history of domestic violence.[2]

The development of the state response to women in domestic violence situations

In the context of this chapter the term 'state' is used restrictively to refer primarily to the legislature, the judiciary and the police.[3] Differences in interpretation of the law may arise between legislators, judges and law enforcers. Judges have been especially conservative in their application of domestic violence legislation (see Dobash and Dobash 1992: 186–7), although there are noticeable rifts in precedent and judicial thinking in cases involving domestic violence and child contact. Also, the police do not act as a homogenous body; while national reports and guidelines may be issued, local police forces and even separate ranks may interpret and act on policy and guidelines in different ways (Stanko 1989). There has been a tendency by the police to take more seriously domestic violence disputes where there are children, and to intervene even less when the woman concerned has no children (or none living with her); (Hanmer 1989: 99).

In Britain the state response to domestic violence can be seen to have gone through a number of phases in recent decades.[4] Activities and concerns emerged in the 1970s, continuing at a more minimal level during the early and mid-1980s, with an increase in activity from the late 1980s. Pressure by feminists has played an important and consistent role throughout.

The issue of domestic violence was placed on the public agenda during the early 1970s, with the establishment of women's refuges and the development of a national Women's Aid refuge movement.[5] The refuge movement highlighted the existence and widespread nature of domestic violence. It effectively challenged the generally accepted view that abuse from a male partner was merely 'a domestic dispute', a private matter between the perpetrator and the woman he was battering or abusing in some other way (Hanmer 1977; Rose 1978; Sutton 1978). Pressure from refuges and other women's groups resulted in the setting up of a Government Select Committee on Violence in Marriage to examine the many areas where the state's response to domestic violence needed radical improvement, specifically the areas of housing, economic and social support, reform of the law and law enforcement. Amongst other issues, the committee's 1975 report noted the problem of police attitudes towards domestic violence, and their general lack of intervention in such disputes at the time (Edwards 1989). There was evidence of tension within the police force between views of domestic violence as either a 'private' and civil matter or as a criminal matter, with some attempts being made to move towards the latter approach. For example the London Metropolitan Police Department reported that:

> Whereas it is a general principle of police practice not to intervene in a situation which existed or had existed between husband and wife in the course of which the wife had suffered some personal attack, any assault upon a wife by her husband which amounted to physical injury of a serious nature is a criminal offence which it is the duty of the police to follow up and prosecute.
>
> (quoted in Edwards 1989: 93)

It is necessary of course to question exactly what was meant here by 'physical injury of a serious nature' and highlight that domestic violence was being seen purely in terms of *physical* attack at that time.

Overall, the Committee's report did suggest some positive recommendations towards state protection for women subject to violence from male partners. These ranged from adequate refuge provision to social security benefits and housing provision. The committee also recommended that the police should review their policies and approach to domestic violence and issue regular guidance:

> Special instructions about this difficult and delicate subject should be given to all new recruits, and regular written guidance should be issued by the Chief Constable in the form of advisory leaflets.
>
> (quoted in Edwards 1989: 132)

Few of these recommendations were implemented, and the Select Committee had virtually no direct effect on the improvement of responses to and services for women. Combined with pressure from the refuge movement, however, it did result in limited legislation and policy changes geared to improving women's safety and welfare rights. Of particular importance was the Domestic Violence and Matrimonial Proceedings Act (1976) placed before Parliament as a private members bill – that is, not as a government priority. Barron (1990: 15) points out that while it provided some important redress it had serious limitations, including 'that no expenditure of public money be required for its enforcement, and that it should be straightforward and non-contentious in order to ensure rapid progress through Parliament'. Even so, the new Act did make a number of important changes to the law on domestic violence. It introduced emergency non-molestation measures and exclusion orders for both married and cohabiting couples. It also gave the police power to arrest a man who broke the non-molestation injunction, a significant breakthrough in terms of potential protection for women but one that until recently has hardly been used in practice (Barron 1990: 16).[6] As indicated earlier, the judges have on the whole tended to interpret domestic violence legislation conservatively, and in this case the courts immediately challenged both the exclusion order and the power of arrest attached to such orders. Through a series of Court of Appeal and House of Lords decisions the judiciary rapidly whittled away the scope of the legislation to allow women merely Band-Aid relief from abuse. The challenge was based partly on a patriarchal concern with men's right to *their* homes, as one judge commented:

> I find it difficult to believe that it could ever be fair, save in most exceptional circumstances to keep a man out of HIS flat or house for more than a few months.
>
> (quoted in Dobash and Dobash 1992: 187)

The judiciary also felt that the power of arrest should not be seen as a 'routine measure', especially if used to provide long term protection. In addition exclusion orders have been difficult to get, they are temporary, and of limited value (*Richards v. Richards 1983*; Hanmer 1989: 92; Law Commission 1989; Hester and Radford 1992: 61–2). As a result of much criticism in this area there are, however, changes being proposed by the Law Commission to both non-molestation and exclusion orders which aim to tackle some of these problems as well as widening the scope of the present legislation. As Hague and Malos point out, however, the changes will still depend on implementation by the judiciary, and 'unless the judiciary and the rest of the legal system take on board the spirit of the legislation' (1993: 98) change will not go far.

Despite the legislative changes there was little shift in police practice or policy until the late 1980s.[7] Research carried out during the mid-1980s showed the continued reluctance of police officers to take domestic violence seriously or to intervene in 'domestic disputes' (Radford 1987; Edwards 1989). Edwards has pointed out that the problem was both one of attitude and of frustration at the difficulty of making meaningful interventions. In a study of police attitudes to domestic violence in London and southeast England it was found, for instance, that:

> Spousal violence, where assault occasioning actual bodily harm was apparent, was considered a private matter, and it was expected that the complainant would in any event withdraw her allegation.
>
> (Edwards 1989: 100)

In other words, the police still regarded violence from men to their female partners as merely 'domestics'. There was little understanding of the difficulties women face in leaving violent men. While the police were often faced with similar problems of complainants withdrawing their complaints in other cases of assault, they still viewed domestic violence situations as different and 'boring' by comparison (Edwards 1989: 102).

Continued criticism of police practice, mainly from feminists (Radford 1987), did however lead to a reassessment and change of approach by the police, and by the London Metropolitan police in particular. A report was produced in 1986, and statements and guidelines issued during the next few years took a more serious attitude to domestic violence, defining it as a criminal act more directly analogous to an assault which occurs in the street (Edwards 1989: 199). An especially important new development was the establishment of police domestic violence units. The first was set up in London in 1987, and by 1989 further units were established in West York-shire, Manchester and Birmingham, staffed largely by female officers and with a remit to respond sensitively and provide support for women who have experienced domestic violence (Hanmer 1989; Home Affairs Committee 1993: xi). It should also be recognized that the setting up of these units occurred in the context of the need by the police to respond to criticism of their handling of the uprisings in the inner cities during 1981 and 1985. It is interesting to note that the early units were based in areas with large black communities subject to coercive policing. Black feminists have consequently been particularly sceptical about domestic violence units (Mama 1989; Southall Black Sisters quoted in Home Affairs Committee 1993).

While the late 1980s saw a reawakening of the state response to domes-tic violence, this developed into an 'explosion of public interest' during the early 1990s, this time 'involving much greater receptivity, indeed activity, by various state institutions' (Morley 1993: 2). There have, for example, been a number of far-reaching inquiries by the government and policy makers; government funding of experimental projects dealing with 'family violence and crime'; the setting up of interagency working groups which include the police; and programmes for batterers as well as the recommendations regard-ing non-molestation orders and ousters already mentioned.

In 1990 the Home Office issued a circular (Circular 60/1990) to all police forces in the country in a concerted attempt to improve responses, particularly

> to ensure that all police officers involved in the investigation of cases of domestic violence regard as their overriding priority the protection of the victim and the apprehension of the offender.
>
> (quoted in Home Affairs Committee 1993)

Evidence suggests that there has been some change, albeit patchy across the country (Hague and Malos 1993: 78–83). The most discernable change has been the setting up of domestic violence units. In London, 62 of the 69 Metropolitan Police Divisions now have domestic violence units, and of the 42 local police forces in the rest of England and Wales, 20 have similar units (Home Affairs Committee 1993: xi). These units offer a service – at times excellent but also limited – for women who have been subject to domestic violence. Some have proven dangerous for the women concerned, however. For example, Vanda Patel was left alone with her violent husband in Stoke Newington police station to 'sort things out' and was subsequently stabbed to death by him (Morley and Mullender 1994).

Despite the limited and uneven progress there has been an increasingly vocalized acceptance of women's right to police protection from violent male partners. Summarizing these changes, the recent report from the government appointed Home Affairs Committee concludes that, while there was some change during the 1970s and 1980s with regard to public awareness and legislation, 'the extent of the problem, far from abating, is perhaps only now beginning to be revealed' (1993: v).

In sum, the state's approach to domestic violence has been primarily of the Band-Aid variety with an emphasis on encouraging short term support. During the 1970s there was a focus on the civil law, but with little interest in how the legislation worked in practice or how it was enforced, with the parallel problem of the judiciary whittling away the scope of the legislation towards temporary injunctions, and non-enforcement by the police through no-criming of domestic violence. The 1980s were largely concerned with how to tackle these problems. Despite the setting up of multiagency forums which include representatives from welfare agencies, the so-called private family law side of state protection of women from domestic violence has however, been largely ignored.

The Children Act and domestic violence

The Children Act was enacted in 1989 and came into force in October 1991. It is a part of the increasing emphasis on so-called family values involving sanctity of the heterosexual nuclear family with an onus on individual responsibility, and the preference for non-intervention which has exemplified the philosophy of the Conservative government in Britain since 1979.

The Act also constitutes an important consolidation exercise, combining both private and public law: private law which specifies the responsibilities parents have in relation to their children, including if they separate or divorce; public law which covers local authority responsibilities for children in need of protection. The Act 'tries to create a uniform and coherent framework for strands in child welfare law which have developed largely independently of each other over some hundreds of years' (Eekelaar and Dingwall 1990: 1). Ironically, given its focus on the protection and well-being of children, the Act is undermining the trend towards state intervention in domestic violence situations. It marks a shift away from protection of women, supposedly towards bettering the welfare of children. In practice this provides greater rights for fathers and facilitates access to female ex-partners by those men who are violent.

The new Act was shaped by a variety of factors including government reviews of the care and custody of children during the 1980s,[8] enquiries into problems relating to child protection in a number of instances where children had died despite social services involvement,[9] and pressure from fathers' rights lobbies for greater access to children (Smart 1989; Eekelaar and Dingwall 1990; Harne and Radford 1994). Within the context of this chapter it is the private law aspect of the Children Act, concerning parents and their children, which is the most important.

The Act has introduced the notion of 'parental responsibility', with married parents both having automatic responsibility for their children. Lone mothers automatically have parental responsibility and unmarried fathers can apply to have parental responsibility. This replaced the former notions of joint and sole custody. In a sense the Act has formalized the shift towards joint custody (with care and control usually to the mother) which was beginning to be discerned by the late 1980s. But there are also distinct differences in that parental responsibility may be awarded to others apart from the biological parents, such as stepfathers or grandparents. Despite the focus on the heterosexual nuclear family the Act allows parental responsibility to be shared by more than two people, and has the capacity to recognize a diversity of family forms (see also Harne and Radford, 1994). A further distinction from earlier legislation is that each holder of parental responsibility can exercise it without consulting the other holder, being able to make decisions about all aspects of the child's welfare and upbringing, including issues like schooling. Parental responsibility is couched in terms of *parents'* responsibilities and duties to their children, rather than as state endowed rights of parents. Eekelaar and Dingwall point out that the use of the term 'responsibility'

> needs to be seen in the context of the general Conservative belief in the desirability of privatizing the responsibility for the care of dependent individuals, including children, and the diminution of any role for the state.
>
> (1990: 21)

Thus the term 'parental responsibility' reflects the current Conservative ideals of individual responsibility and non-intervention. In this framework, parents are deemed responsible individuals who can, between themselves, come to adequate and sensible decisions about their children – even when they are separated by the bitterness of marital breakdown.

Guidance published on the Children Act makes it clear that central to the Act is the view that it is beneficial for children to have contact with both their (biological) parents in the event of divorce, family breakdown or the child going into care. The court can specify where the child will live (residence order), require that the other parent has contact with the child (contact order), disallow certain aspects of parental responsibility (prohibited steps order), or suggest how specific areas of parental responsibility should be carried out (specific issue order). However the courts are, within the remit of the Act, reluctant to make such orders, will only make them when asked, and only if it is considered 'in the best interests of the child' and only if it is preferable to making no order at all. We have found in our interviews with solicitors that since the Children Act courts are indeed less likely to make any orders, and there is less likelihood of a specified order stating when and how contact should take place. Overall, and in the government's spirit of *laissez-faire*, the legislation thus aims to reduce legal involvement in parents' care of their children post-separation. There is also expectation that less reliance on formal court intervention, and the availability of conciliation/mediation for those parents who have difficulty coming to agreement, will reduce conflict between ex-partners during separation/divorce and the negotiation of child contact arrangements (Hester and Radford 1992: 58).

It is worrying that, despite the increasingly well-documented links between child abuse and domestic violence, and links between women's and children's welfare, nowhere does the Children Act refer to circumstances of domestic violence, and there appears to have been no debate about this issue during the development of the legislation (DHSS 1985). Reference could have been made to domestic violence with respect to both child protection (the public law aspect) and to the separation/divorce of parents (the private law aspect). While there has never been a comprehensive incidence study of domestic violence in the UK, it has been estimated that as many as one in three marriages that end in divorce may involve domestic violence (Borkowski *et al.* 1983). A recent survey in London suggests that 1 in 10 women in the borough of Islington are subject to domestic violence (Home Affairs Committee 1993: vii; Mooney 1994). The police figures are of course much lower as they are restricted to reported incidents.[10] Domestic violence is therefore, or should be, a serious consideration when parents separate or divorce. Clearly the period of separation or divorce is likely to be one of potential conflict and tension for parents and their children. In situations involving domestic violence there is even more likelihood of conflict between the parents. Yet as indicated, a basic tenet of the Children Act is that parents are able to negotiate a reasoned outcome for their children's future. A report from the voluntary sector organization Victim Support has pointed out that while such an approach may in general be beneficial 'it is likely that problems will continue to occur when it is applied to families where domestic violence has been a chronic feature' (1992: 57). Furthermore, 'it is an approach that can *make the plight of the abused woman even worse*' (p. 57, our emphasis). The government's Home Affairs Committee Report on domestic violence also concedes that, while appreciating that the Children Act was framed on the basis of reasonable behaviour by parents even when they separate, 'clearly those who perpetrate domestic abuse cannot be expected necessarily to behave in this reasonable way' (1993: xli).

Our research suggests that domestic violence is not generally taken into account when arrangements for children's contact with parents post-separation are made (Hester *et al.* 1994). Furthermore, we have evidence from solicitors that since the implementation of the Act, with its emphasis on contact for children with both parents, ousters and exclusion orders have been even more difficult for women to obtain. Women unaware of the procedural changes have also been surprised where contact arrangements for the children *vis-à-vis* fathers have been tied in with such applications. This has resulted in women having to make very rushed and ill-considered decisions about contact issues.

The notion of parental responsibility suggests greater equality between parents in relation to decisions about their children's lives and welfare. Parental responsibility suggests 'shared parenting', and greater involvement by men in child care which many women, including some feminists, have argued for (Smart 1989). But 'parental responsibility' does not take into account the inequalities and power differences between men and women which undermine this, and in particular the profound inequality and assertion of power by violent men. Publicity surrounding the Children Act to the effect that fathers now have more 'rights' (although that is not the terminology of the legislation) has led to fathers wanting to take up these 'rights'. Professionals surveyed in our study claimed that many more fathers, including perpetrators of domestic violence (and child abuse), are seeking residence and/or contact (if married) than sought custody and/or access in the past. Unmarried fathers are also increasingly applying for parental responsibility and/or contact with their children. While there does seem to have been a worrying decrease in cases going through the courts, the number of contact cases being seen by solicitors and in-court conciliation/mediation have increased.

The importance attached to continued contact causes innumerable safety problems for women and their children. Our study reveals that professionals often perceive women to be obstructive in relation to children's contact with fathers, but in actual fact women will generally try very hard to establish contact by fathers with their children, and usually only attempt to restrict or stop it if they feel the children's, and to a lesser extent, their own, safety is being compromised. While professionals may see women's obstruction and hostility as a main problem in contact cases, we are finding that it is the lack of safety provisions for children in relation to contact that constitutes the underlying problem.[11]

Mothers, violence from fathers and legislation about children

Three key issues concerning parents, children and domestic violence are important to discuss here:

- ideologies of 'mothering' and 'fathering' and their influence on recent legislation and state responses;
- the links between domestic violence and the abuse of children;
- the fact that violence does not necessarily stop when the parents separate, and thus arrangements made post-separation or divorce have important implications for the safety of both women and children.

The links between domestic violence and women as mothers are important. Women's own experience and understanding of violence to themselves is profoundly influenced by their work as mothers and carers. Becoming and being mothers may influence both the onset of violence and women's decisions about terminating the relationship. On the one hand, many women experience systematic violence when they are pregnant or the children are small, at a time when they are likely to be more emotionally and economically dependent on their husbands (Pahl 1985; Hester and Radford 1991). On the other hand, we have found that it is often 'for the sake of the children' that women make decisions about leaving a violent partner, or staying in the relationship. Women may leave when they feel the children are being affected by the violence to themselves, either directly or indirectly. Or they may be reluctant to leave because they feel the financial and material circumstances for the children seem advantageous if they stay rather than leave and become lone parents (see also Christensen 1984; Pahl 1985: 50).

Prior to the Children Act, mothers rather than fathers tended to gain custody, care and control of children upon separation or divorce. This 'maternal preference' was based on the assumption that mothers are more likely to be the main carers of children than fathers. Cases of contested custody were rare. However, if allegations were made by fathers about a mother's poor parenting skills, her competence in mothering could be scrutinized extensively. Fathers who merely expressed an interest in children have, on the other hand almost automatically been designated 'good parents'. This has had some unfortunate and problematic repercussions in domestic violence cases where the impact of ongoing violence on a woman's health and well-being, and her attempt to cope in a relationship with a violent man by using tranquillizers or alcohol have been used against her as evidence of her inability to care properly for her children. We have found that men have used this argument successfully against their ex-wives/partners in disputes over children. We have also found that a woman's positive attempts to escape from a violent man by moving to a refuge may on occasion also be used against her, that a refuge is not seen as suitable accommodation for children. In these ways women's behaviour and mothering is the focus rather than men's violence. Consequently men's violent behaviour is obscured.

Where fathers are seeking contact with their children, their ability to care tends not to be examined in the same detail. Some of the men who are violent to their female partners may at times be caring fathers, but a significant proportion may not be (Johnston 1992). The effect of their violence on the children also needs to be considered, as does the possible continuation of violence after the women chose to end the relationship.

A variety of studies have shown that there are clear links between domestic violence and abuse of children. A number of different studies have indicated physical abuse of children in anywhere between 30 to 70 per cent of domestic violence cases (Straus *et al.* 1980; Bowker *et al.* 1989; Christensen 1990). In Britain it has been estimated by Women's Aid that 'between 20–33 per cent of the children coming to refuges are physically and/or sexually abused by the mother's husband or cohabitee' (Hanmer 1989: 92). It may also be argued that most if not all children living in circumstances of domestic violence are affected in some way through exposure to the 'passive mental maltreatment' of witnessing violence against their mothers (Christensen 1990). Children may be fearful of seeing their father as a consequence. Some children may still want to see the abusive parent, but also want to feel safe. Some children may not want to see the violent father, however, and this should also be accepted. Johnston (1992), from her study in the US, proposes that if children are severely distressed by visits to the abusive parent, or refuses to visit him, visitation should be suspended and reassessed.

We are finding that professionals appear to be creating certain myths in their application of the Children Act. The Act provides a 'welfare checklist' of various factors to consider in order to determine what outcome is in the child's 'best interest'.[12] But professionals are tending to (mis)interpret 'in the best interests of the child' as meaning a child *always* having contact with both parents, even though the Act says this is not the only factor to consider. As a result of professionals' focus on contact, children are being made to have direct contact with the abusive parent even if the child expresses extreme stress. In one recent instance from our research, the child (a girl aged six) was extremely distressed when faced with visiting her father. The social worker attached to the case did not suspend contact while investigating the distress, and advised the mother that if the contact stopped she might lose the child. The social worker organized psychiatric help for the mother on the basis that the mother was the source of the child's fears. It transpired later that the child was being physically abused by the father during contact visits.

In another instance, where the mother was worried that the father's use of drugs would detrimentally affect the child, the court welfare officer recommended that there should none the less be direct contact by the child with the father. The court, however, on the basis of the welfare checklist, decided that it was in the best interests of the child not to have direct contact with the father.

As indicated, violence does not necessarily stop on separation. Our own and other research has shown that the violent male ex-partner will often use situations where he is in contact with his female ex-partner to continue his violence and attempts to exercise control over her. He may indeed seek to create such situations. Contact with the children can be used in this way. It is clear from our research that men are often more interested in gaining access to their ex-partners through the children than they are in seeing the children themselves. Johnston has also pointed out how contact with the children may place women 'at higher risk for continuing abuse' (1992: sec. I, 68). In a recent survey by Women's Aid Federation England (WAFE), it has similarly been found that '50 per cent of the refuges surveyed had evidence that women had been further abused after contact with their ex-partners made necessary by the [Children] Act' (Hague and Malos 1993: 152).

Despite this evidence, men's violence to their female partners has seldom been taken into account in judicial settlements of child contact arrangements post-separation. This is largely because of the belief that any history of 'parental conflict' can and should be set aside from the consideration of the child's current welfare.[13] Clearly this is problematic where the safety of both women and children are concerned.

Domestic violence, child contact and professionals: the case of mediation

To give an example of the role of professionals in contact arrangements, in-court and voluntary sector mediation will be briefly examined. Especially court welfare officers but also voluntary sector mediators are playing an increasingly central role in the process of negotiating contact in cases involving domestic violence.

Before the Children Act, and even more so since it was enacted, there has been an increasing trend in Britain (as in many other western countries) towards the private ordering of child care or related matters on separation or divorce of the parents. This has placed a greater onus on the use of both in-court and voluntary sector conciliation/mediation. In-court conciliation/mediation is carried out by Family Court Welfare Officers, appointed from the probation service, and out-of-court conciliation/mediation is carried out primarily by the Family Mediation Association and National Family Mediation. There tend to be differences in practice between court welfare officers and out-of-court mediators. The role of the mediator, as described by Roberts (1988: 8), is to facilitate communication and the settling of disputes between the ex-partners with the mediator acting as an 'auxiliary' to the parties. Our research shows that court welfare officers in particular may take less of an 'auxiliary' and more of an interventionist role (see also Roberts 1988; James and Hay 1993). There appears to be little control over the methods employed by court welfare officers to bring about 'agreement', and in many of the cases we have looked at, 'agreement' has been coerced. Even so, court welfare officers and out-of-court mediators are at times the same individuals, working in both sectors.

Unlike the United States, in Britain there has been little published debate amongst conciliation/mediation professionals about the impact of domestic violence on the private ordering of child care arrangements.[14] Our research indicates that there is a lack of knowledge about domestic violence and as a consequence inconsistencies in relation to safe practice by many of the professionals involved. Overall there is a trend to minimize both the existence of violence and the effect this might have on clients. These factors undermine the protection of women and children attempting to escape domestic violence (Hester and Pearson 1993).

In many respects the way mediators and court welfare officers (as well as other relevant professionals such as solicitors) ignore and minimize the impact of domestic violence is reminiscent of the attitudes and practice of the police during the 1970s and 80s. Those we have interviewed were inclined to see domestic violence as a private matter, not understanding the power dynamics involved, the detrimental effects of the past history and current threat of violence on women's ability to negotiate with the violent ex-partner. They also had minimal understanding of the difficulties women generally face when leaving violent men. Moreover they often blamed women themselves for the violence, making comments to the effect that 'there must be something in it, women must have been provocative' if men 'have' to hit them. The critical attention which has prompted some change in police practice needs to be extended to all professional groups which are in a position to affect women's safety positively or negatively.

In our study, none of the court welfare officers or voluntary sector mediators interviewed knew with any certainty whether or not their clients had been or were in a violent relationship. They relied mainly on the client's solicitor (if there was one) to tell them about any history of violence, or on the women themselves to mention it during mediation with the expartners. Some felt they could at times deduce that violence had occurred by the way the expartners interacted. However, very few of those interviewed in Britain had any specific mechanism by which to identify that there was previous (or current) violence. This lack of knowledge was compounded by the tendency to ignore or not examine clients' histories prior to conciliation/mediation. Many had been influenced by the American mediator John Haynes's (1993) work, and mentioned how this had led them to focus only on the clients' current and future situations but not on their past.

Of particular concern was the comment made by one court welfare officer that the identification of violence has been made *'even more difficult'* since the Children Act, as there is no longer a 'culture of affidavit' which might indicate a history of domestic violence. Instead there is now 'simply the statement of arrangements' for child contact, which is presented in a more conciliatory manner. This is compounded by solicitors committed to 'agreement' who withhold information on past abuse.

Women may avoid out-of-court mediation if they do not feel safe, and some are counselled or screened out of this process by the mediation service concerned. Despite in-court conciliation/mediation being voluntary, women may feel unable to refuse or avoid it. They may therefore end up being told by the out-of-court service that mediation is inappropriate in their case, only to find that they end up with their violent ex-partner in in-court conciliation/mediation. Our research suggests that compulsory attendance is becoming the norm, albeit unofficially, where ex-partners find it difficult to agree. As one court welfare officer commented: 'The parties actually don't realize it's voluntary. They are told they should attend a meeting before they go to court'. Women whom we interviewed also told of the pressure they felt under to attend at least in-court conciliation/mediation, lest they should otherwise be seen as 'uncooperative' by court officials and judges. Once forced into a meeting, many women in our study felt compelled to agree to contact arrangements which put their own safety at risk.

Conclusion

In recent years there has been a noticeable change in state policies on domestic violence, especially with respect to police policy and practice. However steps towards intervention in the criminal law are being undermined by the implementation of the Children Act, which does not take domestic violence into account, and where the supposed focus on children's welfare – in practice defined as contact with the absent (male) parent – operates to undermine women and children's (limited) safety. This latter trend is compounded by both professionals' lack of awareness and the absence of practical guidelines regarding domestic violence. If the gains made in the arena of the criminalization of domestic violence are not to be further undermined there needs to be a concerted change in relation to policy and practice of professionals concerned with child contact, especially a recognition that domestic violence affects both women and children, and that violence by men against women, however 'private', is criminal behaviour.

Acknowledgement

Thanks to Jill Radford for comments on an earlier draft.

Notes

1 The research, entitled Domestic Violence and Child Contact Arrangements in Britain and Denmark and completed in 1995, has been carried out by Marianne Hester, Lorraine Radford, Julie Humphries, Chris Pearson, Khalida Qaiser and Kandy-Sue Woodfield (in Britain), Maja Føgh and Anne-Mette Kruse (in Denmark). It has been funded by the Joseph Rowntree Foundation, the Nuffield Foundation, the British Council, the University of Aarhus and the Danish Academy of Research. The information received and views expressed in this chapter are, however, those of the authors and not necessarily those of the funding bodies.

   The research involves multiple interviews with 100 women (53 in Britain and 26 in Denmark), and interviews with 75 professionals (83 in Britain and 22 in Denmark) engaged in the process of negotiating child contact: voluntary sector mediators, court welfare officers, solicitors and refuge workers in Britain and equivalent professionals and advisers in Denmark.

   Two central concerns are the safety of women who have experienced violence from male ex-partners, and the safety and welfare of their children.

2 Domestic violence is defined here as ongoing physical, sexual, psychological and/or verbal abuse from the male to the female partner. The vast majority of incidents of domestic violence involve violence from the male to the female partner (see Dobash and Dobash 1992). This is what we focus on here.

3 It should be noted that where legislation and the legal machinery are concerned, Britain is divided into three separate areas: England and Wales, Scotland, and the so-called six counties of Northern Ireland. There are some variations in the laws and legislature between these areas. This article focuses specifically on the situation in England and Wales, which is also the area covered by the major research project on which the article is based.

4 There have also been debates and state responses prior to the 1970s. In the early nineteenth century, for example, there were debates about 'domestic brutality' or 'cruelty', and feminist pressure ensured the enactment of the Married Women's Property Act in the late nineteenth century. See also discussion of 'rough music' – local responses to domestic violence in earlier centuries (Hester 1992).

5 Women's Aid is the main national umbrella group for refuges in Britain and is based on the feminist principles of collectivism, mutual support and self-help.

Women's Aid is now organized as four separate regional affiliations: Women's Aid Federation England, Welsh Women's Aid, Scottish Women's Aid, and Northern Ireland Women's Aid. See Hague and Malos (1993) for details of Women's Aid, especially Women's Aid Federation England (WAFE).

6 As pointed out earlier, we are talking here about the laws and their implementation as applies in England and Wales. There are slight variations with respect to Scotland. Dobash and Dobash (1992) discuss these differences (and provide comparisons with the US). The situation is also different in the so-called six counties of Northern Ireland (see Casey 1987).

7 In England and Wales there are two main types of courts dealing with matrimonial cases: county courts, which deal largely with civil cases, divorce and injunctions, and the magistrates' courts which deal largely with less complex matrimonial cases. The Domestic Violence and Matrimonial Proceedings Act (1976) was to be implemented by the former, and another act, the Domestic Proceedings and Magistrates' Courts Act (1978) brought in similar, albeit even more limited, powers of protection for women through the more accessible magistrates' courts.

8 These reviews include the report by the Social Services Select Committee of the House of Commons leading to a separate *Review of Child Care Law* (1985); and a review by the Law Commission of the legal position of children in private disputes about their care and custody (see Eekelaar and Dingwall 1990: 1).

9 These included in particular reports into the death of Jasmine Beckford (report in 1985), and the way allegations of sexual abuse were handled in Cleveland (report in 1988), and to a lesser extent reports into the deaths of Heidi Koseda (1985), Tyra Henry (1985) and Kimberley Carlile (1985) (See Eekelaar and Dingwall 1990: 1–2).

10 Figures of domestic violence incidents recorded by the police in Islington, London suggests that 1 in 30 women 'was known to the police to be a victim of domestic violence' (Home Affairs Committee 1993: p. vii).

11 If the mother resists contact by the father the court may order a court officer or the police to take the child to the other parent, with the right to enter premises to search and use force if the child is believed to be there. We have already come across an instance of this with respect to a woman staying in a refuge so as to be safe from her violent ex-partner. The police entered the refuge and took the child. Prior to the Children Act breach of access was also an offence, for example *C v. C* (1990) *Fam Law* 220, where the mother was imprisoned for seven days for disobeying the access order to the husband.

12 The welfare checklist consists of the following:
That the courts must have regard, in particular, to

(a) the ascertainable wishes and feelings of the child concerned (considered in light of his [*sic*] age and understanding);
(b) his physical, emotional and educational needs;
(c) the likely effect on him of any changes in his circumstances;
(d) his age, sex, background and any characteristics of his which the court considers relevant;
(e) any harm which he has suffered or is at risk of suffering;
(f) how capable each of his parents, and any other person in relation to whom the court considers the question to be relevant, is of meeting his needs;
(g) the range of powers available to the court under this Act in the proceedings in question.

(Extract from Children Act 1989 section 1(3))

13 *B v. B* (1971) 3 All ER 682; *M v. M* (1973) 2 All ER 281 (quoted in Hester and Radford 1992: 61). There are some exceptions, for example *M v. M*, *The Times*, 22 February 1990, CA.

14 In the US many have reached the conclusion that mediation in domestic violence situations is likely to be disastrous, leaving women and children who have been abused in danger of further violence (Hart 1990; Grillo 1991). Others argue that if, but only if, mediators are trained to understand fully the nature and dynamics of domestic violence, and if mediation policy and practice reflect the needs of these cases, then mediated outcomes may be positive (Magana and Taylor 1993).

In Britain Roberts (1988), is one of the few to mention domestic violence, although the August 1993 issue of *Family Mediation* is devoted to the issue of domestic violence in an attempt to initiate debate (see also Mullender and Morley 1994).

References

Barron, J. (1990) *Not Worth the Paper . . .? The Effectiveness of Legal Protection for Women and Children Experiencing Domestic Violence.* Bristol: Women's Aid Federation England.

Borkowski, M., Murch, M. and Walker, V. (1983) *Marital Violence: the Community Response.* London: Tavistock.

Bowker, L., Arbitell, M. and McFerron, J. R. (1989) On the relationship between wife beating and child abuse. In K. Yllo and M. Bograd (eds) *Feminist Perspectives on Wife Abuse.* London: Sage.

Casey, M. (1987) *Domestic Violence: the Women's Perspective.* Dublin: Women's Aid.

Christensen, E. (1984) *Vold Ties Ikke Ihjel.* Copenhagen: Nyt Nordisk Forlag.

Christensen, E. (1990) Children's living conditions. An investigation into disregard of care in relation to children and teenagers in families of wife maltreatment, *Nordisk Psychologi*, 42, Monograph No. 31.

Department of Health (1989) *Children Act.* London: HMSO.

Department of Health and Social Services (DHSS) (1985) *Review of Child Care Law.* London: HMSO.

Dobash, R. E. and Dobash, R. P. (1992) *Women, Violence and Social Change.* London: Routledge.

Edwards, S. (1989) *Policing 'Domestic Violence'.* London: Sage.

Eekelaar, J. and Dingwall, R. (1990) *The Reform of Child Care Law, a Practical Guide to the Children Act 1989.* London: Routledge.

Grillo, T. (1991) The mediation alternative: process dangers for women, *The Yale Law Journal*, 100: 1545–610.

Hague, G. and Malos, E. (1993) *Domestic Violence, Action for Change.* London: New Clarion Press.

Hanmer, J. (1977) Community action, women's aid and the women's liberation movement. In M. Mayo (ed.) *Women in the Community.* London: Routledge.

Hanmer, J. (1989) Women and policing in Britain. In J. Hanmer, J. Radford and E. A. Stanko (eds) *Women, Policing and Male Violence.* London: Routledge.

Harne, L. and Radford, J. (1994) Reinstating patriarchy: the politics of the family and the new legislation. In A. Mullender and B. Morley (eds) *Children Living with Domestic Violence.* London: Birch and Whiting.

Hart, B. (1990) The further endangerment of battered women and children in custody mediation, *Mediation Quarterly*, 7(3): 317–29.

Haynes, J. (1993) *Alternative Dispute Resolution: The Fundamentals of Family Mediation*. Horsmonden: Old Bailey Press.

Hester, M. (1992) *Lewd Women and Wicked Witches: The Dynamics of Male Domination*. London: Routledge.

Hester, M., Humphries, J., Pearson, C., Qaiser, K., Radford, L. and Woodfield, K. S. (1994) Domestic violence and child contact. In A. Mullender and B. Morley (eds) *Children Living With Domestic Violence*. London: Birch and Whiting.

Hester, M. and Pearson, C. (1993) Domestic violence and mediation: Some recent research findings, *Family Mediation*, summer: 3–6.

Hester, M. and Radford, L. (1992) Domestic violence and access arrangements for children in Denmark and Britain, *The Journal of Social Welfare and Family Law*, 1: 57–70.

Home Affairs Committee (1991) *Third Report: Domestic Violence*, Vol. I. London: HMSO.

Home Affairs Committee (1993) *Third Report: Domestic Violence*, Vol. II. London: HMSO.

James, A. L. and Hay, W. (1993) *Court Welfare in Action*. Hemel Hempstead: Harvester Wheatsheaf.

Johnston, J. R. (1992) 'High-conflict and violent divorcing families: findings on children's adjustment and proposed guidelines for the resolution of disputed custody and visitation', report of a project. Corte Madera CA: Centre for the Family in Transition.

Law Commission (1989) *Domestic Violence and Occupation of the Matrimonial Home*, Working Paper No. 113. London: HMSO.

Magana, H. A. and Taylor, N. (1993) Child custody mediation and spouse abuse: a descriptive study of protocol, *Family and Conciliation Courts Review*, 31(1): 50–64.

Mama, A. (1989) Violence against black women: gender, race and state response, *Feminist Review*, 32: 30–48.

Mooney, J. (1994) *The Hidden Figure: Domestic Violence in North London*. London: Islington Police and Crime Prevention Unit.

Morley, R. (1993) Recent Responses to Domestic Violence Against Women: a Feminist Critique. In R. Page and J. Baldock (eds) Social Policy Review 5: the Evolving State of Welfare. Canterbury: Social Policy Association.

Morley, R. and Mullender, A. (1994) *Preventing Domestic Violence to Women*, Crime Prevention Unit Series, paper no. 48. London: Police Research Group, Home Office.

Mullender, A. and Morley, B. (eds) (1994) *Children Living with Domestic Violence*. London: Birch and Whiting.

Pahl, J. (1985) *Private Violence and Public Policy*. London: Routledge and Kegan Paul.

Radford, J. (1987) Policing male violence – policing women. In J. Hanmer and M. Maynard (eds) *Women, Violence and Social Control*. London: Macmillan.

Richards v. Richards (1983) 2 All E.R. 807.

Roberts, M. (1988) *Mediation in Family Disputes*. Aldershot: Wildwood House.

Rose, H. (1978) Women's refuges: creating new forms of welfare? In C. Ungerson (ed.) *Women and Social Policy*. London: Macmillan.

Smart, C. (1989) Power and the politics of child custody. In C. Smart and S. Sevenhuijsen (eds) *Child Custody and the Politics of Gender*. London: Routledge.

Stanko, E. A. (1989) Missing the mark? Policing battering. In J. Hanmer, J. Radford and E. A. Stanko (eds) *Women, Policing and Male Violence*. London: Routledge.

Straus, A., Gelles, R. J. and Steinmetz, S. K. (1980) *Violence Behind Closed Doors: Violence in the American Family*. New York: Anchor Books.

Sutton, J. (1978) The growth of the British movement for battered women, *Victimology*, 2(3–4).

Victim Support (1992) *Domestic Violence, Report of a National Inter-Agency Working Party*. London: Victim Support.

7

Unreasonable doubt: the outcomes of rape trials

Sue Lees

Various explanations for why men rape have been put forward by psychologists (see Holmstrom and Burgess 1978; Grubin and Gunn 1990; Scully 1990), and feminists (see Brownmiller 1976) and the way it is condoned by the criminal justice system (see Jeffreys and Radford 1984; Adler 1987; Temkin 1987; Ginsberg and Lerner 1989). Feminists in the 1970s contested the way that rape was defined and set up rape crisis groups to both raise awareness of the political significance of rape and to provide services for women survivors (see London Rape Crisis Centre 1984).[1]

This chapter reports on two more recent research projects, the first carried out with Jeanne Gregory[2] (Lees and Gregory 1993) which traces the attrition process by which rape and indecent assault is progressively decriminalized by the judicial system, and the second in which I took transcripts of rape trials to investigate their shortcomings. Building on the insights of radical feminists such as Susan Brownmiller (1976) who argued that rape was 'nothing more or less than a conscious process of intimidation by which all men keep women in a state of fear', and Liz Kelly (1988) who sees rape as one end of a continuum of abusive male sexuality,[3] I examine the way rape is treated by the criminal justice system where, since the passing of the Sexual Offences (Amendment) Act 1976 (Home Office 1976), in some respects the situation has deteriorated.

Background to the research

There is very little research on the workings of the legal system in the area of violence against women. There are two main obstacles: gaining access to police records, court officials and courts and obtaining funding for the research.

Gaining access requires time, patience and energy. Officials employ a variety of delaying tactics, in the hope that researchers will give up and go away. The research project discussed here took two years to negotiate. Islington Council's Police and Crime Prevention Unit provided us with funding through the Department of the Environment's Inner Cities programme. The Islington Police Committee has been at the forefront of a number of crime prevention research initiatives, beginning with the *Islington Crime Survey*, the first local crime survey to investigate the extent of violence against women (Jones *et al.* 1986). The Police and Crime Prevention Unit reacted positively to our initial proposal. Islington has a high proportion of women councillors, many of whom take an active part in promoting safety for women and their support through the Women's Committee was significant.[4] It was a unique combination of an imaginative Police and Crime Prevention Subcommittee and some central government funding for inner city projects that enabled this research to go ahead, not to mention our persistence!

After an arduous process of negotiation,[5] we gained access to police record forms of rape, attempted rape, buggery and indecent assault (of all cases where the complainant was over 16 years) at two London police stations. With the support of two very helpful women police officers who traced many of the forms for us, we analysed all report forms from September 1988 to September 1990 and traced their attrition, the term used to describe the process by which cases are lost or dropped as they go through the various stages from reporting to conviction. Interviews were also conducted with women who reported rape or sexual assault to the police and with representatives from various local professional agencies and volunteer groups concerned with issues of sexual assault, such as rape crisis, victim support, police child protection teams and the Branch Prosecutor of the Crown Prosecution Service.

A number of changes in the judicial treatment of rape have occurred in the past 20 years mainly in response to the campaigning of groups such as the Rights of Women, the Women's Aid Federation, Women Against Rape and rape crisis groups, and in the light of growing evidence of the inadequacy of the judicial system, as highlighted for example even by Detective Inspector Blair (1985). In 1976 the Sexual Offences (Amendment) Act was passed, aimed at limiting reference to a woman's past sexual history and sexual character, and provided complainants with anonymity in press reports. Under section 2 of this Act the defence is required to apply to the judge for permission to cross-examine the complainant regarding her sexual history or sexual character. It is up to the discretion of the judge whether or not this is allowed.[6] At the same time, in response to public outrage at lenient sentences imposed by a number of judges in rape cases, Lord Chief Justice Lane issued new sentencing guidelines (*R. v. Billam* [1986] 1 All ER 986) and took steps to ensure that such cases would in future be heard only by senior members of the judiciary (see Robertshaw 1994). On the legal front in England and Wales, in 1991 the marital rape exclusion was finally abolished by the Law Lords and rape within marriage is now against the law.[7] Several successful actions for damages in civil courts have also been awarded, the first in 1978. The Criminal Justice Act (1994) has made non-consensual buggery (male rape) a crime for the first time[8] and other changes include the abolition of the corroboration ruling and the end of the defendant's right to silence.

Another significant change is that in 1986 the Crown Prosecution Service (CPS) was created and took over responsibility for the prosecution of criminal cases, a task formerly undertaken by the police. It is the CPS who decide whether a case should have a jury trial. (All cases of rape and attempted rape have a first hearing in the magistrates' court). Between 1985 and 1993 the number of cases not proceeded with after an appearance at the magistrates' court increased threefold from 10 per cent in 1985 to 30 per cent in 1993 (see Home Office Statistics 1993).[9] This means that many women who report rape and want to give evidence are denied the right to do so. The CPS are under pressure to keep costs down and the complainant has no right whatsoever to appeal against their decision if they decide the case should not go forward.

On the other hand the improvement in police treatment of rape victims is probably one of the main reasons why the numbers of women reporting has increased. The catalyst to this change was an explosive episode of the BBC television series of *Police* in 1982 in which police officers were seen in a live investigation of a woman reporting rape. This brought the harsh interrogation techniques of rape complainants to the notice of the public and provided the impetus for the police to reform their procedures. As a result of pressure from the Women's National Commission (1985) following the publication of its report on violence against women (1985), the Home Office issued a circular (1993) calling for new police training inputs on rape and sexual assault, the appointment of more women police surgeons and better facilities for the medical examination of women who had been attacked.[10] The number of women reporting rape and attempted rape trebled, although this is an underestimation of the actual rate as we know most women do not report.

A number of recent population surveys have thrown some light on the 'hidden figure' of unreported rapes. The largest random survey of women was carried out in the US by Diana Russell in 1980.[11] Nine hundred and thirty women were interviewed, *41 per cent had been raped at some time in their lives*. Only 9.5 per cent of the non-marital or attempted rape cases were reported to the police. Overall she found a higher rate of rape the higher the social class.[12] In a survey conducted at Cambridge University, it was found that 1 in 5 of 1,500 students surveyed had been victims of rape or attempted rape and 1 in 9 had been raped. Only 1 in 50 had told the police (BBC TV 1992). A recent survey of 2,000 women at Oxford Brookes University showed that 90 per cent of women who had never been the victim of a sexual assault or rape, thought they would report it to the police, yet only 6 per cent who had been raped reported it (El-Faizy 1994). When asked why they did not report, women said they feared an unsympathetic response from the police and had little faith in the judicial system. It appears therefore that even today the vast majority of women who have been sexually assaulted do not even take the initial step of reporting it to the police. Those who do report are merely the tip of the iceberg and yet this tip is further eroded as the criminal justice system runs its course. This evidence stands in sharp contrast to the rhetoric of the politicians and of the media, who give the impression that more women are coming forward to report sexual attacks and that more men are being convicted and receiving their just deserts in the shape of longer sentences.

The widespread condoning of male violence within the legal system must be seen as a reflection of more general societal views. The attrition rate whereby only a tiny proportion of rape offences results in a conviction illustrates this process. When women first report an assault to the police, the report form is filled in and after the initial investigation the case is categorized (broadly speaking as rape, attempted rape, indecent assault or buggery or combinations of these charges). What further action will be taken is also decided. It is at this point that some cases where for various reasons no further action is to be taken, are 'no crimed' which in effect means that the cases are not included in the statistical returns to the Home Office.

The legal definition of rape, focusing on penetration of the vagina, diverts attention away from the coercive and life threatening experience of rape as described by complainants.[13] It is whether penetration has occurred that is all-important. According to Section 1 of the 1956 Sexual Offences Act, rape is defined as penetration of the vagina by the penis without the woman's consent.[14] Included are attempts to rape, which stop before actual penetration occurs. Three issues have to be proved for rape itself. First, that sexual intercourse took place, second, that it was against her will and third, that the defendant did not believe she did not consent or could not have cared less (was reckless as to whether or not she consented).[15] Emission of semen is not required. This definition has been criticized on several grounds. It embraces only penetration of the vagina, not of other parts of the body, and does not cover other forms of sexual coercion such as forced fellatio[16] or cunnilingus, or other intrusions of any object into any part of the woman's body. Such assaults can be just as horrifying.

The process of attrition in the Islington research

The four key attrition points where most cases failed were first when the police decided whether or not to record the case as an offence (i.e. whether to 'no crime' it), second, when the police decide whether or not to refer the case to the CPS, third, whether the CPS proceeds to prosecution or alters the charge through plea bargaining, and fourth, when the jury decides whether or not to convict the defendant of rape.

The high attrition rate in rape and sexual assault cases was well documented in studies undertaken in the early and mid-1980s by Home Office researchers (Chambers and Millar 1983; Wright 1984; Smith 1989; Grace *et al.* 1992). These studies found that a high proportion of reported cases were categorized by the police as 'no crimes' and so were not recorded as offences, and cases were frequently dropped between report and committal (Chambers and Millar 1983). Of those cases that did proceed to court, several resulted in a conviction for a less serious offence and many more resulted in acquittals (Wright 1984; Smith 1989; Grace *et al.* 1992). At each stage in the criminal justice process, cases in which there was some prior acquaintance between the complainant and the suspect were more likely to be dropped or downgraded to a less serious offence than cases of 'stranger' attacks (Smith 1989; Grace *et al.* 1992).

Recording practices

The inadequacy of police recording practices has been identified in a number of recent studies. The Home Office Circular 69 (Home Office 1986), subsequently reinforced in a series of force orders issued by the Metropolitan Police, advised that only false complainants should be 'no crimed'; unsubstantiated complainants and cases where the victim withdrew her complaint *were to remain recorded as crime.* Cases should only be 'no crimed' when they were proven to be mistaken, frivolous or vindictive – in other words inherently malicious. Despite these clear Home Office guidelines, two Home Office studies found this category was widely used; the average no-criming rate was still high although there was considerable variation between forces (Lloyd and Walmsley 1985; Grace *et al.* 1993).

Our findings reflect this high rate of attrition; if anything the rate was even higher than reported elsewhere. One reason for this is that with access to police records, we were able to ensure that all cases of rape and sexual assault against women and girls reported over the two year period were included. This differs from the strategy adopted in the two Home Office studies (Smith 1989; Grace *et al.* 1992) which excluded cases which were 'no crimed' – i.e. not recorded as crimes – by the police during the first month as the analysis was based on the monthly police returns sent to the Home Office. In our study 38 per cent of the cases, over a third of all cases, were 'no crimed'. Reasons varied from the woman's decision not to proceed either due to threats or unwillingness to go to court, to the police regarding the case as lacking sufficient corroboration or viewing the complainant as unreliable. None of these reasons adheres to the police order instructions on no criming. 'No criming' gives the impression that many women were making false allegations, reinforcing the view that women reporting sexual attacks to the police are still not always taken seriously. 'No criming' does occur in other offences besides physical and sexual assault against women but the overall 'no crime' rate is only 3 per cent (Bottomley and Coleman 1981).

Downgrading of offences and plea bargaining

Another reason for attrition is the downgrading of cases by the police and at a later stage through plea bargaining. It appears that the police sometimes downgrade cases of attempted rape to indecent assault. Nineteen cases were downgraded to reflect a less serious offence; two reports of rape and six reports of attempted rape were reclassified as indecent assault. One case of indecent assault became indecent exposure and in the remaining 10 cases the sexual aspect of the crime was removed altogether. Clearly, it is in the interests of the victim to reduce the charge if there is insufficient evidence to proceed with the more serious charge and such decisions have to be made on the basis of experience and judgement. However, some of the cases in which the sexual classification was removed altogether are rather puzzling. They include a case classified simply as robbery, although the suspect had squeezed the victim's breast and put his hand on her inner thigh, and a charge of grievous bodily harm (GBH) in which the attacker had ripped off the victim's T-shirt and bra and put a finger in her vagina, slashing her breasts while threatening to cut them off. In another case classified as common assault, the victim regained consciousness to find the suspect urinating on her.

In several of the cases where the complainant was interviewed, the description of the attack appeared to suggest attempted rape but it was classified as indecent assault. The distinction between rape and indecent assault was often unclear and it is debatable what should constitute the difference. How exactly can intention to rape be measured? Is it genital contact and if so, what kind of contact, or is verbal expression of intent sufficient? Does throwing a woman on the ground or on a bed trying to remove her knickers and then being fought off constitute intention to rape?

Several of the women interviewed described attacks which had been classified as indecent assault but appeared to be as serious as other cases classified as attempted rape. If the woman is knocked off her feet, pinned down, and kissed or groped, this should surely be classified as attempted rape. Consider the following case of Lizzie (not her real name):

> I was attacked in the lobby of a block of flats where I used to live as I came home quite late at night. It was about 2 am in the morning [sic]. I was just about to get into the lift when suddenly a man appeared wearing just a shirt, nothing else and he started moving towards me and he actually had an erection and was masturbating. My first instinct was just to kick. I aimed for his groin and I missed and the next thing I knew he'd thrown me around against the wall and I obviously screamed very loudly but he then covered my mouth and my nose so I couldn't breathe. After a few minutes of struggling we ended up on the floor and I managed to get his hands off my mouth and I decided to talk to him. I told him that I was two months pregnant and that my husband was waiting for me upstairs – and said, 'Please, please, let me go'. He released his grip and I managed to get out and ran into the street. I was looking for a phone and couldn't find one even though if I'd thought about it I knew where one was. I stopped a taxi and got him to take me round the block and asked the taxi driver to come in with me. I phoned the police as soon as I got in.

It transpired that the suspect lived in the same block of flats and over the next weeks Lizzie kept sighting him and was terrified of coming face to face with him. She eventually moved from her flat as she was so terrified of running into him. After seeing him she alerted the police and he was arrested. She spent a day in the police station picking him out of an identification parade. The assailant was already on a suspended sentence for another sexual offence and had since attacked two other women, who had also picked him out of an identification parade. Yet he was not charged with attempted rape but with indecent assault. He was found guilty of two counts of indecent assault (both of which appeared to be attempted rapes) and received only an 18 month sentence to be served on top of the 18 months of his suspended sentence. Lizzie had been terrorized and suffered from nightmares and panic attacks. It appears that if a woman fights back and gets away from her assailant he is unlikely to be charged with attempted rape even if masturbating, has an erect penis, is half-naked, and is pinioning a woman down with his hand over her mouth.

The only case where a woman had reported her separated husband shows how indecent assault cases are often difficult to prove even when the charge is combined with actual bodily harm. Una (not her real name) described what happened:

> I was married for 17 years. I took a lot over the years for the sake of the children. But you get to the point when you think 'that's it'. You can't explain the kind of pressure I was under when I left, phone calls and hassle. I had an injunction as well to keep him away. But he just flipped. I thought he was going to kill me. I'd never seen him like that. He said 'Sleep with me and I'll give you some money'. Then he tried to rape me. I fought and he beat me up. My daughter was in the house and she heard everything. The police arrested him for indecent assault. I said I wanted him arrested for attempted rape. He got off for indecent assault but was found guilty for ABH. I would rather he had been found guilty on the indecent assault than the ABH charge.

It is interesting to consider why the police would wish to downgrade the seriousness of cases in this way. One senior policewoman helped to throw light on this question when she recounted how, on returning to the station from other duties at the end of 1988, she had taken a statement from a rape victim who did not wish to proceed with the case. In accordance with previous practice, she had 'no crimed' the report and was reprimanded for doing so. She was informed that the new guidelines related to rape reports only and was asked if the report could be downgraded to indecent assault; in which case it could then be 'no crimed'.

The Crown Prosecution Service

The third main point of attrition is the Crown Prosecution Service whose lawyers decide whether cases that the police regard as sound go to court. The

Table 7.1   Attrition in rape cases

Total rapes reported	109
Recorded as an offence	60
Detected	44
To CPS	37
To court	30
Convicted	12
Convicted for rape/attempted rape	9

CPS only recommends cases for a hearing if they consider there is a good chance of conviction. The code of practice for the CPS asserts that for prosecution to occur, all cases must have a realistic prospect of conviction. Since few reported rapes result in a conviction, the CPS are unwilling to take cases to court which they think will result in an acquittal. (Informally in rape cases police refer to the CPS's 70 per cent rule for rape.)

The court process

The final point of attrition is due to the imbalances in the trial which make it very difficult to gain a conviction. Of the 109 cases of rape and attempted rape reported between September 1988 and September 1990, only 30 cases reached the Crown Court and in only nine of these cases was the defendant found guilty of rape or attempted rape (see Table 7.1). These all led to prison sentences except one which involved two teenage boys who raped a 13 year old in council care.[17] In almost all cases the men convicted were involved in more than one offence of rape, or with other offences such as burglary or ABH (actual bodily harm) taken into consideration. One of the women I interviewed where the suspect had been found guilty of her attempted rape had only been caught and brought to trial after committing another rape, and this may well be the case elsewhere. Compared to the Home Office study (Grace *et al.* 1992) based on 1985 data where 51 per cent of cases resulted in a prosecution, only 25 per cent of our sample reached court. Of these, in the Home Office sample two-thirds resulted in a conviction, while in our sample only a third did so.

Another relevant factor affecting whether or not cases result in conviction was whether there had been any consensual social contact between the two previously. Six of the convicted men were complete strangers to their victims and in only one case, the case of *R. v. Bogie*, were the man and woman of similar age (apart from the pair rape referred to above of the girl in council care). By further research tracing what happened to cases at the appeal court, the appalling fact transpired that Bogie's five year sentence was reversed on appeal. The complainant could not be contacted to let her know her assailant had been set free. Since this was the only conviction of what is categorized as 'acquaintance' rape, where the two were roughly the same age, it is worth examining in some detail as it illustrates the incredible difficulty of gaining convictions. Even after a jury has found the defendant guilty, it is by no means assured that the sentence will not be reversed on appeal.

This case also raises another form of imbalance in rape trials which concerns the calling of character witnesses regarding the woman's alleged promiscuity, which is allowed at the discretion of the judge. *R. v. Bogie* involved a young woman who reported being raped by a man who had offered her a place to stay after she had locked herself out of a friend's flat where she was staying. She reported the rape to the police, was examined by a doctor and found to be scratched and bruised. The police arrested the defendant who denied the charge. In due course the case went to court.

The judge used his discretion to allow the defendant to call character witnesses and the woman's reputation was called into question. The defence had asked for no fewer than five character witnesses to be called to testify to her general unreliability. During the course of this testimony, again without any application by the defence under section 2 of the 1976 Sexual Offences (Amendment) Act, one of the witnesses declared the complainant to be a 'tart and an easy lay'. Another said she was familiar with customers at the pub and behaved like a frustrated actress. Neither of these were relevant to her truthfulness. The defence then applied under section 2 of the Sexual Offences Amendment Act to cross-examine her about three separate incidents involving her previous sexual behaviour, one of which the judge allowed. In spite of this and the attacks on her credibility mentioned above, the jury found Bogie guilty and he was sentenced to five years.

Bogie then appealed. At the appeal court, the three judges ruled that the judge should not have disallowed the defendant's other character witnesses and therefore quashed the sentence on the grounds that the evidence could have been admitted at common law and the judge was wrong to exclude it. However as Temkin points out, the purpose of the Sexual Offences Amendment Act was not to give statutory authority to the practice of common law but to control it. The appeal was allowed even though the jury had heard a barrage of evidence impugning the complainant's moral and sexual character and was still convinced that she was telling the truth. The appeal court did not spell out the reasons for its decision but what does emerge clearly from the judgement is that the judges took a very dim view of the complainant, were particularly unimpressed by her alleged sexual activities and disloyalty to her boyfriend, and found it remarkable that she was claiming rape at all when, semi-clothed, she had shared a bed with the defendant. The implication of this decision is that the only material question is whether the exclusion of sexual history evidence would be unfair to the defendant, not whether it might be unfortunate for the complainant (Temkin 1993: 14).[18]

In light of the cumulative imbalances in the processes of rape trials, it is unsurprising, perhaps, that the conviction rate is low. In this study in 18 of the cases the defendant was found not guilty or the case was dismissed and in the remaining three cases the defendants were found guilty of indecent assault and the original charge of attempted rape was dropped. Less than 1 in 4 reported cases reached Crown Court and of these 1 in 3 resulted in a conviction. Expressed another way, less than 1 in 10 of those reported to the police resulted in a conviction. Of the 109 cases of rape reported, 100 of the cases had fallen away, leaving only nine cases of rape and attempted rape formally recognized by the criminal justice system to exist. The low conviction rate reverberates down the whole process. The police and CPS censure most cases in the knowledge that very few result in guilty verdicts in the present court system.

Research into the working of the court system

I only accidentally started to attend rape trials. I first became interested in criminal law when working as a probation officer. I came to realize that men who killed their wives were treated more leniently than those who killed strangers and sometimes even more leniently than women who killed husbands after years of violence inflicted on them (Lees 1994). One day when undertaking a small investigation of murder trials, I wandered into a rape trial. In my innocence I imagined there was no way, in the light of the evidence presented, that the defendant would be acquitted. He was, however, discharged. In 1989 I sat in on 10 trials and a further four retrials. By the time seven of the 10 defendants had been found not guilty and another case abandoned, I came to see these trials as a cruel hoax, a travesty of justice, equivalent to a second rape by the judiciary.

The ambivalence of male attitudes towards rape colours everything. Outside the courts, in the listings office at the Old Bailey, I looked at the notice board which contains details of cases coming up. Someone had written in pencil under the charge of ATTEMPTED RAPE, the word SHAME. Shame, that is, that he had not succeeded. On a number of occasions I was tempted to intervene, to try and break through the court officials' insensitivity and call into question their identification with the alleged defendants.

Various court procedures imbalance the trial in favour of the defendant, making it very difficult for jurors to convict even in the light of corroborative evidence. Additionally, all sorts of extraneous factors can be introduced and often involve attacks on the woman's reputation, not limited to sexual past history. These attacks are often used in spite of the 1976 Sexual Offences Amendment Act, and all kinds of irrelevant factors are also brought in by the defence barrister, seemingly to confuse the jury.

The complainant has no representation in court whereas the defendant can consult with his defence lawyer before the case comes to trial and can even employ plainclothes detectives to spy on the complainant in order to try and collect compromising evidence about her. The complainant, as the main prosecution witness, is not allowed even to speak to the prosecution barrister, indeed she may not even know which of the barristers he or she is. The ban on the prosecution barrister consulting with the witness is to prevent the briefing of witnesses, but in a rape trial where often the victim rather than the defendant's reputation is under attack, she needs some representation. Prosecution barristers are often inept at countering myths and prejudices about women, indeed they often share them. In one case, several police officers, including a police surgeon, gave evidence that the woman was shaking with fear and distress, tears were streaming down her face, she wanted to wash herself frequently and was afraid afterwards to go out alone. They all agreed she was in acute distress and showing every sign that she was suffering from what has been identified as the rape trauma syndrome. Yet the prosecution counsel failed even to mention her distress in his summing up. In this case I abandoned my role as participant observer and followed him out of the court and asked him why he had not mentioned her distress. He responded that it was absurd to regard the woman's state as corroborative and dismissed the judge's view as irrelevant. This exemplifies the lack of sympathy between the prosecution counsel and the complainant and the way it can prejudice her case.

Jurors, often faced with all sorts of information about the woman's character which they assume is relevant to the case since it has been presented, can only deal with the conflict between the doubts they have been presented with by the defence and the need to find the defendant guilty beyond any reasonable doubt by presenting a 'not guilty verdict'.

The corroboration warning

The corroboration ruling refers to the common law rules which require a judge to give a warning about the danger of relying on the uncorroborated testimony of two categories of witness, accomplices and complainants in sexual offences. Generally in England the evidence of a single witness, if believed, is sufficient to prove the case against the accused. There are however some exceptions to this rule. With certain sexual offences, such as procuring a woman for the purposes of prostitution, the victim's evidence alone is incapable of securing a conviction. There must be some additional confirmatory evidence which implicates the accused person and tends to confirm his guilt. This is known as the *corroboration requirement*. For other sexual offences, both homosexual or heterosexual, and whether or not consent is an ingredient of the offence, corroboration is not actually required, but until recently the judge is obliged to warn the jury of the danger of convicting solely on the basis of the evidence of the complainant. A welcome change is the abolition of the compulsory nature of this warning in the 1994 Criminal Justice Act but it is likely that some judges will continue to warn the jury in one way or another about the assumed propensity of women to make false allegations.[19] The whole issue of corroboration is directly related to the question of reputation, as if the woman is considered credible then the idea is that corroboration is not necessary.[20]

An equally important issue is how the jury is directed to view corroboration.[21] When the ruling was compulsory during my research, judges argued that it was given totally neutrally but I found that judges frequently embroidered the warning in a most disturbing way. Over and over again they argued that allegations of sexual misconduct are very easy to make and very difficult to disprove. Unlikely reasons why women allegedly make such allegations were often blatantly suggested by judges. The judge would pull this bias against the complainant together in his directions to the jury, often arguing for example, that people lie more about their sexual behaviour than about any other area of human conduct. Here, for example is how Judge Smedley, in the case heard at the Old Bailey on 1 September 1993, gave the corroboration warning by insinuating that women are both irrational and malicious. He said:

> Experience has shown that people who allege sexual offences, whether women, men, boys or girls, for some reason or *no reason at all* tell false stories. Some reasons are obvious. More common in the past was unwanted pregnancy. Also wicked jealousy, spite, or revenge as suggested here may be a motive. Allegations of that kind are relatively easy to make and are difficult for a man to refute. It is difficult for a man to prove she consented.

Some judges are however wholeheartedly opposed to the corroboration ruling. Judge Perleman referred to it as an anachronism, an absolute insult and described how 'I do it because I have to do it and I take a deep breath but I don't like to do it'.[22]

Yet some judges appear, intentionally or unintentionally, to mislead juries rather than clarify the court procedures. Judges often openly state that it is extremely easy, perhaps too easy, for women to bring cases to court, implying that it is their decision rather than the police and CPS's; the Common Sergeant of London illustrates this by reiterating the cliché 'that it is easy for women to make false allegations of rape but difficult for a man to refute them'. The jury are not told that the woman will have spent hours, even days, under police questioning, she will have had a thorough medical examination, she is likely to have had pregnancy and VD tests, she may have spent hours at the police station involved in identification parades, she will have gone to the magistrates' court, she may well have been subjected to threats from the defendant or his friends. Myths about women making false allegations override women's explanations of why they have run naked into the street, cried compulsively, spent the night in police stations for fear of retribution for taking the case to court, changed their name or even moved house. The judge rarely draws the jury's attention to the fact that most women who have been raped cannot face the ordeal they will have to go through if they complain to the police (many, indeed cannot face telling anyone) and that they are often threatened with retaliation if they do go to the police.

Conclusion

The central argument of this chapter is that the criminal justice system is not merely failing to protect women but that the processes involved legitimize male violence. First, sexual behaviour is socially constructed, and supported by group norms. For example, boys and men boast about their sexual exploits and this enhances their social status. Girls and women have to keep quiet about sex to avoid the risks of attacks on their sexual reputation. Second, such social norms not only operate at a group level but also at an institutional level, both within the police and court practices. A rape trial can be seen as a barometer of ideologies of sexual difference, of male dominance and women's inferiority. Current ideology condones and legitimizes male violence. The conduct of rape trials has the manifest function of limiting the degree of violence against the few women who bring cases to court and its latent function is to reinforce male dominance, undermine women's experience and hold their autonomy in check. The public airing of stereotypical views of women reinforces male dominance.

Whether due to an actual increase in rapes or to a greater willingness to report, more women are coming forward, and on the whole, are being treated with greater sensitivity by the police. At the same time, the possibility of gaining a conviction has diminished. It appears from the findings presented here that since the CPS was established in 1986 an even greater proportion of cases are, for one reason or another, being dropped. The total attrition rate for the Home Office study (Grace *et al.* 1992) was 73 per cent compared with 92 per cent in our study. This trend is confirmed by the Home Office's own statistics which show that the conviction rate for cases of rape and attempted rape has fallen from 24 per cent of all cases recorded (excluding those 'no-crimed') in 1985 to 10 per cent in 1993 (*Home Office Statistics* 1993). This means that more women are being subjected to the ordeal of undergoing intensive interrogation, an arduous medical examination, sometimes combined with intimidation from suspects to withdraw the cases, without legal and adequate counselling support, only for the case against their assailant to be abandoned or worse still, to undergo the humiliation of the court appearance to be disbelieved and to see her assailant's innocence proclaimed.

For a legal system to be fair it is of course vital that the rights of the defendant to a fair trial are protected. It is of equal importance that complainants can obtain justice. The conflicting rights of defendants and complainants must be balanced. This is the dilemma of legislation. Women should be enabled to obtain justice without jeopardizing the rights of the accused. In rape trials where issues of acceptable masculinity and femininity are contested, this is not the case. The defendant is too advantaged, allowing men guilty of sexual assault to go free and rape again. The myth of equal justice for all is nowhere more blatantly exposed than in a rape trial. The whole procedure loads the dice against the complainant. Not only her testimony, but her very life up to the moment of making that complaint are brought into question.

The present system is a mockery of justice. The following reforms are long overdue: no criming should cease; the legal definition of rape needs to be widened; the prosecution counsel should be allowed to prepare the case with the complainant as is the case in some American states; the Sexual Offences (Amendment) Act 1976 (Home Office 1976), which had failed to implement in full the recommendations of the Heilbron Committee (1975) designed to restrict the use of sexual history evidence about the complainant, should be tightened up. Where such evidence is permitted, equivalent information about the defendant, including previous convictions, should automatically be allowed. A radical overhaul of the way in which prosecution barristers handle rape cases is needed, including training in the *modus operandi* of rapists and the effects of rape, an opportunity to meet with the complainant before the trial and greater use of expert evidence regarding typical reactions to rape. A proper application of 'similar fact' evidence would mean that where the defendant was accused of more than one sexual assault, the cases could be heard together, thereby reducing the likelihood of the same man being acquitted on several separate occasions as frequently occurs under the present system. Screens should be provided in all courts so the complainant would not have to face her assailant. The lengthy delays in trials coming to court should be cut. There should also be some monitoring of trials and the analysis of acquittal and sentencing rates in different parts of the country.

New South Wales introduced such a package of reforms in the Crimes (Sexual Assault) Amendment Act (1981), which has led to a significantly higher proportion of cases going to trial and a conviction rate of 82 per cent (see Allen 1990: 231). The increased costs involved in improving the judicial treatment of rape are likely to be reimbursed by the avoidance of the appalling emotional aftermath of rape and its effect on men, women and children's lives.

Notes

1 The first rape crisis centre was set up in 1976.
2 Professor of Gender Studies at the University of Middlesex.
3 This continuum extends from sex murders, rape and sexual assault to sexual harassment and flashing to wolf whistling.
4 I was a member of the Women's Committee for some years, and had contacts with a number of councillors.
5 Scotland Yard insisted we wait a year before embarking on the research, and access to the records was withdrawn after an initial agreement, which set the project back 18 months. I think the Chief Superintendents hoped we would eventually give up and go away.
6 As we shall see this piece of legislation appears to have been largely ineffective.
7 In the US, most states have abolished or modified the marital rape exclusion. In Illinois, instead of the prosecution having to prove that the victim did not consent, the defence have to prove 'by word or deed' that she did.
8 Consensual buggery is legalized for over 18 year olds.

9 The proportion of cases recorded by the police as crimes which proceed to trial fell from 31 per cent in 1985 to 19.4 per cent in 1993.

10 See also the results of Holmstrom and Burgess's (1978) research into the rape trauma syndrome.

11 Random samples of women residents of San Francisco were asked about their experiences of incest, extra-familial child sexual abuse, unwanted sex with authority figures, rape by strangers, acquaintances, friends, dates, lovers, ex-lovers, husbands and ex-husbands.

12 Nearly one-half of women whose fathers had upper middle-class occupations were victims of rape or attempted rape at some time in their lives. This compares with a third of women whose father had middle-class occupations and those who had lower-class occupations.

13 Statutory rape refers to rape of children who are too young to give consent, i.e. under 16.

14 The new Criminal Justice and Public Order Act (1994) widens the definition to include male rape (penetration of the anus).

15 The jury has to consider whether a man believed that a woman was consenting; the presence or absence of reasonable grounds for such a belief is a matter to which the jury is to have regard, in conjunction with any other relevant matters, in considering whether he so believed.

16 An amendment to the Criminal Justice and Public Order Act (1994) redefines rape as non consensual anal (as well as vaginal) penetration, but has not widened the definition to include oral sex.

17 One was given a conditional discharge and the other was given 100 hours of community service.

18 Temkin (1993: 14) quotes another three recent cases where the Court of Appeal regarded the woman's sexual history as relevant on quite spurious grounds. In summing up, she concludes 'the willingness of the Court of Appeal to see a wide range of evidence as of relevance to consent means that trial judges who refuse to allow in sexual history evidence do so at considerable risk of a quashed conviction on appeal' (Temkin 1993: 17).

19 Besides the compulsory ruling there are other cases where it is a 'rule of practice' that the jury is warned about the danger of convicting without corroboration (see Wells 1990). Some class of witnesses fit the 'rationale' but not the strict definition of the common law rule, such as people with a motive for giving false evidence, psychiatric patients or those giving evidence of identification. In such cases the judge has to decide whether there is a need for special caution.

20 In *R. v. Horn* (1912) an appeal against conviction of an indecent assault, there was no corroboration of the girl's story. Yet the judge ruled that since the girl was respectable there was no reason why she should concoct such a story and the appeal was dismissed (Criminal Appeals Report). In the case of *R. v. Gardner* (1973), where the defendant and complainant had been sexually acquainted, the defendant was acquitted.

Providing the warning is administered, a conviction cannot be quashed on appeal merely because of the absence of corroboration. But where the warning is not given, the conviction will be quashed by the Court of Appeal even though there is abundant corroborative evidence (Temkin 1987: 133).

21 Only in very few cases is the jury actually forbidden to convict in the absence of corroboration. Until 1988 the unsworn evidence of children was one such category.

22 Panorama Programme, *The Rape of Justice*, September 1993.

References

Adler, Z. (1987) *Rape on Trial*. London: Routledge and Kegan Paul.

Allen, J. (1990) *Sex and Secrets: Crimes Involving Australian Women Since 1880*. Oxford: Oxford University Press.

BBC TV (1992) *Public Eye: Hidden from View, Hidden from Justice*, 14 February.

Blair, I. (1985) *Investigating Rape*. London: Croom Helm.

Bottomley, A. and Coleman, C. (1981) *Understanding Crime Rates*. London: Saxon House.

Brownmiller, S. (1976) *Against Our Will*. Harmondsworth: Penguin.

Chambers, G. and Millar, A. (1983) *Investigating Sexual Assault*. Edinburgh: Scottish Office Central Research Study Unit, HMSO.

El-Faizy, M. (1994) Let down by the law, *The Guardian*, 20 August.

Ginsberg, E. and Lerner, S. (1989) *Sexual Violence Against Women: A Guide to the Criminal Law*. London: Rights of Women Publications.

Grace, S., Lloyd, C. and Smith, L. (1992) *Rape: From Recording to Conviction*. London: Home Office Research Unit.

Grubin, D. and Gunn, J. (1990) *Imprisoned Rapists and Rape*. London: Home Office Research Unit.

Heilbron Committee (1975) *Report on the Advisory Group on the Law on Rape*, Cmnd 6352. London: HMSO.

Holmstrom, L. and Burgess, A. (1978) *The Victim of Rape: Institutional Reactions*. New York: Wiley.

Home Office (1986) *Violence Against Women: Treatment of Victims of Rape and Domestic Violence*. Home Office Circular No. 69. London: Home Office.

Home Office Statistics (1993) (Available from Home Office Research and Statistics Department.) London: HMSO.

Jeffreys, S. and Radford, J. (1984) Contributory negligence: Being a woman. In P. Scraton and P. Gordon (eds) *Causes for Concern*. Harmondsworth: Penguin.

Jones, T., McLean, B. and Young, J. (1986) *The Islington Crime Survey*. London: Gower.

Kelly, L. (1988) *Surviving Sexual Violence*. London: Polity.

Lees, S. (1994) Lawyers' work as constitutive of gender relations. In M. Cain and C. Harrington (eds) *Lawyers in a Postmodern World*. Buckingham: Open University Press.

Lees, S. and Gregory, J. (1993) *Rape and Sexual Assault: A Study of Attrition*. London: Islington Council.

London Rape Crisis Centre (1984) *Sexual Violence: The Reality for Women*. London: Women's Press.

Lloyd, C. and Walmsley, R. (1989) *Changes in rape offences and sentencing*, Home Office Research Study No. 105. London: HMSO.

Robertshaw, P. (1994) Sentencing rapists: first tier courts in 1991–92, *Criminal Law Review*, May: 343–5.

Scully, D. (1990) *Understanding Sexual Violence: A Study of Convicted Rapists*. London: Unwin Hyman.

Smith, L. (1989) *Concerns About Rape*. Home Office Research Study 106. London: HMSO.

Temkin, J. (1987) *Rape and the Legal Process*. London: Routledge, and Kegan Paul.

Wells, C. (1990) Corroboration of evidence in criminal trials, *New Law Journal*, July (20): 1031–2.

Women's National Commission (1985) *Violence Against Women*, report of an Ad Hoc Working Group. London: Cabinet Office.

Wright, R. (1984) A note on the attrition of rape cases, *British Journal of Criminology*, 24(4): 399–400.

Part III

Researching experience and supporting women

8

Sexual experiences and sexual abuse of women with learning disabilities[1]

Michelle McCarthy

Any discussion of research into the sexuality and sexual experiences of people with learning disabilities must begin with an acknowledgement that it is a very underresearched area. There have been a small number of incidence and prevalence studies on the sexual abuse of children and adults with learning disabilities (see for example Dunne and Power 1990; Turk and Brown 1992) and there has been some limited research into the levels of sexual knowledge of adults with learning disabilities (see Timmers *et al.* 1981; Andron 1983).

The distinctive feature of my research is the very detailed nature of the explorations into the actual sexual experiences of women with learning disabilities. This is necessary in my view to avoid making assumptions; the only way to discover what people actually do and how they feel about it is to ask them in detail. My research is based on ethnographic principles, although it does depart from some of ethnography's traditions. For example, there are no elements of participant or direct observation.

The research was carried out in the context of my role as sex education worker for women with learning disabilities (originally funded by a regional health authority, then by an NHS trust). This means in effect that all the information I gained about the women's sexual experiences was gained in the context of educational/counselling sessions and not traditional research interviews. All the women involved were referred by staff (usually direct care staff, social workers, consultant psychiatrists) with the exception of a small number of women who referred themselves.

Because people with learning disabilities can often find it difficult to understand what is being put to them and can find it difficult to make choices, careful attention needs to be paid to seeking *informed* consent to participate in this kind of process. With regards to the women's consent to come to my sessions in the first place, I would explain what it might entail, then they were simply asked if they wanted to come. Almost all said yes. As a member of staff and therefore in a position of authority, it would clearly have been difficult for them to have said no to me. Because of the power imbalance that exists between service providers and service users with learning disabilities, there was little I could do at that stage to decrease this acceptance other than make it explicit that they did not have to see me if they did not want to. Despite the very high levels of compliance, it is important to note that a few women did refuse outright and some found indirect ways of saying no. For example, a few simply did not turn up to sessions, one woman pretended to lose her voice, another ran away from me on our way to the office.

All the information gained from the women was from semi-structured in-depth interviews. Some of the interviews have formed part of my academic research (for MA and PhD). These interviews differed only from the others in that they were taped and transcribed (by me). It was difficult to gain informed consent from the women to take part in this process, as the words and indeed the concepts of 'research' or 'methods' or 'policy' would not have meant anything to the women concerned. Therefore a very simplified explanation was offered such as 'I'm talking to women about sex, so I can learn more about it and to try to make sure women get the help they need. I might want to talk to other people and write about what I learn, but I won't tell them anything personal about you or use your name.' All women with learning disabilities who were asked for their permission for their sessions to be taped agreed.

I tended to see each individual woman on a weekly basis for approximately two to three months, but sometimes for considerably longer than this. Because of the nature of my role I was not in a position to offer very long term support. Although few if any of the women seemed to want to focus the content of our discussion on sexuality issues beyond the length of time I have indicated, very many did want to continue seeing me regularly. Ending work with many of the women was emotional and painful for us both; the women would commonly feel rejected and angry towards me and I would feel upset that I had upset them and *feel* like I had mishandled the process although I don't *think* I did.

Although I have experience of rape crisis counselling, I have never carried out parallel work with women who do not have learning disabilities, so I am not in a very good position to say quite how working with women with learning disabilities on these issues is different or special. However, there are two observations I can make, one with regards to process and the other with regards to content. First, with regards to process, I have found it invaluable to work with visual aids such as pictures showing different sexual acts, images of sexual abuse, aspects of relationships. Because such resources are not common – particularly if you want images that are not racist, sexist or homophobic – a colleague and I developed our own (McCarthy and Thompson 1993). The advantage of visual materials like these is that they can help facilitate communication for people who find it difficult to express themselves verbally and/or who lack a good vocabulary on sexual matters.

Second, with regard to content, the discussion tended to be focused much less on feelings than it might be with other women. One of the features common to many people with learning disabilities is a great difficulty in thinking in abstract terms and understanding abstract concepts. This is, of course, not the same as saying that people with learning disabilities do not have the same feelings as other people (an old-fashioned and terribly damaging misconception) but rather that they might have more trouble understanding and expressing those feelings (for an example of skilled creative work in helping women with learning disabilities express their feelings see Millard 1994).

My work follows many of the principles of feminist research methodology. It focuses on individual women's experiences, but does not pathologize the individual women. Rather I seek to place these women's personal experiences in a wider political context. The overall aim of the research is to contribute to improving the lives of women with learning disabilities.

Feminist researchers and activists have been criticized for having neglected the experiences and contributions of women with disabilities. The disabled feminist and researcher Jenny Morris has written widely about the failure of feminism and feminists to identify with women with physical disabilities (Morris 1991). This criticism is undoubtedly more valid with regard to the academic and theoretical side of feminist work, as many feminist activists *have* tried to make services inclusive and accessible to women with physical disabilities. But if it is true that feminism has at some levels neglected the issues surrounding physical disability, then it is doubly true in relation to learning disabilities. However, this is not to say there are no overlaps between the two spheres. Certainly, feminists working within the learning disabilities field have theorized their work from a feminist perspective – for examples of this see Burns (1993), Williams (1992) and Brown and Smith (1992). Equally some feminists including myself have incorporated our beliefs and principles into our practical work – for an example of truly inspirational practical work with women with learning disabilities from a feminist perspective see the work of the Powerhouse women in East London, who are setting up a refuge for women with learning disabilities[2]. However, outside what is in fact a very small field of work, feminists and feminisms have not traditionally made reference to the experiences of women with learning disabilities nor sought to make events, materials or ideas accessible to them.

Part of what I am hoping to achieve with my work is to bridge some of these gaps and to bring the experiences of a highly marginalized and oppressed group of women into mainstream feminist and sociological thinking. In doing so I hope to highlight some of the commonalities amongst women as well as the differences.

The findings presented here are based on my work with 60 women with learning disabilities, conducted over a four-year period. Their ages ranged from 20–63, the majority had mild or moderate learning disabilities and almost half had additional mental health problems.[3] Three-quarters lived or had lived in long stay hospitals and 25 per cent lived in a variety of community based settings. All but four were white British and the remaining four were black British. There were no differences in the types of experiences the black women related, but I certainly would not draw any conclusions from this partly due to the very small numbers of black women I interviewed and partly because I am not especially skilled or experienced in drawing those factors out. It is an area that needs more work in its own right and Carol Baxter has highlighted the need for culturally sensitive attention to be paid to the sexuality of black people with learning disabilities (Baxter 1994).

What follows is a description of the most common features of the women's sexual experiences; most women I have worked with do not have any way of expressing their sexuality that is autonomous from men's sexuality. Most of the women do not masturbate and the few that do, do not experience this in any positive way. They think it is wrong and bad for them to do it and sometimes report a belief that they will physically harm themselves by it.

None of the women encountered has had any sexual experiences with other women, nor do they know any other women who have. This is despite the fact that many of the women have lived on women-only wards for most or all of their adult lives. However, this is not to say that they are unaware of the possibility of same-sex relationships; most women did know of their existence. Almost without exception they spoke of lesbian sexuality in very negative terms.

The fact that the women's sexual experiences are inextricably linked to men, means the women have no way of understanding any sexual feelings or experiences outside of that context. Sex, then, becomes something that they do, not only *with* men, but *for* men.

An analysis of the kind of sexual activities which take place clearly illustrates for whose benefit the sex is happening. Because people with learning disabilities often lack insight into their situations, it might reasonably be supposed that the women are not really aware of the differences between how they experience sex compared to their male partners. However this is not true; when asked who enjoys sex more, women or men, the vast majority of women are clear that the man likes sex much more than they do, if they like it at all. Those women who say they enjoy sex as much as men usually reveal on further questioning that they mean they like having a boyfriend as opposed to sex itself. No woman with learning disabilities (or any woman, if the question is posed in general terms) has ever said to me that she enjoys sex more than men.

The sex focuses purely on the men's genitals and is almost exclusively penetrative. The process of events in most sexual encounters (as described by both women and men with learning disabilities) is one where, if there is any pre-penetrative stimulation at all, it will be the woman rubbing the man's penis when or until he has an erection, penetration of an unlubricated vagina or anus then follows and sex finishes with the man's orgasm. Although sexual pleasure for women with learning disabilities is conspicuous only by its absence, the significant thing is not merely that the women do not get any sexual pleasure, but also that they do not expect to get any and they often accept discomfort and pain without complaint. Linda Andron, who is one of the few other people to have reported in-depth investigations into the sexual lives of people with learning disabilities confirms this point in her findings (Andron 1983).

In the course of almost all the sexual encounters the women with learning disabilities have described to me, little or nothing happens to arouse the woman. There is little touching, kissing or skin contact. As people with learning disabilities often do not have much private time and space for their sexual encounters, clothes will often be left on. But if anybody does get fully or partially undressed (beyond what is necessary to have intercourse) then it is always the woman. Clothes offer some level of protection and it is never the man who experiences being exposed and vulnerable.

The situation regarding oral sex is also very significant. The vast majority of women with learning disabilities have never experienced a man's mouth on their vagina, but many have limited experience of a penis in their mouth. This particular sexual act arouses very strong and very negative feelings as no other sexual act does, even ones which the women find physically painful such as anal intercourse. Quite why this is the case will form part of my future research, but there is no doubt that this is the one thing which women with learning disabilities say they loathe and refuse to do. How they manage to refuse this and why the men accept this refusal, when this clearly goes against the overall pattern of male control of sex, are aspects for my further research.

Once what actually happens during sexual encounters with women and men with learning disabilities is understood, it is clear that the women will experience little or no physical pleasure from these acts. And it is indeed the case that sexual pleasure is rarely, if ever, reported by women with learning disabilities, who often have difficulty understanding the very concept.

None of the women with learning disabilities I have met have been aware of the existence of the clitoris and its role in women's sexual pleasure (incidentally neither have the men with learning disabilities that my colleagues have worked with.) None of the women have experienced orgasm – one or two of the most able women have said that they have 'come', but in fact have confused this term with the experience of their vaginas becoming wet.

A complicating factor in the sexual lives of people with learning disabilities who live in institutional settings is that there is an expectation on the part of both the men and women that an exchange of (very small amounts of) money, cigarettes, tea, sweets, etc. will take place for sex. This exchange of sex for money or valued items is entirely a one-way exchange – the men pay the women, never the other way around. This reality both reflects the men's power and at the same time compounds it, because the power to pay brings with it the power to direct and control what happens. The exchange of sex for money is found both in casual, or purely sexual, encounters as well as within the context of long established relationships. Within relationships it bears no relation to the quality of affection or love the partners may have for one another – there is simply an expectation within the subculture that the men will pay women for sex.

Both the content and the context of most sexual encounters for most women with learning disabilities make it hard to escape the conclusion that the women do anything other than provide sexual services for men.

Sexual violence

I define sexual violence as any sexual contact which is unwanted and/or un-enjoyed by one partner and is for the sexual gratification of the other. Using the above definition it can be seen from my interviews that there is a truly shocking amount of sexual violence perpetrated against women with learning disabilities, often starting at a very young age, happening over long periods of time and of a most serious nature, including vaginal or anal rape. Other studies of sexual abuse carried out in Britain and abroad confirm that people with learning disabilities are particularly vulnerable to abuse. Brown and Turk (1992) and Crossmaker (1991) have both produced evidence of this, for example.

Also of significance are research studies such as those by Seemanova (1971) and Bovicelli *et al.* (1982) of reproduction by women with learning disabilities and of children born through incest. These studies often mention in passing that women with learning disabilities make up a disproportionately high percentage of women who conceive as a result of incest, up to an astonishing 460 times the number expected by chance.

Just as for women without learning disabilities, there is no one typical kind of sexual violence. Instead it covers a wide range of violations in a wide variety of circumstances. Liz Kelly's concept of a 'continuum of sexual violence' helps to locate the real and social context of sexual abuse against women (Kelly 1988). However when talking to women with learning disabilities, certain kinds of sexual abuse do emerge as very common.

I have already referred to the high levels of incestuous sexual abuse of women with learning disabilities. This commonly takes place both during the woman's childhood and adulthood. Perpetrators are usually fathers, step-fathers, brothers and uncles.

Also common is ongoing sexual violence by men with learning disabilities, often within the context of an established relationship. Brown and Turk's research (1992) in Britain showed that men with learning disabilities make up the biggest single group of known perpetrators of sexual abuse against other people with learning disabilities and my own work confirms this. Overreporting explains this phenomenon to a limited extent, as men with learning disabilities are more likely to be caught and reported than other perpetrators. This is because much of this kind of abuse actually takes place in learning disability services and some men with learning disabilities are not as skilled as other perpetrators in covering up what they have done. However, overreporting is only part of the picture. It is well acknowledged that much sexual abuse relies on opportunity and access to vulnerable people. As men with learning disabilities have the easiest and most legitimate sexual access to women with learning disabilities, they are going to be the people with the most opportunity to abuse, as David Thompson's and my work has illustrated (McCarthy and Thompson 1993). Much of this kind of abuse goes unnoticed by staff, but my experience has been that even when it is pointed out to them, like the police not wanting to involve themselves in 'domestics', staff are often very reluctant to get involved in people's personal relationships. This is more than a little ironic, when you consider that service providers are involved in practically every other aspect of people's private lives.

Not only do service providers inadvertently or deliberately turn a blind eye to abuse, service provision can and does actively contribute to sexual abuse. Whilst I firmly believe that the prime responsibility for any act of abuse lies with the perpetrator of it, opportunities for abuse can be minimized or enhanced depending on the type of service being provided. Large establishments, particularly the large institutions, bring together combinations of people which anyone ought to be able to see are at best undesirable and at worse downright dangerous. For example, men with learning disabilities who have a history of sexual offending are often placed in the same environments as women with learning disabilities who have been sexually abused – with minimal safeguards. The current debate in mental health services regarding mixed wards in hospitals are just as relevant in learning disability services. The difference is that there is not such a strong and articulate user movement in learning disability services, nor is feminist advocacy to create change and debate so apparent in learning disability services.

It is not only direct service provision which can increase the vulnerability of women with learning disabilities to sexual abuse. Societal attitudes about the low status of people with learning disabilities does not help. For example if a man with learning disabilities commits a sexual offence in the community, it is not uncommon for him to be 'taken out of circulation' and sent to a hospital for people with learning disabilities. Here he is unlikely to receive much, if any, specialist treatment for his offending behaviour, but will almost certainly be free to wander around the buildings and grounds with access to some of society's most vulnerable people. My experience of working in these large hospitals is that the men invariably continue to perpetrate sexual abuse, the difference being this time no great fuss is made about it. It is outrageous that women and other men with learning disabilities are sacrificed to ensure the protection of higher status 'normal' people.

I have concentrated so far on the sexual violence towards women with learning disabilities that takes place from men they know. This is because it is the most common form of abuse as revealed to me by the women I have interviewed and also in my wider experience. But I do not want to overlook the fact that sexual abuse by strangers does happen. It is not uncommon to find men who do not have any kind of disability, who seek out women with learning disabilities purely for sex, either within or outside institutional settings.

People are often shocked when they learn of such behaviour and there is often disbelief about the nature and extent of it, but it does happen and it happens more often than any of us would care to believe.

During the search for the body of Jo Ramsden, a woman with Down's syndrome who was sexually assaulted and murdered, the Dorset Police Superintendent in charge of the case took the unusual step of sending a memo to all Social Services Departments in the country saying;

> During this enquiry my officers have been surprised and sickened by the number of men who are prepared to prey on mentally disabled females. We have identified people who have committed very serious offences against these vulnerable people. Police have taken steps to remind persons responsible for the mentally handicapped of their vulnerability in this type of crime. You may feel it is appropriate to issue similar warnings to persons with such responsibilities in your area.
>
> (Dorset Police 1993).

A shocking example of the low status of women with learning disabilities and the consequent low impact on society that sexual crimes against them creates was the BBC news report on the charges brought against Michael Fox. Michael Fox was eventually found guilty of nine counts of abduction and rape of women with learning disabilities. He was charged only with kidnapping Jo Ramsden, as the judge ruled that there was insufficient evidence to try him for her murder. However the police file on Jo has been closed. Despite the magnitude of Fox's crimes, news of the charges brought against him came some 20 minutes into the broadcast, after items on finance, the manufacturing industry and even an item on cruelty to animals. My letter of complaint on this did not even warrant an acknowledgement from the BBC.

Although it needs to be considered separately from other kinds of sexual abuse, it is also important to note that almost all of the long term relationships and marriages between people who do and people who do not have learning disabilities, are in fact between women who do and men who do not have learning disabilities. A good number of these men are very dominating and violent towards their wives, and one can reasonably suspect that they sexually abuse them too.

Strategies for change

I have suggested elsewhere that staff working in learning disability services need to be enabled to develop a more sophisticated understanding of sexuality (McCarthy and Thompson 1995). Simplistic 'common sense' assumptions are often made, for example, that people have sex because they like it. The motivation for engaging in sexual activity is rarely that simple for anyone, and my research with women with learning disabilities shows that it bears no relation to their reality.

The assumption is usually made that if there are any problems with regards to the sexuality of people with learning disabilities then these are inevitably due either to the person's mental limitations and/or to the unusual circumstances in which they live. This needs to be vigorously challenged. Working from a feminist perspective leads one to conclude that much of what is happening between women and men with learning disabilities and to women with learning disabilities by other men has more to do with the construction of gender power relations than anything specifically related to disability. Much of what I have described of the sexual experiences of women with learning disabilities will be very familiar to other women's experiences of sex with men, throughout history and across cultures. It is imperative therefore that the large body of feminist knowledge and skills in working around sexuality and sexual abuse (and in particular the knowledge that the abuser is most likely to be a known and trusted man) needs to be utilized in learning disability services.

Sex education for people with learning disabilities has an important role to play. Women with learning disabilities need to start sharing in some of the benefits of changing attitudes towards women's sexuality that have taken place over the last century. If this is to be achieved they, like other women who are particularly vulnerable to being taken advantage of sexually (e.g. young women) need to be explicitly educated about their own bodies, their own potential for experiencing sexual pleasure and, most importantly, that their role in sex is not just to satisfy men's wishes. This means empowering women to recognize sexual exploitation and abuse and enabling them to find ways of resisting it.

Men with learning disabilities need to be educated into more respectful and appropriate means of sexual expression. This means helping them understand that they have the right not to be sexually abused or exploited themselves, nor do they have the right to do this to others. Services must not tolerate their sexual abuse towards others; a serious challenge now faces services to provide the appropriate treatment and punishment.

The way forward is not going to be easy – it has already become apparent that many people, including some people with learning disabilities themselves, do not want to acknowledge what commonly happens when men and women with learning disabilities have sex. My work and that of my colleague David Thompson has already prompted hostility in a number of quarters. Resistance to acknowledging the reality of people's sexual experiences is strong, not least because it seems like a big step backwards when the rights of people with learning disabilities to be acknowledged as sexual beings have been gained only relatively recently.

Those who work and write about the sexuality of people with learning disabilities are acutely aware that we do so against a background of oppression towards them. Their historical institutionalization and segregation was due to complex reasons, but issues of sexuality were central to this process. Ideas about the supposedly uncontrolled nature of their sexuality sat side by side with ideas about their sexual vulnerability in society. There is a danger in that in highlighting the vulnerability of many women with learning disabilities to sexual abuse and the extent of the sexual abuse that is perpetrated by men with learning disabilities, that these factors will be used by some people to try to prove that what are now rightly considered as old-fashioned and inherently damaging ideas were right after all. There is also the risk that such work will be used to strengthen some of the more general essentialist ideas about women's sexual passivity and men's sexual aggression. I am the last person to want to turn the clock back in these ways and I am concerned about being accused of perpetuating stereotypes. Yet at the same time I do not want to be pressured into keeping quiet, as I believe that does a great disservice to women with learning disabilities in particular. I am hoping to create a space within the learning disability field and within feminism where we can acknowledge what is happening and find ways of changing it.

Notes

1 Learning disabilities or learning difficulties are the preferred terms in Britain for what was previously known as mental handicap. In an international context it can be used interchangeably with developmental disabilities and intellectual impairment.
2 The Powerhouse women can be contacted at PO Box 3680, London, E6 2SD. Tel: 0181 472 2833.
3 Learning disabilities are usually categorized in a range of increasing severity from mild through moderate and severe to profound.

References

Andron, L. (1983) Sexuality counselling with developmentally disabled couples. In A. Craft and M. Craft (eds) *Sex Education and Counselling for Mentally Handicapped People*. Tunbridge Wells: Costello.
Baxter, C. (1994) Sex education in the multiracial society. In A. Craft (ed.) *Practice issues in Sexuality and Learning Disabilities*. London: Routledge.
Bovicelli, L., Otsini, L. F., Rizzo, N., Montacuti, V. and Bachetta, M. (1982) Reproduction in Down's Syndrome, *Obstetrics and Gynaecology*, supplement, 59(6): 135–75.
Brown, H. and Smith, H. (1992) Assertion or assimilation: a feminist view of the normalisation principle. In H. Brown and H. Smith (eds) *Normalisation: A Reader for the Nineties*. London: Routledge.
Burns, J. (1993) Invisible women – women who have learning disabilities, *The Psychologist*, 6(March): 102–5.
Crossmaker, M. (1991) Behind locked doors – institutional sexual abuse, *Sexuality and Disability*, 9(3): 201–19.
Dorset Police (1993) Jo Ramsden Enquiry. In M. Whoriskey *et al. Consenting Adults: Sexual Abuse and Adults with Learning Disabilities*. Glasgow: Enable.
Dunne, T. and Power, A. (1990) Sexual abuse and mental handicap: preliminary findings of a community-based study, *Mental Handicap Research*, 3(2): 111–25.
Kelly, L. (1988) *Surviving Sexual Violence*. Cambridge: Polity Press.

McCarthy, M. and Thompson, D. (1993) *Sex and the 3 R's: Rights, Responsibilities and Realities.* Brighton: Pavilion.

McCarthy, M. and Thompson, D. (1995) No more double standards: Sexuality and people with learning difficulties. In L. Ward and T. Philpot (eds) *Values and Visions: Changing Ideas in Services for People with Learning Difficulties.* Oxford: Butterworth-Heinemann.

Millard, L. (1994) Between ourselves: experiences of a women's group on sexuality and sexual abuse. In A. Craft (ed.) *Practice Issues in Sexuality and Learning Disabilities.* London: Routledge.

Morris, J. (1991) Us and them? Feminist research, community care and disability, *Critical Social Policy,* 11(3) winter: 22–39.

Seemanova, E. (1971) A study of the children of incestuous matings, *Human Heredity,* 21: 108–28.

Timmers, R. *et al.* (1981) Sexual knowledge and behaviours of developmentally disabled adults living in a normalised apartment setting, *Sexuality and Disability,* 4(1): 27–39.

Turk, V. and Brown, H. (1992) Sexual abuse and adults with learning disabilities: preliminary communication of survey results, *Mental Handicap,* 20(June): 44–55.

Williams, F. (1992) Women with learning difficulties are women too. In M. Langan and L. Day (eds) *Women, Oppression and Social Work: Issues in Anti-discriminatory Practice.* London: Routledge.

9

Researching prostitution and violence: towards a feminist praxis

Maggie O'Neill

This chapter explores the narratives of women who have experienced violence whilst working as prostitutes. These narratives are examined within the context of the 'women centred' research I engage in whilst working with and for this group of marginalized and criminalized women.

My work in progress explores (in part) possibilities for women-centred multi-agency approaches to street prostitution which have women prostitutes as key players (see O'Neill 1994). I was commissioned by Safer Cities to undertake a pilot study exploring responses to prostitution in the East Midlands with a view to developing multi-agency initiatives. From the outset I was committed to women's voices being heard and listened to, that the research should be action oriented, with knowledge arising out of the study being 'knowledge for' as 'feminist praxis' (see Stanley 1990), facilitating empowerment, resistance and social change.

The reflexive interrelationship between feminist research, women's lived experience and policy oriented practice is a central theme in my work. I use an ethnographic approach documenting women who work as prostitutes' narratives and lifespan biographies. From this reciprocal and reflexive relationship between methodology, experience and policy oriented feminist practice came a need or rather an urgency to address some of the problems and issues that the women have talked about. These include: high profile policing; high fines; imprisonment due to fine default; drugs use; clients offering more money for unprotected sex; girls from local authority care undercutting the market price and often offering sex without the use of condoms. Particular issues emerged in relation to young women from local authority care who are often under the age of consent; their experiences encompassed coercion by pimps through physical and sexual violence, emotional neediness and, for some, extreme vulnerability. An additional, central and universal concern amongst women working as prostitutes is sexual violence: by clients, pimps, and sometimes lovers. The forms this violence take includes: intimidation, harassment, rape, robbery and assault, and murder.

This chapter is divided into four sections. The first outlines the inter-relationship between research methods, methodology and epistemology in this work. The second explores the routes women and girls take into prostitution. The third documents the experiences of sexual violence women working as prostitutes talked about. The final section links feminist theory, women's lived experience and possibilities for feminist action.

Methodology as feminist praxis

Doing feminist research can be explained more fully by examining the inter-relationship between research methods, methodology and epistemology. Harding (1987: 8–9) suggests that for certain types of research with and for women, the researcher should attempt to locate herself in 'the same critical plane as the overt subject matter'. My engagement with feminist research was fuelled by my interest and commitment to feminist theory and feminist politics and the need to create the intellectual and practical space within the social construction of knowledge for women's voices to be heard and listened to. Feminism and feminist research is about the development and construction of knowledge which writes women into his-story and exploring, challenging, resisting and changing sexual and social inequalities. My involvement is about passionate, feeling involvement in critical tension with reason and rationality. The social construction of such knowledge is founded upon the relationship between women's everyday experience of prostitution as a cultural practice, academic knowledge, political power and social action (O'Neill 1992: 22).

This methodological approach facilitates the central involvement of the women, who are active participants in the social construction of knowledge, empowerment and social change. There is a continuity in my relationship with some of the women because we are currently working together on a number of projects. The emotional nature of a lot of the work I undertake, particularly on-street, meant I became immersed in the range of differing experiences of women working as prostitutes. A major concern is that this work should have some practical outcomes for them.

The lifespan narratives are conducted as guided conversations. I interject as little as possible and usually only gently to encourage where there is a lull or pause. Importance is placed upon the woman's own story, her descriptions, feelings and meanings. Documenting women's experiences through lifespan narratives/biographies becomes political when contextualized within feminist theory/methodology. Feminist research methodologies are ways of envisioning and grounding knowledge and providing ways of locating and contextualizing women's experiences. There are, of course, dilemmas and dangers thrown up by doing this sort of close 'ethnographic' research with any group, but particularly with 'marginalized', 'criminalized' and 'stigmatized' groups. One can become immersed in the intracommunity as well as the interagency politics and lose the critical perspective which is necessary for the development of effective practice. One risks becoming so emotionally involved that relationships become firmly entrenched, and dependency patterns develop. However, relationships of trust take a long time to build and I often feel like I am walking a tightrope between the two possibilities. Researchers are sometimes seen as akin to pimps, coming into the field to take, then returning to the campus, institution or suburb where they write up the data, publish and build careers – on the backs of those they took data from.

Doing close ethnographic work with women who work on the street has implications for the women themselves as well as for the personal safety of the researcher. Taking time and experiences/information from women working can negatively affect her contact with clients and also produce potential hassle from pimps. 'Taking from women' may be perceived by the women themselves as another form of pimping, particularly given the way the media has portrayed female prostitutes. Most documentaries open with a seedy depiction of the deserted, dark street with the 'hooker' in stilettos, fishnets and miniskirt. The message is clear and the stereotype upheld of the dirty, disease ridden prostitute, irresponsible, immoral and probably feeding a drug habit – the whore stigma in operation (Pheterson 1986). Given this level of stereotyping and the concomitant whore stigma it underpins, it is no wonder female street prostitutes are wary of researchers and research 'on' her. No researcher, feminist or otherwise, can avoid engaging with these complex issues.

I have no answers to these dilemmas and difficulties. I do, however, endeavour to take account of the ethical and political dimensions in the social construction of knowledge as well as recognizing and facilitating the shared participation of the women I am working with. The issue of the personal safety of the researcher is illustrated by my own experience whilst accompanying a health outreach worker in the spring months of 1992. We witnessed at very close range a violent assault on a woman prostitute and attended court four times until the case was finally dealt with. This was the last occasion I visited the street as part of my research.

Four of us were standing talking, myself and Kay leaning against her car, Helen and Pat standing in front of us.[1] The conversation was lively and we were laughing. In what seemed like a few seconds, a man strode across the road straight through our group taking Helen with him. He held her by the throat and marched her backwards slamming her against a stone wall (the side of a house). She shouted to him to get off and he began punching her. He had what could have been a knife in his left hand; it glinted in the darkness. Helen maintains he was carrying a gun. He wanted her money. He tore her gold cross and chain off. I shouted, 'We must help, what can we do to help!' Kay argued that we must wait until it was over and then drive her for help; it was too dangerous to intervene. He left as quickly as he came, and reportedly went into a bar bragging about his theft. We drove Helen a little way before she spotted her boyfriend, she got out of the car and rang the police to give a statement. She knew the assailant. He was known for attacking women when he wanted money. We were told that his 'woman' was 'inside' or had left him. Pat refused to give evidence, she was too scared of the consequences, and she felt it wasn't such an unusual incident.

Kay's statement and my own were not taken for three weeks. Finally we were both contacted by the police and statements taken. The assailant was also wanted on other charges; a court case at the magistrates' court would take place as soon as possible. We turned up at the magistrates' court and waited for what seemed like hours; Helen did not arrive. Word was that she had been 'got at'. The assailant elected for 'paper trial' and we were to be sent dates for the Crown Court case. We turned up at the Crown Court on the day of the hearing, anxious that we may meet him face to face. Helen did not arrive. The judge adjourned the case and a new date was set. Again we turned up, again we were sent home. Helen had disappeared. On the final occasion we arrived, Helen again did not – she was serving a sentence for fine default, but it seems the police were unaware of this. We did not have to give evidence. The assailant pleaded guilty and was given a suspended sentence. We left the court as quickly as we could and headed for the nearest cigarette machine and coffee bar. It was over. We felt sick from the nervous tension and sick that the assailant was dealt with in this way, free to assault and rob the next prostitute he met when he needed cash.

An extra dimension to this case is the fact that I live on the edge of the area known as a red light area. I live in a row of Victorian terraced houses and parking is available only on the street. On the nights preceding the first three court cases my car was vandalized. Descriptions of the individuals who were chased away by various neighbours were all similar. The police took this seriously and the assailant was given a 'dressing down' from the judge on the third court appearance for 'intimidating a witness' and was put on curfew, banned from entering the area. My car went undamaged the night before the fourth court date.

This harrowing and frightening incident raises a lot of issues to do with the nature of this research, risks taken or not taken by the researcher and health workers who are committed to outreach work; the extent to which one should get involved; conflict between commitment to the women and to making a stand against this sort of tyranny of violence, and worries about one's safety and the safety of one's younger family members given this level of involvement (given where I live and the fact that I have two small children). Issues about subjectivity and distance are also thrown up. My approach is clearly subjective in scope – it is about care and commitment relating to addressing sexual and social inequalities. This does not mean poorer quality work; I would argue quite the opposite. Nor does it mean that a critical perspective is lost.

There are also issues for the women who are subject to this level of 'acceptable' violence. There is an analogy to be drawn here with the repercussions for women experiencing domestic violence and the extent to which agencies of public order and social control such as the police can ensure her safety. Why did the police and prison not communicate sufficiently so that Helen was able to attend court? However, what punishment would have been meted out to her had she given evidence against her attacker in court?

Taking an ethnographic approach to documenting the voices of women working as prostitutes has resulted in differing forms of documented material. The form and style of the material has been dictated by: environmental factors (on or off-street); timing, whether the interview was early or later in my research (early material is mostly in the form of notes taken on-street and later material is on tape in the form of lifespan narratives); and my relationship with the woman, the tension between trust and risk in each woman's perceptions of and relationship with me as researcher. Records of street encounters are in the form of short notes written in the car, between stops, or from memory when I returned home. In the initial period of research longer off-street interviews were handwritten because the women preferred this method of note taking; and finally longer lifespan narratives were taped conversations lasting between one and a half and three and a half hours. The lifespan interviews were conducted almost two years after I began the initial work, and are evidence of the developing relationships of trust with women in my local area.

Clearly the stigmatization and marginalization of prostitute women is central to any understanding of the ways in which women are processed by the criminal justice system, represented by the media, and enter the public imagination. In October of 1992 a series of reports on two recent rape cases against prostitute women made local news. Consider the following[2]:

> A prostitute broke down in tears as she described how she was allegedly raped at knifepoint by a client . . . She said: 'I asked him for money and he said "of course". That's when he went to his pocket. I bent down to get my handbag to put the money in and the next minute he had a knife at my throat . . . The knife was at my throat. I was frightened.'
> (local evening paper)

The man had carried out a similar attack on a 14-year-old living in care some months earlier but that case was dropped because of lack of corroboration. The man's defence council claimed:

> Two prostitutes with a grudge against a man over money invented stories that he had raped them at knifepoint. He should have known he was playing with fire − he should have known that prostitutes can be as hard as nails and as greedy as you like for money.
> (local evening paper)

The same newspaper periodically publishes a court column in which the names and sometimes addresses of individuals in court on various charges are printed. Local women in court for soliciting offences have experienced harassment, fear and intimidation due to this publicity. This is a central safety issue.

Routes into prostitution

In the course of my research and my work with and for the East Midlands Multi-Agency Forum, I have met and talked with many women engaged in prostitution. Most of these women are resisting poverty for themselves and for their children. These are not the romantic constructions we see in films such as *Pretty Woman*, but ordinary women who have differing access to material resources such as jobs, salaries, education, housing and health services. Additionally some have limited access to emotional resources, such as family, friends and other support networks which provide practical and emotional support, confidence and self-esteem. Some are young women who drift into prostitution on leaving care because of financial problems and their association with the street culture; others are clearly pimped and coerced into prostitution whilst in care through their developing 'romantic' relationships with local pimps. All of these young women have profoundly sad backgrounds: child sexual abuse; physical or emotional abuse; family breakdowns; multiple placements in care. These experiences result in extreme vulnerability and emotional neediness, since their needs have not been met within the organization of residential care despite the work of some very committed staff in residential units.

In my conversations with prostitutes from Britain and other European countries and representatives from the various agencies and institutions working with and for women who work as prostitutes, it appears that economic need is the bottom line for women's entry into prostitution. Prostitution is a resistance and/or a response to poverty. Care leavers are also vulnerable to entering prostitution, particularly given the relationship between homelessness, poverty, emotional and/or material need (see O'Neill 1991b).

The women I have I talked to are mostly white and aged between 14 and 54. All entered prostitution for financial reasons. Many are also influenced by coercion and/or association with friends working as prostitutes. All except one of the women entered prostitution by association; they knew someone else who was working the streets or engaged in prostitution and eventually explored this option in order to earn enough money to live a 'reasonable' existence.

Association/economic need and coercion are often presented as the differing and separate reasons for women's entry into prostitution. This is too simple and does not reflect the complexity of many women's lives. For some women coercion and association led to their entry into prostitution but economic need keeps them there as well as a subculture of similar and significant others. For others, economic need led to their involvement but coercion and subcultural entrenchment keeps them there. The subcultural aspect is an important consideration; a sense of belonging to the network, friends who understand and do not judge, and feeling wanted and needed are centrally related to understanding women's continued involvement in prostitution. It is important that we develop a better understanding of routes into prostitution to unravel the primary, secondary and sometimes two-pronged reasons for women's initial entry. More complex understanding of routes into prostitution is crucial to both developing better support services for women prostitutes and developing or facilitating exit routes (O'Neill 1991a).

For some young women, access to prostitution occurs through contacts made in certain pubs and clubs frequented by pimps. The women were coerced into prostitution in the course of their developing relationship with a pimp. They were 'chatted up', their drinks bought, a few trips made to the town centre window-shopping to look at expensive items. Sometimes the relationship develops as a 'romantic' one and they are subsequently 'persuaded' to 'do' street work in order that their lifestyle can continue since he (the pimp) does not work and has little possibility of paid work given the economic climate and high levels of unemployment in the area. Another story is that it isn't worth the man's while earning because he would have to pay too much of his salary in maintenance for children from past or current relationships. These strategies are commonly reported by women who moved from local authority care into prostitution.

Care has to be taken to try and separate the 'male domestic partner' who supports his partner practically and emotionally and who may be unemployed, from the 'pimp' who manipulates and coerces. Not all male partners do give support. It is very difficult to draw clear boundaries around relationships. Many women not engaged in prostitution may find resonances in their lives in these descriptions. Many of the relationships I have discussed (with heterosexual women) include degrees of support both practical and/or emotional in tension with degrees of emotional, sexual or physical coercion (see Hoigard and Finstad 1992: 160–72). Where exploitation is accompanied by emotional and/or practical support, the exploitative element is experienced to a lesser extent and sometimes articulated within an understanding or acceptance of taken for granted patterns in heterosexual relationships. Many women would not define their domestic partner as a pimp, other women (a small group) see the pimp/prostitute relationships at one end of a continuum in heterosexual relationships with lesser exploitation, coercion at the other end (for example, marriage), but nevertheless still marked by power, control and ownership. Still other women are quite clear that their relationship with men known as pimps is a coercive relationship based solely upon their use value as prostitutes and their earning potential.

Female prostitutes' experiences of sexual violence

I have talked to many women in the course of this research. Some of these are lengthy interviews of up to three hours, others are relatively short conversations on the street. What is indisputable is that sexual violence against women working as prostitutes is endemic. Clients, pimps and domestic partners perpetrate most of it, although sometimes other women are involved or assailants unknown to the women. The violence women have talked about

includes rape and beatings. Women have recounted various experiences ranging from verbal abuse and threats to extreme and brutal violence: being
punched and kicked and battered with the heel of a man's shoe whilst
desperately trying to escape from his flat naked; being kidnapped, raped and
imprisoned; being raped, knifed, stoned and left for dead in the middle of a
major road; and for one under-age girl, being kidnapped from local authority
care, starved and beaten into working for two people – a man and a woman.

Some women maintain that they have experienced very few physical
assaults and attacks because they are good at 'gentling' the men, at 'negotiating' and 'counselling'. However, when referring to the violence they experience or have experienced, they talk about it in a very matter of fact way.
Hoigard and Finstad (1992: 63) also comment on this aspect of the lives of
women working in prostitution.

> I often felt that the women talked about violence in a strange way.
> Bluntly, without any special dramatization, they could relate kidnappings,
> confinements, rapes, and death threats as if these were almost normal
> occurrences . . . In our material the majority of the women had experi-
> enced a great deal of physical violence earlier in life as well: parents
> who hit; institutional personnel who abused them . . . It's possible that
> the women have been so exposed to violence that they have become
> socialized to accept violence as part of life.

Women's stories

In this section I will introduce and locate the women's narratives within the
context of feminist action research as feminist praxis. The women's own
names have been changed to protect their confidentiality as have other minor
details which might allow them to be recognized. All the women are white
and identify as heterosexual.

Angela

Angela was 21 and a mother of two when I first met her in 1990. She had
a male partner who looked after the children whilst she was out working, or
she paid a babysitter. The babysitter did not know she worked as a prostitute;
she thought she worked in a club. Angela had been working intermittently
for about two years, always on the street. She got involved with prostitution
when drinking with her friend in a pub in the middle of the red light area.
They were getting pissed, and wondered if they could 'go' with a bloke for
money, and decided that they could. Both of them were in debt and were
very worried about their situations. They bought some condoms from a
vending machine in the toilet and chatted to two men who were willing to
pay for sex. They took 10 pounds each. I asked how did you know what
to do? Were you scared or worried? Angela answered 'It was easy, I was
pissed . . . I had heard that you just play dead until it is over'. In the course

of my time assisting an outreach worker on-street I saw Angela only three or four times more. I heard that Angela was severely beaten and had her throat cut by a client in February of 1992. She is alive and recovering. I cannot be certain that it is her, for I am going on descriptions by the other women. This incident did not make the local press.

Jane

Jane was about 18 years old, and a single parent when I first met her in January 1991. She had been anally raped and beaten by a client. The police responded quickly and the man was caught. Jane also had fines of about £1,800 which she could not pay. She was evicted from her council flat; she felt this was because she became known as a prostitute. Her belongings were taken and sold to pay her debts. She and her child moved back to live with her mother. Her relationship with her mother was difficult at times; Jane had been in and out of care as a child. After she moved in with her mother Jane continued to work the streets whilst her mother looked after her child. According to Jane her mother did not know for sure she worked 'on-street', but her child had seen her there and had asked her what she was doing. Jane shrugged this off and continued to work. Jane was being pimped by a male pimp.

Karen

Karen was about 20 years old when I first met her in October of 1990. She tried prostitution because she had been given a council flat on leaving care, but did not have the income to heat or furnish it. Karen ran away from four prospective clients until she finally had to go through with it in order to eat. She told me that after about four clients she could 'stomach it', and had been working for about 18 months. Six months prior to my initial conversation with her she had been raped at knifepoint by a client. The police had arrived very quickly and caught the man. He was given two years imprisonment.

Ann

When I interviewed Ann she was working in three part time jobs, had been alcohol free for five years, separated from her husband (a heavy drug user) for one year and had given up all drugs. Ann was also paying for adult education classes. Ann's involvement in prostitution lasted for three and a half years beginning in her fifteenth year whilst living at home and ended when she moved away from her home town to a different area altogether. Ann left home when she was 15 and went to live with friends who supported her through a difficult period at home and who were involved in prostitution. She felt she could not tell any of her school friends or teachers about her family problems and turned to two new friends who gave her much time and support. Ann was sexually harassed and assaulted by her sister's husband from the age of 13 to 15. Her sister and her sister's new husband moved into the family home when Ann was 13, not long after her father died. Ann developed avoidance strategies such as not being left alone with him and telling her mum she would be leaving friend's houses much later than she actually was in order to avoid the lift home in his car. Ann had jumped out of a moving car and had thrown ornaments, breaking a window in her home in order to escape and attract attention to her plight.

The central problem for Ann was that her mum did not listen to her; in fact her mum thought that Ann was the 'problem', not her son-in-law. The family began rationalizing Ann's behaviour; she was lying, seeking attention and making trouble. Understandably Ann began to exhibit 'extreme' behaviour in response to what she saw as 'lack of trust' and was 'devastated at her mum's response'. Ann was labelled as a delinquent and as being 'out of control'. She left home to live with friends about six months after she first began to work as a prostitute. A woman who lived in the local area acted as a madam and organized women and girls for men who mostly lived in the surrounding areas. Ann received a lot of emotional support from her friends and they 'looked out for each other', taking it in turns to wait outside clients' houses in case of problems. However, Ann maintains that she did not 'choose' prostitution. Prostitution brought freedom, money, fun and the ability to leave home. For her, 'choice' and 'control' were exercised by leaving prostitution. She experienced prostitution as a damaging form of work 'trading off sex for the spending power of men', she talked about wanting her self-worth to be more than it was, she felt 'passive' and 'done to'. Prostitution was about being used and she was vociferous in her insistence that money and spending power cannot buy self-esteem. Ann said:

> Everyone should have the right to form relationships without having to pay for it. Everyone should have the right to relationships which are about give and take. This is good for self-respect and self-esteem and confidence[3].

Sarah

The following narrative is from a young girl who works as a prostitute whilst in the care of a local authority. Her situation raises a number of issues around sexual violence for those in the care of the local authority, for example, the extent to which 'carers' perceive sexual violence as 'deserved' and 'deserving'; sexual violence as the 'effect' of an 'immoral lifestyle'; and sexual violence as 'outside' their 'control and ability to care'. This narrative also raises issues about the nature and form of local authority care, whether or not the social and emotional needs of young people are being met, particularly around self-esteem, sexual identity, sexuality and the relationship of one's self to one's body.

Sarah was 14 years old in September 1992. Between the autumn of 1990 and September 1992 she had been in five different care institutions. She was put into voluntary care by her mother at age eight because of family problems. The family split up, her father left, her older brother went to live with her gran, she and her younger brother went into foster care. Sarah had three foster care placements each lasting approximately six months between the ages of eight and 10. In the first placement she remembers 'crying a lot', 'feeling lost', 'unable to understand why she was there', but generally it was a 'good placement'. The second she describes as 'horrible' and the third 'not nice'. Sarah was returned to her mother with her younger brother for a short time. It was during her time at home that she first started to 'work'. Sarah met some girls who she became friends with; she ran away with them as she was not happy at home. She lived with them near the regular beat and soon met a man and a woman whom she later was forced to 'work for'. She was picked up by the police and returned to her mum; however this didn't work out and she was put into care again. She was subsequently kidnapped from care by the two people she met, they told her she must 'work for them' and gave her some 'draw' (marijuana). The woman accompanied her with every client. Sarah was very scared. She was 'slashed and beaten' for trying to run away and she 'wasn't fed properly'. After one week she was picked up by the police, told them what happened and was put back into care.

Whilst in care she decided she would work for herself. She wanted to buy 'draw, cigarettes and clothes'. Sometimes she would sleep at the clients' houses, sometimes a man would drive her to another city to work for about one week at a time. Sarah was introduced to crack by a man she met at a blues party. He showed her how to take it using a Coke can. She became frightened, ran away and found a police station. She was returned to care. Sarah felt that she was moved around so much from care institution to care institution because she was perceived as encouraging other girls to try prostitution. Unhappy, not attending school, chain smoking, Sarah soon ran away again and lived for five months in a rented flat. At this time she was working in prostitution, drinking, taking crack and smoking draw. Later she began to take heroin and was not eating – 'only packets of crisps'. She was picked up (because her mum saw her out on the beat) and returned to care. After this she had a trial period at home with her mum. But the relationship was difficult – 'lots of arguing' – and she was put back into care. Of her mother she said, 'I love her deep down but disrespect her for all the messing about'. Once again she began to work as a prostitute, taking heroin and crack but the person supplying her stopped. She is currently, with the help of a prostitute self-help group and social workers, off heroin and crack and tying to remain so. She is in a community home which is not very comfortable – 'always cold' and 'worn out' furnishings – but she likes it and feels relatively at home.

At first Sarah felt 'rotten and disgusted with old men on top of me'; she talked about how she used to hurt physically and emotionally but that she doesn't now because she had 'cut off her feelings'. She said 'it wasn't too bad at first because the first punter just wanted to look at my breasts'. At the home 'they don't understand why I can't stop, they think I should stop – just like that! Two pounds per week is not enough, I am a smoker, and I am in the circle now'. Sarah has had one abortion, and her social worker took her for a hepatitis B injection. She 'couldn't stand school' and describes herself as 'a loner'. Often she goes 'out to work when I get bored, there is nowhere else to go'. Sarah has been 'beaten, slapped, punched and forced to have sex without a condom' – raped.

Louise

I was 12 when I cut myself up really bad and they put me in touch with social workers . . . and I got the idea of children's homes and care and I thought I would really push to get in one . . . I wish now that I had gone back to my dad and that I would not have got put into care because the minute I was put into care everyone was sniffing and my first day in care I went out for a walk with them and I wanted to be like them and I started taking drugs and didn't have no contact with me mum and dad . . . then I started taking whiz when I ran away from care when I was 15. I met a guy called John and I was with him for two years and he got done for murder . . . Then I left care and . . . I stopped taking drugs for awhile but I started sniffing again . . . and I started injecting . . . I got in with the wrong crowd and I got intro-duced . . . well I was told that prostitution was the in thing and I never could see myself as a prostitute. I thought it was dirty and I just started doing it with my friend . . . it was dead easy money. £250 a time or sometimes you got more . . . at first I felt dirty because a dirty old man is lying on top of me . . . I have had punters that said to me 'you remind me of my daughter' and I said 'God don't do this to me' and the punters told me this and it's like they wanted to have sex with their daughters . . . They probably rape their daughters and they scared me sometimes when they do that . . . Then I started taking crack . . . and then ended up selling my body for rock . . . just doing it for the rock . . . That hurt me when I got raped that time . . . but some men have abused me but it doesn't bother me . . . But a few weeks ago I got attacked and I went to a place where he wanted to do it and he got a knife out. It was on the beat and he wanted to go inside and he wanted oral so he pulled out a knife and cut my throat, well I moved my chin so he cut my chin, I had six stitches. Then he beat me up and made me go down on him and then threw me to the floor and I said, 'Don't, I'm pregnant' . . . I ended up biting him and that did not do anything and he strangled me twice. I remember lying there when he was strangling me and I was struggling all the time I never gave up . . . and I remember hard bricks coming down on my head . . .

The violence recounted above is physical, sexual and psychological. It is misogynistic, about the power of men and men exercising control over women, men taking sexual frustrations out on women working as prostitutes and/or playing out fantasies and desires they would not or could not play out with their regular partners. It is also about damaged women being damaged more. It involves the undermining and marginalizing of prostitute identified women, due in part to the lack of state action against violence against women and the many ways that prostitute women are seen as 'deserving victims' (see Bland 1992). It reinforces and reproduces the 'throwaway' status of women working as prostitutes, women who are seeking to earn the best they can for themselves, their partners and families and for whom prostitution is work; women who are poor, or who have been abused; have come out of care institutions not adequately prepared for independent living; who are emotionally needy and vulnerable and/or are seeking a subculture where they feel they belong.

Feminist research as feminist praxis

Developing social action approaches to women's lived experiences of sexual violence is one way of engaging in feminist praxis and can illustrate the liberating, transformative potential of feminist research as feminist praxis.

In my work, women centred practice, as policy oriented action, arose out of the interrelationship between doing feminist research and women's lived experience. The 'practice' consists of engaging in multi-agency work to address three central issues: routes into prostitution; routes out of prostitution; and support for women who want to work as prostitutes, or for whom there is no other choice of employment, around central needs and problems (see O'Neill 1992).[4] Our multi-agency forum has been meeting regularly to discuss matters relating to these three areas. It aims to facilitate the development of a more coordinated network of services to sex workers which serve educative and empowering functions, as well as fostering greater interagency cooperation and communication. The underlying philosophy to which members are committed is a gender aware approach. This approach will address the ways in which the women and young people involved in sex work can be empowered by developing better services to meet material, economic, social and emotional needs. This will involve connecting experience with theory, practice and policy to develop more positive approaches to service provision, and to ensure that the objectives outlined below meet the aims of the project.

The current objectives to which members are committed are as follows: the development of joint work and interagency cooperation; the development of education and training packages to increase the awareness and understanding of professionals who encounter sex workers, as well as to challenge attitudes; networking with other projects; policy review; monitoring and evaluation, for example discussing the usefulness and practicality of the project as it develops; and finally engaging and assisting in research.

Violence, health, welfare, legal rights, human rights and civil liberties, iniquitous fining systems, the policing of street prostitution are all issues we are grappling with at both a discursive and practical level. The facilitation of social action approaches to prostitution must have women working as prostitutes centrally involved. The problems and needs of prostitutes are the key concerns women working as prostitutes or representing prostitutes bring to our multi-agency working group.

Peer empowerment as feminist practice

These dimensions of methodology, practice and experience are interrelated, woven into my central focus of concern; 'being' a feminist researcher and 'doing' feminist research that has practical implications and possibilities for the women involved as 'subjects' of that research.

In order to expand upon the reflexive interrelationship between feminist research, women's lived experience and policy oriented practice it is, I believe, important to start with the possibilities for women centred approaches to practice/action. Peer group empowerment supported by a multi-agency working group is central to the progress and development of our work. Particularly peer group empowerment as organized and delivered by organizations such as POW!, the Safe Project, ScotPep and others. POW! (prostitute outreach workers) is a peer education organization and registered charity working from the East Midlands and led by Sue Johnson. The Safe Project is a pioneering health education project operating from Birmingham and led by Hilary Kinnell. ScotPep is a peer led education programme based in Edinburgh and led by Ruth Morgan-Thomas. All are health based initiatives and funded largely by health authority funds and operate referral systems to other agencies where necessary. POW! is a key player in the East Midlands Multi-Agency Forum.

Judith Green (1992: 17) provides a useful description of empowerment in relation to the youth service: 'The role of empowering young people, enabling them to make informed and discriminating choices with regard to their own lives, is seen as a major one for youth workers'. Of course this aim must be understood as one which operates within the constraints of the material, ideological and emotional contexts of the lived experience of young people.

What is peer led education leading to peer empowerment in the context of prostitution? Peer led education is a specific social action approach to the needs of women and children engaged in prostitution which starts at grass roots level, at the level of everyday experience involving peer support, education and sharing of knowledge, information and empowerment. Peer empowerment as well as participatory action research has its roots in the women's movement in the development of feminist thought, feminist research and feminist action. Advantages include the development of: greater knowledge and awareness; self-esteem and self-protection; greater confidence which in turn enables the creation of better organized and more accountable support networks to function around the issues of violence, welfare rights, civil liberties, self-protection, counselling and therapeutic services (POW! in O'Neill 1993).

Peer led education and empowerment projects could create the intellectual and practical spaces for the voices of women involved in sex work (who are usually the 'subjects' of research) to be heard and listened to. Listening to these voices is part of the process of understanding that must accompany social change. Creating this space is also part of the 'democratization' process involved in peer education as opposed to a hierarchical model based upon professional and non-professional, teacher and taught, researcher and subject.

For example, POW! gives support, counselling and guidance on health, welfare and legal rights. It provides safe houses and ultimately aims to build a network of women working and not working in prostitution enabling peer support, peer education and peer empowerment. Work such as this must be supported financially, practically and emotionally at local levels via groups such as our multiagency forum and also at national and international levels.

Education and empowerment is not a process operating only between women working as prostitutes, but is reflexive and can include others working with and for them. Certainly peer led techniques could enable agencies working with and for women to better understand the issues, practicalities and emotions involved in doing prostitution. This has been my experience and the experience of those attending our multi-agency forum. Hopefully, this approach could also lead to policy changes around employment, housing, anti-poverty strategies (through greater awareness and lobbying of concerned groups) as well as greater awareness regarding health, safety, and greater empowerment and self-esteem for marginalized groups.

One small but significant example of the possible outcomes of action research and multi-agency working involved our forum taking up the issue (mentioned earlier in the chapter) of the local newspaper printing the names and addresses of women prosecuted for soliciting, with the editor of this paper. His answer was that if the women do not want their names and addresses printed they must say so in court and also fill out a form available in the reception of the newspaper's offices. Since we contacted him, however, there has been no further evidence of names and addresses appearing in print – one small but significant example of the possible outcomes of action research.

Outcomes of a formally organized network (local and national) of feminists and women working as prostitutes, around the issue of peer empowerment, could effect change in woman centred ways. These would include: changes in policing violence against prostitutes (see Mavolwane *et al.* 1989); changes in the way courts deal with women; changes in the activities of the criminal injuries compensation board (who militate against those with criminal records and particularly against female victims of rape and assault); changes in the street culture acceptance and/or toleration of levels of violence towards women; changes in the way the press and media represent prostitute victims of violence; and 'child centred' changes in the form, content and delivery of care to young people in the care of the local authority. These are all changes I look forward to within a coordinated feminist resistance and feminist challenge to sexual and social inequalities, a developing feminist praxis.

Conclusion

The reflexive relationship between methodology, experience and practice aimed at policy change has evolved alongside the development of a relationship of trust and risk with women working as prostitutes within the context of a research process which prioritizes developing 'knowledge for' as feminist praxis. This work is linked to resistance and empowerment: resistance to sexual and social inequalities; self-empowerment, peer empowerment and social knowledge as a form of power. I have highlighted the terrible experiences and high levels of sexual violence against women prostitutes and the dilemmas and ethical concerns for the feminist researcher. This work is part of an emerging model both nationally and internationally, using feminist participatory research methods to work *with* women and children working in the sex industry. The need is to support, struggle and act against male violence against women in order to develop critical praxis via immanent critique.

Acknowledgements

Thanks to Jill, Marianne and Liz for sound editorial support; the chapter is much the better for it. Thanks also to the women who helped in the development of this work. The names of the women who talked to me about routes into prostitution and experiences of sexual violence have been changed to protect confidentiality. I am indebted to Karen Hughes who enabled this work to happen and to all the members of the multi-agency forum.

Notes

1 All the women's names have been changed. Some women chose their own name, others were happy for me to create a new name for them. Not all the women were offered the option of choosing their own name due in part to the realities of researching on-street. During most off-street interviews women chose for themselves. Confidentiality and respect for their personal space was stressed at the outset of the initial pilot study and maintained throughout the later work.
2 Some references have been omitted to preserve anonymity.
3 Ann's narrative is reproduced more fully in 'Women at work: Prostitution and feminism in the context of late modernity', *PHOEBE*, State University New York, Oneonta, NY, Vol. 4, no. 1, spring 1992.
4 This is a grouping of statutory and voluntary agencies including police, social services, city and county council representatives, probation, health authority, solicitors, magistrates, a drug rehabilitation programme, the church and women working as prostitutes and women representing prostitutes.

5 The policing of street prostitution is currently in focus given: the meeting of the all-Parliamentary group on prostitution chaired by Diane Abbott; moves by Birmingham City Council to examine the setting up of zones of tolerance on the Utrecht model; calls from the 'Soliciting for Change' forum, who hosted a national conference in Nottingham, September 1993, to decriminalize prostitution; signs of an increasing relationship between prostitution and drugs, notably crack and crack related problems; the lack of national standards in dealing with street prostitution; and a series of murders in the East and West Midlands against prostitutes, all bearing significant similarities.

Currently in the East Midlands the anti-vice squad operate a three pronged approach to street prostitution. Pimps and kerbcrawlers are prosecuted along with women soliciting on-street. In 1993, 21 pimps were convicted for living off immoral earnings; 141 women were prosecuted for soliciting offences, the offences total 479 cases; and 85 kerbcrawlers were prosecuted. Between January and July 1994 10 juveniles were dealt with by the police. An increase in juvenile prostitution, specifically children from local authority care or having left local authority care and an increase in drug related prostitution with this group is encouraging the police anti-vice and drug squad to work more closely with residential units and senior managers in social services.

With the policing of street prostitution multi-agency action research is a valuable way of working out the key areas for policy oriented practice in a more holistic way and how such action might be enabled in partnership with the major agencies working with and for women and young people engaged in prostitution.

References

Bland, L. (1992) The case of the Yorkshire ripper: mad, bad, beast, or male? In J. Radford and D. Russell (eds) *Femicide: The Politics of Woman Killing*. Milton Keynes: Open University Press.

Green, J. (1992) It's No Game: responding to the needs of young women at risk or involved in prostitution. Leicester: National Youth Agency.

Harding, S. (ed.) (1987) *Feminism and Science*. Milton Keynes: Open University Press.

Hoigard, C. and Finstad, L. (1992) *Backstreets: Money, Prostitution and Love*. Cambridge: Polity Press.

Mavolwane, S., Miller, S., Watson, J. and Cadman, E. (1989) *Policing and Prostitution*. London: Rights of Women.

O'Neill, M. (1991a) *Current Responses to Prostitution: A Multi-agency Response*. Report for Nottingham Safer Cities, Nottingham Trent University.

O'Neill, M. (1991b) 'Routes into prostitution: poverty, homelessness and leaving care', conference paper given to 'Crime, Justice and the Sex Industry', Nottingham Polytechnic, November.

O'Neill, M. (1992) 'Academic power and social knowledge: prostitution, critical theory and feminist praxis'. Paper prepared for the International Conference on Academic Knowledge and Political Power, University of Maryland, College Park, MD, November 20–22.

O'Neill, M. (1993) Prostitution and the state: towards a feminist practice. In C. Lupton and T. Gillespie (eds) *Working with Violence: Dilemmas for a Feminist Practice*. London: Macmillan.

O'Neill, M. (1994) Prostitution and the state: towards a feminist practice. In C. Lupton and T. Gillespie (eds) *Working with Violence*. London: Macmillan.

Pheterson, G. (1986) *The Whore Stigma: Female Dishonor and Male Unworthiness*. Amsterdam: Dutch Ministry of Social Affairs and Employment.

Stanley, L. (1990) *Feminist Praxis*. London: Routledge.

10

Rape crisis centres and 'male rape': a face of the backlash

Terry Gillespie

Introduction

This chapter critically examines issues surrounding the rape of men, or 'male rape' as it has been named, insofar as they interact with, and affect rape crisis centres. Male rape, now recognized as a sexual crime in British law, refers to the non-consensual buggery of a man by another man or men. Rape is a brutal and degrading crime of sexual violence whether perpetrated on a female or a male, adult or child, and one which, whoever the victim, is perpetrated by men. It is important to stress, at the outset, that male rape does not refer to the 'rape' of men by women; rather it is an example of men's sexual violence towards other, less powerful men. My concern here is to examine the extent to which the discourse around male rape has marginalized feminist support services, and rape crisis centres in particular.

Before going further, it is important to point to the distinction made by feminists between the terms 'victim' and 'survivor'. Feminists working in the field of violence against women have preferred to use the term 'survivor' for women who have suffered sexual, emotional and physical violence (Stanko 1985; Kelly 1988; Chapter 2 of this volume). This term is seen as more empowering than that of 'victim', which suggests passivity and loss of autonomy. Positivist victimology has historically sought to locate female survivors of sexual assault as 'victims', at times blaming women for violence perpetrated on them. However, some feminists are seeking to redress the balance by insisting on a critical and progressive victimology which acknowledges the way in which women negotiate processes of powerlessness and oppression in their daily lives (Walklate 1994), including the survival of sexual violence.

While referring to media, police and professional responses to male rape

I intend to use the term 'victim', in the sense of being a victim of a criminal offence. Nevertheless, I also use, and acknowledge the importance of using, the term 'survivor', not least for those who have survived violence. This terminology is now used by some professional bodies and statutory agencies working in the field of rape and sexual assault.

Over the last two decades in Britain and other countries feminists have made a real impact on improving support services for female victims of men's sexual violence and raising awareness of the nature of sexual violence, while deconstructing myths about rape and sexual assault. Despite a history of poor funding and marginalization by statutory and professional bodies, rape crisis centres (RCCs) have nevertheless survived and flourished, offering a range of support services for female survivors of rape and sexual assault.[1]

However, the success of feminist support services was followed by a political and ideological backlash in the late 1980s. This backlash has sought to undermine and marginalize feminist services in a range of ways (Lupton and Gillespie 1994). This has been apparent both in the media and within academia, most notably in the concept of 'post-feminism' and in the kneejerk reaction by right wing ideologues to 'political correctness' or any other acknowledgement of the effectiveness of feminism in changing perceptions and behaviour.

One form of the backlash has been expressed in the promotion of myths: that men are abused as much as, if not more than, women; that women are as violent as men; and that men have been wilfully denied support services enjoyed by female victims of violence and sexual assault. Further, it has been suggested that feminists working in the field of violence against women have lied or fudged the truth about the incidence and prevalence of men's violence against women and children. Admittedly, such views, voiced largely by embittered male libertarian writers (for example in Britain: Lyndon 1993; Thomas 1993) have been largely dismissed as polemical, misogynist, short on empirical evidence and lacking any research base.

Nevertheless, there is still a resistance on the part of statutory agencies and professional bodies to feminist organizations and support groups, seen, in the main, as unprofessional and politically motivated. This antipathy towards feminist services has been reinforced over recent years by burgeoning men's movements, both in Britain and the US. While some men's groups have been supportive of feminism, a few have been overtly hostile, particularly where such groups see themselves as competing directly with feminist organizations for the funding of support services.

This 'face of the backlash' (Rush 1990) has expressed itself largely through unfounded assertions about the hostility of RCCs towards male rape survivors and towards men in general. Meanwhile, the same assertions, frequently cited in the media by key spokespersons for male survivors groups, have been consistently used by professionals working in the field of support for victims of rape and sexual assault as a justification for marginalizing RCCs. In the course of my research into support services for victims of rape and sexual assault, I have found this persistent undermining of feminist organizations generally, and RCCs in particular, astounding, given that such criticisms of the nature and organizational modes of RCCs are based neither on systematic research nor empirical evidence.[2]

Florence Rush points to the backlash against feminist organizations from 'men's rights' groups in the US. For example, she cites Sidney Siller, organizer of the National Organization for Men who 'insists that men are victims of false accusations by disgruntled, angry women in cases of sexual harassment, rape and child molestation' (1990: 169). She became aware in the late 1980s of an organization set up by male rape survivors to raise public awareness of the issues surrounding male rape, citing statistics 'which indicated that a quarter or more of all rape victims in New York City are males' (p. 169).

As with all areas of sexual violence there are methodological problems associated with the prevalence and incidence of male rape. For example, figures cited by survivors' groups and in male rape literature often refer to the incidence of male rape in prisons, based on studies in the US. There has been very little research on male rape in Britain, other than that conducted by Gillian Mezey and Michael King discussed below. However, quite apart from the issue of the validity of statistics on male rape, Florence Rush is sceptical of the implication that rape is 'gender neutral' and that 'male rape' is perpetrated on men by women. As she points out:

> We know, and they know, of course, that it is gay and heterosexual men, not women, who rape men. This fact, however, does not make male rape gender-neutral. Men rape other men because they feminize their victims within heterosexual patterns of dominance and subordination.
> (1990: 169)

In this chapter I focus on issues for feminists surrounding male rape including the gendered nature of men's sexual violence against predominantly female, and also male, victims of rape and sexual assault. In addition, I explore the implications for RCCs of the growth of male rape survivor groups and the wave of public sympathy and police response to this form of victimization.

Male rape and the law

The criminal law in Britain has changed with regard to male rape. The Criminal Justice and Public Order Act (1994) has amended the definition of rape which now includes non-consensual buggery of a male and carries a maximum life sentence for rape of male or female victims alike.[3] Previously, buggery of a male over 16 years of age carried a maximum 10-year sentence (Section 12, Sex Offences Act, 1956).[4] Male rape victims whose cases reach the courts will be granted anonymity in the same way as female victims. At the same time the Act legalizes consensual anal sex between a man and woman (*Pink Paper* 1994). At the least these 'reforms' should introduce anonymity for women who have been non-consensually anally raped. Non-consensual buggery has effectively been redefined as rape, and in the process rape has become 'gender neutral', to use the term favoured by long term campaigners for these changes in the law on sexual offences. Michael King, a senior lecturer in psychiatry at the Royal Free Hospital School of Medicine in London who has conducted research into male rape, was consulted by the Home Office on the legal reforms. For King, 'As well as bringing about gender equality for the offence of rape, this move establishes the principle of the offence in the eyes of the public, who probably don't know enough about it' (*Pink Paper* 1994).

In terms of 'gender neutrality' the recent changes in the law bring Britain in line with Germany, Canada, Holland and some US states. Feminists had long campaigned for changes in the legal definition of rape to broaden out beyond penile penetration, though not necessarily to include men sexually assaulting men. Elaine Ginsberg and Sarah Lerner (1989) argued for a broader definition of rape in an attempt to move the focus away from the issue of consent while retaining its gender specificity. An alternative definition was proposed: 'A man commits rape on a woman if he uses, or intends to use, force, threats, coercion or intimidation to accomplish sexual penetration'; sexual penetration being defined as 'penetration, however slight, of the labia or anus by any part of the body by another, or by any object, or the penetration, however slight, of the mouth by a penis' (1989: 41).

For feminists, while acknowledging the degradation and brutality of male rape, to refer to 'non-consensual buggery' as the same as female rape (i.e. that the crime is gender neutral), is to render invisible the gendered power relations between men and women expressed through men's sexual violence to women. Feminists were concerned that in changing the legal definition of rape, the only gender specific crime in British law would disappear from the statute book.

The change in law was largely a result of campaigning work by gay men's and male rape survivors' groups over the last decade. For Ernest Woollett, a counsellor with and spokesperson for Survivors: 'At last the Government has recognised this offence, which traumatises hundreds of men every year' (*Pink Paper* 1994). Survivors, which receives approximately 400 calls a year from male victims of sexual assault, expects this number to increase with the change in law (*Pink Paper* 1994).[5]

In *Male Rape: Breaking the Silence on the Last Taboo*, Richie McMullen, one of the founders of the UK male rape Survivors group, set up in 1988, argues that in a male dominated culture men don't want to see themselves as 'victims' hence the notion that male rape is the 'last taboo' (McMullen 1990). There is evidence that few women wish to become, or be seen as victims either (Kelly 1988), however, McMullen's statement presumes the 'normality' of female rape, which is not considered taboo, regardless of the fact that many women find it difficult to name their experiences of forced sex as rape (Koss and Harvey 1991).

McMullen had long campaigned for legal reforms so that male rape could be brought into line with female rape in law and be extended to include women raping men. Hence male rape would be defined as either 'non-consensual active (or passive) anal penetration with a male offender(s)' and/or 'non-consensual vaginal penetration with a female offender(s)' (1990: 13). The term 'male rape' is often misinterpreted as referring to women 'raping' or abusing men sexually. However, it is acknowledged that this form of sexual assault is statistically insignificant (Mezey and King 1992).

What is glaringly obvious, both from official statistics and academic studies of rape, together with women's accounts of sexual violence, is that it is overwhelmingly men who rape and sexually abuse other men, women and children. It would be hard to find a crime that is more specifically gendered, yet this important variable appears to be overlooked in criminological and victimology literature. While the issue of gender is acknowledged with regard to the predominantly female victims of rape and sexual assault, and, more recently, with the discovery of males being raped, the issue of the male perpetration of sexual violence is virtually ignored. Florence Rush has stated:

> Gender-neutrality is rooted in the idea that both genders, male and female, are equally oppressed and that any attempt to hold men and male institutions accountable for transgressions against women is no longer fashionable nor acceptable.
>
> This concept has become a useful tool in an attempt to establish that women are as guilty as men for the offenses attributed to them. Professionals and experts tell us that women are also rapists and child molesters, that women batter and sexually harass men and are also the producers and consumers of pornography . . .
>
> True, some small percentage of women sexually abuse children and sexually harass men, but I can safely assure you that if women were the rapists, child molesters, and sexual harassers, the problem of sexual assault would barely exist.
>
> (1990: 170)

Incidence and prevalence of male rape

Where the crime has been the subject of academic study it is frequently suggested that male rape may be even more underreported than female rape (Katz and Mazur 1979; Hillman *et al.* 1990; McMullen 1990; Mezey and King 1992; Dyer 1994). Home Office figures for 1984–89 indicate that offences of buggery increased by 90 per cent and indecent assault of boys by 24 per cent. Eighty-five per cent of male victims of indecent assault were under 15 years, thus there is evidence of widespread sexual abuse of male children by men (Bunting 1992). It is not clear whether the figure of 90 per cent refers specifically to cases of male rape, or whether they are referring to a subset of offences.

The number of male rapes reported to the police has risen as police forces have reportedly developed a more sympathetic approach to male victims.

In 1993, 50 incidents of 'male rape' were reported to the Metropolitan police compared with 27 the previous year (Dyer 1994). However, we need to view these figures in the context of comparable figures for female rape. In the same year there were 1,360 cases of female rape reported to the Metropolitan Police, an increase of 210 on the figures for 1992 (Metropolitan Police Statistics Branch 1994).

The police response to male rape, as with female rape, has, in the past, been hesitant and largely reactive to public and media pressure. The Metropolitan Police have led the way in providing a more victim-sensitive approach and claim to provide the same level of service provision for male and female victims of rape. Nevertheless, it should not be forgotten that it was largely due to campaigns by feminist organizations that police initiatives on the treatment of rape victims emerged during the 1980s. Such initiatives include rape examination suites, the training of specialist women police officers, the recruitment of more women police surgeons and the introduction of more sensitive reporting procedures. While it was, and still is, traumatic for female rape victims to report incidents of sexual violence, male rape victims claimed that they have in the past suffered the additional trauma of homophobia on the part of the police, whether the victim was gay or heterosexual (McMullen 1990; Mezey and King 1992).

While other forces are now offering similar support services, the Metropolitan Police experienced pressure to develop initiatives on male rape following an apparent increase in the number of cases reported in the early 1990s. In 1992 six cases in the London region were reported in the press over a period of three months (Bunting 1992).

The Metropolitan Police, following the publicity surrounding several reported cases, set up a pilot project whereby 26 officers were trained as 'chaperones' to support male rape victims. These specially trained officers would take a statement, accompany the victim for HIV screening and offer long term support where cases went to court. In addition, a support unit, set up primarily to meet the needs of female victims of rape and sexual assault, was being made available for male rape victims. However, from March to October 1992, the unit had dealt with only four cases (Bennetto 1992).

Growing concern about the prevalence of male rape in prisons and penal institutions has led to some astounding claims. For example, Walker (1994) points out that there were 106,590 reported incidents of rape of females in the US in 1991. Citing American studies he confidently goes on to assert: 'But there are twice, probably three times as many rapes of men taking place in American prisons' (Walker 1994). These figures are estimates based on small-scale studies of rape in male prisons. In addition, such figures ignore the vast numbers of female rapes which go unreported (Hanmer and Saunders 1984; Hanmer and Maynard 1987; Kelly 1988). Indeed, they compare reported rapes of women with unreported rapes of men and thus are not comparing like with like. In the context of the lack of any reliable empirical evidence, it should not be assumed that male rape is more underreported than female rape.

Research cited by Dumond (1992) and others suggests that for young male prisoners the chances of avoiding rape are 'almost zero . . . He'll get raped within the first 24 or 48 hours. That's almost standard' (Lerner cited in Dumond 1992: 136). Further, once an inmate has been raped, the chances of revictimization are apparently high and remain so for the length of his sentence. If this is in fact the case, it is a reflection of the brutal and brutalizing regimes of many male penal institutions where it appears that some prison officers choose to ignore or to sanction the sexual abuse of young male offenders. Following cases in the US, a British prisoner is suing the Home Office for negligence as a result of having been raped in his cell in 1991 (Armistead 1994). If this case is successful it may encourage additional complaints against prison authorities. Such fears have clearly stimulated interest, on the part of professional and voluntary agencies alike, in the incidence and prevalence of male rape.

Survivors has strong links with professionals working in the field of male rape and is involved in a two year survey of 10,000 men in institutions, including prisons, the army and university campuses, funded by the Wellcome Foundation (*Pink Paper* 1994). The purpose of this research is to examine the prevalence and incidence of male rape, seen as a growing problem with the increase in young men being incarcerated in penal institutions.

Some of the distinctions drawn between rape of men in penal institutions and that of women demonstrates a lack of awareness of the literature on rape. One example is the claim that 'few female rape victims must repay their rapist for the violence he inflicted upon them by devoting their existence to servicing his every need, but rape victims in the world of prison must' (Rideau and Wikberg, cited in Walker 1994: 14).

This spurious claim is based on the common assumption that women are most frequently raped in isolated incidents by strangers. However, studies of female rape have revealed that women are most commonly raped by men known to them and, further, that they are likely to be subject to repeat victimization. In other words, once the rapist is sure that the woman is not going to report the assault, he is likely to repeatedly rape her over time (Brownmiller 1975; LRCC 1984; Kelly 1988). In this sense, it appears that some rapists are likely to assault their victims repeatedly, whether male or female. Feminists working in support services for female survivors of men's violence are well aware of the levels of repeat victimization in relation to sexual assault including marital rape and domestic violence (Dobash and Dobash 1992).

Male survivor groups and rape crisis centres

As more publicity is accorded to male rape it is probable that there will be a greater demand for support services for male rape victims in both prison and community settings. Given that the majority of RCCs will continue to offer services solely for women, the onus is on men's survivor groups to develop services for male rape victims and to establish and strengthen links with other service providers. In this respect, the London based support group Survivors has already established itself as the primary support group for male rape victims in Britain.

While I would not wish to diminish the important work undertaken by the Survivors organization, it is worrying that its spokespersons have at various times expressed ambivalent views about RCCs in interviews with the media. On the one hand, they acknowledge the contribution and work of feminist groups in putting men's violence, rape and sexual abuse on to the public agenda and the setting up of support services for women, while, on the other hand, they repeatedly assert that RCCs have been unhelpful, indeed hostile, to male survivors who have called telephone counselling lines for support.

Martin Dockrell, the co-founder with Richie McMullen of Survivors, stated in a television documentary on male rape, 'Men who have been raped suffer the same trauma as female victims' (Sampson 1991). While he respects the right of RCCs to remain 'women-only structures' he believes they should help male victims too. Meanwhile, Gillian Mezey and Michael King have said:

> There is little evidence that the gender of therapist is important in influencing the victim's rate of recovery: the requirement of many RCCs that only women deal with female rape victims is based more on political rather than scientific considerations.
>
> (1992: 137)

Gillian Mezey's statement ignores the research which shows consistently that women who have been raped or sexually assaulted by men prefer to talk to women counsellors (Kelly 1988; Foley 1994). It would appear that her argument is in itself politically motivated, given her advocacy both of men's support groups and victim support schemes (Gillespie 1994).

Richie McMullen, however, highlights the expertise of RCC workers and states that male survivor groups need to learn from them in terms of developing caring services and responses and also 'in learning how to put the male case' (1990: 85), an acknowledgement that RCCs have been successful in winning resources for service provision in a difficult financial climate.

Nevertheless, male rape survivor groups frequently refer in the press to RCCs as 'extreme unhelpful' organizations. For example, a male rape victim refers to phoning his local RCC, 'but they refused to help because I was a man'. (Sampson 1991). Again, Richie McMullen, cited in *Company* magazine: 'When I was raped my first instinct was to ask London RCC for help but they just slammed the phone down on me' (Kirsta 1991), while Stuart Turner has asserted that: 'It is possible that some of the anti-male rhetoric associated with female RCCs, in which men are cast only in the role of aggressor, is serving to add to the isolation of the male victim of sexual assault' (Mezey and King 1992: 82). Writing in the *British Medical Journal*, Michael King states that: 'There is a great need for the specialised rape services already catering for women to include men as well' (King 1990).

These extracts are just a selection of comments critical, in varying degrees, of RCCs, which cumulatively amount to gross generalizations about the organizational modes and policies of centres. There appears to be a contradiction between, on the one hand, criticisms of the supposed 'political, rather than scientific' stance of RCCs in wishing to retain service provision 'for women, by women' and the demand that such organizations, seen at one and the same time as both professional yet 'anti-men', should extend services to men. This hostility towards, or apparent jealousy of, feminist organizations is reflected in the men's movement in the US.

A male rape survivor, Fred Pelka, supports fears about a backlash against autonomous women's groups providing services for female rape survivors:

> It's true that the vast majority of rape crisis counsellors are women, that the entire stop-rape movement is an extension of the women's movement. For the record, though, I have never felt any hostility in response when calling a rape crisis center, this in spite of the fact that rape crisis centers are often plagued by 'hotline abusers' – men who call to masturbate to the sound of a female voice . . . Some male survivors even blame women for the denial and homophobia they encounter after the assault. They openly resent the (pitifully few) resources available to female survivors, as if any help women receive is at the expense of men.
>
> (1992: 11)

Male survivors frequently argue in the media that they prefer to speak to female counsellors. They claim to feel safer talking to a woman and Richie McMullen endorses this apparent 'need'. London RCC states, however, that its women only policy is designed to promote a feeling of safety among those who contact the service. Male callers are referred to Survivors: 'The women who work here don't want to counsel men. We are not the right people to do it' (Sampson 1991).

The right people to do it are more likely to be male rape survivors who would appear to enjoy the support and backing of professional groups who, in turn, have not in the past been as keen to support feminist services for female victims of sexual violence. It is unrealistic to expect RCCs, already overstretched and underfunded, to offer counselling on masculinity to gay and heterosexual men who have been sexually assaulted. However, it appears that men who have been sexually assaulted want to talk to women, not other men and therein lies the problem for RCCs, already experiencing pressure to extend service provision in the face of funding difficulties.

Rape crisis centres and survival

My ongoing research into service provision for rape victims is focused primarily on support services for female victims of rape and sexual assault. The research has explored the interagency relationship between RCCs, who have been at the forefront of working with sexual violence since the 1970s in

Britain, victim support schemes (VSSs), who have moved steadily since the mid-1980s into the area of provision for sexual crime 'victims', and the police. The research has been concerned mainly with the survival and development of RCCs in the context of a protracted, difficult economic and political climate for the funding of voluntary groups in Britain during the 1980s and early 1990s. However, despite these difficulties, which have in any case been spread unevenly, RCCs in Britain, like other feminist organizations, have continued to survive and indeed grown in number over the last decade (Lupton and Gillespie 1994).

In my survey of RCCs in 1989, the majority reported being overstretched, underresourced and facing increasing demand for services from women. A particular element of the research is an examination of the various organizational modes of RCCs and it has been interesting to see how RCCs have responded to these pressures. Centres were asked about their policy of dealing with male callers but were not asked for numbers of men calling. The majority of centres continue to run support services solely for women. All 38 centres responding to the survey had a policy of referring male callers to appropriate agencies and survivor groups. Twenty-four centres provided counselling support for male partners or close friends of women who had been sexually abused. Interestingly, 15 of the 38 centres left decisions about counselling sexually abused males to individual counsellors. Only two centres had set up separate services specifically for male clients, one of which had done so for eight years; during this time, however, they had not received a single call from sexually abused males.

At least two centres have set up joint services for female and male survivors using separate buildings for male and female users. One centre received specific funding from the regional health authority to set up a male rape service following pressure from male rape survivors. However, for at least one of these centres, this expansion of service provision to men has been problematic. Issues of concern to RCC workers include whether male counsellors should be trained by female counsellors; negotiating the demand for more female counsellors to provide services for men; the issue of appropriate counselling models; negotiating the power relations between male and female counsellors; and ensuring that the quality of service provision for female rape victims is maintained. One particular centre, which has been the focus of an in-depth case study, had actually received fewer calls from men in 1993/4 than in 1991/2 with numbers of male callers declining from 17 in 1991/2 to six in 1993/4 (or 2 per cent of their total calls).

Since the extensive media coverage of, albeit a small number, of male rape cases in the London region, referred to earlier in this chapter, it has become apparent that RCCs are experiencing pressure to extend service provision to men, both from statutory services, who are also often funding bodies, and who may be on the management or executive committee of RCCs, and also from male survivors of sexual assault. While RCCs are generally supportive of the need for male rape survivor groups, they do not on the whole wish to divert hard won resources and to dissipate energies needed for running female support services in the pursuit of setting up separate services for men. Centres do not, in any case, receive many calls from genuine male rape survivors. Part of this resistance appears to stem from the numbers of hoax or abusive calls that many RCCs receive from men. Moreover, rape is often perceived differently by, and certainly has different meanings for, women and men.

Rather than expressing hostility towards men, several of the RCCs in the survey reported good working relations with local male survivors groups. Incidentally, many centres also report in positive terms on initiatives towards effective multiagency working with local statutory groups, including the police (Gillespie 1994).

There is, however, some concern expressed by RCCs over the funding of separate support services for victims of male rape, with fears that centres may find themselves competing for funding with male groups. Most local authorities have a fairly limited resource allocation for victim support, which may have to be divided among a number of groups, including victim support schemes. Within the context of a rationalization of resources for voluntary groups generally, tied in with changes in the structures and functions of local authorities, the movement to set up a network of male rape survivor groups may, in the long term, pose problems for RCCs.

It would appear inevitable that, given the recent changes in the law concerning male rape, increased pressure will be placed on RCCs to provide services for men. Indeed campaigners from the Survivors group have already expressed the 'hope that Rape Crisis Centres around the country will improve their service to male victims' (*Pink Paper* 1994). Similarly, Michael King asserts that 'rape crisis centres for women and victim support schemes that counsel victims of crime will need assistance to widen their remit and make greater provision for men who have been sexually assaulted' (Mezey and King 1992: 11).

It is disappointing to note that literature on male rape (Mezey and King 1992) continues to reflect a rather narrow view of the nature and work of RCCs. In comparing VSSs and RCCs as the primary service providers for rape victims in the voluntary sector in Britain, Gillian Mezey and Michael King, for example, are unsympathetic to RCCs which, they claim 'regard rape as a manifestation of societal power inequality and misogyny rather than the product of individual pathology' (1992: 134). VSSs, on the other hand, 'have less of a political emphasis in their interpretation of rape. . . . and they offer an immediacy, frequency and duration of support not provided by rape crisis centres' (1992: 134). This is not necessarily the case as the level of service provision offered by VSSs to victims of rape and sexual assault varies regionally (Gillespie 1994). Mezey and King go on to assert that 'Unlike rape crisis centres, they [VSSs] encourage collaboration with the victim's social network, including police and other professional workers' (1992: 135). Given the tremendous amount of time and energy expended by RCC workers in order to encourage interagency networks and collaborative relationships with both statutory and voluntary agencies (Gillespie 1994), and the fact that most

RCCs do talk to women's supporters be they partners, relatives or friends and encourage women to find support from their social networks, these assertions are unfounded, misguided and potentially damaging to RCCs.

A recent survey found that rape crisis counsellors are highly trained, more so than counsellors in VSSs whose training is broad-based, covering support services for all crime victims (Charities Evaluation Services 1993). The CES report found that initial training for paid staff in RCCs varied from 30–420 hours per person (average, 97 hours), while volunteer staff averaged 61 hours initial training with some programmes providing up to 500 hours (CES 1993: 19).

Importantly, RCCs also offer a completely confidential service to rape survivors, unlike some of their counterparts in VSSs (Gillespie 1994). The latter take referrals directly from the police, use male as well as female counsellors in supporting female rape victims and cannot guarantee confidentiality, due to their close collaboration with the police together with the ethos of their service provision.

The effects of rape on female and male victims

Most of the studies on the psychological effects of rape, summarized in Mezey and King (1992) use the post traumatic stress disorder model to understand and respond to the effects of sexual violence on predominantly female victims. Female and male victims of sexual assault alike can suffer a range of responses, both in the short and long term, including guilt, feeling dirty, sleeplessness, nightmares, flashbacks and suicidal feelings. Victims often also feel anger towards the perpetrator/s, however this is rarely acknowledged in psychiatric and medical models of rape trauma.

Burgess and Holstrom's work (1979) has been particularly influential with their suggestion of an identifiable rape trauma syndrome (RTS), a model which many RCCs and male survivors groups find useful in helping survivors of rape and sexual assault (however, for a critique of this model see Kelly 1988; Foley 1994; and Kelly *et al.* 1994). The work that has been done on treating male rape survivors suggests that men suffer the same range of symptoms as women when victimized (Mezey and King 1992). However, in addition to these symptoms, men reportedly experience a 'crisis of masculinity' whether they identify themselves as heterosexual or homosexual. For example Groth and Burgess found in the case of male rape victims in prison, that in addition to the reactions normally associated with RTS, many experienced anxieties about their masculinity and feared repeat victimization (cited in Dumond 1992). Similarly, Cotton and Groth found that:

> In addition to the trauma experienced by the male victim, which is similar to the female victim of sexual assault, the experience may be more devastating, since the victim is devalued in regard to the two primary sources of the male identity: sexuality and aggression.
>
> (Dumond 1992: 143)

Dumond has identified three cycles of victimization in cases of male rape including revictimization which occurs both within the prison setting and in the general community, and refers to the revenge wishes that some 'embittered, angry and violent' male rape victims may experience and which may find expression in the desire to sexually assault others, including women and children (1992: 146).

One British study (Mezey and King 1989) argues that rape is 'worse' for male victims because they had felt their masculinity to be threatened and had felt the assault to be life-threatening. In this latter respect male rape victims do not differ markedly from female victims of sexual assault who often feel that their lives were threatened during the assault (LRCC 1984; Kelly 1988). Referring to this study, Dyer reports that 'male victims were even more likely than female to blame themselves and suffer crippling guilt' (Dyer 1994). Suggestions that rape is 'even worse' for male than female rape victims are clearly questionable, given the difficulties in any case in measuring and comparing subjective feelings.

For Zsuzanna Adler, 'it is arguable that adult male victims of sexual assault may, in some respects, have even more formidable obstacles to overcome in reporting and substantiating sexual victimization than do their female counterparts' (Mezey and King 1992: 117). Male rape victims, as indicated above, are frequently portrayed as fearful of the homophobia of the police. Rape is considered to be 'even worse' for men as victims since it may prompt confusion about their sexual orientation, but, again, women also express conflicts in relation to sex and sexuality.

Gillian Mezey and Michael King argue that 'the stigma for men may be even greater, however, in a society which expects its male members to be self-sufficient physically and psychologically' (1992: 10). Meanwhile, Richie McMullen takes this argument to its logical conclusion by asserting that, without support, men who have been raped are 'in real danger of becoming revenge rapists, thus creating more and more problems which, like it or not, will have an impact on the wider community' (1990: 23).

There is, as yet, nothing in the research literature to support this claim, while it is an underhand way of holding women, and specifically RCCs, accountable for the actions of men who choose to sexually assault women, children or other men. It would be difficult to imagine similar levels of argument resulting in public sympathy and professional concern were female victims to act vengefully towards the perpetrators of sexual violence. However, women are not supposed to suffer the same degree of trauma; as Richie McMullen has stated, 'Although rape of a woman disgusts us it remains a confirmation of gender. Rape of a man brings his gender into question' (Kirsta 1991). This appears to contradict his assertion elsewhere that 'as soon as people can take on board that it is not to do with gender, there can be an understanding of these issues. A victim is a victim' (Sampson 1991).

Richie McMullen seems to be exemplifying the confusion which exists around the issue of gender and rape. For women to be raped by men is deemed 'normal' while for men it is abnormal, an experience which 'feminizes' men, and one which is viewed as somehow more shocking and horrifying. Yet, in these extracts, he ignores the fact that the perpetrators of sexual violence are men. It is men who are raping women and men. So a rape victim is not merely a victim; a victim of sexual assault, whether male or female, is a victim of the gendered power relations between women and men, acted out in everyday life. Indeed, in describing how male rape victims can move from being 'victim to survivor to victor', McMullen equates the powerlessness experienced by male victims as feeling 'less than a man; more like a woman; effeminate; a legitimate target for abuse; deserving; cowardly; responsible and guilty' (1990: 67). Again, it is difficult to imagine female rape victims viewing themselves as 'victors', a masculine term which serves to emphasize how rape has different meanings for women and men.

It appears from the research on male rape, both within institutional settings such as prisons (Mezey and King 1992) and in community studies (Mezey and King 1989), that the victim is frequently 'feminized' and, as such, 'his attacker's sense of masculinity is preserved or even heightened' (Mezey and King 1992: 69; see also Bennetto 1992). Such fears of 'feminization' on the part of male rape victims highlight gendered differences in relation to rape and, further, point to difficulties with regard to demands that RCCs extend services to men. Presumably men who have been raped would not be comfortable discussing their concerns about masculinity and feminization with female rape counsellors.

Gender is an inherent issue in the area of rape and sexual assault and is both central to an understanding of the prevalence and incidence of male and female rape and, at the same time, problematic theoretically and practically. While the gender of male rape victims has become the focus of much academic research, there is a danger of neglecting the practical and emotional needs of the vast majority of female rape victims. Such neglect and obfuscation can have material effects on the level of service provision for female survivors of men's sexual violence.

Conclusion

I have argued in this chapter that male rape, like female rape, is a crime of sexual violence and one which can have long term effects on its victims. These effects may be differentiated along gender lines, however not enough is known about the incidence or prevalence of male rape. Not enough is known either about female rape, while we are indebted to feminist academics and organizations for highlighting its vastly underreported nature. It is, therefore, a matter of some concern that a national survey of 10,000 men is being funded to discover the nature and extent of male rape, while no similar study has been conducted on the incidence and prevalence of female rape.

Despite the status of RCCs as the established and acknowledged specialist service providers for female rape survivors (CES 1993; Gillespie 1994), centres are characterized consistently as hostile, unprofessional and politically motivated organizations. As Fred Pelka has noted:

> The men's movement claims that rape is a 'gender-neutral issue', and thus has nothing to do with sexism. What is ironic about all this is that what little acknowledgement there is of male victimisation generally comes from the *women's* stop-rape movement. To the extent that male survivors *can* tell their stories, it is because of the foundation laid down by feminists. So this woman-bashing is as ungrateful as it is gratuitous.
>
> (1992: 40)

While it would clearly be ridiculous to .claim that the apparent increase in cases of male rape is in itself part of an anti-feminist backlash, nonetheless the castigation of RCCs in the media by key spokespersons can be seen as part of an attempt to marginalize and vilify both feminist organizations and analysis.

I have suggested in this chapter that there are a number of valid reasons why it is not appropriate for feminist RCCs to counsel male rape survivors. The publicized and unfounded criticisms by men's support groups of RCCs suggests a considerable degree of anger towards women, who are at times blamed for men's trauma following sexual assault. Given that men who have been sexually assaulted by other men claim that one of the most traumatizing effects of rape is feminization, it is difficult to see why they claim benefit from support by women if they hold women and femininity in such low regard. In addition, I would question the basis on which women are assumed to be the appropriate people to offer counselling to men on issues of masculinity which, men frequently claim, has been undermined by the experience of male rape.

Women and RCCs should not be coerced through being held accountable for revictimization by 'revenge rapists'. It is the responsibility of the Home Office and prison authorities, rather than RCCs, to ensure the safety of its inmates and provide appropriate services for victims of male rape where assaults have occurred in penal institutions.

Further, there are contradictions inherent in claims by professionals on the one hand, such as Gillian Mezey who argues that 'scientifically' the gender of counsellors providing support services is irrelevant to the victim, and, on the other hand, the demands by male rape survivors, supported by such professionals, that RCCs extend services to provide counselling for men who 'need' to talk to women about their experiences of sexual assault by other men. One cannot say that RCCs who wish to provide women-only services are politically motivated, while male rape survivor groups' campaigns for women's support groups to extend services to men are neutral.

Developing services for men who need or want them should not be achieved at the expense of what is now 20 years of developing knowledge and expertise within the rape crisis movement. Services for men who have been sexually assaulted should develop in similar ways to those for women, responding to levels of need and service use. The discussion also needs to move beyond the unhelpful stereotyping and baiting of RCCs into serious engagement with the similarities and differences in meaning and impact rape has on women and men, and how these are both a product and reproduction of gendered power relations.

Provision for male rape victims, in both prison and community settings, should not be allowed to undermine the policy and practice of feminist RCCs which continue to offer the most experienced support services for the overwhelming numbers of female survivors of men's sexual violence.

Notes

1 Rape crisis centres are also referred to as sexual assault centres in other countries, while, in Britain, they are distinct from sexual assault referral centres which operate alongside police and medical services (Foley 1994 and Chapter 11, this volume).

2 In 1989 I conducted a national survey of RCCs in England and Wales. Of 59 centres sent a postal questionnaire, 38 centres responded. The survey covered a range of issues pertinent to the effective delivery of quality services for female victims of rape and sexual assault. To this end, questions were asked about: the type of service(s) provided; the duration and content of training programmes for paid and volunteer workers; the interface with statutory and voluntary agencies working in related fields of victim support; the organizational modes and service philosophies of centres.

The research is ongoing and has more recently focused on a longitudinal case study of a centre which has adopted managerialist structures (Gillespie 1994), and which has set up joint services for male and female victims of sexual assault.

3 The legal definition of rape of women in British law still refers specifically to penile penetration of the vagina thus excluding oral rape or penetration by objects other than the penis. These are covered under 'other sexual offences' and, apart from anal rape, none carry a potential life sentence.

4 The Criminal Law Revision Committee (1980) recommended that the sentence for non-consensual buggery for women and men should be equalized upwards to life imprisonment, and that the maximum sentence for 'consensual' buggery with a girl or boy under the age of 13 should be life imprisonment, and with a girl or boy over 13 years and under 16 years should be five years' imprisonment.

5 It is difficult to estimate the numbers of calls received from abused men by the Survivors support group as published figures vary markedly according to the source. Figures cited include: 100 per month (Kirsta 1991), 250 per month (Boseley 1991), 400 per year (*Pink Paper* 1994), 800 per year (Bunting 1992).

References

Armistead, C. (1994) Sentenced to silence, *Guardian*, 21 July: 15.

Bennetto, J. (1992) Gang rape of men 'seldom by gays', *Independent on Sunday*, 18 October.

Boseley, S. (1991) End to silence on male rape, *Guardian*, 24 April: 23.

Brownmiller, S. (1975) *Against Our Will: Men, Women and Rape*. New York: Bantam Books.

Bunting, M. (1992) Confronting last taboo of male rape, *Guardian*, 24 August.

Burgess, A. and Holstrom, L. (1979) *Rape Crisis and Recovery*. Bowie: Brady.

Charities Evaluation Services (CES) (1993) *Review of the Needs of Rape Crisis Centres (and Related Services), Interim Report*. London: CES.

Dobash, R. E. and Dobash, R. P. (1992) *Women, Violence and Social Change*. London: Routledge.

Dumond, R. W. (1992) The sexual assault of male inmates in incarcerated settings, *International Journal of the Sociology of Law*, 20: 135–57.

Dyer, C. (1994) Rape law helps male victims, *Guardian*, 12 July.

Foley, M. (1994) Professionalising the response to rape. In C. Lupton and T. Gillespie (eds) *Working with Violence*. Basingstoke: Macmillan.

Gillespie, T. (1994) Under pressure: Rape crisis centres, multi-agency work and strategies for survival. In C. Lupton and T. Gillespie (eds) *Working with Violence*. Basingstoke: Macmillan.

Ginsberg, E. and Lerner, S. (1989) *Sexual Violence Against Women: A Guide to the Criminal Law*. London: Rights of Women.

Hanmer, J. and Maynard, M. (eds) (1987) *Women, Violence and Social Control*. Basingstoke: Macmillan.

Hanmer, J. and Saunders, S. (1984) *Well-founded Fear: A Community Study of Violence to Women*. London: Hutchinson.

Hillman, R. J. *et al.* (1990) Sexual assault of men: a series, *Genitourinary Medicine*, 66: 247–50.

Katz, S. and Mazur, M. A. (1979) *Understanding the Rape Victim: A Synthesis of Research Findings*. New York: John Wiley and Son.

Kelly, L. (1988) *Surviving Sexual Violence*. Cambridge: Polity Press.

Kelly, L., Regan, L. and Burton, S. (1994) Syndromes and disorders: the dangers of medicalizing the impacts of sexual violence in legal cases. *Rights of Women Bulletin*, autumn/winter: 2–6.

King, M. (1990), Male rape: victims need sensitive management, *British Medical Journal*, 301, 15 December: 1345.

Kirsta, A. (1991) Male rape, *Company Magazine*. May: 46–8

Koss, M. P. and Harvey, M. R. (1991) *The Rape Victim: Clinical and Community Interventions*. London: Sage.

London Rape Crisis Centre (LRCC) (1984) *Sexual Violence: The Reality for Women*. London: Women's Press.

Lupton, C. (1994) The British refuge movement: the survival of an ideal. In C. Lupton and T. Gillespie (eds) *Working with Violence*. Basingstoke: Macmillan.

Lupton, C. and Gillespie, T. (1994) *Working with Violence*. Basingstoke: Macmillan.

Lyndon, N. (1993) *No More Sex War: The Failures of Feminism*. London: Mandarin.

McMullen, R. J. (1990) *Male Rape: Breaking the Silence on the Last Taboo*. London: Gay Men Press.

Metropolitan Police Statistics Branch (1994) Performance Information Bureau (unpublished information).

Mezey, G. and King, M. (1989) The effects of sexual assault on men: a survey of 22 victims, *Psychological Medicine*, 19: 205–9.

Mezey, G. and King, M. (eds) (1992) *Male Victims of Sexual Assault*. Oxford: Oxford University Press.

Pelka, F. (1992) Raped: a male survivor breaks his silence, *On the Issues*, spring: 8–11.

Pink Paper (editorial) (1994) Peers recognize male rape as crime, 336, 15 July: 1.

Rush, F. (1990) The many faces of backlash. In D. Leidholdt and J. G. Raymond (eds) *The Sexual Liberals and the Attack on Feminism*. Oxford: Pergamon Press.

Sampson, V. (1991) Against their will, *Guardian*, 23 July: 17.

Stanko, E. A. (1985) *Intimate Intrusions? Women's Experiences of Male Violence*. London: Routledge and Kegan Paul.

Thomas, D. (1993) *Not Guilty: Men, the Case for the Defence*. London: Weidenfeld and Nicolson.

Walker, M. (1994) Meat on the table, *Guardian*, 21 July: 14.

Walklate, S. (1994) Can there be a progressive victimology? *International Review of Victimology*, 3(1/2): 1–15.

11

Who is in control?: changing responses to women who have been raped and sexually abused

Marian Foley

In 1986 the first sexual assault centre (SAC) in England opened in Manchester. At the time I was a paid worker for Manchester Rape Crisis (MRC) and remember my own and other women's reactions. Our concerns were primarily political; we feared that women using the SAC would be put under intense pressure to report to the police even if they did not want to; that the politics of the SAC reduced women's responses to rape to a medical 'condition'; that the needs of women using the SAC had not been properly thought out. We also feared that the SAC represented a move by professionals to take over a sphere of work that feminists had been providing for many years. For some of us the SAC represented a threat not only to MRC, but all rape crisis centres (RCCs). Our response was to send a letter out to all RCCs outlining our concerns and making them aware that what was currently happening in Manchester could easily be replicated elsewhere. At that time we were clear that SACs were a potential threat to the future existence of feminist RCCs.

This threat has never materialized and SACs have never (to date) really taken off in Britain. Nine years on, as a volunteer for MRC and a worker for a SAC development project, the tensions between feminist and non-feminist services for women who have experienced rape and sexual assault are still as critical to me as they were in 1986. It was this strength of feeling that made me apply for my current post. I hoped that my knowledge of the limitations of the British model of SACs combined with my experience of working for a RCC would help me to push for a very different type of service provision. The irony that I'm now working with representatives from organizations such as the police and Victim Support who have traditionally been antagonistic to RCCs is not lost on me. Being in such a position has also enabled me to explain the importance of RCCs and to push for better funding. It has also meant that like many other feminists working in non-feminist organizations, I have sometimes felt both compromised and isolated. There has been a positive side; being a development worker has given me time to reflect on what women want and how it can be provided. This process has made me reconsider some of the ways in which some RCCs could also be improved. It is with all this in mind I want to revisit and reflect on the issues raised by SACs and alternatives to RCCs.

RCCs have a long history of providing services for women since 1974 in North America and 1976 in England. The first RCC in England opened in London, providing a 24-hour telephone line as well as individual, legal and medical support. Campaigning was a fundamental aspect of their work and feminists campaigned to raise the issues around rape; to challenge the ortho-doxy which blamed women and excused men; to push for changes in the way the police, courts and other professionals treated women who had re-ported rape. Women pooled their skills and experiences to provide a service which responded to women's needs, rather than defining for them what those experiences and responses should be. This process taught those of us doing this work a great deal, we drew on existing theories and understanding of rape and junked them when they did not fit what we were being told and created our own political analysis of rape. RCCs were never just about service provision but about making the fundamental connection between practice and theory and translating that into campaigning for social change (Anna 1988). The service informed the campaigning and the campaigning informed the service. Women's personal distress became the focus for collec-tive action and collective change. Rape had to be understood in a political and social context which encouraged, condoned and excused male violence against women. This context also influenced public responses to rape, what services were available and how women understood and responded to their experiences (Roberts 1989).

Campaigning for change clearly brought RCCs into conflict with es-tablished organizations and explains their historical distrust of the police and professionals and the hostility that the police and professionals have displayed to RCCs. Despite this hostility, feminist campaigns for changes in police practice were successful in that the development of police rape victim exam-ination suites and improved training for police officers on rape, were largely a response to feminist criticism. Rape victim examination suites were an attempt by the police to improve the physical environment in which women reporting rape were medically examined and interviewed. The introduction of SACs can be perceived as the next step on from these suites but actually although this was true in the case of the Northumbria police it certainly was not the case in Manchester. The Greater Manchester Police were not quick to respond to changes in police practice and the SAC represents their first attempt at improvement rather than the natural progression of existing services.

At the same time this public interest in rape and rape services created a shift in some RCCs from Women's Liberation groups, to service providers, with workers and management committee members.

The development of SACs in England

In November 1986 the Greater Manchester Police (GMP) opened the first SAC in the country, which is now known as the St Mary's Centre. This centre is situated on the ground floor of a large maternity hospital close to Manchester city centre. It is comprised of a suite of rooms which include an interview room, counselling room, medical examination suite and bathroom with shower facilities. In terms of facilities the Manchester SAC was similar to the best existing rape victim examination suites already in operation in many police forces, with two notable exceptions. First, the St Mary's facilities were open to women regardless of whether or not they had reported the offence to the police and second the centre employed women counsellors to provide a counselling service. In these two respects the SAC represented a new development in services provided by the police by extending the scope beyond the immediate investigation of the crime, to include aftercare services for women provided by nurses. As a 'new' police development (in England) the centre generated a great deal of interest from the media and from other police forces across the country.

The Manchester SAC is a joint collaboration between the Greater Manchester Police (GMP), Greater Manchester Police Authority (GMPA) and Central Manchester Health Authority (CMHA) with the bulk of the funding coming from the GMPA. The SAC represents a convergence of police and medical needs which obviously overlap in relation to forensic medical examinations. It is not therefore surprising that as early as 1982 a woman police surgeon working for the GMP wrote a letter to *The Times* suggesting the setting up of a SAC which she followed up in a seminar paper in 1984 (Roberts 1984). As far as the GMP were concerned the SAC met a number of police purposes, the main one being dispelling what they viewed as women's 'unwarranted scepticism' of police procedures (Greater Manchester Police 1986), in order to increase the reporting of rape and sexual assault. The centre also offered improved forensic medical facilities; aftercare service that the police viewed as victim-friendly and could refer to, thus avoiding MRC; enhanced police credibility. Its establishment shifted the debate on rape away from the police and into the realm of medical intervention (Foley 1991). Those involved in establishing the SAC saw it as a unique venture which would act as a model for other police forces (Greater Manchester Police 1988).

As a model for service provision the SAC did generate a great deal of interest from many police forces, interagency working groups and local authorities across the country including Northumbria, West Yorkshire, Leicester, Merseyside and Hammersmith and Fulham. What has happened as a result of this interest has varied depending on: whether or not financial support has been forthcoming; responses of local feminist groups; and whether individual feminists in local government and the voluntary sector have been able to use this interest to create something different for women.

Northumbria police did succeed in setting up two SACs in Newcastle and Sunderland which offer a similar service to Manchester SAC. Other police forces such as Strathclyde, West Yorkshire and Leicester, whilst showing an interest in the SAC model, have not as yet adopted it. This is probably due to a combination of factors. SACs are very expensive. This, coupled with the fact that police forces have already invested money in rape victim examination suites, do not make SACs a financially viable alternative in times of financial constraints. In some cases the interest in SACs has been explored and a different type of service provision opted for. For example, Hammersmith and Fulham Council looked into the idea of setting up a SAC and opted for The Sanctuary, a community based counselling and support service for women in the borough. This project is housed in a quiet residential street and offers telephone, individual counselling and group work. The fact that SACs have not taken root does not mean that concerns expressed by RCCs were premature or unfounded. On the contrary, existing SACs and the interest generated in them represent sites of struggle between professionals and existing RCCs; struggles which were ultimately about the assertion of professional expertise in an area of work which had up until that point been largely left in the hands of feminists.

Exclusion and marginalization of rape crisis centres

RCCs have traditionally been marginalized or completely excluded from entering the debates around the policing of rape and sexual assault and services including the establishing of SACs. The working party set up to establish the Manchester SAC made no attempt to consult with feminist organizations already undertaking support work with women who have experienced rape or sexual assault. In fact MRC only found out about the proposal by chance. MRC then wrote to the police, health authority, Dr Roberts (a local police surgeon) and St Mary's hospital where the SAC was to be based for clarification, consultation and to be kept informed of future developments. All subsequent contact with the SAC working party was initiated by MRC and although this contact allowed MRC to put forward their views, no formal consultation ever took place. Similarly Leicester RCC only became aware that a SAC working group had been meeting when Leicestershire health authority sent them a background paper on the type of service they would like to see established. This paper made it clear that the working party already had had several meetings (Leicester Rape Crisis 1992).

This deliberate exclusion and marginalization of RCCs from the debate around services which they were already providing is not simply about professional versus the voluntary sector. Victim Support, although a voluntary organization, is Home Office funded and has not been excluded from these debates. The issues at stake were professional control and the lack of respect and acknowledgement for the work undertaken by feminist organizations. Underpinning this was a belief that feminists have nothing of value to contribute to discussions or debates about new services. This has sometimes been hidden under the rhetoric of multi-agency working, the need to acknowledge service providers and the need for complementary services. However, as Terry Gillespie (1994) points out, there is a significant subtext within the rhetoric. This language hides an unease with, if not hostility to, a feminist analysis of male violence. Excluding feminists provided an opportunity for professionals to accept the need for services whilst at the same time redefining the issues involved, arguing that they, not 'unprofessional' or 'amateur' autonomous women's groups, should be providing such services. For example, two prominent members of the Manchester SAC wrote papers on the need for SACs in which they acknowledged the work of RCCs and survivors' groups but saw their existence as the negative outcome of professionals' lack of interest in this area and questioned whether such groups were the right people to be doing this work (Roberts 1984). A telling point was their representation of feminist RCCs as anti-men and anti-police. Feminist critiques of the way in which rape complaints are responded to throughout the criminal justice system, from initial reports, through to the minority which proceed to trial, were reduced to a simplistic anti-police stance. The commitment of RCCs to enable informed choices for women is reduced to the suggestion that RCCs discourage women from reporting, unlike victim support who are viewed as police-friendly and with whom the police are happy to work (Duddle 1985).

Complementary or competing services

In an interview with an assistant chief constable in the GMP, it was argued that the SACs are able to offer complementary services to RCCs, and that since SACs cater more for police needs to some extent a division of labour has or can develop (Foley 1991). SAC referrals come predominantly from the police with self-referrals constituting approximately a third of all total referrals. Since SACs are fundamentally a police resource it is not surprising that police referrals are higher than self-referrals and that SACs predominantly deal with women who have recently been raped or sexually assaulted. RCCs by contrast only take self-referrals which are often from women who were attacked some time ago. This division is however by no means always so clear cut and both organizations may work with the same women. Women who may have initially gone to the SAC subsequently contact an RCC for counselling and women unable to get through on an RCC phone line may contact the SAC or even think that they are the same organization. However, these broad divisions of work are to some extent reflected in different pots of money being made available to both organizations which has meant that competition for funding between the two services has been avoided. This is not to suggest that both groups receive equal levels of funding as SACs have much greater financial backing than local RCCs. What it does mean is that those currently funding RCCs are less able to argue that there is a duplication of services. This distinction between the two services may become less clear in the future as SACs develop new areas of work, for example the Manchester SAC has advertised for a sessional counsellor to offer telephone and individual counselling to women who have experienced child sexual abuse. In the future, competition for funding is likely to occur; in Northumbria the staffing costs have been met by the police authority with the help of urban programme funding for an initial three year period only. A working party has been established to secure long term funding from other sources.

The fact that organizations offer different services should not be taken to indicate that the only area of potential tension is funding. Organizations can provide different and complementary services and still be in intense conflict over who has the authority to define the issues at stake. As I have mentioned above, the SAC in Manchester met a very practical need in enhancing conditions for women reporting rape and sexual assault to the police. But attaching counsellors to the centre was also clearly motivated by a dislike of feminist alternative provision. The SAC was set up both to meet a particular police need and to provide an alternative service provision to MRC. The SAC provision has also been presented as a 'better' option (SAC 1988), better being defined in terms of claims to professionalism based on formal qualifications. Nor is the SAC in Manchester unique, for many of the services provided (or suggested) not only offer alternative services but an alternative definition of the problem.

Medical services versus medicalization of rape

Often little distinction is made between the forensic medical examination of women following an assault, the medical services that women require and the medicalization of rape. Instead the three different elements are often lumped together as if they were all one and the same, whereas they are completely different processes.

The forensic medical examination concerns the collection of evidence. The purpose is to verify that sexual assault has taken place, to discover signs of force and any other forensic evidence. This examination is used to establish that a crime has taken place and to, where it is possible, indicate who committed it. This is seen as an essential part of the criminal investigation.

Medical services encompass not just assessing any physical damage which a sexual assault can result in, but also other possible consequences. Manchester SAC currently offers pregnancy testing, morning-after contraception and sexually transmitted diseases testing (STDs). The SACs in Newcastle and Sunderland decided not to offer STD testing on the grounds that if a woman had contracted an STD before she was raped, this information could be requested by the defence barrister and used to argue in court that she was a woman of loose moral standing. In their view STD clinics offered women more protection. This provides a useful example of when the needs of the criminal justice system and the aftercare needs of women can be in tension.

The medicalization of rape is a process whereby a social and political issue is redefined as an individual problem requiring treatment. Pathologizing women's experiences of male violence has been addressed in relation to rape trauma syndrome (Kelly 1988, 1989), battered women's syndrome (Edwards 1989) and incest (Armstrong 1990). Giving women's reactions to rape a medical label is not confined to providing a neat label for a cluster of symptoms, it frames how rape and women's responses to it are understood. It stipulates what 'recovery' means, how it is to be judged and who has the authority to assess it and what happens to women who are deemed not to have recovered. Feminist RCCs have always sought to contextualize service provision for individual women within a political framework which sought to challenge traditional orthodoxy which blamed women and excused men, and to combine service provision with fighting to end male violence against women. Professional alternatives such as SACs in England seek to provide services which sever women's individual experiences of violence from the broader political contexts of our lives and respond to those experiences from within the realm of medicine. This medical model of rape involves patching women up without acknowledging the conditions which cause and condone rape. The sexual politics of male violence is negated through the use of gender neutral language which goes to considerable lengths to avoid recognizing that rapists are men.

The medical model defines certain aspects of women's responses to rape as problematic and in need of intervention. For example, whereas feminists would view a dislike or mistrust of men as a realistic response to men's violence, the medical model defines a return to sexually active heterosexuality as goal of successful treatment. This version of what constitutes normal recovery disallows women abstaining from sex (Heller 1990) or women positively choosing to become lesbians (Kelly 1988) as positive coping strategies. This results in women's unwillingness to reconcile themselves to abusive men and/or their behaviour being treated as the problem, even an element in mental illness. Thus women's, not men's, behaviour becomes the focus, women's responses to rape, rather than men's enactment of it, the problem.

Current challenges to RCCs

Securing core funding has always been one of the biggest challenges facing RCCs in Britain, with many groups struggling to provide a service on short term funding from a variety of sources (Gillespie 1994). The situation is getting worse in the current economic and political climate. Government cutbacks in public spending have left local government and statutory bodies in financial difficulty. Local authorities' attempts to rationalize have focused on what they perceive as duplication of services and laying down stricter funding criteria. Accountability to funders is increasingly modelled on private enterprise and business practice. Most voluntary groups who are in receipt of funding now have to agree and sign contracts, which are quasi-legal agreements. Whilst not necessarily a bad thing, the way this has been implemented means groups are expected to conform and perform as if they were private businesses, reflected in the language of 'performance indicators', 'outputs,' 'cost effectiveness' and 'quality assurance'. It is within this context that RCCs are having to compete for funding. These new requirements, with competition from alternative service providers, have put RCCs under increasing pressure to 'professionalize' their own service. Some RCCs have moved away from collective working and adopted more hierarchical structures, some have sought formal counselling qualifications and training and some have included men as service users (see Gillespie, Chapter 10, this volume). RCCs are attempting to secure funding at a time when rape has in many respects become a forgotten issue. In the early 1980s feminists were putting intense pressure on the police and the criminal justice system to improve the ways in which women reporting rape were dealt with. This pressure, combined with a number of high profile cases widely reported in the media, resulted in police forces making a number of improvements in the way in which rape cases were handled. These included training women police officers to take statements, women-only squads, attempts to recruit more women police surgeons, rape victims' examination suites and SACs. These were an improvement although implementation is still variable and patchy. The police view that they've now 'got it right' around rape and can move on to other issues is disputed by many of us involved in rape crisis work.

Since these developments there has been a curious silence about rape as a public issue, as if there is nothing more to say and nothing more to do. The exception to this has been the furore about what has come to be known as 'date' rape. 'Date' rape in the early 1990s has become a new sight of struggle. The phrase itself trivializes, implying rape is no more than impolite sex, thus denying its violence. 'Date' rape is explained in terms of mutual miscommunication. By disconnecting it from other forms of sexual violence, it has become possible for traditional woman-blaming analyses to be reworked and reinstated. Although rape in marriage has formally become a crime through precedent rather than legal reform, rape by a man you know (especially if you have gone out with him) is increasingly trivialized and in effect decriminalized.

The irony is that as this public and political silence around rape continues, the number of reported rape grows, and evidence is emerging that it is actually harder to get a conviction now than it was 10 years ago. The number of convictions has remained constant over that period whilst reported rapes have increased four-fold (Lees 1996).

This lack of debate about rape and sexual assault alongside the increasing growth of 'counselling' services and training courses also has an impact on the internal structure of RCCs. It seems to be increasingly difficult to attract volunteers who are committed to the feminist politics of RCCs. Instead we attract women who are on counselling courses and need practical experience. This causes all sorts of difficulties not only in keeping our frontline service going, but in terms of the ability of groups to evaluate their service critically and discuss and debate the issues currently facing us. Sometimes our own organizations mirror what is happening outside and we ourselves seem to have nothing more to say about rape, and become increasingly preoccupied with other forms of sexual violence.

A wider concern is the defining of rape crisis in terms of service provision alone, separated from feminist concerns to end sexual violence and male control of women. There have been other internal difficulties in the rape crisis movement which have not been openly discussed. Two of these concern internal support and the tensions inherent in being an employer with responsibility for managing paid workers and working collectively. Anyone involved in providing services for women who have experienced violence knows it is very difficult work, and that those doing it need support. But we seem to spend an increasingly disproportionate amount of time on internal support to the detriment of the service. Many women's organizations have had an ambivalent position in relation to paid workers. On the one hand, we have wanted to be good employers. On the other, we have abdicated responsibility for dealing with bad or indifferent workers. We continue to lack a coherent feminist ethos and practice for managing paid workers.

There are a number of external challenges facing RCCs in terms of funding; competition from alternative service providers both professional and voluntary such as victim support; a retrenchment of many of the old definitions of rape; pressure to professionalize and conform; the move towards contracting services; a political climate which is hostile to feminism. This makes the future for RCCs uncertain and difficult but there is nothing unusual in this. Susan Schecter reminds us: 'We have won what we have now because we, or others before us, have struggled for it. It was NOT given to us' (1981: 102). The battle we all face is the need to develop strategies which make it possible for the feminist agenda to reverberate through other non-feminist organizations; to make them take on our political agenda rather than us taking on theirs. To establish this and to ensure our own survival RCCs need to network and build alliances with other groups and organizations.

References

Anna, T. (1988) Feminist responses to sexual abuse: the work of the Birmingham Rape Crisis. In M. Maguire and M. Pointing (eds) *Victims of Crime, a New Deal?* Milton Keynes: Open University Press.

Armstrong, L. (1990) Making an issue of incest. In D. Leidhort and J. G. Raymond (eds) *The Sexual Liberals and the Attack on Feminism*. New York: Pergamon Press.

Duddle, M. (1985) The need for sexual assault centres in the United Kingdom, *British Medical Journal*, 290: 771–3.

Edwards, S. (1989) *Policing Domestic Violence – Women, the Law and the State*. London: Sage Publications.

Foley, M. (1991) 'Rape: a feminist analysis of recent public service provisions for women with particular reference to the sexual assault referral centre', unpublished PhD thesis, Salford University.

Gillespie, T. (1994) Under pressure: rape crisis centres, multi-agency work and strategies for survival. In C. Lupton and T. Gillespie (eds) *Working with Violence*, Basingstoke: Macmillan Press Ltd.

Greater Manchester Police (1986) *Chief Constable's Report*. Greater Manchester Police, Force Administration.

Greater Manchester Police (1988) *Chief Constable's Report*. Greater Manchester Police, Force Administration.

Heller, V. (1990) Sexual liberalism and survivors of sexual abuse. In D. Leidhort and J. G. Raymond (eds) *The Sexual Liberals and the Attack on Feminism*. New York: Pergamon Press.

Kelly, L. (1988) *Surviving Sexual Violence*. Cambridge: Polity Press.

Kelly, L. (1989) 'The professionalisation of rape', *Rights of Women Bulletin*, spring: 8–11.

Lees, S. (1996) *Carnal Knowledge*. London: Penguin.

Leicester Rape Crisis (1992) Personal correspondence.

Roberts, C. (1989) *Women and Rape*. London: Harvester Wheatsheaf.

Roberts, R. (1984) 'The Case for a Sexual Assault Referral Centre in Manchester', unpublished paper.

Schechter, S. (1981) The future of the battered women's movement. In F. Delacoste and F. Newman (eds) *Fight Back! Feminist Resistance to Male Violence*. London: Routledge and Kegan Paul.

Sexual Assault Centre (SAC) (1988) Progress Report. Manchester: St Mary's Hospital.

12

Close to home: the experience of researching child sexual abuse

Jo Moran-Ellis

Introduction

The researcher as a person

Since the 1980s there has been a growth in the academic attention paid to the *experience* of doing research and the impact of that experience on data collection, analysis and presentation. The positioning of the researcher as a person who is gendered and has their own particular origins has come to be seen as an important, albeit often invisible, component in the research process (Oakley 1986; Stanley 1990; Stanley and Wise 1993; Wilkins 1993).

Exploration of the contribution of the researcher as an individual to the research process has largely taken place through an examination of the impact of the researcher on the collection of data. The implications that have flowed from this have been primarily framed as methodological or analytical. Anne Oakley (1981), for example, examined how her identity as a woman and a feminist had implications for her use of interview techniques and methodologies. Her experiences of researching women's transitions to motherhood led her to argue that the techniques associated with interviewing 'subjects' objectified and manipulated them in morally insupportable ways. She contested the masculine paradigm of objectivity and proposed instead that a non-hierarchical relationship between the researcher and the researched should be aimed for, and that interviewers should be prepared to contribute aspects of themselves to the interview relationship alongside the contribution from research participants. Anne Oakley's response to the personal contradictions she experienced as a woman interviewing other women was to propose a change to how data is collected.

Pettigrew (1981) exemplifies another response to the experience of doing research. In a reflective paper she analyses how her identity as a gendered subject influenced her opportunities for pursuing her research amongst Sikhs in the Punjab. She explores how, in seeking to study rural land-owning Jats, her role as a woman in that community and more specifically her status as a wife of a Sikh ultimately shaped both her research question and her understanding of power-relations amongst the group she studied. Through reflection on her experiences of attempting to gain access and her own personal experiences she concludes that researchers should attempt 'an analysis of their fieldwork *experiences* . . . [because] their data is gathered through interaction, as persons with other persons' (p. 77; my emphasis).

Renate Duelli Klein (1983) has also argued that a consciously feminist methodology has to include a means by which the researcher can incorporate her own experiences as a woman and a worker into both the doing of research and a sharing of her subjectivity with research participants. More recently Liz Stanley and Sue Wise (1993) reiterated and strengthened their arguments for the analytic use of personal and research experience in a feminist sociology in relation to the gathering and analysing of data as well as in theorizing.

So in varying ways these writers have drawn attention to the consequences and effects of the researcher being a person with a personal identity, a personal history and personal reactions to the events and encounters that come out of doing research. On the whole the research that has prompted these reflections has been qualitative, although Liz Stanley and Sue Wise point out that, irrespective of research method,

> [r]esearch is a process which occurs through the medium of a person – the researcher is always and inevitably *in* the research. This exists whether openly stated or not; and feminist research ought to make this an open presence.
>
> (Stanley and Wise 1993: 175; original emphasis)

Research as a lived experience

In this chapter I want to reflect on another potential consequence of the researcher being a person – namely the impact of the research on researchers themselves: on their lives, and on them as individuals. Specifically I aim to explore this impact within the context of researching topics that may have great personal meaning for the researcher. This examination of the lived consequences of researching in a demanding or sensitive area is derived from my own experiences of researching child sexual abuse, and in particular from a contemplation of the impact on my own life of my engagement with this issue in the first child sexual abuse research project I worked on. The project itself was a telephone survey of police forces' and social services' arrangements for investigating child sexual abuse referrals (Moran-Ellis *et al.* 1991; Moran-Ellis and Fielding 1996).

My aim is to illustrate the consequences for me of 'doing' research on sexual abuse. The structure and nature of my life has no doubt influenced the structure and nature of my lived experience; I write this as a white woman who has young children and who lives with a man. Furthermore I draw on support from men as well as women in my personal life. When the nature of academic work requires me to be away from home for periods of time my children are in the care of their father. All these aspects of my personal life have become arenas within which the repercussions of my engagement with issues related to child sexual abuse have been felt.

Although the material effect of researching sensitive topics may be different for others, I would argue that the potential for the research to impact on the researcher's life in domains that are outside the academic sphere is always present. As such the personal reactions one has to doing the research may have ramifications not only for approaches to data collection and analysis, but also for how the individual organizes and shapes their own life.

Accounting for myself

In this narrative concerning how researching child sexual abuse came to affect me personally I will recount a number of events that had particular significance for me during and after being a researcher on the project. Whilst some of them caused me distress or provoked a need for support, and others caused me anger, they all provoked much thinking about the work of research and its relationship to other parts of my life or my experiences as a woman and as a mother. I am not attempting to provide an accurate detailed account of all my experiences of researching child sexual abuse, rather I am aiming to demonstrate through a selective account how my work came to be troubling and challenging for me in a number of domains in my life.

Inevitably, through the operation of selective recall and selective inclusion or exclusion of anecdotes in this account, a *version* of reality is created, but it is a version that resonates with my remembered and current experiences and so is in that sense as 'accurate' a version as can be achieved through the medium of writing (see Stanley 1992). The coherence that may seem to be present is certainly something I have imposed in the process of writing – the experience of the described events, and others not included here, was often more chaotic and puzzling than I can convey in this medium.

A first encounter with a difficult topic

As I indicated earlier, my first in-depth engagement with child sexual abuse occurred when I was employed as research officer on a survey of organizational responses to child sexual abuse referrals. The interviews were semi-structured and conducted over the telephone with workers at middle management level: child protection coordinators and detectives in charge of police child protection investigative teams. I was not exposed to face-to-face contact with children who had been abused, the parents of those children or even workers who had the most frequent contact with these situations.

However, I did hear many harrowing anecdotes in the course of the interviews and the hearing of these anecdotes became one of the central parts of my experience of being a researcher in this field.

I was employed on the project in 1989/90 when the aftermath of Cleveland was much in the public domain, so I was aware of the major issues around sexual abuse but not familiar with either the scope and extent of it, or more pertinently the extent to which the majority of perpetrators were male. The process of becoming familiar with the literature around child sexual abuse had great salience for me, since it exposed me to knowledge (albeit sparse) about the prevalence, incidence and nature of child sexual abuse in a way that I had not encountered before.

Auto/biography

The repercussions of my experiences were manifested in both my private and my work life. The slight sense of exposure I am experiencing in revealing my feelings in a public domain via this chapter suggests to me that this continues to be the case.

In sifting through my memories over the past five years, and looking back at various notes I have made over that time there are four or five events that stand out in my mind as having been particularly significant. These are only examples of a range of encounters I had, but they have come to symbolize moments of coalescence of my fears and concerns, my children's own vulnerability and my own limited means to protect them. These significant events occurred in a number of settings and provoked responses in me in a variety of ways. I have chosen to reflect on three categories of notable events: those related to basing a career on researching child sexual abuse; those that created an interaction for me between the 'facts' of sexual abuse and my working life; and those that created an interaction between my growing awareness and consciousness about sexual abuse and my personal life. These notable events raised, and still raise, questions for me about how I can incorporate what I know about sexual abuse with what I can do about it personally and politically.

Careers of abuse

Midway through the telephone interviewing project I went to a conference on child sexual abuse for academics and practitioners. During the course of one paper I became increasingly uncomfortable with the tenor of the questions being asked, particularly by men; there seemed to me to be an element of salaciousness in them. Simultaneously, I recognized that I too felt a type of prurient curiosity about the case material that some speakers were presenting. My disquiet grew as I thought about how we all were making academic and professional careers out of the socially institutionalized damage of children. I realized that I had been objectifying sexual abuse as an academic topic, and as something that happened to children I did not know and was perpetrated by men I would not meet. The subjectivity of sexual abuse and its relevance to me as a woman was forced on me at that conference by hearing papers describing case studies. I felt an urge to leave or to stand up and shout or to strike out in anger but in reality I sat there and did nothing. I chose instead to suppress what I felt and ignore the implications for me.

Later, as I looked around the audience, I was overwhelmed by the feeling that perhaps in this audience there were men present who were abusing their children. The majority of perpetrators of sexual abuse are men (see for example Finkelhor 1984, 1986; Baker and Duncan 1985) but beyond that it is impossible to identify or predict which men will sexually abuse children. I felt that whilst it might well be that none of the men at the conference were abusers, equally any of them could be. This collision between the academic research findings and what they might mean in reality was almost intolerable.

Anger and isolation

At the same conference, I was in conversation with a group of probation officers when one of them said that he and his colleagues were finding that large numbers of young male offenders with whom they worked were sexually abused by their mothers, and that they suspected this was only the tip of the iceberg. He went on to suggest that women abused boys in subtle hard-to-detect ways: being overphysical when changing their nappies, touching their genitals inappropriately later on, making their sons get into bed with them when they are older. The suggestion was that a significant proportion of mothers were satisfying their own sexual needs on the bodies of their sons. My initial reaction was a desire to say 'Show me how that compares with men who anally fuck their sons, orally rape them, make them take part in pornography; who do the same to their daughters, tear and bruise and split their children's mouths, anuses and vaginas; who then blame the children for being seductive, or their "wives" for being unavailable'. I felt anger and frustration in the face of what seemed like a diversion away from recognizing male violence. Wherever there is a power imbalance, the weak are vulnerable; some women do independently sexually abuse children, and some parents work out their sexual desires and inclinations on their children in subtle ways, but this does not detract from the extent of male sexual violence. I did try to say some of this, politely (for after all we were in a public place, and I am a polite woman), but he did not listen. He seemed to have his own theory; that women do it just as much as men, and the effects are just as damaging even if the actions are not necessarily as invasive or assaultive.

At this point I felt lonely and in need of support. Conferences can be lonely places, and this was not a feminist event. I looked at all men with suspicion: were they perpetrators? Were they apologists for perpetrators? The effect of these encounters on me was such that after the conference I avoided male company at work and in my social life. I also stopped discussing my work with anyone for a while. I felt despondent about the possibility of the sorts of social changes which might reduce or eliminate the occurrence of child sexual abuse.

Pain by proxy: who can you talk to?

A year later, as the research project neared completion, I had been reading some graphic accounts of sexual abuse in the research literature, and going over some of the qualitative data from the telephone interviews relating to medical examinations and forensic evidence. I felt appalled by what I was finding out, and I felt much pain by proxy for the children who had been subjected to what amounts to physical as well as emotional and sexual assault. I could barely contemplate the pain they had felt, these unknown children of all ages from babyhood to adolescence. And yet I found I couldn't not think about it. It was hard to talk to anyone about the details, I could barely name them out loud (how then did the children ever manage to tell?). My co-researcher, who had been a social worker, was supportive and yet perhaps not really able to understand my emotional state. Her own experiences of working with sexually abused children had moved her beyond these initial reactions. The person in charge of the project was sympathetic but we were all busy and lacked opportunities to spend any substantial amounts of time together where we could debrief.

My need to talk about the realities and details of sexual abuse grew and, feeling very much in need of support, I spent some time with a close (male) friend talking about all the details, expressing my incomprehension as to how people (men) could do such dreadful things in the name of their own pleasure, and (what felt most chilling of all to me), how these things were being done by 'ordinary' men. His reaction was to argue that perpetrators must be psychiatrically abnormal, or perverted, and that 'normal' men could not do the type of things I had described. This developed into an argument and, rather than finding support, I was presented instead with all the rationalizations about perverts, strangers and sick men. I felt overwhelmed by the power of the image of the pervert, and saw how this served to excuse men from reflecting on their own behaviour, their own sexuality, and their power. In the course of the argument I had direct experience of how these theories of abnormality are sustainable in the face of questions that might undermine them; for example why is it virtually impossible to predict which men will sexually abuse (see Corby 1993)?

The image of the perpetrators of sexual abuse as mentally abnormal or perverted men is not supported by research (see Macleod and Saraga 1988; Hearn 1990). However, as an explanation of the occurrence and prevalence of sexual abuse, it is both pervasive and comforting since it locates responsibility for sexual abuse in a few dangerous strangers. This then absolves society, patriarchy and/or masculinity of any inherent responsibility for the sexual abuse of children, and hence of any responsibility for stopping it. It also makes children more vulnerable since protective efforts on a universal

level are aimed at alerting them to the danger strangers may present and not
the danger that may come from people they trust.

   Even now, I feel diffident about expressing how I feel. Am I overstat-
ing the case? Am I simply overanxious? Each rereading of the research
literature makes me feel more sure that one of the central issues is that sexual
abuse, sexual violence against children, is largely perpetrated by men who are
not sick or perverts, but I am aware of the reactions this provokes, especially
in men who feel betrayed and distrusted by this. Trying to reconcile an
understanding of sexual abuse with trusting people on an individual basis has
sometimes been problematic for me. I find that it is difficult to discuss these
issues with men since they become offended by the implied suspicion, which
is then a barrier to exploring how men can reflect on their own behaviour
and attitudes in a way that facilitates the safety of children. I tend to not
discuss it except with my partner, and it is interesting to reflect on how little
public discussion there is about what adults can do to protect children in
terms of the *adults* altering their own behaviour and perspectives.

Close to home

Two years later, in a different job, I attended another academic conference
on child abuse. In the last two years my male partner had lost his job and
taken up full time parenting, staying at home to look after our three children.
One night at the conference dinner I became engaged in a conversation with
a group of women about the nature of heterosexual relationships, the effects
and implications in women's lives of living in the same household as a male
partner, and how male sexual abusers exploit these sorts of social structures.
More precisely, what we talked about was how women seem to be expected
to protect their children from the men in their lives, and yet cannot carry
on their own lives without relying on those men for childcare some of the
time. Our collective research knowledge had led us all to see how often
sexual abusers exploit trust and opportunity, using the times when women
are absent from the home (for whatever reason: shopping, working, leisure,
education) to perpetrate abuse and silence children with threats. Furthermore,
this is done in a way that can make it quite invisible to women (Hooper
1992). In the course of this conversation, one woman asked: 'While you are
here at this conference dealing with sexual abuse, who is looking after your
children?' The answer was 'my male partner'. I felt panic rise up in me; I
wanted to go home straight away and check on them but I was abroad, a
plane or boat trip away. I did not (and do not) doubt my partner as the
person he is but at the same time I was overwhelmed by the fact that he is
a man and the children were young. I left the table and phoned home – I
realized I was monitoring how long he took to answer, how he sounded.
When I spoke to the children, I tried to gauge whether they were OK, were
they just missing me, was that all? I did not (don't) believe that he would
abuse them, and when I got home after the conference they seemed the
same as they ever were: noisy, laughing, annoying, loving. They were OK

(I think) but I realized that although my trust of my male partner is mainly founded on knowing him, it also requires a leap of faith.

Responding in the personal domain

All the events I have described here have been a confrontation for me between the realities of sexual abuse and the realities of patriarchy. The work by Finkelhor (1986), Hooper (1992), Stanley (1993), and others (see for example *Feminist Review* 1988; Corby 1993) has shown that the majority of perpetrators are male; that children are silenced through fear and specifically with threats; that perpetrators exploit the trust that women place in them and yet structurally women may be manoeuvred into dependency and trust on men for some childcare; that sexual abuse is either generally denied or theorized in lay terms as an act perpetrated by perverts or other abnormal men.

The cumulative effect on me of reading this research and working in this area has been to raise some profound questions about my personal life. Have I brought my children up in a way that would enable them to tell me about things they were uncomfortable with? Have I judged their father correctly? We have been through a lot of soul-searching together about sexual abuse, about what I would do if he abused our children (are threats any use in controlling someone who is structurally more powerful than me?), about how to build an atmosphere of respect and privacy and autonomy in our home. About how to maintain loving tactile relationships with the children within very clear boundaries. My paid work also entails me leaving my children in the care of others for quite long periods of time. In the way my life is at present their father is my main domestic resource: who else would look after my children for those long periods of time if not their father? Who would see to them when I have to work late? These issues and problems with child care are the sort that many women have to contend with. Solutions to dependency on men and specifically on male partners may not be easily found or organized, or may require more change than can be contemplated at particular times.

In contrast to a number of my friends who are not involved in this work, I sometimes feel overvigilant about my children, more wary of men who are a part of their lives. I feel inclined towards drawing up more rules about acceptable and non-acceptable behaviours in our household.

On a personal level, staying in my current household has seemed a reasonable option given the trust and faith I have in my partner. And to some extent I have realized that at certain points I have become immune to the horrors of sexual abuse (one way of coping with that knowledge, and something that can easily happen when a topic is 'professionalized'), and at other times I have pushed it very much to the back of my mind. There were two events which I will discuss below that made me realize that I had dealt with the turmoil created by my exposure to sexual abuse research by distancing and objectifying the 'facts'. This strategy became apparent to me because I was shocked about being shocked 'after all this time'.

Being shocked: a route out of professional distance

More recently I attended a seminar given by Beatrix Campbell about children and society where she talked about Cleveland and its aftereffects as well as current media representations of children. She reminded us that babies as young as six seeks are sexually abused. I felt shocked and sick. Just after this I was working in my office, reading accounts of children's 'disclosures' of sexual abuse (Richardson 1991). I read their descriptions which used words like 'knife' and 'razor' to describe the pain of sexual or anal intercourse. I felt shocked and acutely disturbed by this and went out of my office needing someone to talk to, but at the same time unable actually to describe to anyone else what I had read. Reflecting on my emotional reactions I realized that I had to some extent become immune to the realities of sexual abuse. Recapturing a sense of shock and outrage through hearing or reading accounts of abuse had reduced this professional distance from the subject and hopefully prevented me from becoming totally immune to the realities of sexual abuse.

I am left, though, with some doubt as to whether I am entitled to have felt the emotions and anxieties I have described. Have I just been indulging in a vicarious type of suffering to which I have no legitimate claim? Perhaps. On the other hand, if the personal is political then the political is also personal. What I have recounted here has been specific to my research into sexual abuse, and some of the impact of my exposure to research and theorizing in this area has resulted from the way it has raised questions and doubts in my own life. However, my conversations with women working around issues of rape and domestic violence suggest that looking at the incidence, prevalence, nature and context of those arenas of violence has had similar impacts on their lives.

Conclusion

In the course of the research project I struggled with coming to terms with child sexual abuse in the context of my own life, and this is a process that continues still. I received support from the project supervisor and my co-researcher but at times I felt alone and exposed, and overwhelmed with anxiety about the safety and vulnerability of my own children in all arenas of their lives. I found that the impact of researching sexual abuse occurred in a number of different arenas: heterosexual motherhood, family, teaching, researching, academe. In short, researching sexual abuse changed my life to some degree because it changed me, and that was not something I had anticipated happening.

I realize that my questions and concerns arise partly out of the actuality of what constitutes my life, and for other women different questions and concerns will be pertinent. The point I wish to draw attention to, is that researching areas of violence can impact on the researchers' life extensively, and that the effect may be to call into question the very way in which one constructs one's life. One response can be to use this effect as part of a framework to analyse research data, draw conclusions, and programme action. However, the actual means by which this can be done can be unavailable or at the very least difficult to utilize.

My own problem with using my experiences reflexively was that the semi-structured questionnaire I used directed the data analysis in a way that left little room for a reflexive interpretation of it. Possibly this lack of opportunity for reflexive analysis amplified the repercussions for me in a negative way. The main location in which I have been able to use my experiences has been in my personal life. For example I have tried to instigate rules and considerations in my household that enhance my children's safety and recognize their potential vulnerability in open and supportive ways. I have also aimed to develop a culture of respect for privacy and individuality regardless of age or status. Whether or not these actions are successful is another question, but it has given me a way of working with and through my experiences in a positive way.

With regards to my colleagues, friends and acquaintances, I remain confrontational in the face of theories about 'perverts' and 'dangerous strangers' being the main perpetrators of abuse. I am also unyielding about adults taking responsibility for their actions and behaviour however uncomfortable or unfair it may be for them. In relation to the issue of women who sexually abuse children I am exploring how far power is the issue to be addressed without losing sight of the extent to which perpetrators of sexual abuse are most often male and most often trusted figures in the child's life rather than people not known to them. Mostly I remain angry and political in a feminist sense.

What did emerge from my experiences in the work setting was a strong feeling that researchers working in sensitive areas need emotional support and that this support should be part of the context within which the research is conducted. I would like to conclude by proposing some guidelines for ensuring that this emotional support is available to researchers and others working in these areas such as support administrative staff.

Looking forward: two suggestions for the research process

Support

Emotional support for researchers working in the area of violence against women and children is something that one might expect to occur when feminists are engaged in research. However, we may not always be working in supportive groups or have access to each other. I propose that all research that is concerned with violence against women or children should have, as part of the method and as part of the process of conducting research, a clear mechanism for giving support to all staff engaged on the project, including support/administrative staff as well as researchers. I would go so far as to say that no research proposal should be approved by a funding body unless it has this support clearly built into the structure, and that in refereeing such research proposals this is a point that should be made.

Utilizing reflection

By supporting workers engaged in research into violence against women and children we can ease some of the emotional pain that this work can bring. In doing this we can also attend to the nature of that pain and our impulse strategies for dealing with it as another source of data which can illuminate and contextualize how women who are subject to violence may also react, or how situations of violence can be perpetuated. If these processes are illuminated further, then counter-strategies can be developed.

I have resisted an impulse to deny or apologize for some of the emotional experiences I had during the research since I feel this would constitute 'coming to terms' with sexual abuse. Violence against women and children must never be accepted. Instead reflecting on and reviewing our reactions to what we encounter through our research as well as our everyday lives can be incorporated into working to end these oppressions. Ignoring something that is painful is an effective strategy but it does not lead to the situation being changed.

References

Baker, A. and Duncan, S. (1985) Child sexual abuse: a study of prevalence in Great Britain, *Child Abuse and Neglect*, 9: 457–67.

Corby, B. (1993) *Child Abuse: Towards a Knowledge Base*. Buckingham: Open University Press.

Duelli Klein, R. (1983) How to do what we want to do: thoughts about feminist methodology. In G. Bowles and R. Duelli Klein (eds) *Theories of Women's Studies*. London: Routledge and Kegan Paul.

Feminist Review (1988) *Family Secrets: Child Sexual Abuse*, special issue, 28, spring.

Finkelhor, D. (1984) *Child Sexual Abuse: New Theory and Research*. New York: Free Press.

Finkelhor, D. (1986) *A Sourcebook on Child Sexual Abuse*. Newbury Park, CA: Sage.

Hearn, J. (1990) Child abuse and men's violence. In The Violence Against Children Study Group (eds) *Taking Child Abuse Seriously*. London: Unwin Hyman.

Home Office (1976) *Sexual Offences (Amendment) Act*. London: HMSO.

Hooper, C. (1992) *Mothers Surviving Child Sexual Abuse*. London: Routledge and Kegan Paul.

MacLeod, M. and Saraga, E. (1988) Challenging the orthodoxy: towards a feminist theory and practice, *Feminist Review*, 28, spring: 16–55.

Moran-Ellis, J., Conroy, S., Fielding, N. and Tunstill, J. (1991) *Investigation of Child Sexual Abuse – An Executive Summary*. Guildford: University of Surrey, Sociology Department.

Moran-Ellis, J. and Fielding, N. (1996) A national survey of the investigation of child sexual abuse, *British Journal of Social Work* (in press).

Oakley, A. (1981) Interviewing women: a contradiction in terms. In H. Roberts (ed.) *Doing Feminist Research*. London: Routledge and Kegan Paul.

Oakley, A. (1986) Interviewing women: a contradiction in terms? In A. Oakley, *Telling the Truth About Jerusalem*. Oxford: Basil Blackwell.

Pettigrew, J. (1981) Reminiscences of fieldwork among the Sikhs. In H. Roberts (ed.) *Doing Feminist Research*. London: Routledge and Kegan Paul.

Richardson, S. (1991) The continuum of disclosure. In S. Richardson and H. Bacon (eds) *Child Sexual Abuse: Whose Problem?* Birmingham: Venture Press.

Stanley, L. (ed.) (1990) *Feminist Praxis: Research, Theory and Epistemology in Feminist Sociology*. London: Routledge.

Stanley, L. (1992) *The Auto/Biographical I: Theory and Practice of Feminist Auto/Biography*. Manchester: Manchester University Press.

Stanley, L. (1993) On auto/biography in sociology, *Sociology*, 27(1): 41–52.

Stanley, L. and Wise, S. (1993) *Breaking Out Again: Feminist Ontology and Epistemology*. London: Routledge.

Wilkins, R. (1993) Taking it personally: a note on emotions and autobiography, *Sociology*, 27(1): 93–100.

Index

FEMICIDE
THE POLITICS OF WOMAN KILLING

Jill Radford and Diana E. H. Russell (eds)

The first of its kind – and a classic. This book should be required reading for everyone: college students and their professors, policy makers, and businesspeople, lawyers and judges, police officers and members of the clergy. It raises our consciousness and inspires resistance to femicide.

Phyllis Chesler

While the issues of date rape and sexual harassment have finally entered into mainstream discourse, femicide, the most brutal form of sexist behaviour, has yet to be widely acknowledged and understood. In this wide-ranging study, more than 40 contributors document and describe the phenomenon of femicide as it occurs across continents and cultures, analyse the roles that our social values and institutions play in perpetuating it, and articulate the actions that can be taken to combat it. *Femicide: The Politics of Woman Killing* is at once a disturbing testimony to the many women who have been victims of femicide and an act of resistance.

Contents
Part 1: Femicide is as old as patriarchy – Part 2: The patriarchal home – Part 3: Femicide and racism – Part 4: The mass media, pornography, and Gorenography – Part 5: Femicide and travesties of justice – Part 6: Women fighting back against femicide – Summary and conclusion – Sources – Index.

400pp   0 335 15178 7 (Paperback)

MAKING VIOLENCE SEXY
FEMINIST VIEWS ON PORNOGRAPHY

Diana E. H. Russell (ed.)

A crucially important collection of feminist voices challenging the pornocrats. Even if you read nothing else on the subject, read this.

(Robin Morgan)

Making Violence Sexy is a courageous book that chronicles women's resistance to pornography over the last twenty years. It does this in a collection of feminist articles, including testimonies by victims/survivors of pornography that together make a convincing case for the view that pornography (as distinct from erotica) causes harm to women, including acts of violence.

This book will appeal to students and lecturers of women's studies and sociology, political activists, public officials, social scientists, legal and medical professionals – those who consider it a form of discrimination against women. Women's studies teachers will find it a welcome addition to their required reading lists, and those working against sexual violence will appreciate it as a primary, up-to-date, and comprehensive source and inspiration.

Contents
Introduction – Part I: Survivors of pornography – Part II: Overview – Part III: Feminist research on pornography – Part IV: Feminist strategies and actions against pornography – Notes – References – Index.

320pp   0 335 19200 9 (Paperback)

POWER IN STRUGGLE
FEMINISM, SEXUALITY AND THE STATE

Davina Cooper

What is power? And how are social change strategies shaped by the ways in which we conceptualize it? Drawing on feminist, poststructuralist, and marxist theory, Davina Cooper develops an innovative framework for understanding power relations within fields as diverse as queer activism, municipal politics, and the regulation of lesbian reproduction. *Power in Struggle* explores the relationship between power, sexuality, and the state and, in the process, provides a radical rethinking of these concepts and their interactions. The book concludes with an important and original discussion of how an ethics of empowerment can inform political strategy.

Special features:
* brings together central aspects of current radical, political theory in an innovative way
* offers a new way of conceptualizing the state, power and sexuality

Contents
Introduction — Beyond domination?: productive and relational power — The politics of sex: metaphorical strategies and the (re)construction of desire — Multiple identities: sexuality and the state in struggle — Penetration on the defensive: regulating lesbian reproduction — Access without power: gay activism and the boundaries of governance — Beyond resistance: political strategy and counter-hegemony — Afterword — Bibliography — Index.

192pp   0 335 19211 4 (paperback)   0 335 19212 2 (hardback)